Canadian Perspectives
on Advanced Practice Nursing

Canadian Perspectives on Advanced Practice Nursing

SECOND EDITION

Edited by Eric Staples, Roger Pilon,
and Ruth A. Hannon

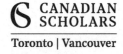

CANADIAN
SCHOLARS

Toronto | Vancouver

Canadian Perspectives on Advanced Practice Nursing, Second Edition
Edited by Eric Staples, Roger Pilon, and Ruth A. Hannon

First published in 2020 by
Canadian Scholars, an imprint of CSP Books Inc.
425 Adelaide Street West, Suite 200
Toronto, Ontario
M5V 3C1

www.canadianscholars.ca

Library and Archives Canada Cataloguing in Publication

Title: Canadian perspectives on advanced practice nursing / edited by Eric Staples, Roger Pilon, and
    Ruth A. Hannon.
Names: Staples, Eric, 1958- editor. | Pilon, Roger, 1966- editor. | Hannon, Ruth A., editor.
Description: Second edition. | Includes bibliographical references and index.
Identifiers: Canadiana (print) 20200330799 | Canadiana (ebook) 2020033106X | ISBN 9781773382173
    (softcover) | ISBN 9781773382180 (PDF) | ISBN 9781773382197 (EPUB)
Subjects: LCSH: Nursing—Canada—Textbooks. | LCSH: Nurse practitioners—Canada. |
    LCGFT: Textbooks.
Classification: LCC RT41 .C36 2020 | DDC 610.730971—dc23

Cover design by Em Dash Design
Page layout by S4Carlisle Publishing Services

20   21   22   23   24   5   4   3   2   1

Printed and bound in Ontario, Canada

Canada

Contents

Foreword

The year 2020 finds us celebrating nursing and midwifery globally, spurred by the two-hundredth anniversary of the birth of Florence Nightingale, the great social reformer and a founder of modern nursing and health care. The world of advanced practice nursing (APN) will gather in Halifax, Nova Scotia, and the thirtieth anniversary of the founding of the Canadian Association of Advanced Practice Nurses (CAAPN) will be marked in 2021. The timing could not be better for the release of the second edition of *Canadian Perspectives on Advanced Practice Nursing*, a record on the state of APN in Canada.

Clinical nurse specialists (CNSs) and nurse practitioners (NPs) make up the two streams of advanced practice nursing in Canada. The first CNSs in Canada were hired during the 1970s by legendary nurse administrator Dorothy Wylie, who was then the director of nursing at Sunnybrook Health Sciences Centre in Toronto, Ontario. In a subsequent decade of leadership as the vice-president for nursing and patient care at the Toronto General Hospital in Toronto, Ontario, beginning in 1978, Wylie would go on to champion and help shape the role, which has gone on to be established across the country.

The broad spread of NPs in Canada is a newer phenomenon, emerging from the investments in health care reform initially laid out in the First Ministers' Meeting Communiqué on Health (2000) in Ottawa, Ontario. Committing to supporting improvements in primary health care and multidisciplinary teams across the provinces and territories, the federal government went on to allocate $800 million to the Primary Health Care Transition Fund during the years 2004–2006. The Canadian Nurses Association (CNA) was awarded $8.8 million from that fund for two years of work to put all the structures in place to integrate nurse practitioners into Canada's health care systems. Within short order, the role was established in all 13 Canadian provinces and territories, the title was protected, and common entry-to-practice examinations established. Today there are over 6,000 NPs deployed and making a difference across Canada. For those who sometimes feel change in health care systems is slow to come, I often say, "Stand back and take a look at the story of NPs—a hugely disruptive change in the health care landscape with 10 years, basically start to finish, and we will never look back."

In nearly every poll over the past 20 years, the people of Canada have accorded higher trust and respect to nurses than any other professional group. And we know from at least one poll that Canadians trust information coming from nursing associations more than any other source. These are tremendous pillars of power for Canadian nursing. They reflect more than a century of work in nursing education, the development of expected competencies in the different regulated categories, and rigorous nursing regulation. In many cases major steps forward have been spearheaded by strong professional nursing associations such as the CNA, who are charged with advancing the profession at large in the interest of the public. These laudable outcomes are the envy of every other profession. It is up to us to use that power and influence wisely as we advocate to achieve the quadruple aim through value-based health care.

At its 1982 annual meeting, CNA members voted that the association should work with partners to establish a baccalaureate degree as the minimum education for entry to practice for registered nurses by the year 2000. That standard is now implemented in all jurisdictions other than Quebec. The year 2020 marks 60 years since the first Canadian graduate degree program in nursing was established at Western University in London, Ontario. A graduate degree is now the minimum education for entry to APN across Canada, and many APNs also hold doctoral degrees. A significant body of science has made plain that advanced nurses clearly deliver better health care outcomes, better quality and safety of care, and a better value for dollars invested—all in ways that are as satisfying or more satisfying to the public than traditional models of care. These roles represent wins all around for the public, for health care teams, and for health systems budgets.

Together, all these undergirding structures have helped to position Canadian nurses in 2020 among the best educated and most respected nursing workforces in the world. This second edition of *Canadian Perspectives on Advanced Practice Nursing* should be the go-to book for information on the state of the art in APN. Dr. Eric Staples, Dr. Roger Pilon, and Dr. Ruth A. Hannon have laid out the story of these roles in Canada, starting with history and evolution of the roles and concluding with commentary on the future of APN. In between, they weave the full story of these roles, placing a strong focus on the current state of advanced practice with updates from the first edition in the areas of APN role competencies, specialty roles, and specific issues related to APN, including health policy, impacts and outcomes of advanced practice, and global perspectives.

Importantly and usefully, this second edition provides an extensive discussion of the interactions between broad social determinants of health and APN. As we collectively grapple with ways to respond meaningfully in health care to the 94 calls for action issued by the Truth and Reconciliation Commission of Canada—arguably the most prominent topic of discussion in every region of Canada in 2020—Section II of the book opens by speaking about Indigenous populations. The story goes on to address some of our most vexing challenges in delivering universal health care and better health care outcomes for urban and rural/remote populations, migrant populations, and those who identify as LGBT2SQ. These are valuable additions to the story of APNs in Canada and will also be helpful to readers in other countries, many of whom are affected by these same issues.

With the infrastructure for APN well established in Canada, it falls on us now to create the conditions that ramp up these roles to create large-scale returns on investments. This second edition of *Canadian Perspectives on Advanced Practice Nursing* is a valuable guide to nurses, whether considering pursuing an advanced practice role or already well established in the role; administrators of teams deploying APNs; and of course those who educate and study these nurses. Perhaps most critically, this book should be in the hands of decision makers and those responsible for developing formal public policy who may be asking, "What exactly do they do? If they want to be doctors, why don't they just go to medical school? Why should

I hire an APN? What will I get for the dollars I invest?" This book answers these questions and represents a critical addition to the canon as the definitive Canadian textbook on APN.

Michael J. Villeneuve, MSc, RN, FAAN
Chief Executive Officer, Canadian Nurses Association, Ottawa, Ontario

Canadian Contributors

Michelle Acorn, DNP, NP-PHC/Adult, MN/ACNP, ENC(C), GNC(C), Samuel H. and Maria Miller Fellow
Provincial Chief Nursing Officer
Ontario Ministry of Health and Long-Term Care, Toronto, Ontario
Adjunct Faculty, Lawrence S. Bloomberg Faculty of Nursing
University of Toronto, Toronto, Ontario

Cynthia Baker, RN, PhD
Executive Director
Canadian Association of Schools of Nursing, Ottawa, Ontario
Professor Emerita
Queen's University, Kingston, Ontario

Marilyn Ballantyne, RN(EC), PhD
Chief Nurse Executive and Clinician Investigator
Holland Bloorview Kids Rehabilitation Hospital, Toronto, Ontario
Adjunct Professor, Lawrence S. Bloomberg Faculty of Nursing
University of Toronto, Toronto, Ontario

Line Beaudet, RN, PhD
Advanced Practice Nurse, Neurosciences
Principal Scientist, Centre de recherche du Centre hospitalier de l'Université de Montréal
Associate Professor, Faculty of Nursing
Université de Montréal, Montreal, Quebec

Jennifer Beaveridge, MScN, DNP, NP-F
Family Nurse Practitioner and Regional Department Head/Director of Nurse Practitioners
Vancouver Coastal Health, North Vancouver, British Columbia
Clinical Lead/Adjunct Professor, Family Nurse Practitioner Program, School of Nursing
University of Northern British Columbia, Prince George, British Columbia
Adjunct Professor, University of British Columbia, Vancouver, British Columbia

Monique Benoit, BA (Sociology), MA (Sociology), PhD (Sociology)
Professor, Department of Nursing
Université du Québec en Outaouais, Saint-Jérôme, Quebec
Adjunct Professor, School of Nursing
Laurentian University, Sudbury, Ontario

Elaine Borg, RN, LLB
Legal Counsel
Canadian Nurses Protective Society, Ottawa, Ontario

Denise Bryant-Lukosius, RN, BScN, CON(C), MScN, PhD
Associate Professor, School of Nursing, Inaugural Chair, Alba DiCenso Professorship in Advanced Practice Nursing, and Affiliate Member, Department of Oncology, Faculty of Health Sciences, McMaster University, Hamilton, Ontario

David Byres, DNP, MSN, BSN (Hons), RN, CHE
Adjunct Professor, School of Nursing
University of British Columbia, Vancouver, British Columbia
Adjunct Assistant Professor, School of Nursing
University of Victoria, Victoria, British Columbia

Marcia Carr, RN, BN, MS, GNC(C), NCA
Clinical Nurse Specialist Consultant and Nurse Continence Advisor
Carr CNS Consulting, Delta, British Columbia

Michelle Carter, RN, BSN, MScN, BSc
Clinical Nurse Specialist, Psychiatry
St. Paul's Hospital, Vancouver, British Columbia
Adjunct Professor, School of Nursing
University of British Columbia, Vancouver, British Columbia

Jamie Churchill, RN, MSc, PNP
NP-Pediatrics, Neurology
McMaster Children's Hospital, Hamilton, Ontario

Laurie Clune, RN, PhD
Associate Professor, Faculty of Nursing
Vice Chair, Research Ethics Board
University of Regina, Regina, Saskatchewan

Joanna Dickinson, NP-PHC, MSc
Wellness Lead, Syl Apps Youth Centre
Oakville, Ontario

Cheryl Forchuk, RN, PhD
Beryl and Richard Ivey Research Chair in Aging, Mental Health, Rehabilitation, and Recovery
Distinguished Professor, Arthur Labatt Family School of Nursing
Scientist and Assistant Director, Lawson Health Research Institute
Professor, Department of Psychiatry, Schulich Medicine & Dentistry
Western University, London, Ontario

Jennifer Fournier, NP-PHC, MHS, PhD
Adjunct Professor, School of Nursing
Laurentian University
Sudbury, Ontario
Proprietor, AllureRX, Sudbury, Ontario

Steve Gagné, RN, MScN, CCNC(C)
Advanced Practice Nurse, Critical Care
Associate Scientist, Centre de recherche du Centre hospitalier de l'Université de Montréal
Associate Clinical Nurse Specialist, Faculty of Nursing
Université de Montréal, Montreal, Quebec

Doris Grinspun, RN, MSN, PhD, LLD (hon), O.ONT
Chief Executive Officer
Registered Nurses' Association of Ontario, Toronto, Ontario

Ruth A. Hannon, NP-PHC, MHA, MSFNP-BC, DNP
Teaching Professor, School of Nursing
McMaster University, Hamilton, Ontario

Roberta Heale, NP-PHC, DNP, PhD
Professor, School of Nursing
Laurentian University, Sudbury, Ontario

Kathleen F. Hunter, PhD, RN, NP-Adult, GNC(C), NCA
Professor and Coordinator, MN Entry to Practice as an NP Program, Faculty of Nursing
Adjunct Professor, Faculty of Medicine and Dentistry, Division of Geriatric Medicine
University of Alberta, Edmonton, Alberta

Laura Johnson, RN, MN, NP, DNP
Independent Contractor, Bayshore Home Health
Winnipeg, Manitoba

Mary Ellen Labrecque, RN(NP), PhD
Assistant Professor and Director, Nurse Practitioner Programs
College of Nursing, University of Saskatchewan, Saskatoon, Saskatchewan

Sandra Lauck, RN, PhD
Clinical Associate Professor and St. Paul's Hospital and Heart & Stroke Foundation Professorship in Cardiovascular Nursing
University of British Columbia, Vancouver, British Columbia

Lucie Lemelin, RN, PhD
Associate Professor and Director of Graduate Nursing Programs, Department of Nursing
Université du Québec en Outaouais, Saint-Jérôme, Quebec

Janet Luimes, RN(NP), MScN
Assistant Professor, Academic Programming
College of Nursing, University of Saskatchewan, Saskatoon, Saskatchewan

Jane MacDonald, RN, MN, NP(F)
Interior Health Authority
Vernon, British Columbia

Mary-Lou Martin, RN, MScN, MEd
Clinical Nurse Specialist, Mental Health, Forensic Program
St. Joseph's Healthcare, Hamilton, Ontario
Associate Clinical Professor, School of Nursing
McMaster University, Hamilton, Ontario

Ruth Martin-Misener, NP, PhD
Professor and Director, School of Nursing
Assistant Dean, Research, Faculty of Health
Dalhousie University, Halifax, Nova Scotia

Mary McAllister, RN, BScN, MHSc, PhD
Associate Chief of Nursing, Advanced Practice Nurses
The Hospital for Sick Children, Toronto, Ontario

Ken McDonald, RN, BScN, MScN
Clinical Nurse Specialist, Mental Health & Substance Use
Fraser Health Authority, Vancouver, British Columbia

Gloria McInnis-Perry, RN, PhD
Associate Professor, Faculty of Nursing
University of Prince Edward Island, Charlottetown, Prince Edward Island

Lynn Miller, DNP, NP
Strategy Policy Consultant
Nova Scotia College of Nursing, Bedford, Nova Scotia

Brenda Mishak, RN(NP), PhD, CCHN(C)
Assistant Professor, Academic Programming
College of Nursing, University of Saskatchewan, Saskatoon, Saskatchewan

Josephine Muxlow, RN, MS, CPMHN(C)
Clinical Nurse Specialist Mental Health
Professional Practice Support Directorate
Indigenous Services Canada, First Nations & Inuit Health Branch, Atlantic Region
Halifax, Nova Scotia
Adjunct Professor, School of Nursing
Dalhousie University, Halifax, Nova Scotia

Carole Orchard, RN, EdD
Professor Emerita, Arthur Labatt Family School of Nursing
Western University, London, Ontario

Tammy O'Rourke, RN, BS, MS, PhD, NP
Assistant Professor, Faculty of Health Disciplines
Athabasca University, Athabasca, Alberta

Pierre Pariseau-Legault, RN, PhD, LLM
Associate Professor, Department of Nursing
Université du Québec en Outaouais, Saint-Jérôme, Quebec

Monica Parry, NP-Adult, MEd, MSc, PhD, CCN(C)
Associate Professor, Lawrence S. Bloomberg Faculty of Nursing
University of Toronto, Toronto, Ontario

Joanna Pierazzo, RN, PhD
Associate Professor and Assistant Dean, Undergraduate Nursing Programs
Faculty of Health Sciences School of Nursing
McMaster University, Hamilton, Ontario

Roger Pilon, PhD, NP-PHC, CCNE
Associate Professor and Director, School of Nursing
Assistant Professor, Northern Ontario School of Medicine
Laurentian University, Sudbury, Ontario

Jennifer Price, RN, BNSc, MScN, ACNP, CCN(C), PhD
Chief Nursing and Professional Practice Executive
Women's College Hospital, Toronto, Ontario

Susan L. Ray, RN, CNS/APN, PhD (deceased)
Associate Professor/Associate Scientist, Arthur Labatt Family School of Nursing
Western University, London, Ontario

Josette Roussel, RN, MSc, MEdl, inf. aut.
Executive Advisor
Canadian Nurses Association, Ottawa, Ontario

Angela Russolillo, PhD, MSc, RPN
Practice Consultant and Researcher, Mental Health Substance Use
Providence Health Care, Vancouver, British Columbia

Sara Ryan, NP-PHC, MN
NP-Cannabis Clinic
North Star Wellness, Toronto, Ontario

Esther Sangster-Gormley, PhD, RN, ARNP (Florida, US)
Associate Professor and Associate Dean
Faculty of Human and Social Development
University of Victoria, Victoria, British Columbia

Isabelle Savard, BScN, MScN, NP-Primary Care
Associate Professor, Department of Nursing
Université du Québec en Outaouais, Saint-Jérôme, Quebec
NP-Primary Care, Centre Sida Amité, Saint-Jérôme, Quebec

Monakshi (Mona) Sawhney, NP-Adult, PhD
Assistant Professor
School of Nursing and Department of Anesthesia and Perioperative Medicine
Queen's University, Kingston, Ontario
NP-Adult, North York General Hospital, Toronto, Ontario, and Kingston Health Sciences
Centre, Kingston, Ontario

Andrew Sharpe, BBA, BSc, BN, NP-PHC, MN
NP-PHC, Transgender Health Clinic
London InterCommunity Health Centre, London, Ontario
Lecturer, Fanshawe College, London, Ontario
Lecturer and Clinical Instructor, Nipissing University, North Bay, Ontario

Mary Smith, NP-PHC, PhD
Assistant Professor
Faculty of Health Sciences School of Nursing
Queen's University, Kingston, Ontario

Eric Staples, RN, BAA(N), MSc, ACNP (cert.), DNP, Samuel H. and Maria Miller Fellow
Independent Nursing Practice Consultant, Ancaster, Ontario

Shannon Sweeney, NP-PHC, MScN
NP-PHC, East End Community Health Centre, Toronto, Ontario

Amanda Symington, RN(EC), BSc, BScN, MHSc
NP-Pediatrics, Neonatal Intensive Care Unit, Niagara Health
St. Catharines General Hospital, St. Catharines, Ontario

Paul Tylliros, NP-PHC, MScN
NP, Waasegiizhig Nanaadawe'iyewigamig Clinic, Kenora, Ontario

Don Versluis, BScN, MSc, PHC-NP, DNP
NP-PHC, Niagara Health
St. Catharines General Hospital, St. Catharines, Ontario
Clinical Instructor, Ontario Primary Health Care Nurse Practitioner Program
Faculty of Health Sciences School of Nursing, McMaster University, Hamilton, Ontario

Françoise (Frankie) Verville, RN(NP), MN, AGD
Program Head/Faculty, Collaborative Nurse Practitioner Program
Saskatchewan Polytechnic, Regina, Saskatchewan
Graduate Adjunct Professor, Faculty of Nursing
University of Regina, Regina, Saskatchewan

Michael J. Villeneuve, RN, MSc
Chief Executive Officer
Canadian Nurses Association, Ottawa, Ontario

Bernadine Wallis, RN, BN, MEd
Instructor, Helen Glass Centre
College of Nursing, Faculty of Health Sciences
University of Manitoba, Winnipeg, Manitoba

Rosemary Wilson, NP-Adult, PhD
Associate Professor, School of Nursing
Queen's University, Kingston, Ontario
NP-Adult, Kingston Health Sciences Centre, Kingston, Ontario

Amy Wright, MScN, PhD, NP-Pediatrics, NCC-BC, CNeoN(C)
Neonatal Nurse Practitioner, Neonatal Intensive Care Unit
McMaster Children's Hospital–Hamilton Health Sciences, Hamilton, Ontario
Assistant Professor, Lawrence S. Bloomberg Faculty of Nursing
University of Toronto, Toronto, Ontario

Vanessa Wright, NP-PHC, MScN
NP-PHC, Crossroads Clinic
Women's College Hospital, Toronto, Ontario

Erin Ziegler, PhD, NP-PHC
Assistant Professor, Daphne Cockwell School of Nursing
Ryerson University, Toronto, Ontario

Kevin Zizzo, NP-Pediatrics, MN, GDipNPAC
NP-Pediatrics, MyPediatricNP, Woodstock, Ontario
Clinical Professor, School of Nursing
McMaster University, Hamilton, Ontario
Adjunct Lecturer, Lawrence S. Bloomberg Faculty of Nursing
University of Toronto, Toronto, Ontario

Preface

It was humbling to be asked by Canadian Scholars to produce a second edition of *Canadian Perspectives on Advanced Practice Nursing*. It is rewarding to see that the book has been so well received across the country since its publication in 2016.

For the second edition, and for succession planning, we brought on Dr. Roger Pilon to act as second editor. We were aware that the advanced practice nursing (APN) landscape in Canada had advanced since the first edition, and that much of the content was in need of updating. Our goal in revising the textbook was not only to update the content of the existing chapters, but also to add more breadth and depth by introducing topics that would showcase what advanced practice nurses (APNs) across Canada are currently doing.

This textbook is intended for graduate nursing students, practicing APNs in all APN roles, educators, leaders, and policy-makers in nursing. It provides a view of the APN roles in Canada, the unique contribution each makes, and the practice competencies associated with advanced skills that are distinct to APN. The textbook can be useful to practicing APNs in updating their knowledge while they are working in a continuously changing health care environment. For educators, the textbook serves as an educational curricular resource. Continuing from the inaugural edition, the textbook provides application, in the form of case studies and critical thinking questions, and promotes faculty and student discussions when looking at the essentials for APN roles and practice competencies that are relevant to any APN context across the country.

Canada is a vast country; there are many similarities, but there are also many differences across jurisdictions related to APN education, titling, title protection, integration, legislation, and regulation. The contributors to this textbook come from across the country and have backgrounds in academia, practice, health policy, and professional nursing organizations, provincially and nationally. They were chosen to represent, share, and demonstrate the essential components of APN practice from their distinctly Canadian perspectives.

The organization of the textbook into sections follows the same structure as the inaugural edition. The biggest addition to the textbook is Section II, which provides an APN lens on the social determinants of health and the contributions APNs are making with Indigenous, inner-city, rural and remote, LGBT2SQ, and migrant populations.

Efforts were made to reduce unnecessary repetition, but some was left as it provides context, informs, reinforces, and often substantiates discussions across the chapters as they relate to concepts and APN role content, which provides for consistency as the textbook progresses from Section I to Section V.

We would like to encourage readers to examine, apply, compare, and contrast the concepts that both clinical nurse specialist and nurse practitioner contributors have put forward in the book as this will add to the evidence of the importance of APN roles in Canada. As a growing and significant component of our evolving health care system, APNs are demonstrating their advocacy in the face of some challenges in health care delivery. Clearly, APN is essential to improving the health and lives of Canadians and that more APNs will be needed in the future.

Best wishes to APN students, graduates, and educators as you utilize this textbook to help guide your practice in a complex and ever-changing health care system.

Eric Staples, Roger Pilon, and Ruth A. Hannon

Acknowledgements

The origin of this textbook grew out of a simple question from an advanced practice nursing (APN) student: "Why don't we have an APN textbook in Canada?" A collaborative effort ensued to meet this need. We are honoured that the first edition received such acceptance across the country, and it has become the definitive textbook on APN in Canada for graduate nursing students preparing to become advanced practice nurses (APNs). There continues to be a need in providing this unique perspective and we are pleased to present the second edition, which examines Canadian APN roles in a period of accelerated health care change and innovation.

There are many people to thank for their role in the completion of this textbook. First, we'd like to thank the contributing authors in both editions who have shared their expertise and practice. Each contributor was selected for a section in which they could contribute from their individual perspective, range of knowledge, and experience. Each chapter can therefore stand on its own yet contributes a significant component to the whole.

We would like to thank Canadian Scholars for believing in and supporting us throughout this project. A special thank you to Katherine Kurowski for her expertise, support, assistance, and patience while we strove to meet deadlines. It was a pleasure to work with her on this project.

We thank our families, friends, colleagues, and each other in supporting, understanding, encouraging, and pushing us forward, which made completing the book a reality.

Finally, we would like to thank APN students and APNs—past, present, and future—who are the reason this textbook exists, and we dedicate this textbook to you. We hope this textbook helps you in your journey of lifelong learning and discovery. If it succeeds in doing this, our mission has been a success!

Eric Staples, Roger Pilon, and Ruth A. Hannon

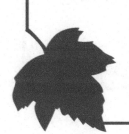

SECTION I

The Evolution of Advanced Practice Nursing in Canada

This section is an overview of the evolutionary timeline of advanced practice nursing (APN) within a Canadian context from early beginnings in outpost settings to the present. Highlights of this section include the strides that have been made in developing and integrating the clinical nurse specialist (CNS) and nurse practitioner (NP) roles, including new rules in Quebec that will see an expansion of practice for NPs. The plethora of Canadian research related to APN demonstrates advanced practice nurses have a valued role in the health care system, particularly in decreasing wait times and improving access to care. Educational, regulatory, legal, and credentialing influences are discussed that have acted as facilitators and barriers to the CNS and NP roles. The Canadian APN framework and other advanced practice frameworks, utilized or developed in Canada, are highlighted to illuminate the evolution of APN in Canada.

Chapter 1

Historical Overview of Advanced Practice Nursing in Canada

Eric Staples, Ruth A. Hannon, and Susan L. Ray

ERIC STAPLES is an Independent Nursing Practice Consultant. He was a graduate of the first postgraduate Acute Care Nurse Practitioner (ACNP) certificate program in Ontario in 1995 from the University of Toronto, and has held Assistant Professor roles at Dalhousie University, Halifax, Nova Scotia, where he was involved in implementing the Advanced Nursing Practice stream in 1998; McMaster University, Hamilton, Ontario, as NP Coordinator in the Ontario Primary Health Care Nurse Practitioner (PHCNP) Program; and the University of Regina, Regina, Saskatchewan. Eric serves or has served on several CASN committees related to NP education, preceptorship, prescribing, and the development of the position statement on doctoral education in Canada. He was the lead developer and editor for the inaugural edition of *Canadian Perspectives in Advanced Practice Nursing*, published in 2016 and in French in 2017.

RUTH A. HANNON is a Teaching Professor in the School of Nursing at McMaster University, Hamilton, Ontario. She also practices as an NP-PHC at Caroline Family Health Team (FHT) in Burlington, Ontario. Ruth was an inaugural editor of *Canadian Perspectives in Advanced Practice Nursing*, published in 2016 and in French in 2017.

SUSAN L. RAY was an Associate Professor and Associate Scientist at the Arthur Labatt Family School of Nursing, Western University, London, Ontario, and, having completed the Tertiary Care NP certificate at Western University, was a CNS-Mental Health in London, Ontario. Susan was a visionary for this textbook but passed away after a short battle with cancer during the initial stages of the book. Susan was a prolific researcher in areas such as the impact of psychological trauma on contemporary peacekeepers, military personnel, veterans, and military families, PTSD and homeless veterans, male survivors of sexual abuse/incest, the immigrant/refugee population, and survivors of natural disasters.

<table>
<tr><td>

KEY TERMS

acute care nurse practitioner
(ACNP)
advanced practice nursing
(APN)
clinical nurse specialist (CNS)
nurse practitioner (NP)
primary health care nurse
practitioner (PHCNP)

</td><td>

OBJECTIVES

1. Appraise the origins of advanced practice nursing (APN) in Canada.
2. Explore the development of the clinical nurse specialist (CNS) role.
3. Explore the development of nurse practitioner (NP) roles.

</td></tr>
</table>

Introduction

In order to fully understand and appreciate advanced practice nursing in Canada, it is necessary to investigate the historical evolution of the roles that today define a level of nursing practice that utilizes extended and expanded clinical competencies, experience, and knowledge that include, but are not limited to, the assessment, diagnosis, planning, implementation, and evaluation of patient care. **Advanced practice nursing (APN)**, as defined by the Canadian Nurses Association (CNA), is

> ... an umbrella term for registered nurses (RNs) and nurse practitioners (NPs) who integrate graduate nursing educational preparation with in-depth, specialized clinical nursing knowledge and expertise in complex decision-making to meet the health needs of individuals, families, groups, communities and populations. (2019, p. 13)

In practice, APNs accomplish this by demonstrating that they analyze and synthesize knowledge, critique, interpret and apply theory, participate in and lead research from nursing and other disciplines, use their advanced clinical competencies, and develop and accelerate nursing knowledge and the profession as a whole. Unlike the **clinical nurse specialist (CNS)** role, the **nurse practitioner (NP)** additionally has regulatory authority to autonomously diagnose, prescribe, order, and interpret diagnostic tests for their clients (CNA, 2019).

This chapter highlights the development of APN roles in Canada from early beginnings to the present day and examines the CNS and NP roles in the context of the socio-political, educational, regulatory, legislative, and economic environments that have shaped them. Chapter 2 will explore the unique historical context of APN in the province of Quebec.

Early Beginnings of Advanced Practice Nursing

Nurses in expanded roles have safely accepted responsibilities traditionally taken by family and general practitioners in rural and remote areas of Canada for over 100 years (Hodgkin,

1977). The demand for nurses to work in these underserviced areas was a result of the chronic shortage of physicians in remote areas of Canada. They were known as outpost nurses and were introduced by religious organizations to improve primary health care services for underserviced populations (Kaasalainen et al., 2010; Kulig et al., 2003). The first formally educated nurses to work in Canada arrived from England as part of the Grenfell Mission (Higgins, 2008; Kulig et al., 2003). Wilfred Grenfell, a British medical missionary, led the Grenfell Mission with the intent to provide the earliest medical services in Labrador and northern Newfoundland (Higgins, 2008). Before the Mission, essentially no health care resources or formally educated nurses existed in these remote rural areas. Demand for nurses to work in underserviced areas of Canada continued to grow following the Grenfell Mission, as nurses in expanded roles accepted responsibilities traditionally held by family and general practitioners (Hodgkin, 1977). These early beginnings of APN have been noted, but largely remain unrecognized within the Canadian health care system (McTavish, 1979).

Evolution of the Clinical Nurse Specialist Role

In 1943, Reiter first introduced the term *nurse clinician* to describe nurses with advanced knowledge and clinical skills capable of providing a high level of patient care (Davies & Eng, 1995; Hamric, Spross, & Hanson, 2009; Lusk, Cockerham, & Keeling, 2019; Montemuro, 1987). After World War II, the term *specialist* was one of the first terms used to describe what the CNS is today.

In the aftermath of two world wars, the federal government encouraged the building of hospitals, and by 1960 most nurses (59%) worked in hospitals, compared with 25% in 1930 (Haines, 1993). Guided by this change in environment, current CNS practice grew to span the continuum of care from pediatric to adult, including long-term and acute care settings such as in-patient units, critical care units, and hospital-based clinics (Bryant-Lukosius et al., 2010; Mayo et al., 2010). Clinical nurse specialists now provide an advanced level of nursing practice through the integration of in-depth knowledge and skills as a clinician, educator, researcher, consultant, and leader (CNA, 2009a) in a variety of clinical specialties, including oncology (Ream et al., 2009), cardiology (Avery & Schnell-Hoehn, 2010), acute and critical care (Jenkins & Lindsey, 2010; Wetzel & Kalman, 2010), gerontology (Smith-Higuchi, Hagen, Brown, & Zeiber, 2006), and mental health (Mayo et al., 2010). Three substantive areas of CNS practice, identified by Lewandowski and Adamle (2009), include the management and care of complex and vulnerable populations, the education and support of interdisciplinary staff, and the facilitation of change and innovation within health care systems.

It was in the 1960s, when a shortage of skilled nurses combined with increasing complexity in health care and technology became the driving force for the introduction of the CNS role into the Canadian health care system. The changes to modern health care following World War I and World War II generated a need for more advanced and specialized nurses with the knowledge and skills to support nursing practice at the bedside (CNA, 2003; Kaasalainen et al., 2010).

By the 1970s, decentralization of political and administrative authority, consumer participation, a shift in emphasis to community-based care and increased emphasis on health care outcomes, combined with physician shortages, a trend toward specialization by physicians, and baccalaureate-level preparation for nurses, created an impetus to critically examine the scope of nursing practice (MacDonald, Herbert, & Thibeault, 2006). The University of Toronto introduced a master's degree program in nursing in 1970 and although it was not specifically designed to educate or produce CNSs, the program focused on clinical specialization.

There has been a consensus in the literature that the minimum level of education required for CNS practice should be a master's degree (CNA, 2009a, 2009b; DiCenso et al., 2010b). This level of educational preparation has been found to influence the extent to which CNSs practice at an advanced level and how they implement their roles. For example, CNSs holding a master's degree can influence patient and population health, nursing practice, and health care systems because they are more likely to implement a range of role activities that are consistent with the national framework for advanced nursing practice. These activities include caring for the most complex patients; working with specific populations; working with staff, patients, and families to develop a plan of care; and policy and program development. In contrast, clinical practice that is focused on the direct care of individuals is the major focus for baccalaureate-prepared CNSs (Schreiber et al., 2005a, 2005b).

By 1986, most practicing CNSs were prepared at the graduate level (Montemuro, 1987). Beaudoin, Besner, and Gaudreault (1978) argued that the CNS role was more in keeping with nursing values than the NP role, which they described as an extension of medicine because of the medical role functions it incorporated. Stevens (1976) agreed and added that the CNS role contributed vastly in attempts to not only professionalize nursing, but to substantiate its existence as an independent profession. However, there are currently no mandatory credentials, educational requirements, nor title protection for CNSs in Canada (Profetto-McGrath, Negrin, Hugo, & Smith, 2010).

The CNA released its first position statement on the CNS role in 1986, describing it as

> ... an expert practitioner who provides direct care to clients and serves as a role model and consultant to other practicing nurses. The nurse participates in research to improve the quality of nursing care and communicates and uses research findings. The practice of the clinical nurse specialist is based on in-depth knowledge of nursing and the behavioural and biological sciences ... A CNS is a registered nurse who holds a master's degree in nursing and has expertise in a clinical nursing specialty. (p. 1)

Following this report, Ontario and British Columbia released two provincial statements on the CNS role. Both statements identified the major components of the CNS role as clinical practice, education, research, consultation, and leadership/change agent. Over time, the CNA has put forth many iterations of definitions of the CNS role (1978, 1986) but these components of the CNS role remained constant throughout subsequent iterations of CNA position statements on the CNS role (CNA, 2003, 2009a, 2014, 2016).

In 1989, one of the most significant developments in advancing the CNS role across Canada was the formation of a national interest group, initially called the Canadian Clinical Nurse Specialist Interest Group (CCNSIG). Leaders within this group worked closely with CNSs from other provinces to help develop their own provincial organizations as well as organize conferences to advance their professional practice. In 1991, CCNSIG became an associate group of the CNA. CCNSIG was renamed in 1998 to the Canadian Association of Advanced Practice Nurses (CAAPN) for the purpose of including other types of APNs (Kaasalainen et al., 2010). Since that time, CAAPN has disbanded into two national groups. The CNS arm of CAAPN rejoined the CNA as the Clinical Nurse Specialist Association of Canada in 2015. Most provinces have CNS associations that are linked to provincial professional nursing bodies where intra-provincial CNS networking and shared issues can be maintained.

Unlike that of the NP, the CNS role has continued to formally exist over the last 40 years; however, hospital budget cutbacks in the 1980s and 1990s led to the elimination of many of these positions (DiCenso & Bryant-Lukosius, 2010). CNS role development and implementation were often challenged by issues related to role ambiguity, lack of involvement or recognition in the organizational structure, and lack of administrative support (Davies & Eng, 1995; Montemuro, 1987).

In early 2000, interest in the CNS role returned, with the intent to bring clinical leadership back into health care environments. Emphasis on helping staff nurses apply evidence to practice was necessary as this leadership was lacking due to reductions in nurse executive and nurse educator positions (Kaasalainen et al., 2010). Currently, the most significant challenges facing the CNS role in Canada include a lack of common vision and understanding of the CNS role, limited access to CNS-specific graduate education programs, and the continued lack of title protection or credentialing (DiCenso et al., 2010a).

Based on the Canadian Institute for Health Information (CIHI; 2010), there were about 2,227 CNSs in Canada in 2008, and the largest numbers of CNSs were found in British Columbia, Quebec, and Ontario. However, the true number of CNSs is unknown because current CNS estimates are based mostly on self-report. Kilpatrick et al. (2013) found that about 1:5 who identify themselves as a CNS have a baccalaureate degree as their highest level of education, and that estimate is most probably considerably low.

CNSs have played an important part in the delivery of advanced nursing services in Canada (Kaasalainen et al., 2010). In several Canadian studies, CNSs described how they promote evidence-based practice (Pepler et al., 2006), influence clinical and administrative decision making (Profetto-McGrath et al., 2007), and integrate research, education, and leadership expertise to improve patient care at three levels—individual patients and nurses/health care providers, the clinical unit, and the organization (Schreiber et al., 2005a, 2005b).

However, their full integration into the health care system will require high-quality research evidence. To date, very little research has been conducted on CNSs in Canada (Bryant-Lukosius et al., 2010; Kilpatrick et al., 2013; Staples & Ray, 2016), but over the next decade, research will play a critical role in forecasting the evolution, needs-based deployment, and impact of the CNS role in Canada.

In recognition of the valuable contributions of the CNS role in Canada, CNA (2014) published the *Pan-Canadian Core Competencies for the Clinical Nurse Specialist* framework, which defines core competencies for CNS practice. The purpose of the framework was to clarify the CNS role and demonstrate its contribution to health care and facilitate role utilization. As well, this framework provides the most updated definition of the CNS role. The current pan-Canadian framework (CNA, 2019) defines the CNS as:

> A registered nurse with advanced nursing knowledge and skills in making complex decisions who holds a master's or doctoral degree in nursing with expertise in a clinical nursing specialty. The CNS role reflects and demonstrates the characteristics and competencies of APN within the RN scope of practice. ... The CNS is an agent of change who brings value to clients, practice settings and organizations to improve safety, promote positive health outcomes and reduce costs. (p. 45)

The framework may be of great value for CNSs, nurse researchers, regulators, and leaders in further defining, integrating, and evaluating the CNS role's scope and influence across diverse practice settings in response to population health needs, and a changing practice and health care landscape.

Evolution of the Nurse Practitioner Role in Primary Health Care

The earliest **primary health care nurse practitioners (PHCNPs)** began practicing in northern Canada over 100 years ago as outpost nurses (Kaasalainen et al., 2010; Kulig et al., 2003; Staples & Ray, 2016). In 1967, the first nursing education programs in Canada for educating midwives and outpost nurses were started at Dalhousie University in Halifax, Nova Scotia. By 1971, other NP programs had been developed at McMaster University, Hamilton, Ontario, and McGill University, Montreal, Quebec, that focused on preparing "family practice nurses" to work in urban settings. The University of British Columbia and Memorial University, St. John's, Newfoundland, followed soon after with similar programs. Six more universities—Alberta, Manitoba, Western Ontario, Toronto, McGill, and Sherbrooke—followed by 1972. The Kergin Report, published in 1970, was highly influential in the development of curriculum for the new programs, which focused on preparing clinically trained nurses (CTNs) to practice in isolated settings (Hazlett, 1975).

In 1972, Boudreau's report, commissioned by the Department of National Health and Welfare and released by the Committee on Nurse Practitioners, strongly recommended that the implementation of the NP role be of the highest priority in meeting primary health care needs of Canadians (Boudreau, 1972). Based on this report, pilot and demonstration projects were initiated across Canada. The evaluation of these projects was favourable: 93% of NPs found employment, more time was reported being spent with patients, and NPs reported role satisfaction (Scherer, Fortin, Spitzer, & Kergin, 1977; Spitzer & Kergin, 1975). Chenoy, Spitzer, and Anderson (1973) found that patients supported nurses being involved in primary health care promotion activities, but in some situations still preferred a physician.

Research also supported the role of NPs in pediatric settings (McFarlane & Norman, 1972), outpatient clinics (King, Spaulding, & Wright, 1974; Ramsay, McKenzie, & Fish, 1982), and emergency settings (Vayda, Gent, & Paisley, 1973). However, in northern Newfoundland and Ontario, outpost nurses were still responsible for providing primary health care to communities in clinics that focused on preventative health and for treating episodic illnesses (Dunn & Higgins, 1986), and the evaluation of one pilot project of four NPs in rural Saskatchewan showed mixed results with the conclusion that role implementation was dependent on specific community needs (Cardenas, 1975).

Two distinct streams of educational programs developed across the country; those continuing to prepare the outpost nurses that provided health services in remote areas of northern Canada, and those that focused on developing nurses with primary health care skills to work in family practices and community nursing settings (Nurse practitioners—the national picture, 1978). The length and educational level of these programs varied; outpost programs were typically two years in length at the post-diploma level while NP programs were eight months in length at the post-baccalaureate level. Debate about educational requirements for NP practice was an issue during the early 1970s. There were several recommendations for baccalaureate education for NPs (Buzzell, 1976) and graduate education for CNSs (Boone & Kikuchi, 1977). A nationwide consensus was achieved in the 1970s determining that additional education beyond a baccalaureate or diploma level was required to prepare nurses for NP roles (Donald et al., 2010). Collaborative practice became an essential expectation of the PHCNP role and integral to defining role functions. Arguments for increased standardization of NP education, however, continued to be debated up until the last decade, when graduate education for all APN roles was deemed necessary (Canadian Nurse Practitioner Initiative [CNPI], 2006b; Schreiber et al., 2005a, 2005b).

Family physicians were not initially interested in NP practice (Kilpatrick et al., 2010), but by 1973, the CNA and the Canadian Medical Association (CMA) released a joint statement on the role of the NP signalling medical support and co-operation in revisiting the need for the NP role. Several provincial nursing groups, as well as NPs, were prolific during this time, working to legitimize expanded nursing roles (Cardenas, 1975). Lalonde's report in 1974 was instrumental in linking the concepts of primary health care and the influence of the determinants of health on societal health and well-being, and the impact of the expanded RN role in health promotion and disease prevention (Lalonde, 1974).

Despite these efforts, by the 1980s, NP education program implementation ceased due to a perceived oversupply of physicians; weak support from medicine, nursing, and policy-makers; little public awareness; lack of funding; and a failure to develop regulation, legislation, and remuneration processes (CIHI, 2006). Although this initial attempt to implement NP roles failed, interest in an expanded role for RNs continued across Canada, and NPs continued to work in several provinces, including Ontario and Saskatchewan, in urban community health centres, northern nursing stations, and First Nations/Indigenous communities. When a perceived undersupply of physicians and a shift to primary health care led to a renewal of the health care system in the 1990s, the role of the NP was again revisited (Collins & Hayes, 2007; Staples & Ray, 2016).

Provincial nursing groups, including former graduates of ceased NP education programs, continued to lobby government for NPs' legitimization, and in the early 1990s, were instrumental in creating new initiatives with Ontario's Ministry of Health and Long-Term Care (MOHLTC) as part of the government's primary health care reform strategy. This eventually resulted in the re-establishment of NP university education programs in 1995 and the Expanded Nursing Services for Patients Act, which was passed in 1998. This legislation gave NPs registered in the new extended class with the College of Nurses of Ontario the authority to practice within a broader scope of practice by adding three controlled acts: communicating a diagnosis, prescribing a limited range of drugs, and ordering certain diagnostic tests, X-rays, and ultrasound (Registered Nurses' Association of Ontario [RNAO], 2013).

During the latter part of the 1990s and into the early 2000s, federal and provincial government reports called for primary health care reform and identified the unique role of nurses in improving timely access to health care delivery services (Kirby, 2002; Romanow, 2002). Provincial and federal governments began investing in primary health care infrastructure and in the establishment of interprofessional health care teams (Butcher, 2015). Reform efforts were fuelled by unprecedented federal and provincial investments in primary health care infrastructure and interdisciplinary health care teams, leading to a countrywide emphasis on enhancing health promotion and improving equitable health care access and quality (Hutchison, 2008). This context prompted the revival of governments' interest in the PHCNP role and initiated the second wave of PHCNP role implementation, supported by legislation, regulation, remuneration mechanisms, and funded education programs. Foundational to implementing the role was the abundant research that strongly demonstrated PHCNPs as effective, safe practitioners who positively influenced patient care, as well as provider and health care system outcomes (Dierick-van Daele et al., 2010).

Many provinces introduced university-based education programs and legislation to support the renewal of PHCNPs and improve access to primary care amid the growing concerns about shortages of doctors and burgeoning interests in developing team-based approaches to health care delivery. In Ontario, the MOHLTC, in conjunction with the Council of University Programs in Nursing, announced a new NP initiative in 1994 as part of broader efforts to improve access to primary health care, supported by a newly funded, 10-university consortium education program in 1995 (CIHI, 2006; DiCenso et al., 2010a; Nurse Practitioners' Association of Ontario [NPAO], 2011; Staples & Ray, 2016).

Other provinces and territories followed suit, with some developing programs at the post-diploma or post-baccalaureate level and others at the master's level (CNPI, 2006c). As of 2008, a graduate degree from an approved graduate-level PHCNP program became the recommended educational standard, both in Canada and internationally (CNA, 2008; International Council of Nurses [ICN], 2008). By the end of 2014, all PHCNP programs across Canada were at the graduate and/or post-graduate level with the newest NP program being a Collaborative

Nurse Practitioner Program between the Schools of Nursing at Saskatchewan Polytechnic, formerly the Saskatchewan Institute of Applied Science and Technology (SIAST), which had a long reputable history of preparing NPs at the post-baccalaureate level, and the University of Regina (Saskatchewan Collaborative Programs in Nursing, 2015; Staples & Ray, 2016; University of Regina [UR] & SIAST, 2013).

Nursing leaders, realizing that a national integrated approach was required for continued sustainability of the role, proposed the development of a Canadian APN framework. The CNPI, funded federally by Health Canada and sponsored by CNA, was instrumental in developing literature related directly to practice, education, legislation, implementation, and social marketing of the NP role across Canada (CNA, 2008). Accomplishments of this group included the development and later revision of the *Canadian Nurse Practitioner Core Competency Framework* (CNA, 2010), which identified the core competencies required for all NPs in practice, regardless of individual clinical specialization; the Canadian Nurse Practitioner Examination (CNPI, 2006b); the *Implementation and Evaluation Toolkit for Nurse Practitioners in Canada* (CNPI, 2006a); and frameworks for practice, education, legislation, and regulation (CNPI, 2006c).

Prior to the CNPI, each provincial/territorial regulatory body had its own examination for licensing/credentialing PHCNPs. In 2005, CNA, in collaboration with all nursing regulatory bodies except Quebec, announced the first national examination, the Canadian Nurse Practitioner Examination (CNPE). This also marked a change led by CNA from care-based licensure/credentialing to a population-based focus that was called Family/All Ages.

Today, although there is no national definition for the PHCNP role, it is understood that they provide primary health care services to individuals, groups, and families across the lifespan and work in a variety of community-based settings (DiCenso, Paech, & IBM Corporation, 2003; DiCenso et al., 2007). The focus of their practice is health promotion, illness prevention, the diagnosis and treatment of episodic conditions and injuries, and the monitoring and managing of stable chronic conditions (DiCenso et al., 2003; Sidani, Irvine, & DiCenso, 2000a; Way, Jones, Baskerville, & Busing, 2001). PHCNPs utilize an evidence-informed holistic approach that emphasizes health promotion and community partnership development and practice that complements rather than replaces physicians.

Patient satisfaction with the PHCNP continues to be high (Heale & Pilon, 2012). Heightened awareness of the NP role has made the Canadian public more comfortable with NPs and most are willing to see an NP instead of their physician for health care needs (Harris/Decima, 2009). PHCNP, also referred to as NP-Family/All Ages, is the fastest-growing advanced practice nursing role in Canada.

Evolution of the Nurse Practitioner Role in Acute/Tertiary Care

While PHCNP programs were being phased out and closed in the 1980s, there was a rising interest for an APN role in acute/tertiary care settings. Government cutbacks in medical school funding had led to decreased numbers of medical residency positions. Compounded by an exodus of medical graduates to the United States (US), Canadian physicians were experiencing increased workloads in acute care settings. Health care administrators, medical directors, and nurses described a lack of continuity in patient care, leading to a growing concern regarding the rising acuity in acute/tertiary patients and the increasing complexity of care delivery. Additionally, in neonatal intensive care units (NICU), a concern for maintaining a high standard of newborn care in the face of these economic and workforce issues generated the development of a post-graduate diploma NP program at McMaster University, Hamilton, Ontario, in 1986 (Paes et al., 1989).

The role title that evolved from this program was that of the neonatal nurse practitioner (NNP). The introduction of the NNP in Ontario was based on comprehensive needs assessments (DiCenso, 1998; Paes et al., 1989). These included surveys that were conducted to delineate the role (Hunsberger et al., 1992), evaluations of the graduate-level education program that was developed (Mitchell et al., 1995), a randomized controlled trial to evaluate the effectiveness of the role (Mitchell-DiCenso et al., 1996), and assessments of team satisfaction with the role (Mitchell-DiCenso, Pinelli, & Southwell, 1996). Around this time, the term *CNS* was also attached to the NP title: CNS/NP. This was a deliberate action aimed to legitimize the non-clinical advanced practice role domains that included education, research, and leadership (DiCenso, 1998; Hunsberger et al., 1992).

The term *acute care nurse practitioner* (ACNP) was first coined in the US to describe NPs working in critical care areas (Kleinpell, 1997). In Canada, the term was adopted in the mid-1990s for NPs working in specialty disciplines within acute care settings (Simpson, 1997). Also known as specialty or specialist NPs, ACNPs provide advanced nursing care for patients who are acutely, critically, or chronically ill with complex conditions (CNA, 2008).

The ACNP program at the University of Toronto began in 1993 and was the first NP program to offer post-graduate level education outside of neonatology (Simpson, 1997). Some provinces continue to offer generalist graduate ACNP programs, for example, in an adult-focused specialty discipline (CNA, 2008), where the knowledge and skills specific to the desired clinical specialty are obtained through both graduate education and preceptored clinical learning placements.

Neonatology, however, was the most specialized acute care program in the English-speaking provinces (Rutherford & Rutherford Consulting Group Inc., 2005). In Quebec, the ACNP was the first NP role formally introduced into the health care system and remains the most specialized acute care program (Ordre des infirmières et infirmiers du Québec [OIIQ], 2009). Acute care NPs in Quebec are authorized to practice only in the clinical specialty areas, such as neonatology, nephrology, cardiology, and primary care, in which they are prepared (Allard & Durand, 2006; OIIQ & Collège des médecins du Québec [CMQ], 2006), and specialty preparation and certification are required for using the title *specialized* (Bussières & Parent, 2004).

Acute care NP programs and roles were also developed and introduced at the University of Western Ontario, London, Ontario, and the University of Calgary, Calgary, Alberta, and focused on specialty areas within hospitals in response to the shortage of medical residents and lack of continuity of care for seriously ill patients (Pringle, 2007).

In contrast to the PHCNP programs, all ACNP educational programs were developed at the graduate or postgraduate level throughout Canada (Alcock, 1996; Faculté des sciences infirmières, Université de Montréal, 2008; Roschkov et al., 2007). The first wave of graduates from these programs specialized in neonatal ICU, cardiology/cardiovascular, oncology, gerontology, and nephrology. Kilpatrick et al. (2010) found that internal politics influenced the selection of these specific specialty areas over primary health care, specifically one specialist in the university teaching hospitals who was responsible for lobbying in support of educating ACNPs focused on these areas.

Canadian and international literature agree on the components of the ACNP role (Almost & Laschinger, 2002; Royal College of Nursing [RCN], 2008; Sidani & Irvine, 1999). Both the CNS and NP roles share the core competencies with other types of APN roles, that is, direct patient care, research, education, consultation, and leadership activities (CNA, 2009b, 2019; Schreiber et al., 2005a). Studies have also demonstrated the effective and safe practice of ACNPs in a variety of clinical settings, such as emergency rooms, in-patient settings, NICU, outpatient and ambulatory clinics, based on a range of patient and health care system identified outcomes (i.e., patient health status, quality of care, patient or provider satisfaction, health care system costs, and length of stay). Acute care NPs contribute to the delivery of complex (D'Amour et al., 2007), patient-centred care and can utilize both pharmacological and non-pharmacological approaches. Additionally, ACNPs promote patient self-care abilities, improve symptom management, and increase patients' abilities to perform activities of daily living (Sidani, 2008; Sidani et al., 2006a). RNs, physicians, administrators, and ACNPs have all reported that the ACNP role has led to improvements in the continuity of care for acutely ill patients (van Soeren & Micevski, 2001).

Although ACNPs engage predominantly in direct patient-focused care activities, diagnostic activities, care planning, and coordination (Sidani et al., 2000b) are non-clinical activities that are generally performed with, or for the benefit of, nursing or other organizational staff. In Quebec, it is recommended that 70% of ACNP practice constitute direct clinical activities and 30% in non-clinical activities such as leadership, education, and research (OIIQ & CMQ, 2006). Clearly identifying ACNP non-clinical activities are important because these activities distinguish this role's strong combined clinical and leadership focus. It is this unique combination that enables ACNPs to contribute effectively to the improvements of patient care quality, and health care provider and system outcomes (Irvine et al., 2000).

Many ACNPs, however, have difficulty integrating all the domains or competencies of their APN role, given their patient care responsibilities (D'Amour et al., 2007; Staples & Ray, 2016). The struggle to balance direct clinical and non-clinical functions has created high, even unrealistic expectations of the ACNP role, and confusion with the similar role functions of the CNS. Griffiths (2006) highlighted the importance of clearly articulating and defining each role's purpose and scope of practice, since the overlap of role function may be significant between CNSs and ACNPs in the same medical discipline, given that they both have graduate-level education and share many care coordination functions (Sidani et al., 2006a, 2006b; Williams & Sidani, 2001).

There is also a discrepancy between the expectations of administrators and the expecta-tions of physicians regarding the amount of time ACNPs spend in direct patient care acti-vities. Physicians believe that the ACNPs' time should be devoted predominantly to direct clinical practice, whereas administrators have recognized the importance of protecting the time ACNPs spend engaging in leadership, education, and research aligned with their role because these activities support nursing practice within the organization (Kilpatrick et al., 2010). This situation stems from neonatology, when CNS and NP roles were purposefully combined in order to distinguish and legitimize non-clinical nursing activities (DiCenso, 1998; Hunsberger et al., 1992).

The exploration of nursing administrators' roles and perspectives when introducing an ACNP role within the health care team by Reay, Golden-Biddle, and Germann (2006) found that nursing administrators faced three major challenges: task reallocation, manage-ment of altered working relationships, and management of the team in an evolving situation. Successful implementation of ACNPs into health care teams was reliant on administrators' ability to clearly communicate ACNP role expectations (van Soeren & Micevski, 2001), pro-vide a clear vision of the ACNP role to both ACNPs and team members, and support ACNP roles across the organization (Reay, Golden-Biddle, & Germann, 2006).

The development of detailed role descriptions (Cummings, Fraser, & Tarlier, 2003), with input from ACNPs (Nhan & Zuidema, 2007) and open dialogue between administrators and team members, promotes a greater understanding of the ACNP role (Wall, 2006) and helps to define clear expectations of the ACNP role (Rosenthal & Guerrasio, 2009). These strate-gies have increased job satisfaction and assisted the facilitation of ACNP integration into the health care team (Cummings et al., 2003).

Notoriously, physicians have had the final say on whether or not they will accept the implementation of an ACNP in their practice (D'Amour et al., 2007), directly affecting the ability of ACNPs to work to their full scope of practice (McNamara et al., 2009). Disagreement related to the scope of ACNP practice has created interprofessional barriers that impede the development of the role in Quebec (D'Amour et al., 2007; D'Amour, Tremblay, & Proulx, 2009; Desrosiers, 2009; McNamara et al., 2009; OIIQ, 2009). Professional territoriality has been highlighted in acute care–setting literature. Some medical residents have expressed concern about losing control of patient care decisions and competing with ACNPs for oppor-tunities to perform medical skills (D'Amour et al., 2007; Fédération des médecins résidents du Québec, 2003a, 2003b, 2003c, 2004).

Findings regarding nurses' views of ACNP roles, however, are mixed. D'Amour et al. (2007) reported that in Quebec, RNs expressed concern over a perceived increase in hierar-chy within the nursing profession following the introduction of ACNP roles. Other studies (Harwood et al., 2004; Mitchell-DiCenso, Pinelli, & Southwell, 1996) found that nurses had a positive view of the ACNP role because ACNPs were a ready source of patient information, attended to team members' concerns about patients in a timely manner, improved commu-nication among team members, and provided consistency in patient care because they were always visible unlike medical residents, who are clinically rotated. The results vary, in part due to the length of time nurses had been exposed to ACNPs prior to the study being conducted, since further studies demonstrated that nurses did not feel their roles were threatened by the introduction and integration of ACNPs (Irvine et al., 2000).

Until 2008, ACNPs, now referred to, in keeping with the CNPE population-based focus, as NP-Adult and NP-Pediatrics (CNA, 2010), were not licensed/credentialed and, therefore, were not included in the regulatory data. However, the number of ACNPs increased between 2003 and 2007 in all provincial jurisdictions by 5% (CIHI, 2008). Roots and MacDonald (2008) conducted an exploratory study on NPs and stakeholders to identify the factors influencing NP role implementation in British Columbia, and they reported a mismatch between NP education and available positions. For example, some NPs educated in primary health care were working in acute care or with specialized populations. Schreiber et al. (2005a) found that APNs in British Columbia needed to engage in both formal and informal education opportunities to further role development.

After CAAPN was disbanded around 2016, NPs who had been part of CAAPN came together and re-emerged in 2017 as the Nurse Practitioner Association of Canada. Most provinces also have NP associations that are linked to the provincial professional nursing bodies where intra-provincial NP networking and shared issues can be maintained.

Unfortunately, access to clinical specialty education in Canada is very limited. This is notable because specialty education is significant in developing role confidence, job satisfaction (Bryant-Lukosius et al., 2007), self-confidence, and the ability to solve complex problems (Richmond & Becker, 2005). Researchers (CNA, 2006; D'Amour et al., 2007; DiCenso & Bryant-Lukosius, 2010; OIIQ, 2009) question the long-term survival of ACNP roles without stable funding and salaries that clearly recognize their scope of practice and the level of responsibility involved once they have been successfully incorporated into the health care delivery organization.

Research on the role of ACNPs demonstrates that ACNPs can improve patient health (i.e., symptom management and ability to perform activities of daily living); enhance quality of care and patient or provider satisfaction; and reduce health care system costs and length of hospital stay (Sidani, 2008; Sidani et al., 2006a; Staples & Ray, 2016; Wilson, 2016). In addition, ACNPs have been found to improve the continuity of care for acutely ill patients (van Soeren & Micevski, 2001). The status of ACNP roles continues to evolve across the nation and ongoing leadership and research continue to be vital to the enhancement and the integration of these roles into the Canadian health care system.

Conclusion

Nurses have practiced in several expanded roles across Canada for over a century. The role that began with outpost nurses—world war "nurse clinicians" and "specialists"—has undergone an intense evolution and emerged as the CNS, PHCNP, NP, ACNP, and other streams of APN that are visible today.

An updated definition of the CNS role (CNA, 2014) provided direction for role clarity and ongoing role integration across practice settings within a changing health care environment.

There continues to be only one definition for all NP roles in Canada that focuses on the required educational preparation and experience required to autonomously practice within a regulated scope of practice. Through the integration of in-depth knowledge and skills, each of the APN roles provides an advanced level of nursing practice that is diverse and spans all aspects of clinical practice.

Although NNPs were the first to be termed ACNPs in Canada, ACNPs are found in all areas of practice and predominantly engage in direct patient care activities, diagnostic activities, care planning, and care coordination. However, the continued sustainability of CNS and NP roles, once they have been successfully incorporated into the health care system, without stable funding and salaries that recognize both their scope of practice and level of responsibility is in question. Ongoing leadership and continued research are required to enhance the development and integration of all APN roles into the Canadian health care system.

Critical Thinking Questions

1. Compare and contrast the roles of CNS and NP.
2. What has been the impact of the CNS and NP roles in the delivery of health care services?
3. Can you trace the introduction of either the CNS or NP role within your organization?
4. What have been the facilitators and barriers of implementing APN roles in Canada?

References

Alcock, D. S. (1996). The clinical nurse specialist, clinical nurse specialist/nurse practitioner and other titled nurse in Ontario. *Canadian Journal of Nursing Administration, 9*(1), 23–44.

Allard, M., & Durand, S. (2006). L'infirmière praticienne spécialisée : Un nouveau rôle de pratique infirmière avancée au Québec [The specialized nurse practitioner: A new role for advanced nursing practice in Quebec]. *Perspective Infirmière: Revue Officielle de l'Ordre des Infirmières et Infirmiers du Québec, 3*(5), 10–16.

Almost, J., & Laschinger, H. K. (2002). Workplace empowerment, collaborative work relationships and job strain in nurse practitioners. *Journal of the American Academy of Nurse Practitioners, 14*(9), 408–420.

Avery, L. J., & Schnell-Hoehn, K. N. (2010). Clinical nurse specialist practice in evidence-informed multidisciplinary cardiac care. *Clinical Nurse Specialist, 24*(2), 76–79.

Beaudoin, M. L., Besner, G., & Gaudreault, G. (1978). Praticienne? Clinicienne? [Practitioner? Clinician?]. *Infirmière Canadienne, 20*(12), 23–25.

Boone, M., & Kikuchi, J. (1977). The clinical nurse specialist. In B. LaSor & R. Elliott (Eds.), *Issues in Canadian nursing* (pp. 101–112). Scarborough, ON: Prentice-Hall.

Boudreau, T. J. (1972). *Report of the committee on nurse practitioners.* Ottawa, ON: Department of National Health and Welfare.

Bryant-Lukosius, D., Carter, N., Kilpatrick, K., Martin-Misener, R., Donald, F., Kaasalainen, S., ... DiCenso, A. (2010). The clinical nurse specialist role in Canada. *Canadian Journal of Nursing Leadership, 23*(December), 140–166.

Bryant-Lukosius, D., Green, E., Fitch, M., Macartney, G., Robb-Blenderman, L., McFarlane, S., … Milne, H. (2007). A survey of oncology advanced practice nurses in Ontario: Profile and predictors of job satisfaction. *Canadian Journal of Nursing Leadership, 20*(2), 50–68.

Bussières, J., & Parent, M. (2004). Histoire de la spécialisation en santé au Québec—1re partie [History of health specialization in Quebec—Part 1]. *Pharmactuel, 37*(1), 39–50.

Butcher, M. (2015). Ontario's first nurse practitioner-led clinic. In C. Mariano (Ed.), *No one left behind: How nurse practitioners are changing the Canadian health care system* (pp. 21–34). Victoria, BC: Friesen Press.

Buzzell, E. M. (1976). Baccalaureate preparation for the nurse practitioner: When will we ever learn? *Nursing Papers, 8*(3), 2–9.

Canadian Institute for Health Information (CIHI). (2006). *The regulation and supply of nurse practitioners in Canada: 2006 update.* Ottawa, ON: CIHI. Retrieved from https://secure.cihi.ca/free_products/The_Nurse_Practitioner_Workforce_in_Canada_2006_Update_final.pdf

CIHI. (2008). *Regulated nurses: Trends, 2003 to 2007: Registered nurses, licensed practical nurses, registered psychiatric nurses.* Ottawa, ON: CIHI. Retrieved from https://secure.cihi.ca/free_products/nursing_report_2003_to_2007_e.pdf

CIHI. (2010). *Regulated nurses in Canada: Trends of registered nurses, 2005 to 2009.* Ottawa, ON: CIHI. Retrieved from https://secure.cihi.ca/free_products/nursing_report_2005-2009_en.pdf

Canadian Nurses Association (CNA). (1978). *Position statement: Clinical nurse specialist.* Ottawa, ON: CNA.

CNA. (1986). *Position statement: Clinical nurse specialist.* Ottawa, ON: CNA.

CNA. (2003). *Position statement: Clinical nurse specialist.* Ottawa, ON: CNA.

CNA. (2006). *Report of 2005 dialogue on advanced nursing practice.* Ottawa, ON: CNA.

CNA. (2008). *Advanced nursing practice: A national framework.* Ottawa, ON: CNA.

CNA. (2009a). *Position statement: The clinical nurse specialist.* Ottawa, ON: CNA.

CNA. (2009b). *Position statement: The nurse practitioner.* Ottawa, ON: CNA.

CNA. (2010). *Canadian nurse practitioner core competency framework.* Ottawa, ON: CNA.

CNA. (2014). *Pan-Canadian core competencies for the clinical nurse specialist.* Ottawa, ON: CNA. Retrieved from http://cna-aiic.ca/en/news-room/news-releases/2014/canadian-nurses-association-launches-core-competencies-for-clinical-nurse-specialists

CNA. (2016). *Position statement: Clinical nurse specialist.* Ottawa, ON: CNA.

CNA. (2019). *Advanced practice nursing: A pan-Canadian framework.* Ottawa, ON: CNA. Retrieved from https://www.cna-aiic.ca/-/media/cna/page-content/pdf-en/advanced-practice-nursing-framework-en.pdf

Canadian Nurse Practitioner Initiative (CNPI). (2006a). *Implementation and evaluation toolkit for nurse practitioners in Canada.* Ottawa, ON: CNA. Retrieved from https://nurseone.ca/~/media/nurseone/files/en/toolkit_implementation_evaluation_np_e.pdf

CNPI. (2006b). *Nurse practitioners: The time is now: A solution to improving access and reducing wait times in Canada.* Ottawa, ON: CNA. Retrieved from http://www.npnow.ca/docs/tech-report/section1/01_Integrated_Report.pdf

CNPI. (2006c). *Nurse practitioners: The time is now. Technical reports.* Ottawa, ON: CNA.

Canadian Nurses Association (CNA), & the Canadian Medical Association (CMA). (1973). *The joint committee on the expanded role of the nurses: Statement of policy.* Ottawa, ON: CNA/CMA.

Cardenas, B. D. (1975). The independent nurse practitioner. Alive and well and living in rural Saskatchewan. *Nursing Clinics of North America, 10*(4), 711–719.

Chenoy, N. C., Spitzer, W. O., & Anderson, G. D. (1973). Nurse practitioners in primary care. II. Prior attitudes of a rural population. *Canadian Medical Association Journal, 108*(8), 998–1003.

Collins, P. A., & Hayes, M. V. (2007). Twenty years since Ottawa and Epp: Researchers' reflections on challenges, gains and future prospects for reducing health inequities in Canada. *Health Promotion International, 22*(4), 337–345.

Cummings, G. G., Fraser, K., & Tarlier, D. S. (2003). Implementing advanced nurse practitioner roles in acute care: An evaluation of organizational change. *Journal of Nursing Administration, 33*(3), 139–145.

D'Amour, D., Morin, D., Dubois, C., Lavoie-Tremblay, M., Dallaire, C., & Cyr, G. (2007). *Évaluation de l'implantation du programme d'intéressement au titre d'infirmière praticienne* [Evaluation of the implementation of the incentive program as a nurse practitioner]. Montreal, QC: Ministère de la Santé et des Services sociaux du Québec.

D'Amour, D., Tremblay, D., & Proulx, M. (2009). Déploiement de nouveaux rôles infirmiers au Québec et pouvoir médical [Deployment of new nursing roles in Quebec and medical power]. *Recherches sociographiques, 50*(2), 301–320.

Davies, B., & Eng, B. (1995). Implementation of the CNS role in Vancouver, British Columbia, Canada. *Clinical Nurse Specialist, 9*(1), 23–30.

Desrosiers, G. (2009). Toutes les infirmières sont importantes, mais alors, pourquoi encore parler des infirmières praticiennes spécialisées? [All nurses are important, but then why talk about specialized nurse practitioners?]. *Le Journal, 6*(3), 2.

DiCenso, A. (1998). The neonatal nurse practitioner. *Current Opinion in Pediatrics, 10*(2), 151–155.

DiCenso, A., Auffrey, L., Bryant-Lukosius, D., Donald, F., Martin-Misener, R., Matthews, S., & Opsteen, J. (2007). Primary health care nurse practitioners in Canada. *Contemporary Nurse, 26*(1), 104–115. doi: 10.5172/conu.2007.26.1.104

DiCenso, A., & Bryant-Lukosius, D. (2010). The long and winding road: Integration of nurse practitioners and clinical nurse specialists into the Canadian health-care system. *Canadian Journal of Nursing Research, 42*(2), 3–8.

DiCenso, A., Bryant-Lukosius, D., Bourgeault, I., Martin-Misener, R., Donald, F., Abelson, J., … Harbman, P. (2010a). *Clinical nurse specialists and nurse practitioners in Canada: A decision support synthesis.* Ottawa, ON: Canadian Health Services Research Foundation.

DiCenso, A., Martin-Misener, R., Bryant-Lukosius, D., Bourgeault, I., Kilpatrick, K., Donald, F., … Charbonneau-Smith, R. (2010b). Advanced practice nursing in Canada: Overview of a decision support synthesis. *Nursing Leadership, 23*(Special Issue), 15–34.

DiCenso, A., Paech, G., & IBM Corporation. (2003). *Report on the integration of primary health care nurse practitioners into the province of Ontario.* Toronto, ON: MOHLTC.

Dierick-van Daele, A., Steuten, L., Metsemakers, J., Derckx, E., Spreeuwenberg, C., & Vrijhoef, H. (2010). Economic evaluation of nurse practitioners versus GPs in treating common conditions. *British Journal of General Practice, 60*(570), e28–e35.

Donald, F., Martin-Misener, R., Bryant-Lukosius, D., Kilpatrick, K., Kaasalainen, S., Carter, N., … DiCenso, A. (2010). The primary healthcare nurse practitioner role in Canada. *Nursing Leadership, 23*(December), 88–113.

Dunn, E. V., & Higgins, C. A. (1986). Health problems encountered by three levels of providers in a remote setting. *American Journal of Public Health, 76*(2), 154–159.

Faculté des sciences infirmières, Université de Montréal. (2008). *Une maîtrise, quatre options* [One master's degree, four options]. Montreal, QC: Université de Montréal.

Fédération des médecins résidents du Québec. (2003a). *Avis consultatif de la FMRQ déposé dans le cadre des activités du comité conjoint consultatif paritaire OIIQ-CMQ concernant l'infirmière praticienne en cardiologie-volet chirurgie cardiaque* [FMRQ advisory opinion submitted within the framework of the activities of the joint OIIQ-CMQ consultative committee concerning the nurse practitioner in cardiology-cardiac surgery]. Montreal, QC: Fédération des médecins résidents du Québec.

Fédération des médecins résidents du Québec. (2003b). *Avis consultatif de la FMRQ déposé dans le cadre des activités du comité conjoint consultatif paritaire OIIQ-CMQ concernant l'infirmière praticienne en néonatologie* [FMRQ advisory opinion submitted within the framework of the activities of the joint OIIQ-CMQ consultative committee concerning the nurse practitioner in neonatology]. Montreal, QC: Fédération des médecins résidents du Québec.

Fédération des médecins résidents du Québec. (2003c). *Avis consultatif de la FMRQ déposé dans le cadre des activités du comité conjoint consultatif paritaire OIIQ-CMQ concernant l'infirmière praticienne en néphrologie* [FMRQ advisory opinion submitted within the framework of the activities of the joint OIIQ-CMQ consultative committee concerning the nurse practitioner in nephrology]. Montreal, QC: Fédération des médecins résidents du Québec.

Fédération des médecins résidents du Québec. (2004). *Avis consultatif de la FMRQ déposé dans le cadre des activités du comité conjoint consultatif paritaire OIIQ-CMQ concernant la création du rôle de l'infirmière praticienne spécialisée en cardiologie-volet cardiologie médicale au Québec* [FMRQ advisory opinion submitted within the framework of the activities of the joint OIIQ-CMQ consultative committee concerning the creation of the role of nurse practitioner specializing in cardiology-medical cardiology component in Quebec]. Montreal, QC: Fédération des médecins résidents du Québec.

Griffiths, H. (2006). Advanced nursing practice: Enter the nurse practitioner. *Nursing BC, 38*(2), 12–16.

Haines, J. (1993). *The nurse practitioner: A discussion paper*. Ottawa, ON: CNA.

Hamric, A. B., Spross, J. A., & Hanson, C. (2009). *Advanced nursing practice: An integrative approach* (4th ed.). Philadelphia, PA: W. B. Saunders.

Harris/Decima. (2009, August 13). *Canadians very comfortable with expanded role for nurse practitioners*. Ottawa, ON: Harris/Decima.

Harwood, L., Wilson, B., Heidenheim, A. P., & Lindsay, R. M. (2004). The advanced practice nurse–nephrologist care model: Effect on patient outcomes and hemodialysis unit team satisfaction. *Hemodialysis International, 8*(3), 273–282.

Hazlett, C. B. (1975). Task analysis of the clinically trained nurse (C.T.N.). *Nursing Clinics of North America, 10*(4), 699–709.

Heale, R., & Pilon, R. S. (2012). Nurse practitioner clinics: Exploration of client satisfaction. *Canadian Journal of Nursing Leadership, 25*(3), 43–55.

Higgins, J. (2008). *Grenfell Mission: Newfoundland and Labrador heritage*. St. John's, NL: Memorial University of Newfoundland.

Hodgkin, K. (1977). The family practice nurse. *Canadian Medical Association Journal, 116*(8), 829–830.

Hunsberger, M., Mitchell, A., Blatz, S., Paes, B., Pinelli, J., Southwell, D., … Soluk, R. (1992). Definition of an advanced nursing practice role in the NICU: The clinical nurse specialist/neonatal practitioner. *Clinical Nurse Specialist, 6*(2), 91–96.

Hutchison, B. (2008). A long time coming: Primary healthcare renewal in Canada. *Healthcare Papers, 8*(2), 10–24.

International Council of Nurses (ICN). (2008). *The scope of practice, standards and competencies of the advanced practice nurse*. Geneva, CH: ICN.

Irvine, D., Sidani, S., Porter, H., O'Brien-Pallas, L., Simpson, B., McGillis Hall, L., ... Nagel, L. (2000). Organizational factors influencing nurse practitioners' role implementation in acute care settings. *Canadian Journal of Nursing Leadership, 13*(3), 28–35.

Jenkins, S. D., & Lindsey, P. L. (2010). Clinical nurse specialists as leaders in rapid response. *Clinical Nurse Specialist, 24*(1), 24–30.

Kaasalainen, S., Martin-Misener, R., Kilpatrick, K., Harbman, P., Bryant-Lukosius, D., Donald, F., ... & DiCenso, A. (2010). A historical overview of the development of advanced practice nursing roles in Canada. *Nursing Leadership, 23*(Special Issue), 35–60.

Kilpatrick, K., DiCenso, A., Bryant-Lukosius, D., Ritchie, J. A., Martin-Misener, R., & Carter, N. (2013). Practice patterns and perceived impact of clinical nurse specialist roles in Canada: Results of a national survey. *International Journal of Nursing Studies, 50*(11), 1524–1536.

Kilpatrick, K., Harbman, P., Carter, N., Martin-Misener, R., Bryant-Lukosius, D., Donald, F., ... DiCenso, A. (2010). The acute care nurse practitioner role in Canada. *Nursing Leadership, 23*(December), 114–139.

King, B., Spaulding, W. B., & Wright, A. D. (1974). Problem-oriented diabetic day care. *The Canadian Nurse, 70*(10), 19–22.

Kirby, M. (2002). *The health of Canadians—The federal role. Final report.* Ottawa, ON: Parliament of Canada. Retrieved from http://www.parl.gc.ca/content/sen/committee/372/soci/rep/repoct02vol6-e.htm

Kleinpell, R. M. (1997). Acute-care nurse practitioners: Roles and practice profiles. *American Association of Clinical-Care Nurses (AACN) Clinical Issues, 8*(1), 156–162.

Kulig, J., Thomlinson, E., Curran, F., Nahachewsky, D., Macleod, M., Stewart, N., & Pitblado, R. (2003). *Nursing practice in rural and remote Canada: An analysis of policy documents.* Prince George, BC: University of Northern British Columbia. Retrieved from http://ruralnursing.unbc.ca/reports/jkulig/FinalReportweb.pdf

Lalonde, M. (1974). *A new perspective on health of Canadians: A working document.* Ottawa, ON: Government of Canada. Retrieved from http://www.phac-aspc.gc.ca/ph-sp/pdf/perspect-eng.pdf

Lewandowski, W., & Adamle, K. (2009). Substantive areas of clinical nurse specialist practice: A comprehensive review of the literature. *Clinical Nurse Specialist, 23*(2), 73–90.

Lusk, B., Cockerham, A. Z., & Keeling. A. W. (2019). Highlights from the history of advanced practice nursing in the United States. In M. F. Tracey & E. T. O'Grady (Eds.), *Hamric and Hanson's advanced practice nursing* (6th ed., pp. 10–15). St. Louis, MO: Elsevier.

MacDonald, J., Herbert, R., & Thibeault, C. (2006). Advanced practice nursing: Unification through a common identity. *Journal of Professional Nursing, 22*(3), 172–179.

Mayo, A. M., Omery, A., Agocs-Scott, L. M., Khaghani, F., Meckes, P. G., Moti, N., ... Cuenca, E. (2010). Clinical nurse specialist practice patterns. *Clinical Nurse Specialist, 24*(2), 60–68.

McFarlane, A. H., & Norman, G. R. (1972). A medical care information system: Evaluation of changing patterns of primary care. *Medical Care, 10*(6), 481–487.

McNamara, S., Giguère, V., St-Louis, L., & Boileau, J. (2009). Development and implementation of the specialized nurse practitioner role: Use of the PEPPA framework to achieve success. *Nursing and Health Sciences, 11*(3), 318–325.

McTavish, M. (1979). The nurse practitioner: An idea whose time has come. *Canadian Nurse, 75*(8), 41–44.

Mitchell, A., Watts, J., Whyte, R., Blatz, S., Norman, G., Southwell, D., ... Pinelli, J. (1995). Evaluation of an educational program to prepare neonatal nurse practitioners. *Journal of Nursing Education, 34*(6), 286–289.

Mitchell-DiCenso, A., Guyatt, G., Marrin, M., Goeree, R., Willan, A., Southwell, D., … Baumann, A. (1996). A controlled trial of nurse practitioners in neonatal intensive care. *Pediatrics, 98*(6), 1143–1148.

Mitchell-DiCenso, A., Pinelli, J., & Southwell, D. (1996). Introduction and evaluation of an advanced nursing practice role in neonatal intensive care. In K. Kelly (Ed.), *Outcomes of effective management practice* (pp. 171–186). Thousand Oaks, CA: Sage.

Montemuro, M. A. (1987). The evolution of the clinical nurse specialist: Response to the challenge of professional nursing practice. *Clinical Nurse Specialist, 1*(3), 106–110.

Nhan, J., & Zuidema, S. (2007). Nurse practitioners in the northern Alberta renal program. *Canadian Association of Nephrology Nurses and Technologists Journal, 17*(2), 48–50.

Nurse practitioners—the national picture. (1978). *The Canadian Nurse, 74*(4), 13.

Nurse Practitioners' Association of Ontario (NPAO). (2011). *NP history in Ontario.* Toronto, ON: NPAO. Retrieved from http://npao.org/nurse-practitioners/history/

Ordre des infirmières et infirmiers du Québec (OIIQ). (2009). *Les infirmières praticiennes spécialisées : Un rôle à propulser, une intégration à accélérer. Bilan et perspectives de pérennité* [Specialized nurse practitioners: A role to propel, an integration to accelerate. Assessment and prospects for sustainability]. Montreal, QC: OIIQ.

Ordre des infirmières et infirmiers du Québec (OIIQ), & Collège des médecins du Québec (CMQ). (2006). *Lignes directrices sur les modalités de la pratique de l'infirmière praticienne spécialisée* [Guidelines for the practice of the nurse practitioner]. Montreal, QC: OIIQ/CMQ.

Paes, B., Mitchell, A., Hunsberger, M., Blatz, S., Watts, J., Dent, P., … Southwell, D. (1989). Medical staffing in Ontario neonatal intensive care units. *The Canadian Medical Association Journal, 140*(11), 1321–1326.

Pepler, C. J., Edgar, L., Frisch, S., Rennick, J., Swidzinski, M., White, C., … Gross, J. (2006). Strategies to increase research-based practice: Interplay with unit culture. *Clinical Nurse Specialist, 20*(1), 23–31.

Pringle, D. (2007). Nurse practitioner role: Nursing needs it. *Canadian Journal of Nursing Leadership, 20*(2), 1–5.

Profetto-McGrath, J., Negrin, K. A., Hugo, K., & Smith, K. B. (2010). Clinical nurse specialists' approaches in selecting and using evidence to improve practice. *Worldviews on Evidence-Based Nursing, 7*(1), 36–50.

Profetto-McGrath, J., Smith, K. B., Hugo, K., Taylor, M., & El-Hajj, H. (2007). Clinical nurse specialists' use of evidence in practice: A pilot study. *Worldviews on Evidence-Based Nursing, 4*(2), 86–96.

Ramsay, J. A., McKenzie, J. K., & Fish, D. G. (1982). Physicians and nurse practitioners: Do they provide equivalent health care? *American Journal of Public Health, 72*(1), 55–57.

Ream, E., Wilson-Barnett, J., Faithful, S., Fincham, L., Khoo, V., & Richardson, A. (2009). Working patterns and perceived contributions of prostate cancer clinical nurse specialists: A mixed-method investigation. *International Journal of Nursing Studies, 46*, 1345–1354.

Reay, T., Golden-Biddle, K., & Germann, K. (2006). Legitimizing a new role: Small wins and micro processes of change. *Academy of Management Journal, 49*(5), 977–998.

Registered Nurses' Association of Ontario (RNAO). (2013). *Expanded role for RNs = greater access to care for patients.* Toronto, ON: RNAO. Retrieved from https://rnao.ca/news/media-releases/2013/04/15/expanded-role-rns-greater-access-care-patients

Richmond, T. S., & Becker, D. (2005). Creating an advanced practice nurse–friendly culture: A marathon, not a sprint. *American Association of Critical-Care Nurses Clinical Issues, 16*(1), 58–66.

Romanow, R. J. (2002). *Building on values: The future of health care in Canada—Final report.* Ottawa, ON: Commission on the Future of Health Care in Canada.

Roots, A., & MacDonald, M. (2008, September 17–20). *3 years down the road: Exploring the implementation of the NP role in British Columbia, Canada.* Poster presentation at the 5th International Council of Nurses, International Nurse Practitioner/Advanced Practice Nursing (INP/APN) Conference in Toronto.

Roschkov, S., Rebeyka, D., Comeau, A., Mah, J., Scherr, K., Smigorowsky, M., & Stoop, J. (2007). Cardiovascular nurse practitioner practice: Results of a Canada-wide survey. *Canadian Journal of Cardiovascular Nursing, 17*(3), 27–31.

Rosenthal, L., & Guerrasio, J. (2009). Acute care nurse practitioner as hospitalist: Role description. *American Association of Critical-Care Nurses Advanced Clinical Care, 20*(2), 133–136.

Royal College of Nursing (RCN). (2008). *Advanced nurse practitioners: An RCN guide to the advanced nurse practitioner role, competencies and programme accreditation.* London, UK: Royal College of Nursing.

Rutherford, G., & Rutherford Consulting Group Inc. (2005). *Education component: Literature review report.* Ottawa, ON: CNA/CNPI.

Saskatchewan Collaborative Programs in Nursing. (2015). *Nurse practitioners—Improving health care in communities.* Regina, SK: Saskatchewan Polytechnic and University of Regina. Retrieved from http://www.sasknursingdegree.ca/cnpp/

Scherer, K., Fortin, F., Spitzer, W. O., & Kergin, D. J. (1977). Nurse practitioners in primary care. VII. A cohort study of 99 nurses and 79 associated physicians. *Canadian Medical Association (CMA) Journal, 116*(8), 856–862.

Schreiber, R., MacDonald, M., Pauly, B., Davidson, H., Crickmore, J., Moss, L., ... Regan, S. (2005a). Singing from the same songbook: The future of advanced nursing practice in British Columbia. *Canadian Journal of Nursing Leadership, 8*(2), 1–14.

Schreiber, R., MacDonald, M., Pauly, B., Davidson, H., Crickmore, J., Moss, L., ... Hammond, C. (2005b). Singing in different keys: Enactment of advanced nursing practice in British Columbia. *Canadian Journal of Nursing Leadership, 6,* 1–17. Retrieved from http://www.longwoods.com/content/19026

Sidani, S. (2008). Effects of patient-centered care on patient outcomes: An evaluation. *Research and Theory for Nursing Practice: An International Journal, 22*(1), 24–37.

Sidani, S., Doran, D., Porter, H., LeFort, S., O'Brien-Pallas, L., Zahn, C., ... Sarkissian, S. (2006a). Processes of care: Comparison between nurse practitioners and physician residents in acute care. *Canadian Journal of Nursing Leadership, 19*(1), 69–85.

Sidani, S., Doran, D., Porter, H., LeFort, S., O'Brien-Pallas, L., Zahn, C., & Sarkissian, S. (2006b). Outcomes of nurse practitioners in acute care: An exploration. *Internet Journal of Advanced Nursing Practice, 8*(1). Retrieved from https://ispub.com/IJANP/8/1/12232

Sidani, S., & Irvine, D. (1999). A conceptual framework for evaluating the nurse practitioner role in acute care settings. *Journal of Advanced Nursing, 30*(1), 58–66.

Sidani, S., Irvine, D., & DiCenso, A. (2000a). Implementation of the primary care nurse practitioner role in Ontario. *Canadian Journal of Nursing Leadership, 13*(3), 13–19.

Sidani, S., Irvine, D., Porter, H., O'Brien-Pallas, L., Simpson, B., McGillis Hall, L., ... Redelmeir, D. (2000b). Practice patterns of acute care nurse practitioners. *Canadian Journal of Nursing Leadership, 13*(3), 6–12.

Simpson, B. (1997). An educational partnership to develop acute care nurse practitioners. *Canadian Journal of Nursing Administration, 10*(1), 69–84.

Smith-Higuchi, K. A., Hagen, B., Brown, S., & Zeiber, M. P. (2006). A new role for advanced practice nurses in Canada: Bridging the gap in health services for rural older adults. *Journal of Gerontological Nursing, 32*(7), 49–55.

Spitzer, W. O., & Kergin, D. J. (1975). Nurse practitioners in primary care: The McMaster University educational program. *Health Care Dimensions,* (Spring), 95–103.

Staples, E., & Ray, S. L. (2016). An historical overview of advanced practice nursing in Canada. In E. Staples, S. L. Ray, & R. A. Hannon (Eds.), *Canadian perspectives on advanced practice nursing.* Toronto, ON: Canadian Scholars' Press.

Stevens, B. J. (1976). Accountability of the clinical specialist: The administrator's viewpoint. *Journal of Nursing Administration, 6*(2), 30–32.

University of Regina (UR), & Saskatchewan Institute of Applied Science and Technology (SIAST). (2013). *Collaborative nurse practitioner program proposal.* Regina, SK: UR/SIAST.

van Soeren, M. H., & Micevski, V. (2001). Success indicators and barriers to acute nurse practitioner role implementation in four Ontario hospitals. *American Association of Critical-Care Nurses (AACN) Clinical Issues, 12*(3), 424–437.

Vayda, E., Gent, M., & Paisley, L. (1973). An emergency department triage model based on presenting complaints. *Canadian Journal of Public Health, 64*(3), 246–253.

Wall, S. (2006). Living with grey: Role understandings between clinical nurse educators and advanced practice nurses. *Canadian Journal of Nursing Leadership, 19*(4), 57–71.

Way, D., Jones, L., Baskerville, B., & Busing, N. (2001). Primary health care services provided by nurse practitioners and family physicians in shared practice. *Canadian Medical Association Journal, 165*(9), 1210–1214.

Wetzel, C., & Kalman, M. (2010). Critical care clinical nurse specialist. Is this role for you? *Dimensions of Critical Care Nursing, 29*(1), 29–32.

Williams, D., & Sidani, S. (2001). An analysis of the nurse practitioner role in palliative care. *Canadian Journal of Nursing Leadership, 14*(4), 13–19.

Wilson, R. (2016). The nurse practitioner: Adult. In E. Staples, S. L. Ray, & R. A. Hannon (Eds.), *Canadian perspectives on advanced practice nursing.* Toronto, ON: Canadian Scholars' Press.

Chapter

2

Advanced Practice Nursing in Quebec

Monique Benoit, Roger Pilon, Isabelle Savard, Lucie Lemelin, and Pierre Pariseau-Legault

Monique Benoit is a Full Professor at the Université du Québec en Outaouais (UQO) in the Department of Nursing, Saint-Jérôme, Quebec. She is also an Adjunct Professor at Laurentian University School of Nursing, Sudbury, Ontario. She is a sociologist with an interest in health care and much of her research has focused on the nursing profession. She teaches qualitative methodologies for nursing research as well as public and community health at the undergraduate and graduate levels at UQO.

Roger Pilon is an Associate Professor and Director at Laurentian University, School of Nursing; Assistant Professor at the Northern Ontario School of Medicine; and an NP-PHC in Sudbury, Ontario. His areas of research include Indigenous and francophone health, primary health care, and the integration of NPs into practice. Roger was one of the first primary health care nurse practitioners (PHCNPs) to be recognized in the province of Ontario in 1998. Since leaving full-time practice in 2008 to begin his academic career, Roger has maintained an active clinical practice in a local francophone community health centre and a First Nation community funded by the Aboriginal Healing and Wellness Strategy.

Isabelle Savard is an Associate Professor in nursing at the UQO in the Department of Nursing, and an NP-Primary Care (PC) in Saint-Jérôme, Quebec. After being an emergency nurse for several years, she practiced as an NP in a general primary health care practice for five years and completed a master's in public health from the London School of Hygiene and Tropical Medicine before making the leap into an academic career. She continues to provide direct patient care in a community-based organization, where she cares for stigmatized patients outside the mainstream health care system. Her research interests focus on access to primary health care, community and public health, care for people in vulnerable situations, and the role of advanced practice nurses.

Lucie Lemelin is an Associate Professor at the UQO and Director of Graduate Nursing Programs at the UQO in the Department of Nursing, Saint-Jérôme, Quebec. She teaches the epistemology of nursing and pediatric care at the undergraduate and graduate levels. Her research focuses on health promotion, specifically for children. She is involved in the implementation of advanced practice nursing in Quebec.

PIERRE PARISEAU-LEGAULT is an Associate Professor at the UQO in the Department of Nursing, Saint-Jérôme, Quebec. He currently teaches mental health nursing, crisis intervention, as well as health law and ethics for advanced nursing practice. His current research explores the marginal spaces in which so-called vulnerable people live and studies the particularities of relational work in a context of coercion. He also studies how different norms (legal, professional, social) contribute to the legitimacy of health care interventions.

KEY TERMS

advanced practice nurses (APNs)
colony nurse
primary health care nurse practitioner (PHCNP)
scope of practice
specialized nurse practitioner

OBJECTIVES

1. Introduce the historical context with respect to advanced practice nursing (APN) in Quebec.
2. Describe conditions that have facilitated the integration of the APN/nurse practitioner (NP) role in recent years.
3. Identify the challenges encountered with the integration of APNs/NPs in the province of Quebec.
4. Review some of the catalysts that have helped to advance and better integrate the APN/NP role.

Introduction

In recent years, Quebec's health care system has slowly been making room for **advanced practice nurses (APNs)**. There are two categories of APNs: the clinical nurse specialist (CNS) and nurse practitioner (NP) roles. The CNS role, which emerged in the 1970s, was created in response to an increased complexity of patient care in the hospital setting. These nurses were tasked with providing clinical consultation, guidance, and leadership to nursing staff who were responsible for the care of these complex patients. In contrast, the NP role was created in order to provide care that was for the most part unavailable in rural and remote regions of the country (Canadian Nurses Association [CNA], 2019). For the purpose of this chapter, the focus will only be on the evolution of the NP role in the province of Quebec.

In Quebec, NPs are referred to as infirmières praticiennes spécialisées (IPS). Although considered a model of innovation in health care, the role of the NP has seemingly unsettled the established order in Quebec, particularly when it comes to primary health care (Jean et al., 2019). Unfortunately, up until now, the role of NPs in Quebec has had much less autonomy than other provinces and territories across Canada (Contandriopoulos et al., 2017), and the evolution and integration of the role has been at a much slower pace in contrast to the rest of the country (Benoit et al., 2017).

Nurse practitioners in this province are expected to work within interprofessional collaboration teams with doctors and other health care workers. They are found mainly in subsidized private clinics such as family medicine groups (groupe de médecine familiale [GMF] or groupe de médecine familiale universitaire [GMF-U]), which are primarily staffed and controlled by doctors. The reason that Quebec NPs work mainly in the GMF model is in part due to an apparent lack of political will and a framework that is aimed mostly at achieving ministerial targets for "medical" care. These primary health care models also happen to be the main structures in which first-line care is provided. NPs in this context enrol their patients under a physician to help them reach their targets. Past provincial governments have apparently never favoured other clinical models in which physicians were not at the head as this would have an impact on the targets currently being measured by the ministry (Santé et Services sociaux Québec, 2020).

Recently there have been new and innovative non-physician-led models of care created in Quebec. For example, Services À Bas Seuil d'Accessibilité (SABSA), a clinic that offers low-threshold service accessibility, is a multi-stakeholder initiative that works with vulnerable populations who have difficulty in obtaining care within the conventional network. This model was formed in 2011 by five founding members who felt challenged by the magnitude of the epidemic of hepatitis C virus and human immunodeficiency virus (HIV/AIDS) among vulnerable populations in the city of Quebec. In this model of care, walk-in clinic users do not meet with a physician but rather with a **primary health care nurse practitioner (PHCNP)**, who is authorized to order diagnostic tests and, among other things, prescribe medications. Unfortunately, given the scarcity of these types of models of care, NPs in Quebec are much less likely to work in interprofessional settings such as SABSA. The NPs who are fortunate enough to work within these types of interprofessional settings can perform many of the competencies of APNs, such as collaboration, consultation, and leadership (Carter, Dabney, & Hanson, 2019).

Unlike their counterparts in other provinces and territories, Quebec NPs still do not have the authority to make diagnoses. However, Bill 43, adopted and sanctioned by the minister of Health and Social Services of Quebec on March 17, 2020, will, among other things, allow Quebec NPs to diagnose diseases, based on their specialty. Despite these new developments, which seem to indicate that progress has been made, the terms of application of this law remain to be defined, and it is hoped that Quebec will be able to catch up with the development of the NP role compared to the rest of Canada.

The existence of these political, organizational, and administrative barriers helps to explain why Quebec has lagged in the development of more autonomous and independent roles for NPs. Ultimately, the government of Quebec has the power to provide NPs with the necessary means to meet the current health care needs of the population.

In order to fully understand and appreciate NPs' place in the Quebec health care system, this chapter will provide some historical context, describe some recent changes that have helped to promote the integration of NPs, identify some of the existing pitfalls encountered in the integration of NPs, explain how the expansion of the NP role can act as a catalyst for advancement and provide hope for better access to health care in the future, and show that NPs continue to seek role clarification, particularly in the area of diagnosis, in the event of a possible future emancipation from Quebec's medical law.

Historical Overview of Advanced Practice Nursing in Quebec

> In Canada, the roots of advanced practice nursing can be traced to the efforts of outpost nurses who worked in isolated areas such as the Northwest Territories, Labrador and Newfoundland during the early 1890s. ... These early beginnings of advanced practice nursing have been accepted but largely unrecognized within the Canadian health care system. ... Since the 1960s, advanced practice nursing roles have become more formalized within Canada. (Kaasalainen et al., 2010, p. 36)

In Quebec some trace the creation of the NP role to the colony nurses who, in the 1930s, developed an original model of care and practice that seemed effective in helping to cope with the economic crisis of that era. This was later followed by the "*Grande Noirceur*," during which Quebec was hit hard by great misery and poverty (Rousseau & Daigle, 2013). Given their relative isolation in remote areas, nurses who practiced during this period had very few resources and frequently went without running water or electricity. These nurses often had to cross rivers or use roads that had been closed during the winter. Since the government refused to pay for any form of transportation and because very few even had access to a horse, they often travelled by dogsled, by carts pulled by oxen, or even by foot (Daigle, 2018).

During this period, the Quebec government offered families who had been affected by the economic crisis land to develop the more remote regions of the province. These families established the regions of Abitibi, the lower St-Laurent, and the Basse-Côte-Nord. The government was required to provide these settlers with basic health care services, which included assistance with giving birth, as well as minor surgeries, vaccination, etc. This was how medical services to the settlers were established and included a total of 174 colony nurses, living in clinics and providing ongoing health care services in areas of Quebec where physicians did not want to practice.

At that time, nurses were often torn between poor standards and the tensions between medicine and the nursing profession, the latter often being ill-asserted and poorly represented. Over time, nurses took on tasks and performed substitute functions normally done by physicians, and while physicians refused to work in these areas, they still maintained control over nurses since they had been tasked by the government to provide them with training. This model would continue to exist until the end of the 1960s, at which time public health services were still in their infancy. The friction between nurses and physicians developed in part as a result of the differences in models of care between urban and remote areas. Ultimately, the role of the colony nurse disappeared partly due to the pressure of powerful organized groups, such as physicians, who saw this model of care as a precedent that questioned the division of powers and competencies between nurses and physicians at a time when public investment in health care was growing dramatically (Contandriopoulos et al., 2016).

The colony nurse model had created solutions for health care delivery to populations where no physician services existed. This environment provided an opportunity for nurses to demonstrate that they could practice independently and function outside the dominant medical and pharmaceutical models of care (Rousseau & Daigle, 2013). It would take many years before nurses could once again practice in a more expanded role. This occurred with the arrival of the local community service centres, which were promoting an interprofessional model where tasks would be shared among various health care providers such as physicians, nurses, and social workers. This new model of care was established in both urban and rural areas.

Integration of NPs in Quebec

In the early 1970s, training programs were developed for expanded nursing practice in Quebec. The scope of practice was then established, without legal title, in the far north of Quebec, where medical services were once again lacking. This is not unlike several other Canadian provinces (Kaasalainen et al., 2010). These nurses were required to be sufficiently autonomous, competent, and knowledgeable in order to respond to various health care problems, most often hundreds of kilometres away from the nearest hospital or medical support.

Although Quebec family physicians initially did not take an interest in the practice of NPs (Rousseau & Daigle, 2013), in 1973, the Canadian Nurses Association (CNA) and the Canadian Medical Association published a joint statement to establish increased responsibilities for NPs in order to support the health of populations (Kaasalainen et al., 2010). The Lalonde Report in 1974 also had an impact on the expanded roles of nurse graduates in the promotion and prevention of disease (Staples & Ray, 2016).

It wasn't until the 1990s, with the help of a pilot project in neonatology at the Montreal Children's Hospital and the Sainte-Justine University Hospital Centre, that a new APN role emerged in Quebec. This initiative was similar to one developed in Ontario by neonatal nurse practitioners, who would take on functions normally reserved for physicians (Allard & Durand, 2006).

The beginning of the 21st century marked the introduction of the NP role. Unlike the rest of Canada and other countries, Quebec seemed to focus on developing training programs for NPs based in hospital settings and in specialty areas rather than in primary health care and community settings. This approach helps to explain why Quebec included the term *specialized* in the title of specialized nurse practitioner to designate the *infirmières praticiennes spécialisées* (IPS; Association des infirmières praticiennes spécialisées du Québec [AIPSQ], n.d.).

The development of the NP role was in response to several challenges facing the Quebec health care system with respect to an aging population and an increase in chronic diseases and comorbidities. The increasing number of hospitalizations, a decrease in hospital beds available, and a declining number of medical staff also appeared to facilitate discussions for the development of the NP role. The creation of the NP role also included the CNS role in prevention and infection control, as well as several nurses who had studied at the graduate and doctoral levels in a variety of other advanced fields of practice and specialties (Ordre des infirmières et infirmiers du Québec [OIIQ], 2016).

The implementation of NPs was supported by the Ordre des infirmières et infirmiers du Québec (OIIQ) and various medical associations in cardiology and nephrology (Allard & Durand, 2006). The objectives were to increase access to quality health care and ensure continuity of care, with the expectation of lowering costs within the health care system. Medical specialists played an important role in NP implementation. The NP specialist roles, that were hospital based, were in fact requested by certain medical specialists in this province. Examples of specialities where NPs were being requested included cardiology, neonatology, and nephrology. There were, however, other specialty areas where there seemed to be less or no interest in the NP role (Kaasalainen et al., 2010).

Modifications to the Code of Professionals and Delegated Acts

Bill 90, which brought significant changes to the professional code, was passed in June 2002. This legislation was a critical element in the recognition of NPs in Quebec, leading to changes that influenced the Québec Nurses Act and facilitated the emergence of a new APN role for nurses, that of the NP. Table 2.1 provides examples of the activities that were delegated to NPs in 2003 by Bill 90. Amendments to the Québec Nurses Act resulted in the first group of NPs that would later be introduced into the health care system in 2005.

Creation of Nurse Practitioner Education Programs

It was in the wake of legislative changes such as Bill 90 that academic institutions were invited to create and provide the necessary programs to educate and prepare NPs to practice in Quebec. One of the first university training programs dedicated to the training of NPs began in the fall of 2002 at the Université de Montréal with programs specializing in cardiology and nephrology. This was later followed by the Université Laval in the winter of 2003.

The first training program for PHCNPs began simultaneously in the fall of 2007 at the Université de Montréal and Université Laval. The initial practice guidelines for NPs were adopted by the OIIQ in 2008. These were subsequently revised and updated in 2013, 2018, and again in 2019. The first certification examination developed by the OIIQ was held in 2009.

It is important to note that from the beginning, NP practice and the development of practice standards were controlled not only by the OIIQ but also by the Québec Medical College (CMQ). For the NP role to advance and be officially recognized in the province, the OIIQ was required to allow the CMQ's input in the development of NP practice standards and their scope of practice. This would become the only province or territory in Canada in which

TABLE 2.1: Delegated Medical Activities under Bill 90, Article 36.1 of the Québec Nurses Act

Delegated Medical Acts	Examples
Prescribing diagnostic examinations	Blood cultures, complete blood count, blood group (cross-group), coagulogram, bleeding time, thromboplastin time, lipid status (i.e., total cholesterol, LDL, HDL, triglycerides, etc.), parathyroid hormone, culture of various body fluids, electrocardiogram, Holter and telemetry, abdominal ultrasound, chest X-ray
Using diagnostic techniques that are invasive or at risk of causing harm	Lumbar, bladder, and arterial puncture
Prescribing drugs and other substances	Analgesics, certain antibiotics and anticonvulsants, intravenous solutions, topical antifungals, local anaesthetics, immunosuppressants, bronchodilators, ophthalmic drops for examinations, vitamins, electrolyte supplements, erythropoietic substances, sodium bicarbonate, phosphorus chelators
Prescribing medical treatments	Parenteral nutrition, transfusion of blood products, installation of a gastric or urinary catheter, assisted ventilation mode, epicardial cardio-stimulation, oxygen therapy and modification of respiratory parameters, modification of hemodialysis treatment or peritoneal dialysis
Using techniques that are invasive or entail risks of injury	Insertion and removal of a chest tube, ascites puncture, endotracheal intubation and extubation, removal of temporary cardio-stimulation (epicardial or endo-venous) sound, pleural puncture, cardioversion, defibrillation

Source: Benoit, M., Pilon, R., Savard, I., Lemelin, L., & Pariseau-Legault, P. (2020). Adapted from OIIQ. (2006). *Practice guidelines for the specialized nurse practitioner.* Quebec, QC: OIIQ. Retrieved from https://aipsq.com/infirmieres-praticiennes-specialisees/historique/au-quebec

another profession was involved and given authority in determining the practice of another discipline. This was essentially unprecedented but necessary at the time if the NP role was ever to become established in Quebec.

Finally, in 2018, after several sustained efforts, legislative changes with respect to the supervision of NP practice in Quebec were introduced. This move toward legislative change was intended to broaden the existing scope of practice of the different NP specialties in

Quebec. The adoption of this new regulation would also enable the expansion of new classes of NP specialties such as adult (currently limited to nephrology and cardiology), mental health, and pediatric care.

In the wake of the proposed legislative changes, many universities in the province were quick to respond to the need that these new classes of NP specialties would create. In 2017, one of the first training programs for NPs in adult care began at the Université de Montréal and the Université Laval. At the same time, training programs for NPs in mental health were now being offered at Université du Québec Network, Université de Montréal, and McGill University and in pediatric care, as well as primary health care, at the Université de Québec en Outaouais and McGill University. Universities in Quebec have always responded positively to the government's request for NP education in spite of insufficient resources. The current expectation is that a total of 2,000 NPs will be educated and added to the health care system by 2024–2025. Recently, in a controversial move, the OIIQ decided to abolish the certification examination and chose to test only NPs' legal and role knowledge and skills, relying on university programs to evaluate other skills and competencies to practice (OIIQ, 2019).

Fortunately, the recent adoption of Bill 43, which calls for major legislative changes concerning the practice of NPs in Quebec, will directly lead to the end of medical supervision of NPs since their practice will no longer be regulated by the Medical Act but exclusively by the Nurses Act. This would ultimately allow NPs to diagnose diseases. This bill will require the amendment of 9 laws and 24 regulations, and delays are anticipated before its implementation (Government of Québec, 2020).

Funding

In 2003, to support the implementation of NPs, the provincial government injected $9 million into the creation of 75 NP positions in three specialty areas: cardiology, neonatology, and nephrology. A portion of this budget was dedicated to scholarships for NP students to support them during their training. In 2017, the government invested a further $25 million toward NP education and training with a goal of implementing up to 2,000 NPs in Quebec's health care system by 2024–2025.

In addition to funding for NP positions, there has also been funding made available to physicians in private practice to encourage the integration of these APNs within the health care system. To date, for each primary health care NP working in a private clinic such as GMFs, the partnering family physicians receive altogether $30,000 annually for the partnership. They have also been provided with one-time funding of $5,000 per new NP to help pay for office equipment and other operational costs (Santé et Services sociaux Québec, 2011). In public facilities, such as Centre Local de Services Communautaires (CLSCs), the partnering family physicians of an NP can also receive compensation depending on their salary scheme. To date, medical specialists are not included in such funding agreements and therefore receive no compensation for collaborating with NPs. There is no funding for NPs working in public institutions such as hospitals. However, depending on the type of salary structure, some family physicians can be compensated for certain collaboration arrangements.

Challenges Encountered with the Integration of Nurse Practitioners

As previously discussed, Bill 90 was first introduced in 2002. It would take another three years before the province would see any movement on the implementation of NPs. One of the main issues was the resistance from the Québec Medical College (CMQ) to accept the role of the specialized nurse practitioner (Roy, Cauchy, & Von Hlatky, 2010). However, as a result of a health care system in crisis, the door was finally opened to the sharing of five of the six delegated medical acts, which historically had been limited to physicians. Given that the CMQ believed that medicine belonged exclusively to physicians, this new bill would be subject to several conditions. As a result, the first practice guidelines were drafted jointly by the OIIQ and the CMQ and included a number of restrictions relating to the prescription of medications, radiological examinations, and diagnostic tests, to name a few. In addition to the CMQ's role in regulating the profession, they also insisted on having input in the structure and delivery of educational programs. This led to a delay in opening admissions to NP programs. The CMQ insisted on additional courses, which, at the outset, threatened to cancel training programs altogether (Roy, Cauchy, & Von Hlatky, 2010). These examples of ongoing medical resistance to the training and regulation of NPs has slowed the implementation of this new profession.

In 2005, the first agreement between the OIIQ and the CMQ established guidelines for training programs and practice. This agreement applied to three areas of specialty: cardiology, neonatology, and nephrology. In the latter part of 2005, following the initiative of nine founding NP members from nephrology and cardiology, the Association of Specialized Nurse Practitioners of Québec (AIPSQ) was created. Their mission was to intervene and advocate on behalf of NPs who, up until this point, had had limited input into how the profession would look. Their goal was to become the voice of NP and represent their interests with various decision-making bodies. The AIPSQ also had a goal to create a network of professionals that would allow for exchanging and sharing information on the experiences of the implementation of this new role.

The year 2006 marked a milestone with the first certification examinations for the specialties of cardiology, neonatology, and nephrology. There were 17 NPs in this first cohort to pass the examination. At this time some initial steps were taken by a joint advisory committee of the OIIQ and the CMQ to create the PHCNP role. The purpose of this committee was to make recommendations with respect to the locations of practice, the terms and conditions of partnerships with general practitioners, and the scope of the medical activities that could be performed by NPs. The committee was also tasked to consider the academic requirements, including the clinical placements. Discussions with the CMQ continued as a result of the work carried out by a working group consisting of the OIIQ and the Quebec family physicians' federation (FMOQ). These groups jointly examined a model of collaboration between family doctors and NPs that would aim to improve accessibility and follow-up of clients with chronic health care problems.

In 2007, the AIPSQ expanded their mandate to include the first cohorts of primary health care NP students as well as Quebec nurses who had graduated from Ontario NP programs and were seeking equivalency in order to practice in Quebec as NPs. The AIPSQ now represents all the Quebec NPs who have chosen to be members, regardless of their area of specialty.

Quebec's Delay in Developing the Role of Nurse Practitioners

It is unclear why there have been so many delays in the implementation and integration of the APN role in the province of Quebec (Jean et al., 2019). Some have suggested that the medical establishment was the cause (Fédération interprofessionnelle du Québec [FIQ], 2016). Still others have suggested that issues related to training and lower pay may be responsible for the delays (Plourde, 2019). Finally, some believe that the problems ultimately exist as a result of a disorganized health care system (Jean et al., 2019). Regardless, several administrative and organizational barriers, including a lack of political will, have led to a structural paralysis and problematic development and implementation of APNs in Quebec.

In Quebec, the concept of APN and the role of NPs are not well known. In addition to issues at the health care systems level, there is also a need for a better understanding of the role and scope of practice of APNs such as NPs (Côté et al., 2018). Titles such as super-nurse and mini-doctor are commonly used in this province, which has done little to promote or better understand the role. These characterizations have only perpetuated the notion of APNs or NPs as physician replacements rather than as autonomous and self-regulated health care providers (Côté et al., 2018).

A full integration of the NP role within the Quebec health care system will require not only financial support from the government but also the support and coordinated efforts on the part of nursing and medical associations, professional organizations, and the community. Finally, there will need to be support from health care service organizations and administrators who can provide the environments and resources required for NPs to practice.

Nurse Practitioner Role Expansion

The 2018 change in regulations sought to expand the NP scope of practice and create new areas of specialty, which was followed by the adoption of new practice guidelines in July 2019. This was followed by the tabling of Bill 43 in 2019, which proposed to amend the Nurses Act and other provisions to promote access to health care services.

Adopted on March 17, 2020, this bill will allow NPs to diagnose diseases, according to their field of specialty. The implementation of these legislative changes could take some time since it involves amending many related laws and regulations. Until these changes occur, NPs are only able to identify common health conditions and initiate treatment for six chronic conditions. This new bill also includes major amendments that will see the regulation of the practice of NPs return to the exclusive control of the OIIQ.

It remains unclear how the proposed changes will be implemented, but if passed in its current form this new bill will allow NPs to finally diagnose patients. For the time being, when NPs detect that a patient is suffering from one of the six chronic diseases approved in the 2018 regulations, they have the authority to initiate treatment, but they are prohibited from making a definitive diagnosis. These patients must be assessed by a physician to confirm a diagnosis. Clearly this limitation to NP practice has an impact on the timeliness and access to health care. Until this bill is fully implemented, NPs will be required to maintain the status quo.

Conclusion

This chapter has reviewed the historical journey of APNs, specifically NPs, in the province of Quebec. Compared to the rest of Canada, there continues to be a number of political and systemic reasons for a slower implementation and integration of the APN role in the Quebec health care system. The passing of Bill 43, when fully implemented, will remove many barriers to practice for NPs in this province. It is clear that greater autonomy over education, scope of practice, and regulation will ultimately result in improved access to quality health care services in Quebec.

Critical Thinking Questions

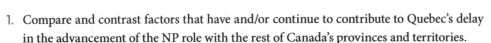

1. Compare and contrast factors that have and/or continue to contribute to Quebec's delay in the advancement of the NP role with the rest of Canada's provinces and territories.
2. How would you characterize the public discourse and current perception of the NP practice in Quebec?
3. Should the popular term *super-nurse* continue to be used to describe NP practice in Quebec?
4. Who should be involved in NP education and supervision? Physicians, nurses, or both? Provide justification utilizing evidence to support your position.

References

Allard, M., & Durand, S. (2006). L'infirmière praticienne spécialisée : un nouveau rôle de pratique infirmière avancée au Québec [The specialized nurse practitioner: A new role for advanced nursing practice in Quebec]. *Perspective infirmière, 3*(5), 10–16. Retrieved from http://www.anfiide-gic-repasi.com/wp-content/uploads/2014/07/Infirmiere-praticienne-sp%C3%A9cialis%C3%A9e-Quebec-perspective_infirmiere_2006_10_16.pdf

Association des infirmières praticiennes spécialisées du Québec (AIPSQ). (n.d.). *Au Québec : Infirmières praticiennes spécialisées au Québec* [In Quebec: Specialized nurse practitioners in Quebec]. Quebec, QC: AIPSQ. Retrieved from https://aipsq.com/infirmieres-praticiennes-specialisees/17-historique

Benoit, M., Pilon, R., Lavoie, A. M., & Pariseau-Legault, P. (2017). Chevauchement, interdépendance ou complémentarité? La collaboration interprofessionnelle entre l'infirmière praticienne et d'autres professionnels de santé en Ontario [Overlap, interdependence or complementarity? Interprofessional collaboration between the nurse practitioner and other health professionals in Ontario]. *Santé publique, 29*(5), 699–706.

Canadian Nurses Association (CNA). (2006). *E-nursing strategy for Canada*. Ottawa, ON: CNA. Retrieved from https://www.cna-aiic.ca/~/media/cna/page-content/pdf-en/e-nursing-strategy-for-canada .pdf?la=en

CNA. (2019). *Advanced practice nursing: A pan-Canadian framework*. Ottawa, ON: CNA. Retrieved from https://cna-aiic.ca/-/media/cna/page-content/pdf-en/apn-a-pan-canadian-framework.pdf?la= en&hash=E1387634D492FD2B003964E3CD4188971305469E

Carter, M., Dabney, C., & Hanson, C. (2019). Collaboration. In M. F. Tracy, & E. T. O'Grady (Eds.), *Hamric and Hanson's advanced practice nursing* (6th ed., pp. 286–309). St. Louis, MO: Elsevier.

Contandriopoulos, D., Brousselle, A., Breton, M., Sangster-Gormley, E., Kilpatrick, K., Doubois, C.-A., … Perroux, M. (2016). Nurse practitioners, canaries in the mine of primary care reform. *Health Policy, 120*(6), 682–689. Retrieved from https://www.sciencedirect.com/science/article/pii/ S016885101630077X?via%3Dihub

Contandriopoulos, D., Perroux, M., Lardeux, A., Bégin, M.-C., Chiasson, A., Clément, S., … Radermaker, M. (2017). *Primary healthcare nurse practitioners (PHCNPs) practice in Canada*. Montreal, QC: Politiques Connaissances Santé. Retrieved from https://www.pocosa.ca/wp-content/ uploads/2017/05/IPSen.pdf

Côté, N., Freeman, A., Jean, E., Pollender, H., & Binette, S. (2018). *Les facteurs contributifs à l'optimisation de la pratique de l'infirmières praticienne spécialisée en soins de première ligne : Enjeux de collaboration interprofessionnelle, d'intégration de rôle et de sens de travail* [Contributing factors to optimizing the practice of primary care nurse practitioners: Challenges of interprofessional collaboration, integration of role, and sense of work]. Laval, QC: Centre de recherche sur les soins et les services de première ligne de l'Université Laval, Institut universitaire de santé et de services sociaux de première ligne, Université Laval Centre intégré universitaire de santé et de services sociaux de la Capitale-Nationale, 50. Retrieved from http://www.cersspl.ca/fileadmin/user_ upload/documentations/fichiers/Les_facteurs_contributifs_a_l_27optimisation_de_la_pratique_ de_l_27IPSPL-Rapport_Final_01.pdf

Daigle, J. (2018). *Infirmière de colonie : Conférence de Johanne Daigle. Organisée par la Société d'Histoire Les Rivières* [Colony nurse: Lecture by Johanne Daigle. Organized by the Les Rivières History Society]. Quebec, QC: Bibliothèque Aliette-Marchand.

Fédération interprofessionnelle du Quebec (FIQ). (2016). *Pratique professionnelle des infirmières : « Pour le bien des patients, le corporatisme des médecins doit cesser »* [Professional nursing practice: "For the sake of patients, the corporatism of doctors must stop"]. Retrieved from http://www. fiqsante.qc.ca/2016/09/27/pratique-professionnelle-des-infirmieres-pour-le-bien-des-patients-le- corporatisme-des-medecins-doit-cesser-regine-laurent/

Government of Québec. (2020). *Amendement au Projet de Loi No 43. Loi modifiant la loi sur les infirmières et les infirmiers et d'autres dispositions afin de favoriser l'accès aux services de santé* [Amendment to Bill 43. An act to amend the Nurses Act and other provisions to facilitate access to health services]. Quebec, QC: Government of Québec. Retrieved from http://www.assnat.qc.ca/Media/Process.aspx? MediaId=ANQ.Vigie.Bll.DocumentGenerique_157765&process=Default&token=ZyMoxNwUn8i kQ+TRKYwPCjWrKwg+vIv9rjij7p3xLGTZDmLVSmJLoqe/vG7/YWzz

Jean, E., Sevilla Guerra, S., Contandriopoulos, D., Perroux, M., Kilpatrick, K., & Zabalegui, A. (2019). Context and implementation of advanced nursing practice in two countries: Exploratory qualitative comparative study. *Nursing Outlook, 67*(4), 365–380.

Kaasalainen, S., Martin-Misener, R., Kilpatrick, K., Harbman, P., Bryant-Lukosius, D., Donald, F., … DiCenso, A. (2010). A historical overview of the development of advanced practice nursing roles in Canada. *Nursing Leadership, 23*(Special Issue), 35–60.

Ordre des infirmières et infirmiers du Québec (OIIQ). (2006). *Practice guidelines for the specialized nurse practitioner.* Quebec, QC: OIIQ. Retrieved from https://aipsq.com/infirmieres-praticiennes-specialisees/historique/au-quebec

OIIQ. (2016). *Pratique infirmière avancée : Réflexion sur le rôle de l'infirmières clinicienne spécialisée* [Advanced nursing practice: Reflection on the role of the clinical nurse specialist]. Montreal, QC: OIIQ. Retrieved from http://www.anfiide-gic-repasi.com/wp-content/uploads/2014/07/8456-reflexion-role-ics.pdf

OIIQ. (2019). *Nouvel examen professionnel des IPS* [New NP professional examination]. Montreal, QC: OIIQ. Retrieved from https://www.oiiq.org/en/pratique-professionnelle/exercice-infirmier/NPs/etudiante

Plourde, A. (2019). *Ces faits que la FMOQ préfère ignorer* [Facts that the FMOQ prefers to ignore]. Montreal, QC: Institut de recherche et d'informations socioéconomiques. Retrieved from https://iris-recherche.qc.ca/blogue/ces-faits-que-la-fmoq-prefere-ignorer

Rousseau, N., & Daigle, J. (2013). *Infirmières de colonie : Soins et médicalisation dans les régions du Québec 1932–1972* [Colony nurses: Care and medicalization in the regions of Quebec 1932–1972]. Laval, QC: Presses de l'Université Laval.

Roy, M., Cauchy, C., & Von Hlatky, K. (2010). *Résistance médicale : Émission Enquête de Radio-Canada (Vidéo)* [Medical resistance: CBC Radio investigation program (Video)]. Retrieved from https://www.youtube.com/watch?v=hGJiz2gx71Y&feature=youtu.be

Santé et Services sociaux Québec. (2011). *Soutien financier pour l'intégration des infirmières praticiennes spécialisées en soins de première ligne (NPS-SPL) et des candidates NPS-SPL, Normes et pratiques de gestion, tome II, répertoire* [Financial support for the integration of nurse practitioners specializing in primary care and graduate NP: Standards and management practices, volume II, directory]. Quebec, QC: Santé et Services sociaux Québec. Retrieved from http://msssa4.msss.gouv.qc.ca/fr/document/d26ngest.nsf/1f71b4b2831203278525656b0004f8bf/a529f5a39a4cd801852578c300616bc9/$FILE/2011-013_Circulaire%20(2011-06-06).pdf

Santé et Services sociaux Québec. (2020). *Accès aux services médicaux de première ligne : Cibles d'amélioration de l'accès aux services de première ligne* [Access to front-line medical services: Targets to improve access to front-line services]. Quebec, QC: Santé et Services sociaux Québec. Retrieved from https://www.msss.gouv.qc.ca/professionnels/documents/cibles-medecins/Entente.pdf

Staples, E., & Ray, S. L. (2016). A historical overview of advanced practice nursing in Canada. In E. Staples, S. L. Ray, & R. A. Hannon (Eds.), *Canadian perspectives on advanced practice nursing* (pp. 2–22). Toronto, ON: Canadian Scholars' Press.

Chapter

3

Advanced Practice Nursing Education in Canada

Cynthia Baker, Eric Staples, and Roger Pilon

CYNTHIA BAKER is the Executive Director of the Canadian Association of Schools of Nursing (CASN) in Ottawa, Ontario. CASN is the national voice of nursing education in Canada. She is a Professor Emerita at Queen's University, Kingston, Ontario, where she was Director, School of Nursing, and Associate Dean, Faculty of Health Sciences. Prior to Queen's University, Cynthia was directrice, École des sciences infirmières at l'Université de Moncton, Moncton, New Brunswick.

ERIC STAPLES is an Independent Nursing Practice Consultant. He was a graduate of the first postgraduate Acute Care Nurse Practitioner (ACNP) certificate program in Ontario in 1995 from the University of Toronto, and has held Assistant Professor roles at Dalhousie University, Halifax, Nova Scotia, where he was involved in implementing the Advanced Nursing Practice stream in 1998; McMaster University, Hamilton, Ontario, as NP Coordinator in the Ontario Primary Health Care Nurse Practitioner (PHCNP) Program; and the University of Regina, Regina, Saskatchewan. Eric serves or has served on several CASN committees related to NP education, preceptorship, prescribing, and the development of the position statement on doctoral education in Canada. He was the lead developer and editor for the inaugural edition of *Canadian Perspectives in Advanced Practice Nursing*, published in 2016 and in French in 2017.

ROGER PILON is an Associate Professor and Director at Laurentian University, School of Nursing; Assistant Professor at the Northern Ontario School of Medicine; and an NP-PHC in Sudbury, Ontario. His areas of research include Indigenous and francophone health, primary health care, and the integration of NPs into practice. Roger was one of the first primary health care nurse practitioners (PHCNPs) to be recognized in the province of Ontario in 1998. Since leaving full-time practice in 2008 to begin his academic career, Roger has maintained an active clinical practice in a local francophone community health centre and a First Nation community funded by the Aboriginal Healing and Wellness Strategy.

KEY TERMS

advanced practice nursing
    (APN)
education trends
educational programs
integration

OBJECTIVES

1. Trace the evolution of education for advanced practice nursing (APN) in Canada in relation to trends in health care delivery.
2. Examine contextual factors influencing education programs for APNs.
3. Discuss barriers and facilitators of future APN education trends.

Introduction

Future directions of a phenomenon are often best understood by examining the historical forces that have shaped it. Health professional education has the mandate of preparing graduates for anticipated future health care system realities. At any point in time, it reflects the actual and perceived trends of the day. The purpose of this chapter is to identify education trends that are emerging in advanced practice nursing (APN) education in Canada and the forces that have influenced its development. The evolution of APN education in Canada is traced, and the contextual forces driving this evolution are examined in order to capture directions for the future. Chapter 2 discusses in depth the development of education programs for APN in Quebec.

Education Programs for Advanced Practice Nursing

Canadian schools of nursing have introduced a succession of educational programs to prepare nurses for advanced practice roles as primary health care nurse practitioners (PHCNPs), clinical nurse specialists (CNSs), and nurse practitioners (NPs) in acute care settings. Each of these roles has encountered contextual challenges that affected their subsequent continuity.

There are several challenges when it comes to APN education in Canada, including, but not limited to, geography, population diversity, and variations in health policies throughout the 13 provinces and territories. In addition, a lack of specialized education programs and a shortage of qualified faculty also contribute to the challenges with respect to APN education (Bryant-Lukosius et al., 2014).

Evolution of Advanced Practice Nursing Education

Dalhousie University, Halifax, Nova Scotia, opened the ground breaking Outpost Nursing Program in 1967 that launched APN in Canada (Martin-Misener et al., 2010). In contrast with the United States (US), however, the subsequent growth of education for APN was slow and discontinuous for several decades (DiCenso & Bryant-Lukosius, 2010a, 2010b). Programs were often developed in response to time-limited, period-sensitive contextual demands and soon waned or disappeared as the particular contextual reality changed. Furthermore, until recently there have been considerable inconsistencies in the academic level of the completion qualifications and the length of the programs.

Nurse Practitioners in Primary Health Care

Immediately after the Outpost Nursing Program was first launched at Dalhousie University, programs emerged across Canada. These programs focused on the clinical education of registered nurses to provide primary health care in isolated settings in the north (Martin-Misener et al., 2010). Later programs preparing NPs to work in urban settings also followed Dalhousie's Outpost Nursing Program, first at McMaster University, Hamilton, Ontario, and at McGill University, Montreal, Quebec (Haines, 1993).

During the 1990s, interest in the PHCNP role resurfaced within provincial governments. DiCenso et al. (2007) attributed this to a combination of factors, including cutbacks in medical residency positions, a need to offset rising costs with greater fiscal efficiency, and government interest in shifting care from hospitals to the community. Thus, some of the same factors that led to the elimination of CNS positions in acute care settings prompted a renewed attention to potential benefits of revitalizing the NP role.

In 1995, the Ontario provincial government funded a Council of Ontario University Programs in Nursing (COUPN) consortium of 10 nursing schools to develop and deliver a post-baccalaureate program for PHCNPs in English and French (Cragg, Doucette, & Humbert, 2003). The program was developed and offered jointly by the 10 (now nine) member schools of nursing using distance delivery methods across consortium sites, and supported by face-to-face didactic learning activities and clinical practicums. This provincial COUPN consortium continues to educate the majority of PHCNPs who graduate in Ontario.

The COUPN program was initially created as a one-year post-baccalaureate certificate program in response to government requirements. It included course content related to roles and responsibilities, health promotion, and health system delivery. Due to the short time frame, the emphasis was on the additional medical knowledge and skills needed to diagnose and treat illness in primary health care (PHC). Advanced nursing knowledge was part of the education of CNSs and ACNPs. Over time, the COUPN consortium members decided it was essential to transition the PHCNP program to a graduate level despite government resistance, and to integrate APN competencies into the role. Curriculum development was carried out to bring all the NP certificate courses to a graduate level, and in 2008/2009, each of the consortium member schools incorporated the revised and shared PHCNP courses with each school's core graduate courses into a two-year graduate nursing program. A one-year graduate diploma, comprised of the core PHCNP courses, can still be obtained at most of the consortium sites for nurses who have already completed a graduate nursing degree.

Clinical Nurse Specialists

While the PHCNP role was vanishing in Canada during the 1970s, positions for CNSs began to emerge in urban hospitals in response to a different set of contextual factors. Advances in health care science and technology were rapidly increasing the complexity of nursing care during the decade, bringing a need for specialized nurses with greater knowledge and skills to support the bedside nurse in providing clinical care (Bryant-Lukosius et al., 2014; Kaasalainen et al., 2010).

This new CNS role was understood to require deeper and more advanced nursing knowledge built on what nurses had learned in their entry-to-practice programs rather than on supplementary medical knowledge about the diagnosis and treatment of diseases. In contrast with PHCNPs, the CNS has consistently required a graduate degree in nursing. Role definitions of the CNS included completion of a graduate degree in nursing among its defining attributes, and this is still the case.

Although CNSs typically required a graduate degree in nursing, educational programs were not specifically designated for it. This may be due to the range and diversity in the clinical expertise associated with the role; however, the introduction of CNSs had an important impact on graduate nursing programs in general, and later with the development of graduate NP programs. The CNS role increased nurses' interest in graduate nursing studies, and in advancing nursing-specific clinical knowledge. Moreover, the CNS role prompted the development of graduate nursing programs that offer clinical nursing specializations (Alcock, 1996).

The first CNS program in Canada was introduced at the University of Toronto, Toronto, Ontario, in 1970 (Montemuro, 1987), and many graduate nursing programs have since developed with a clinical focus. Despite the initial growth of positions for CNSs, fiscal efficiencies introduced in the early 1990s, during a period of health care reform, resulted in the elimination of many of these positions. The lack of role-specific graduate nursing education has also been identified as a contributing factor (Martin-Misener et al., 2010). While there has been some renewed interest in the CNS role in recent years (Canadian Nurses Association [CNA], 2014), this has not translated into the development of sustained nursing education programs in this area.

Nurse Practitioners in Acute Care

Although interest in the PHCNP role had disappeared, universities began to introduce programs for a new type of NP in the latter half of the 1980s to work in acute care settings. The first program was opened at McMaster University, Hamilton, Ontario, in 1986 for neonatal nurse practitioners (NNPs), and in 1993, the University of Toronto, Toronto, Ontario, introduced an acute care NP (ACNP) program for tertiary care settings (Kaasalainen et al., 2010).

Initially, NPs in acute care settings were called expanded role nurses (ERNs), blended CNS/NPs, or APNs. Several years after their introduction, they became known as ACNPs, a term borrowed from the US, where it had been adopted initially to designate NPs working in critical care units (Simpson, 1997). Since 2010, there has been a steady decline in NNP education programs, which has an impact on the supply of NNPs. Currently there are only two NNP programs in Canada: University of Alberta, Calgary, Alberta, and McGill University, Montreal, Quebec. The program at McMaster University, Hamilton, Ontario, closed in 2014, and Dalhousie University, Halifax, Nova Scotia, briefly reopened their program for three cohorts in 2017. Compounding a shortage of NNPs, the workforce has witnessed increased retirement, and given the small numbers, it is difficult or perhaps not financially feasible for universities to continue to offer programs for such small cohorts (Bryant-Lukosius et al., 2014). Perhaps alternative approaches to NNP education will need to be considered in the future.

Schools of nursing delivered the ACNP programs at the graduate or postgraduate level, in line with the education for the CNS role and in contrast with programs for the PHCNP. These programs represented something of a hybrid, educating nurses for a blended CNS and NP role. They were based on the premise that graduates needed to learn components of the CNS role as well as the more medical components of the NP role (Bryant-Lukosius et al., 2014; Kaasalainen et al., 2010). Graduates of these programs were unregulated and were enabled through physician-approved medical directives and protocols (Nurse Practitioners' Association of Ontario [NPAO], n.d.).

The initial contextual factors that identified the stimulus for the creation of ACNP education programs included a shortage of pediatric residents (Paes et al., 1989), a need to address the lack of continuity of care for seriously ill patients (Pringle, 2007), and the need to deliver increasingly complex care in acute care settings (Hravnak et al., 2009). While the NNP programs were highly specialized, most ACNP programs were generic except for those in the province of Quebec (see Chapter 2). Students obtained the specialized knowledge and skills of a given specialty in the selection of their clinical placements and in individualized learning activities.

Nurse Anaesthetist

In 2009, the University of Toronto, Toronto, Ontario, introduced a postgraduate diploma for nurse anaesthetists. This initiative was funded by the Government of Ontario as a potential solution to wait times for surgery resulting from a shortage of anaesthetists. Although a small number of nurses graduated from the program, it has been discontinued because the nurse anaesthetist role did not materialize in the Canadian health care system in contrast with the US, where it is well established.

Expansion of Nurse Practitioner Education

The introduction of Ontario's COUPN consortium program marked a revival of interest in educating NPs in primary health care throughout Canada. An environmental scan conducted by the Canadian Association of Schools of Nursing (CASN) in 2011 found that there had been progressive increases in the number of programs for NPs in Canada between 2000 and 2009, and programs were being offered in all provincial/territorial jurisdictions except Prince Edward Island, Nunavut, and Yukon. In 2019, CASN reported that 28 schools of nursing, representing a quarter of the schools in Canada, offered one or more NP programs. From 2011–2012 to 2012–2013, the numbers increased by 89.3% with 568 students entering nurse practitioner programs across the country. Figure 3.1 demonstrates the number of students entering nurse practitioner programs across Canada over the past five years.

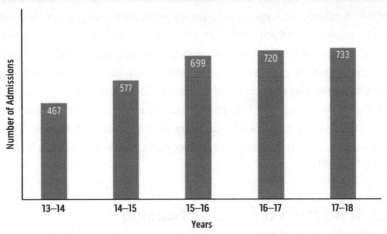

FIGURE 3.1: Admissions to Nurse Practitioner Programs 2013–2014 to 2017–2018

Source: CASN. (2019). *Registered nurses education in Canada statistics: 2017–2018.* Ottawa, ON: CASN. Retrieved from https://www.casn.ca/wp-content/uploads/2019/12/2017-2018-EN-SFS-DRAFT-REPORT-for-web.pdf. Reprinted with permission.

This expansion of NP education is reflected in the growth of licensed NPs since 2007. In 2011, the Canadian Institute for Health Information (CIHI) reported that between 2007 and 2011, the number of licensed NPs doubled from 1,344 to 2,777, and by 2013 the number had risen to 3,655. Between 2017 and 2018, there was an 8% increase, the highest growth among all regulated nursing groups in Canada, to 5,697 NPs (CIHI, 2019). Unfortunately, this data does not provide a full picture of enrolment trends for APNs. There is no information on the education of CNSs because of the lack of role-specific programs to survey. Moreover, as they are not licensed, there are no statistics on their numbers in the health care system (Bryant-Lukosius et al., 2010).

Current State of Advanced Practice Nursing Education Preparation

Consensus across Canada is that the minimum education preparation for all APN roles is a graduate nursing degree. Combined with a theoretical foundation in nursing from baccalaureate education, APN promotes nursing research, generates new knowledge, mobilizes knowledge through knowledge translation, and incorporates new knowledge into clinical practice. The combination of graduate nursing education and clinical expertise in a specialty practice area (i.e., primary health care, wound care, acute care, pediatrics, neonatology) allows nurses to develop the specific competencies required for APN (CNA, 2019).

Regulatory bodies across Canada have established measurable standards by which NP education programs are assessed and evaluated for program approval status. Resources to support APN education are available from CASN. In 2012, CASN published the *Nurse Practitioner Education in Canada: National Framework of Guiding Principles and Essential Components*. Later, the *National Nursing Education Framework* (CASN, 2015) was established that identified fundamental expectations for all graduate nursing programs, regardless of stream or specialization, and provided clarity of the value added of a graduate nursing degree built upon baccalaureate-level nursing education. National guidelines are provided that integrate professional and academic expectations, which assist in developing, reviewing, evaluating, or modifying nursing programs and curricula (CNA, 2019).

All APN education programs benefit from accreditation to promote excellence in identifying strengths and opportunities for program improvement and provide APN educators with information where further program development, medication, and/or where resources are needed (CNA, 2019).

Impact of Advanced Practice Nursing Education Expansion

The expansion of NP education, the increased employment opportunities for graduates, and policy and legislative infrastructure development have created a momentum forward as well as a new set of challenges. There is a movement toward increased clarity in the educational expectations for APNs and better integration of APNs in the interprofessional, health care system. Given the historical vulnerability of advances in nursing practice to contextual changes, calls continue for further articulation and optimum alignment of roles with evolving health system realities.

There are innovative practice opportunities and emerging APN specialties evolving all the time. Some recent examples include NPs who specialize in treating chronic pain, prescribing medical cannabis, or providing cosmetic services. Arslanian-Engoren (2019) states that "the future of advanced practice nursing depends on the extent to which practice meets the needs and priorities of society, health care systems, and the public policy arena" (p. 60). Given the ongoing and rapid changes in the health care system, we should expect to see an increasing number of NPs who choose to set up innovative practices in a variety of settings.

Despite external barriers, the trend has been to ground education for all types of NPs in an advanced nursing model at the graduate level. In 2011, CASN published the results of a task force on NP education in response to nursing demands for further development of national educational standards. The resulting framework supported the growing consensus that NP programs be at the graduate level, and that this graduate education provide a broad-based nursing education that addresses core competencies for all APNs (clinical, research, leadership, and consultation and collaboration). Table 3.1 demonstrates the number of NP programs available in Canada. Data related to the level of program are no longer being reported by CASN.

NPs also appear to be integrating their extended scope of practice skills in an advanced nursing perspective. A recent research synthesis and study comparing NPs and physician assistants (PAs) in Canada found both were appreciated by clients, but offered a different approach. The NPs utilized knowledge and autonomous decision-making skills in analytical

TABLE 3.1: Nurse Practitioner Programs by Province/Territory

	Canada	NL	PE	NS	NB	QC	ON	MB	SK	AB	BC	NT	NU	YT
Nurse Practitioner Programs (all levels)	28	1	1	1	2	4	10	1	2	3	3	0	0	0

Source: CASN. (2019). *Registered nurses education in Canada statistics: 2017–2018.* Ottawa, ON: CASN. Retrieved from https://www.casn.ca/wp-content/uploads/2019/12/2017-2018-EN-SFS-DRAFT-RE-PORT-for-web.pdf. Reprinted with permission.

activities associated with primary health care (Wong & Farrally, 2013). In addition, they incorporated an emphasis on population health and prevention, the social determinants of health, and the effects of illness on the lives of clients and families in their practice. The researchers attribute this to an education base embedded in a nursing model. The PAs, with an education grounded in a medical model and trained to be assistants, were less focused on autonomous decision making and analytical processes, and concentrated more on a technical orientation.

While the debate in Canada has been about a graduate-level requirement, in the US it has been about the Doctor of Nursing (DNP) as the entry to practice degree level for NPs. The American Association of Colleges of Nurses (AACN) adopted this position in 2004, and it recently reported that 348 DNP programs were enrolling students at schools of nursing nationwide and an additional 98 DNP programs were in the planning stages. From 2017 to 2018, the number of students enrolled in DNP programs increased by 89% to 32,678, and the number of graduates increased by 86% to 7,039 (AACN, 2019).

Extensive discussion and debate about whether or not the DNP should be introduced in Canada has taken place at the annual CASN Graduate Study Forum in 2010, 2011, and 2012. This forum is attended primarily by nursing faculty responsible for graduate studies in Canadian universities, and the deans and directors of CASN member schools. The consensus position that emerged in 2011 concluded that, at that time, the DNP was not supported by CASN, but there was recognition that it may be in the future. On the other hand, the CNA (2010) supports two doctoral education streams and believes the DNP supports leadership roles in policy, administration, and practice settings. With differing opinions, no alternatives have been proposed until recently. For the fall of 2021, the Lawrence Bloomberg Faculty of Nursing at the University of Toronto, Toronto, Ontario, announced it will be offering Canada's first Doctor of Nursing (DN) program, and at least one other university is working on developing a professional doctorate program.

Age-Based Nurse Practitioner Roles

In 2010, changes in nursing regulation had an impact on the ACNP designation and ACNP education programs. The nursing regulatory bodies in Canada established the following streams for NP registration: Family/All Ages (also referred to as PHC), Adult, and Pediatrics, organizing NP roles into age-based population categories being served, rather than on a specialization or setting. Despite this broad generalist approach, the more narrowly specialized NNP continues to be recognized. In addition, the Ordre des infirmières et infirmiers du Québec (OIIQ) retained a specialization focus rather than an age-based framework. NPs in Quebec are designated as infirmières praticiennes spécialisées (IPS; specialized nurse practitioners [SNP]) and tend to work in one of the following specialities: PHC, adult, mental health, neonatology, or pediatrics (OIIQ, 2020).

Doctoral Preparation of Advanced Practice Nurses

Currently in Canada, the only nursing doctoral degree that can be awarded is the Doctor of Philosophy (PhD) in nursing. Only 18.6% of universities offer a PhD, and admissions to doctoral programs have remained stable over the past five years. Admissions to doctoral programs decreased by 1% between 2016/2017 to 2017/2018, and doctoral program graduates decreased by 32.7% over the same period (CASN, 2019).

The Canadian Nurse Practitioner Initiative in 2006 indicated that faculty who were engaged in clinical practice were best able to teach NPs, but they were also expected to have a PhD. There has been, for some time, a shortage of nursing faculty who possess both current practice and a PhD (Martin-Misener et al., 2010). Additionally, doctorally prepared NP faculty are challenged in maintaining a practice while meeting the teaching, research, publication, and service criteria for tenure and promotion. Typically, the practice portion of the role is not considered or given scholarly merit when it comes to tenure and promotion.

While there is consensus in Canada about a graduate-level preparation for APNs, in the US, it has been about the Doctor of Nursing Practice (DNP) as the entry to practice degree level for NPs. Some Canadian APNs are pursuing this credential in the US. While this level of education is seen as beneficial to clients, health care systems, and the advancement of the profession, it is not currently required for APN in Canada. The primary difference between the PhD and DNP is in focus; the PhD primarily prepares nurse researchers, while the DNP prepares nursing leaders who are expert in knowledge translation in the practice setting (Acorn, Lamarche, & Edwards, 2009; Tung, 2010; Villeneuve & MacDonald, 2006).

Continuing Education for Advanced Practice Nursing

While APNs bring clinical expertise to their positions, they graduate as novices in their new advanced roles. Like all nurses, there is an expectation that APNs are committed to lifelong learning through reflective practice and measurement of performance outcomes to identify learning needs and opportunities for professional growth and development.

Ongoing learning is "essential given the importance of basing care on current best practices and developing and maintaining specialist knowledge" (DiCenso & Bryant-Lukosius, 2010a, p. 31). APN programs have identified several learning modalities for continuing education that remove barriers such as travel, financial, and distance limitations. Leadership is required at all organizational and health care system levels to support continuing APN professional development (CNA, 2019). "Without the support, protected time, and resources to participate in education, research and leadership activities, APNs risk job dissatisfaction and lose the opportunity to develop and/or disseminate new nursing knowledge" (DiCenso & Bryant-Lukosius, 2010a, p. 25). It has been further recognized that supported continuing professional development is key to recruitment and retention (Little & Reichert, 2018). This, in turn, enhances APN domains of practice and optimizes competence and confidence (CNA, 2019). There are numerous opportunities for APNs to improve their practice and improve the health of Canadians through CNS and NP special interest groups, professional nursing associations, universities and colleges, CASN, and CNA.

An example of addressing a continuing education need came about when the eligibility to prescribe controlled drugs and substances was implemented across the country. This brought a new set of challenges and opportunities for increasing optimum NP integration in both acute care and primary health care services. Practicing and future NPs needed to learn about the specific complexities of controlled drugs and substance prescription, their potential for misuse and abuse, and the array of skills required for good prescribing practices (Kamarudin et al., 2013). Prior to lifting the regulation to prescribe controlled drugs and substances, the Government of Canada (2012), on recommendation by the minister of health, proclaimed the New Classes of Practitioners Regulations under the Controlled Drugs and Substances Act in the *Canada Gazette*, Part II, which removed federal barriers that NPs would face in prescribing controlled drugs and substances.

Interprofessional collaboration is a key component of health system integration. Martin-Misener et al. (2010) reported that the need for interprofessional education for APNs has been consistently flagged in the literature. There has been a growing emphasis on interprofessional collaboration among other health professions in Canada in recent years. Team members' understanding, recognition, and acceptance of roles, however, is a necessary condition for interprofessional collaboration. This appears to be increasing for the NP. Wong and Farrally (2013) reported, for example, that a key element of the NP role in the practice setting is to act as a liaison between the medical plan of care and the interprofessional plan of care. Thus, the trend appears to be an increasing integration of APNs in the interprofessional team.

Continuing education programs for practicing NPs and curricular modifications to address these learning needs have been implemented to assist NPs in their ability to respond autonomously to client needs. In recent years, for example, Canadians have inquired about prescriptive medical cannabis given the current culture of increased access after Canada legalized recreational marijuana, and, in some instances, NPs have incorporated this into their practices.

Articulation of Education and Licensure Streams

Prior to the introduction of NP licensure, education programs were classified into primary health care and acute care streams. As noted earlier, except for Quebec, three licensure streams have been identified: Family/All Ages, Adult, Pediatrics; the highly specialized NNP is also recognized. While many NPs in Canada deliver primary health care services, 41% were reported to be employed in acute care specialty settings (Wong & Farrally, 2013). In contrast, the CNS role is not licensed, does not require role-specific education, and tends to be less understood than the NP role.

The alignment of NP education with licensure requirements, health system service demands, client needs, and graduate employment patterns has created challenges in Canada. Issues revolve around designing program streams to fit an intersection of age-based care with an optimum set of acute and/or primary health care service competencies, and an optimum set of generalist and/or specialist competencies.

As the CNS role does not include components from the medical scope of practice, regulatory bodies do not license it. It is less well understood than the NP role and, as noted earlier, lacks a designated education program. Recently, however, the CNA (2014) has developed competencies for the role in order to facilitate a better understanding of it within the service delivery sector and as a guide to nursing education.

It is worth noting that articulation of APN streams created issues in the US and resulted in a proliferation of categories and inconsistencies across jurisdictions. The Advanced Practice Registered Nurse (APRN) Joint Dialogue Group (2008) published a consensus model that was developed over four years to tackle this problem. Known as LACE (legislation, accreditation, certification, education), it is endorsed by over 40 US nursing organizations and is being progressively implemented in individual US states. The model defines four APRN roles: nurse anaesthetist, nurse midwife, CNS, and NP. In each of these roles, the APRN must be educated in one of six population foci: family/individual across the lifespan, adult-gerontology, neonatal, pediatrics, women's health/gender-related, and psychiatric-mental health. Further specialization within a foci and role is optional but must be based on APRN role/population-based competencies. Specialties are recognized and represent a more focused area of education and practice within a role. Examples include oncology, nephrology, and palliative care.

Currently, US licensing examinations, for some of the NP foci, are used by Canadian regulating bodies and are approved for one or more of the three streams recognized in Canada. It is too early to know if other LACE foci or other APN roles, such as the nurse anaesthetist, will eventually be adopted in Canada.

Conclusion

Although APN was introduced in Canada a half century ago, the roles and the education programs for these roles have been vulnerable to sudden contextual changes. While this vulnerability persists, the needs of an aging population, the associated disease burden, increasing complexity of care, and the demands for fiscal constraints are likely to support the trend of a growing number of APNs in the health care system.

There have been tensions over the years between a generalized education and a specialized practice, and between a context-specific education program and a shifting environment.

Although these issues are unresolved, considerable progress has been made in the last two decades in articulating APN roles, competencies, and educational requirements and this trend is likely to continue. In the last few years there appears to be increased discussion about a move toward a generalist entry into practice for NPs across Canada.

A solid body of evidence, spanning five decades, shows the value APNs bring to the health care system, and this is increasingly being recognized. There appears to be contextual support for a continuation of the current trend of a fuller contribution and a greater integration of APNs in health care services and as members of interprofessional health care teams.

Critical Thinking Questions

1. How are current contextual factors influencing the evolution of APN in Canada?
2. What factors have influenced the lack of education programs designated for CNSs in Canada, and has this lack had an impact on the role?
3. Is there a misalignment between the curricula of education programs for APNs and their employment settings in the health care system?
4. What has contributed positively to the evolution of APN in Canada, and why?

References

Acorn, S., Lamarche, K., & Edwards, M. (2009). Practice doctorates in nursing: Developing nursing leaders. *Nursing Leadership, 22*(2), 85–91.

Advanced Practice Registered Nurse (APRN) Joint Dialogue Group. (2008). *Consensus model for APRN regulation: Licensure, accreditation, certification & education.* Washington, DC: American Association of Colleges of Nurses. Retrieved from http://www.aacn.nche.edu/education-resources/APRNReport.pdf

Alcock, D. (1996). The clinical nurse specialist, clinical nurse specialist/nurse practitioner, and other titled nurse in Ontario. *Canadian Journal of Nursing Administration, 9*(1), 23–44.

American Association of Colleges of Nursing (AACN). (2019). *DNP fact sheet.* Washington, DC: AACN. Retrieved from https://www.aacnnursing.org/News-Information/Fact-Sheets/DNP-Fact-Sheet

Arslanian-Engoren, C. (2019). Conceptualizations of advanced practice nursing. In M. F. Tracy & E. T. O'Grady (Eds.), *Hamric and Hanson's advanced practice nursing: An integrative approach* (6th ed., pp. 25–60). St. Louis, MO: Elsevier.

Bryant-Lukosius, D., Carter, N., Donald, F., Harbman, P., Kilpatrick, K., Martin-Misener, R., … Valaitis, R. (2014). *Report on advanced practice nursing (APN) in Canada for the global summit.* Retrieved from https://fhs.mcmaster.ca/ccapnr/documents/CanadianReportGlobalAPNSummit2014June12FINAL.pdf

Bryant-Lukosius, D., Carter, N., Kilpatrick, K., Martin-Misener, R., Donald, F., Kaasalainen, S., … DiCenso, A. (2010). The clinical nurse specialist role in Canada. *Nursing Leadership, 23*(Special Edition), 140–146.

Canadian Association of Schools of Nursing (CASN). (2015). *National nursing education framework.* Ottawa, ON: CASN. Retrieved from https://www.casn.ca/wp-content/uploads/2014/12/Framwork-FINAL-SB-Nov-30-20151.pdf

CASN. (2019). *Registered nurses education in Canada statistics: 2017–2018*. Ottawa, ON: CASN. Retrieved from https://www.casn.ca/wp-content/uploads/2019/12/2017-2018-EN-SFS-DRAFT-REPORT-for-web.pdf

Canadian Institute for Health Information (CIHI). (2019). *Nursing in Canada, 2018*. Ottawa, ON: CIHI. Retrieved from https://www.cihi.ca/en/nursing-in-canada-2018

Canadian Nurses Association (CNA). (2010). *Toward 2020: Visions for nursing*. Ottawa, ON: CNA.

CNA. (2014). *Pan-Canadian core competencies for the clinical nurse specialist*. Ottawa, ON: CNA. Retrieved from https://www.cna-aiic.ca/~/media/cna/files/en/clinical_nurse_specialists_convention_handout_e?la=en

CNA. (2019). *Advanced practice nursing: A pan-Canadian framework*. Ottawa, ON: CNA. Retrieved from https://www.cna-aiic.ca/-/media/cna/page-content/pdf-en/apn-a-pan-canadian-framework.pdf

Cragg, C. E., Doucette, S., & Humbert, J. (2003). Ten universities, one program: Successful collaboration to educate nurse practitioners. *Nurse Educator, 28*(5), 227–231.

DiCenso, A., Auffrey, L., Bryant-Lukosius, D., Donald, F., Martin-Misener, R., Matthews, S., & Opsteen, J. (2007). Primary health care nurse practitioners in Canada. *Contemporary Nurse, 26*(1), 104–115.

DiCenso, A., & Bryant-Lukosius, D. (2010a). *Clinical nurse specialists and nurse practitioners in Canada: A decision support synthesis*. Ottawa, ON: CHSRF. Retrieved from http://www.ensp.fiocruz.br/observarh/arquivos/Estudo%20Especial%20sobre%20a%20Pratica%20da%20Enfermagem%20%20%20Canada.pdf

DiCenso, A., & Bryant-Lukosius, D. (2010b). The long and winding road: Integration of nurse practitioners and clinical nurse specialists into the Canadian health-care system. *Canadian Journal of Nursing Research, 42*(2), 3–8.

Government of Canada. (2012). *Framework for designating additional classes of practitioners under the new classes of practitioners regulations*. Ottawa, ON: Government of Canada.

Haines, J. (1993). *The nurse practitioner—A discussion paper*. Ottawa, ON: CNA.

Hravnak, M., Kleinpell, R., Magdic, K., & Guttendorf, J. (2009). The acute care nurse practitioner. In A. Hamric, J. Spross, & C. Hanson (Eds.), *Advanced practice nursing: An integrated approach* (pp. 403–436). St. Louis, MO: Saunders.

Kaasalainen, S., Martin-Misener, R., Kilpatrick, K., Harbman, P., Bryant-Lukosius, D., Donald, F., & DiCenso, A. (2010). A historical overview of the development of advanced practice nursing in Canada. *Journal of Nursing Leadership, 23*(Special Issue), 35–60.

Kamarudin, G., Penm, J., Chaar, B., & Moles, R. (2013). Educational interventions to improve prescribing competency: A systematic review. *British Medical Journal Open, 3*(8). doi: 10.1136/bmjopen-2013-003291

Little, L., & Reichert, C. (2018). *Fulfilling nurse practitioners' untapped potential in Canada's health care system: Results from the CFNU pan-Canadian nurse practitioner & retention study*. Ottawa, ON: CFNU.

Martin-Misener, R., Bryant-Lukosius, D., Harbman, P., Donald, F., Kaasalainen, S., Carter, N., … DiCenso, A. (2010). Education of advanced practice nurses in Canada. *Journal of Nursing Leadership, 23*(Special Issue), 61–87.

Montemuro, M. A. (1987). The evolution of the clinical nurse specialist: Response to the challenge of professional nursing practice. *Clinical Nurse Specialist, 1*(3), 106–110.

Nurse Practitioners' Association of Ontario (NPAO). (n.d.). *The history of nurse practitioners*. Toronto, ON: NPAO. Retrieved from http://npao.org/nurse-practitioners/history/#.VQHckI7F-84

Ordre des infirmières et infirmiers du Québec (OIIQ). (2020). *Infirmière praticienne spécialisée ou infirmier praticien spécialisé (IPS)* [Specialized nurse practitioner or specialized nurse practitioner (SNP/SNP)]. Montreal, QC: OIIQ. Retrieved from https://www.oiiq.org/en/acceder-profession/decouvrir-la-profession/ possibilites-de-carriere/infirmiere-praticienne-specialisee-ou-infirmier-praticien-specialise-ips-

Paes, B., Michell, A., Hunsberger, M., Blatz, S., Watts, J., Dent, P., ... Southwell, D. (1989). Medical staffing in Ontario neonatal intensive care units. *Canadian Medical Association Journal, 140*(11), 1321–1326.

Pringle, D. (2007). Nurse practitioner role: Nursing needs it. *Nursing Leadership, 20*(2), 1–5.

Simpson, B. (1997). An educational partnership to develop acute care nurse practitioners. *Canadian Journal of Nursing Administration, 10*(1), 69–84.

Tung, T. K. C. (2010). In support of doctor of nursing practice education in Canada. *Topics in Advanced Practice Nursing eJournal, 11*, 1–4.

Villeneuve, M., & MacDonald, J. (2006). Toward 2020: Visions for nursing setting the stage for the future. *The Canadian Nurse, 102*, 22–23.

Wong, S., & Farrally, V. (2013). *The utilization of nurse practitioners and physician assistants: A research synthesis.* Vancouver, BC: Michael Smith Foundation for Health Research. Retrieved from http://www. msfhr.org/sites/default/files/Utilization_of_Nurse_Practitioners_and_Physician_Assistants.pdf

Chapter 4

The Integration of Advanced Practice Nursing Roles in Canada

Michelle Acorn and David Byres

MICHELLE ACORN is a dually certified nurse practitioner (Adult and Family/All Ages) and currently the provincial Chief Nursing Officer in Ontario. Her expertise spans over 30 years of diverse integration across multiple health care sectors. She is an adjunct lecturer with the University of Toronto, Lawrence S. Bloomberg Faculty of Nursing, Toronto, Ontario. Michelle is an involved executive leader at the provincial and national levels.

DAVID BYRES is a registered nurse with significant experience in health policy, practice, and operations. He is an Adjunct Professor with the University of British Columbia School of Nursing, Vancouver, British Columbia, and Adjunct Assistant Professor with the University of Victoria School of Nursing, Victoria, British Columbia.

KEY TERMS

advanced practice nursing
  (APN)
clinical nurse specialist (CNS)
integration
nurse practitioner (NP)

OBJECTIVES

1. Appraise the integration of advanced practice nursing (APN) in Canada.
2. Explore the integration of nurse practitioner (NP) roles in Canada.
3. Highlight the integration of clinical nurse specialist (CNS) roles in Canada.

Introduction

This chapter reflects on the progress achieved with the integration of advanced practice nursing (APN) roles in Canada. While the clinical nurse specialist (CNS) and the nurse practitioner (NP) are established APN roles within Canada, a historical and innovative practice and leadership lens will demonstrate the successes and challenges impacting optimal integration for both clinical and non-clinical APN role dimensions, which ultimately leverage role sustainability.

Advanced Practice Nursing Pan-Canadian Integration Progress Report

The year 2020 marks 10 years since the *Canadian Journal of Nursing Leadership*'s special issue on APN was published. In a 2016 special issue that focused on APN roles in Canada, Martin-Misener and Bryant-Lukosius reflected on the many advancements for APN integration since 2010. The Canadian Nurses Association (CNA) led the development of position statements and briefing notes to enhance clarity about APN roles and competencies along with a public education campaign that included NPs and CNSs.

The Canadian Council of Registered Nurse Regulators (CCRNR) engaged in a national practice analysis to work toward a regulatory standard harmonization. The Canadian Nurse Practitioner Initiative and the Canadian Association of Schools of Nursing achieved master-level NP education in 2015. The APN Research Chair at McMaster University School of Nursing, Hamilton, Ontario, came to an end in 2011 after an impactful 10 years. The Canadian Centre for Advanced Practice Nursing Research (CCAPNR) emerged and continues to make substantial contributions in APN research capacity building and knowledge translation. Two CCAPNR research priorities targeted the practice patterns of CNSs in Canada and an economic evaluation of APN roles.

The diversity of APN roles across various settings and innovative models of care in Canada were also highlighted in the same issue. In Ontario, APN integration success included the development of a CNS framework for optimizing role capacity at the Centre for Addictions and Mental Health and the implementation of NP-Led Clinics to improve primary care access and chronic disease care. In Alberta, a community-initiated NP rural practice was implemented. New insights regarding stakeholder communication in health regions in British Columbia assisted in facilitating the integration of an evidence-informed framework for NP roles among hospital administrators in Ontario (Martin-Misener & Bryant-Lukosius, 2016). In British Columbia, patient care networks are being established using family practitioners and NPs with a recent announcement of funding to support the integration of 200 NPs into primary care (Government of British Columbia, 2018). Further progress and continued momentum for leadership by APNs, educators, regulators, and policy-makers are needed. Research about and by CNSs is under-represented compared to NPs. Canada can learn from our global APN leaders to enhance APN integration (Martin-Misener & Bryant-Lukosius, 2016).

Canadian Landscape: Role Integration of the Clinical Nurse Specialist

CNSs are APNs who contribute at a systems level to the quality and safety of patient care and can reduce health care costs when fully deployed and all role dimensions are implemented. Kilpatrick et al. (2014) further highlighted the experiences of CNSs in a Canada-wide survey documenting challenges in identifying and tracking CNS role data. An alarming 25% were no longer or had never practiced as a CNS. Almost half of the CNSs no longer practicing were younger than 50 years of age, representing a loss of a highly skilled APN workforce. Lack of role clarity, the inability to find employment, the inability to implement all the CNS role competencies, and lack of supportive leadership were key barriers that are potentially modifiable by nursing leaders in organizations and regulatory bodies (Kilpatrick et al., 2014).

Mechanisms to identify and track CNSs in Canada are needed to support effective workforce integration. The lack of mandatory graduate-level credentials in education requirements for CNSs and lack of title protection create challenges. For example, Quebec regulates the title of Infection Control CNS and New Brunswick identifies CNSs on their annual registration renewals at a graduate level (Kilpatrick et al., 2014). Furthermore, issues in fulfilling CNS clinical mandates are challenging given that Canadian CNSs spent only 22% of their work time in clinical practice, while another 40% reported that their role did not focus on direct patient care (Kilpatrick et al., 2014).

CNSs provide important leadership for the nursing profession and the health care system. Key challenges to full integration of the CNS include fluctuating role prominence; a broadening evidence base and need for rapid knowledge translation to the care setting; lack of common vision and understanding of the CNS role; lack of credentialing and title protection; and funding vulnerability (Bryant-Lukosius et al., 2010a, 2010b; CNA, 2016). Role facilitators include integration of evidence to guide practice and decision making, expert support and consultation, and executing change to improve patient outcomes at a system level (CNA, 2016).

Although some APNs are doctorally prepared nurses, both CNSs and NPs, the role of clinician-scientist within nursing continues to experience limited uptake compared to medicine. In an advanced practice clinician-scientist role, APNs work in both clinical practice as well as academic settings. Further examination of this role—to bridge practice and research—may be important both in the pursuit of advanced practice nursing roles that produce clinically relevant research and assist in the translation of that knowledge into nursing practice (Mackay, 2009).

Canadian Landscape: Role Integration of the Nurse Practitioner

Canada lags behind other countries in integrating NP roles. In the United States there are 248,000 NPs licensed to practice with an NP-to-population ratio of 1:1,314 people, in contrast to Canada, where there are 5,697 NPs or a ratio of 14:100,000 people (Statistics Canada, 2019). NPs in Canada work across primary care, acute care, and complex settings, including public health, home and community care, long-term care, and within correctional facilities. In Canada, NPs are regulated in all 13 provinces and territories and are positioned to meet the ever-growing complexity and needs of the health care system (CNA, 2019).

There has been significant harmonization and expansion of the legal scope of NP practice across Canada. All jurisdictions have authorized NPs to independently perform comprehensive health assessments; communicate a medical diagnosis (except in Quebec, where the role continues to evolve); order laboratory tests; order and interpret diagnostic imaging tests (with some exceptions for CT scans and MRIs); independently refer to a specialist physician (restricted to primary care in Quebec); prescribe massage therapy, acupuncture, and physiotherapy (except in Quebec); and order home oxygen and insulin syringes/blood glucose monitors (except in Quebec), among other things (CNA, 2019).

In 2017, the scope of practice for NPs was optimized through changes to federal legislation/regulation and policy that granted them the authority to, among other things, participate in medical assistance in dying; order controlled drugs and substances in compliance with provincial and territorial regulations; and certify people for the medical expense tax credit, the child care expense deduction, the student disability tax credit, and the disability savings plan (CNA, 2019).

The legislated authority of NPs still differs across jurisdictions, which impedes full practice integration. Examples include the need for collaborative agreements with physicians; clauses in legislation that veto decision-making authority on NP practice; internal processes that may limit changes to NP-authorized practices; and lists or restrictions on diagnostic test ordering, diagnosing, prescribing, and managing specific conditions (Duff, Fehr, Pathak, & Pylypowich, 2018).

Some provinces have granted NPs the legislated authority to admit and discharge patients from hospitals. However, local hospital bylaws may prevent this privilege or authority, therefore limiting the NP's ability to practice in facilities as well as leadership roles such as medical directors or attending/most responsible provider roles. The various legislative acts or jurisdictional limits lead to underutilized NP education and skill along with duplication of services by a physician. Similarly, mental health care is limited by the inability to perform involuntary admissions for psychiatric assessment, or restrictions on opioid replacement therapies (Duff et al., 2018).

It is vital that jurisdictions continue to support the implementation and transportability of NP roles across Canada to optimize access to primary and specialized care. In support of this, several jurisdictions have increased the number of NP educational seats and employment positions available within their province/territory. Other strategies that have been implemented across Canada to support the NP role include bundle legislation, medical bylaws, NP advisory committees, and Right-touch regulation. Strategies may be inconsistently supported between different stakeholder groups within each province/territory (i.e., regulatory bodies, employers, unions). Therefore, NP integration across Canada should focus on the strategies that will have the greatest uptake and effect for their specific province/territory (Duff et al., 2018). Nurse practitioner care provision has seen significant improvements through allowances for autonomous and accountable practice. In an effort to capitalize on health human resourcing, provincial legislative and regulatory changes have enabled and empowered NPs to improve access to quality care (Acorn, 2015a).

In 2016, the CCRNR produced new entry-level competencies for NPs in Canada as a result of the 2015 practice analysis study of NPs. The report showed that differences in NP practice lies in client population needs and practice contexts, including age, developmental stage, health condition, and complexity of clients. These NP competencies have been adopted by nursing regulatory bodies in all Canadian jurisdictions (except Quebec) and across three streams of practice, that is, Family/All Ages, Adult, and Pediatrics (CNA, 2019). Nationally, a debate continues with respect to entry to practice education for NPs and whether to educate NPs as generalists or to provide specialized education within certain practice streams such as primary care, acute care, or pediatrics.

In 2018, 11 Canadian jurisdictions submitted NP data that profiled 5,697 NPs representing 1.8% of the 303,146 registered nurses in Canada (Canadian Institute for Health Information [CIHI], 2019). A 2018 survey conducted by the Canadian Federation of Nurses Unions (CFNU) showed that:

- 92% of NPs were employed in clinical practice
- 94% were employed in nursing (an increase of 82% since 2007)
- 72.4% worked full-time
- 16.8% worked part-time
- 4.4% worked on a casual basis (Little & Reichert, 2018)

The NP field continues to be female-dominated, with only 7.4% of NPs (422) being male. Approximately 32% of NPs were 50 years of age or older (CIHI, 2019). The supply of NPs in Canada has more than tripled from 1,393 in 2007 to 5,274 in 2017 (CIHI, 2019). Educational preparation of NPs in Canada varies, with 85.5% having a graduate degree, followed by 9.0% with a baccalaureate degree, and 4.2% with a post-baccalaureate diploma. Only 1.3% of NPs were educated at the doctoral level. Almost 96% of NPs were educated in Canada, while the other 4.4% (252) were educated internationally (CIHI, 2019). A provincial breakdown found that Newfoundland and Labrador has 168 NPs; Nova Scotia, 182; New Brunswick, 130; Quebec, 509; Ontario, 3,206; Saskatchewan, 228; Alberta, 529; British Columbia, 465; Yukon, 8; and Northwest Territories and Nunavut, a combined 50 NPs (CIHI, 2019).

In 2018, the CFNU released the results of a bilingual Pan-Canadian NP Retention and Recruitment Study. The report indicated that 18% of NPs in Canada provided services in both English and French. The study identified five themes that drive NP retention and recruitment:

- salary/compensation
- legislative barriers to full scope of practice
- funding for NP positions
- expanded employment settings for NPs
- improved opportunities for continuing education/professional development

Salary and benefits, which vary widely across the country, were identified as the top source of dissatisfaction, with 44% of NPs dissatisfied with their overall compensation. The CFNU study reported that NP salaries do not reflect their additional education, scope of practice, responsibility, and accountability. The study also highlighted that limited stakeholder understanding of the NP role and scope of practice limits the full utilization of NP skill sets to enhance interprofessional care. Over a quarter (26%) of NPs reported not working to their full scope of practice, with the highest rates in the hospital setting (33%). Further barriers preventing NPs from working to full scope included federal/provincial/territorial legislation, regulations, and employer policies. However, independent, holistic, and collaborative models of care were shown to support NP job satisfaction and retention (CFNU, 2018).

Title protection for NPs continues to be inconsistent across Canada. While the title NP and its variants are protected in most provinces and territories, several still do not provide this protection (5 of 13). Title protection is important to the successful integration of NPs across the country as it impacts role clarity, especially when delineating between advanced practice nursing roles (i.e., NP and CNS), as well as between the different classes of registered nurses (i.e., RN and RN[EC]). Lack of title clarity for APNs among health care providers and the public leads to ambiguous role expectations and confusion about the scope of practice of an NP versus a CNS. This lack of title clarity in turn can impact public awareness and acceptance of these advanced practice nursing roles and their effect on the health care team (Donald et al., 2010).

The notion that NPs in primary health care can practice only in the community, and that NPs in adult or pediatrics are authorized to practice only in tertiary care settings, is unnecessarily restrictive (Acorn, 2015a; Hurlock-Chorostecki & Acorn, 2017; Hurlock-Chorostecki, van Soeren, & Goodwin, 2008; van Soeren & Hurlock-Chrostecki, 2009; van Soeren, Hurlock-Chorostecki, & Reeves, 2011). There is an increasing understanding that generalist and specialist NP knowledge is portable and responsive to care needs across diverse settings.

While there has been funding targeted to increase some advanced practice nursing roles in several jurisdictions, APN funding in acute care often comes from health care agencies' general nursing funding envelope. Shrinking budgets and lack of specific funding limit opportunities to introduce new APN roles and innovative models of care delivery (Bryant-Lukosius et al., 2014). Other integration barriers include failure to utilize all APN role components; a growing evidence base indicating that a lack of national regulatory standardization leads to scope of practice limitations; variability in team acceptance of NPs due to lack of understanding of NPs' scope, skill, and education; and funding vulnerability. Role facilitators include clear role communication, tailored messages to stakeholders, supportive leadership, and stable funding (Kilpatrick et al., 2010). Strengthening the role of APNs across Canada to improve patient access and outcomes could be assisted by a pan-Canadian approach to regulation and education like the national licensing framework for physicians currently being debated in Canada (Picard, 2019).

Integration of Boundary Work Competencies

Boundary work, defined as "crossing the boundaries between the nursing and medical professions," started with the introduction of cardiology NPs in health care teams at two academic hospitals in Quebec (Kilpatrick et al., 2012, 2013). The findings of a case study revealed that boundary work involves a micro-level process, including creating space, loss of valued function, trust, interpersonal dynamics, and time. The development of trust between key members and co-location of team members for projects and medical and nursing leadership are important. NPs improve communication and collaboration among team members. Kilpatrick et al. (2010) insightfully highlighted the significant shifting boundaries with NPs' privilege and power to prescribe and their impact on the development of medical activities included in the NP scope. The loss of exclusivity of prescriptive authority for physicians as a unique contribution to the team narrows the competence gap that sets the medical profession apart from other health care groups. Overlapping activities and evolving scopes of practice in health care are necessary to give safe and innovative care to patients (Kilpatrick et al., 2010). NP roles share both medical and nursing activities that may result in some boundary turf wars for full integration (Acorn, 2015a). With the evolution of RN prescribing in Canada being implemented in multiple jurisdictions, both RN and CNSs can impact improving access but while shifting nursing practice boundaries.

Ontario showcased NP hospital admission and most responsible provider/practitioner (MRP) management, capitalizing on synergizing advanced practice nursing and medical expertise to optimize access to hospital care. The term is not legally defined; however, the MRP refers to the provider who has primary responsibility and accountability for the care of a patient within the hospital (Ontario Hospital Association [OHA], 2012). The definition of the MRP encompasses primary responsibility and consistent care assumed by the NP across the care trajectory during admission, treatment, diagnostics, diagnosis, prescribing, and discharge (Acorn, 2015a). Many other countries do not have restricting hospital legislation and leave the decision to hospital policies (Acorn, 2015a; Registered Nurses Association of Ontario [RNAO], 2012). Ultimately, hospital professional staff bylaws, credentialing, and privileging will require amendments to be inclusive of NPs (OHA, 2012; RNAO, 2012).

Accountability and reporting structures for NPs currently align with the medical advisory council of privileged staff. Leveraging the role of the chief nurse executive (CNE) to oversee NP and CNS nursing quality of care in hospitals is paramount (OHA, 2012; RNAO, 2012). The CNE holds a strategic role to leverage senior executive nursing leadership and support infrastructures for nursing success and sustainability. The CNE role ensures NP appointments and performance reviews are relevant for patient needs and appropriate for the NP role (OHA, 2012; RNAO, 2012).

The Nurse Practitioner as Most Responsible Provider/Practitioner for Patient Care

The MRP must be clearly established and communicated. Responsibilities for patient care upon admission include taking comprehensive histories; ordering diagnostic tests; prescribing medications and treatments; rendering provisional diagnosis; providing regular care monitoring; providing documentation during hospital care until discharge; ensuring on-call coverage; ensuring thorough completion of medical record upon discharge; and linking to relevant community primary care providers and resource services or referrals to specialists for transfer of accountability and responsibility (Acorn, 2015a; OHA, 2012; RNAO, 2012).

A hybrid range of APN models of care delivery exist, including where NPs function in a consultative model like CNSs; they may support admission and treatment in a shared care dyad with a physician colleague. NPs involved in shared care may also discharge the patient with prescriptions, necessary referrals, and linkages to community resources (Acorn, 2015a). To date, only a few Ontario hospital organizations are leading early adopters designating NPs as the formal MRP. The Lakeridge Health NP-Led Hospital Model of Care in Whitby, Ontario, was the first pioneering hospital to showcase care delivered by NPs as the MRP and granted full admitting rights through organizational supports since July 2012 (RNAO, 2012). Evidence of the NP-as-MRP role, and its positive impact on patient care, exists in pockets of primary health and hospital care in Canada. However, NP hospital roles have been evaluated only in the context of consultation and shared care. A mixed methods pilot study examining qualitative NP satisfaction surveys and quantitative data related to the total number of admissions and discharges in a community hospital in Ontario demonstrated that NPs were able to function as the MRP in providing hospital care from admission through to discharge with high patient, family, and staff satisfaction, and quality of care (Acorn, 2015a).

Enabling, empowering, and embracing the contributions of NPs working at full scope as the MRP were valuable for full integration (Acorn, 2015a). NPs functioning in the MRP role strive for patient-centred care, quality, experience, and favourable outcomes. Enabling and empowering APNs to be champions of change for optimal patient and organizational success leverages their knowledge and leadership capacity. This is not about NP trail-blazing; rather, it is about capitalizing on APNs as health human resourcing. This is not about the transference of power, namely important prescriptive, diagnostic, and admission privileges and authorities. It is about the power to deliver safe, quality care and optimize care accountabilities. NP competence and population needs should be the driver of meaningful change (Acorn, 2015a). Hurlock-Chorostecki and Acorn (2017) revealed that five years after the NP-as-MRP model of care in Ontario hospitals was implemented, minimal uptake in the adoption or integration of the role had occurred.

Integration of Title Protection for Advanced Practice Nurses in Canada

Transforming health care through professional education and experience is paramount for integration. Advanced practice nursing continues to evolve to meet primary care and complex health care system needs, yet doctorally prepared nurses (i.e., Doctor of Philosophy [PhD] or Doctor of Nursing Practice [DNP]), including CNSs and NPs, can be limited in using the title *doctor* when practicing clinically due to professionally restrictive statutes in some jurisdictions. There are 886 nurses registered with doctorate education, 74 of these are NPs (CIHI, 2019). In 2003, Alberta proclaimed that the use of the title *doctor* by an RN or NP can be used in academic or social settings or in conjunction with the delivery of nursing practice (Acorn, 2015b).

Some APNs in Canada are denied the ability to use the academic title of *doctor*; however, momentum and professional equality will be drivers for recognition change (Acorn, 2015b). The title *doctor* represents an academic credential and is not limited to a professional program, and no one discipline owns the title. In the health arena, the term *doctor* is no longer limited to medicine. Recognition of doctoral-educated nurses facilitates equity within the health care system while furthering credibility and legitimacy. The desired outcome is parity with other professional disciplines that have established practice doctorates as the standard entry into practice (Acorn, 2015b).

A driver and solution for delivering safe, quality care should be enabling APNs to be champions of change for optimal patient and organizational success. Care should not be defined by geography, profession, or title restrictions. Legally recognizing nurses who have obtained doctoral education by authorizing the title *doctor* for health provider parity, value, and respect is another key step in advancing health care integration. Removing the barriers for professional title protection is key for transforming professional change (Acorn, 2015b).

Conclusion

Implications for practice and scholarship reveal that enabling, empowering, and embracing advance practice nurses to function at their maximal scope of practice can be valuable and transform the health care system continuum. Full implementation, integration, and sustainability for models of care is a research-rich area for exploration utilizing both CNSs and NPs. Experiences and lessons learned require further policy supports and study to enrich the building of advanced nursing knowledge that further informs and leverages full system integration, realizing that full integration is dependent on the desire and ability to enact the full scope and value-added role of APN.

Critical Thinking Questions

1. What have been the key facilitators and barriers to full APN integration in Canada?
2. Do you feel that both CNSs and NPs can be equally integrated into the health care system?
3. Identify three strategies to facilitate integration further and how these would be beneficial.

References

Acorn, M. (2015a). Nurse practitioners as most responsible providers: Impact on care for seniors admitted to an Ontario hospital. *International Journal of Nursing and Clinical Practices Open Access,* 2(126). http://dx.doi.org/10.15344/2394-4978/2015/126

Acorn, M. (2015b). Title protection policy for doctoral nursing education in Ontario, Canada. *International Journal of Nursing and Clinical Practices (Open Access),* 2(116). Retrieved from https://www.graphyonline.com/archives/IJNCP/2015/IJNCP-116/

Bryant-Lukosius, D., Carter, N., Donald, F., Harbman, P., Kilpatrick, K., Martin-Misener, R., ... Valaitis, R. (2014). *Report on advanced practice nursing (APN) in Canada for the global summit.* Hamilton, ON: CCAPNR.

Bryant-Lukosius, D., Carter, N., Kilpatrick, K., Martin-Misener, R., Donald, F., Kaasalainen, S., & DiCenso, A. (2010a). The clinical nurse specialist role in Canada. *Nursing Leadership, 23*(Special Issue), 140–166.

Bryant-Lukosius, D., Martin-Misener, R., Donald, F., Bourgeault, I., Kilpatrick, K., & Harbman, P. (2010b). Factors enabling advanced practice nursing role integration in Canada. *Nursing Leadership, 23*(Special Issue), 211–238.

Canadian Federation of Nurses Unions (CFNU). (2018). *Fulfilling nurse practitioners' untapped potential in Canada's health care system.* Ottawa, ON: CFNU. Retrieved from https://nursesunions.ca/wp-content/uploads/2018/06/CFNU_UntappedPotential-Final-EN.pdf

Canadian Institute for Health Information (CIHI). (2019). *Nursing in Canada, 2018: A lens on supply and workforce.* Ottawa, ON: CIHI. Retrieved from https://www.cihi.ca/sites/default/files/document/regulated-nurses-2018-report-en-web.pdf

Canadian Nurses Association (CNA). (2016). *Position statement: Clinical nurse specialist.* Ottawa, ON: CNA. Retrieved from https://www.cna-aiic.ca/-/media/cna/page-content/pdf-en/clinical-nurse-specialist-position-statement_2016.pdf?la=en&hash=C89816295FE2F53808E0DEDC0595FE376552EAE1

CNA. (2019). *Advanced practice nursing: A pan-Canadian framework.* Ottawa, ON: CNA. Retrieved from https://www.cna-aiic.ca/-/media/cna/page-content/pdf-en/apn-a-pan-canadian-framework.pdf

Donald, F., Bryant-Lukosius, D., Martin-Misener, R., Kaasalainen, S., Kilpatrick, K., Carter, N., & DiCenso, A. (2010). Clinical nurse specialist and nurse practitioners: Title confusion and lack of role clarity. *Nursing Leadership, 23*(Special Issue), 189–201.

Duff, E., Fehr, C., Pathak, S., & Pylypowich, A. (2018). Optimization of nurse practitioner practice in Canada. Health Canada, Ottawa, ON. Unpublished.

Government of British Columbia. (2018). *Creating new opportunities for nurse practitioners as part of team-based care.* Victoria, BC: Government of British Columbia. Retrieved from https://news.gov.bc.ca/releases/2018HLTH0034-000995

Hurlock-Chorostecki, C., & Acorn, M. (2017). Diffusing innovative roles within Ontario hospitals: Implementing the nurse practitioner as the most responsible provider. *Nursing Leadership, 30*(4), 60–66.

Hurlock-Chorostecki, C., van Soeren, M., & Goodwin, S. (2008). The acute care nurse practitioner in Ontario: A workforce study. *Nursing Leadership, 21*(4), 100–116.

Kilpatrick, K., DiCenso, A., Bryant-Lukosius, D., Ritchie, J., & Martin-Misener, R. (2014). Clinical nurse specialists in Canada: Why are some not working in the role? *Nursing Leadership, 27*(1), 62–75.

Kilpatrick, K., Harbman, P., Carter, N., Martin-Misener, R., Bryant-Lukosius, D., Donald, F., & DiCenso, A. (2010). The acute care nurse practitioner role in Canada. *Nursing Leadership, 23*(Special Issue), 114–139.

Kilpatrick, K., Lavoie-Tremblay, M., Lamothe, L., Ritchie, J. A., & Doran, D. (2013). Conceptual framework of acute care nurse practitioner role enactment, boundary work, and perceptions of team effectiveness. *Journal of Advanced Nursing, 69*(1), 205–217.

Kilpatrick, K., Lavoie-Tremblay, M., Ritchie, J. A., Lamothe, L., & Doran, D. (2012). Boundary work and the introduction of acute care nurse practitioners in health care teams. *Journal of Advanced Nursing, 68*(7), 1504–1515.

Little, L., & Reichert, C. (2018). *Fulfilling nurse practitioners' untapped potential in Canada's health care system: Results from the CFNU pan-Canadian nurse practitioner & retention study.* Ottawa, ON: CFNU.

Retrieved from https://nursesunions.ca/wp-content/uploads/2018/06/CFNU_UntappedPotential-Final-EN.pdf

Mackay, M. (2009). Why nursing has not embraced the clinician-scientist role. *Nursing Philosophy, 10,* 287–296.

Martin-Misener, R., & Bryant-Lukosius, D. (2016). Guest editor's reflections on progress in the development of advanced practice nursing in Canada. *Nursing Leadership, 29*(3), 6–13.

Ontario Hospital Association (OHA). (2012). *Enabling nurse practitioners to admit and discharge: A guide for hospitals.* Toronto, ON: OHA. Retrieved from http://www.oha.com/CurrentIssues/keyinitiatives/PhysicianandProfessionalIssues/Physicians/Resources/Documents/Final%20-%20NP%20Guide.pdf

Picard, A. (2019, January 4). Why isn't there a single medical license for all doctors in Canada? *Globe and Mail.* Retrieved from https://www.theglobeandmail.com/canada/article-why-isnt-there-a-single-medical-licence-for-all-doctors-in-canada/

Registered Nurses Association of Ontario (RNAO). (2012). *Nurse practitioner utilization toolkit.* Toronto, ON: RNAO. Retrieved from http://rnao.ca/resources/toolkits/np-toolkit

Statistics Canada. (2019). CANSIM Table 051-0005. Ottawa, ON: Statistics Canada. Retrieved from https://www150.statcan.gc.ca/t1/tbl1/en/tv.action?pid=1710000901

van Soeren, M., & Hurlock-Chorostecki, C. (2009). *The integration of specialty nurse practitioners into the Ontario healthcare system.* Toronto, ON: NPAO. Retrieved from http://npao.org/nursepractitioners/specialty-project/

van Soeren, M., Hurlock-Chorostecki, C., & Reeves, S. (2011). The role of nurse practitioners in hospital settings: Implications for interprofessional practice. *Journal of Interprofessional Care, 25*(4), 245–251.

Chapter

5

Canadian Research on the Impact and Outcomes of Advanced Practice Nursing Roles

Ruth Martin-Misener and Denise Bryant-Lukosius

RUTH MARTIN-MISENER is a Professor and the Director of the School of Nursing and Assistant Dean, Research, at the Faculty of Health, Dalhousie University, Halifax, Nova Scotia. She is also the Co-Director of the Canadian Centre for Advanced Practice Nursing Research (CCAPNR) at McMaster University, Hamilton, Ontario, and an Affiliate Scientist with the Nova Scotia Health Authority as well as the Maritime Strategy for Patient-Oriented Research Support Unit. The focus of her research is evaluation of the implementation and outcomes of the nurse practitioner role and innovative interprofessional team-based models in primary and long-term care. Ruth has been involved in developing and evaluating policy for nurse practitioner regulation, education, and practice in Canada for more than 20 years and is the recipient of several awards, including induction as a Fellow in the American Academy of Nursing in 2019.

DENISE BRYANT-LUKOSIUS is an Associate Professor in the School of Nursing and Department of Oncology and Co-Director of the Canadian Centre for Advanced Practice Nursing Research (CCAPNR) at McMaster University, Hamilton, Ontario, and Adjunct Associate Professor in the School of Nursing at Hong Kong Polytechnic University, Hong Kong, China. At McMaster University, she is a scientist in the Escarpment Cancer Research Institute and inaugural holder of the Alba DiCenso Chair in Advanced Practice Nursing. She is cross-appointed to the Juravinski Hospital and Cancer Centre in Hamilton, Ontario, as a Clinician-Scientist and Director of the Canadian Centre of Excellence in Oncology Advanced Practice Nursing. Dr. Bryant-Lukosius has led national and international research and numerous education, mentorship, and knowledge translation initiatives to improve the health care systems integration of clinical nurse specialist and nurse practitioner roles.

KEY TERMS

clinical nurse specialist (CNS)
cost effectiveness
nurse practitioner (NP)
value-based health care

OBJECTIVES

1. Review historical milestones in the development of Canadian advanced practice nursing (APN) research.
2. Describe Canadian frameworks for evaluating APN roles.
3. Summarize Canadian research evaluating APN impact and outcomes in four health services areas: primary health care, emergency and ambulatory care, long-term/home care, and acute/hospital care.
4. Identify opportunities for Canadian APN research.

Introduction

Value-based health care is a new focus of reform in Canada and many countries around the globe. At its core, value-based health care is about focusing on the outcomes that matter most to patients and the costs required to achieve those outcomes, with value growing when beneficial outcomes are achieved at a lower cost (Canadian Foundation for Healthcare Improvement [CFHI], 2018; Porter, 2010). The Institute for Healthcare Improvement's (IHI) Triple Aim and Quadruple Aim are frameworks used to guide thinking about value-based health care (IHI, 2019). For example, the Canadian Nurses Association (CNA; 2019) used these frameworks to summarize a sample of advanced practice nursing (APN) research in their *Advanced Practice Nursing: A Pan-Canadian Framework* document.

Research and evaluation have been integral to the introduction and implementation of APN roles in Canada. The two recognized APN roles, clinical nurse specialist (CNS) and nurse practitioner (NP), were introduced at similar times in the late 1960s to mid-1970s (Bryant-Lukosius et al., 2010; Donald et al., 2010). However, there are considerable differences in the nature and magnitude of the research and evaluation accompanying role introduction and development of these two roles. The introduction of the NP role was accompanied by two randomized controlled trials (RCTs) examining role effectiveness of NPs in primary care (Chambers & West, 1978; Spitzer et al., 1974) and one RCT of neonatal NPs (Mitchell-DiCenso et al., 1996). In contrast, research about the CNS role did not materialize until the mid-1990s and used primarily descriptive designs (Bryant-Lukosius et al., 2010).

Although the initial wave of NP implementation failed, the resurgence of interest in the role in the mid-1990s continued to gain momentum and today NPs are a rapidly growing health professional group in Canada (Canadian Institute for Health Information [CIHI], 2019). The federally funded Canadian Nurse Practitioner Initiative (CNPI; 2006a), led by the CNA, contributed to this in several important ways. These included the development of evidence-based technical papers that influenced policy changes, laying the foundation for standardized approaches to education and regulation as well as development of a Research and Evaluation Framework and Toolkit (CNPI, 2006b). No such attention or resources were directed at the CNS role until recently when the CNA (2014) led the development of national CNS competencies. While some progress has been made, full integration of CNS and NP roles into the Canadian health care system has yet to be achieved and lags behind other developed countries with similar APN experience (Lamb et al., 2018). Contemporary evidence relevant to the Canadian context about the outcomes and impact of CNS and NP roles is essential for informing health care policies and influencing effective health care decision-making about their optimal use and sustainability.

Recognizing this, the Canadian Health Services Research Foundation (CHSRF) commissioned a synthesis of Canadian literature published between 1970 and 2009 with an explicit purpose to further the integration of these roles (DiCenso et al., 2010). The synthesis found 224 papers focused on NPs, 44 on CNSs, and another 53 focused on a general APN role (DiCenso et al., 2010). The 2010 synthesis revealed stark differences in the volume of research and evaluation focused on NPs and CNSs and fuelled subsequent national research about CNSs (Kilpatrick et al., 2013) described in a later section of this chapter.

The APN Research Chair

The APN Research Chair program, held from 2001 to 2011 by Dr. Alba DiCenso, had a highly influential capacity-building impact that facilitated substantial growth in the amount of research and evaluation conducted about APN roles. Funded by the CHSRF and Canadian Institutes of Health Research, APN Research Chair program trainees included 24 graduate students (6 MSc, 16 PhD, 2 DNP), four post-doctoral fellows, three junior faculty, and one career scientist. The Chair program secured more than $3.5 million to fund 48 APN-focused studies and resulted in 236 peer-reviewed publications and 21 book chapters, and 605 oral and 182 poster peer-reviewed presentations at national and international conferences (Bryant-Lukosius et al., 2017). Landmark accomplishments included completion of a decision-support synthesis of APN in Canada culminating in 10 articles in a special issue of the *Canadian Journal of Nursing Leadership* in 2010; a national mixed-methods study examining the role of NPs in long-term care settings (Carter et al., 2016; Kaasalainen et al., 2013; Martin-Misener et al., 2015a; Ploeg et al., 2013; Sangster-Gormley et al., 2013) and systematic reviews of the cost effectiveness of NPs and CNSs (Bryant-Lukosius et al., 2015; Donald et al., 2014, 2015; Kilpatrick et al., 2014, 2015; Marshall et al., 2015; Martin-Misener et al., 2015b). In addition to the systematic reviews conducted, this team completed an analysis of the quality of economic papers identifying weaknesses and areas for improvement in future research (Lopatino et al., 2017). For these extensive accomplishments, in 2014 Dr. DiCenso was inducted as a member of the Order of Canada for her research in evidence-based nursing and her contributions to the development of NPs.

The APN Research Chair Program trainees have gone on to develop research centres and assume research chair positions. For example, Dr. Bryant-Lukosius established the Canadian Centre of Excellence in Oncology APN and also holds the Alba DiCenso Chair in Advanced

Practice Nursing at McMaster University, Hamilton, Ontario, and Dr. Kelley Kilpatrick holds the Susan E. French Chair in Nursing Research and Innovative Practice at McGill University, Montreal, Quebec.

Several of the trainees from the APN Research Chair Program decided to continue their collaboration developed through the program and formed a national research centre, the Canadian Centre for Advanced Practice Nursing Research (CCAPNR). Now almost 10 years old, CCAPNR continues to be a productive centre that has made significant contributions to research and evaluation of APN roles in Canada and internationally.

Canadian Frameworks for Evaluating APN Role Introduction, Implementation, and Sustainability

The Participatory, Evidence-based, Patient-focused Process for guiding the development, implementation, and evaluation of APN (PEPPA) framework was developed by Dr. Bryant-Lukosius and Dr. DiCenso in 2004 at McMaster University. Since its publication in 2004, it has been widely used by researchers, clinicians, and students in Canada and around the globe to guide the introduction of APN roles and advanced roles in other professions (Boyko Carter, & Bryant-Lukosius, 2016). Boyko, Carter, and Bryant-Lukosius found that between 2004 and 2014, the PEPPA framework paper was cited 284 times by researchers and authors with a policy background. A cursory search in March 2020 indicated the citation number had increased to 369. The impact of this framework on APN role introduction and implementation in Canada and around the globe is far-reaching and extensive.

Building on the Donabedian structure, process, outcome model, the PEPPA Plus framework was developed by Bryant-Lukosius (2016) in collaboration with colleagues from the Institute of Nursing Science, University Basel, and University Hospital Basel in Basel, Switzerland (see Figure 5.1). The PEPPA Plus framework provides an in-depth approach to evaluating APN roles at introduction, implementation, and long-term sustainability stages of role development (Bryant-Lukosius et al., 2016). Since its publication in 2016, it has already been cited 78 times, demonstrating utility and relevance.

The Nursing Role Effectiveness Model (NREM) was designed to evaluate the nurse and patient structures and processes that impact nursing care (Doran, Sidani, Keatings, & Doidge, 2002; Irvine, Sidani, & Hall, 1998). Sidani and Irvine (1999) proposed an adaptation of the NREM to develop a framework to evaluate the acute care NP. Curnew and Lukewich (2018) used the NREM to guide a scoping review of nursing roles, including NPs, within primary care in Atlantic Canada.

Outcomes and Impacts of APN Roles in Canada

To explore the current landscape of Canadian APN literature, this section discusses Canadian research that examines outcomes and impacts of NP and CNS roles. A convenience search of CINAHL and Medline was conducted using the following keywords: *nurse practitioner, clinical nurse specialist, advanced practice nursing, outcomes, impact, effectiveness,*

FIGURE 5.1: PEPPA Plus Framework

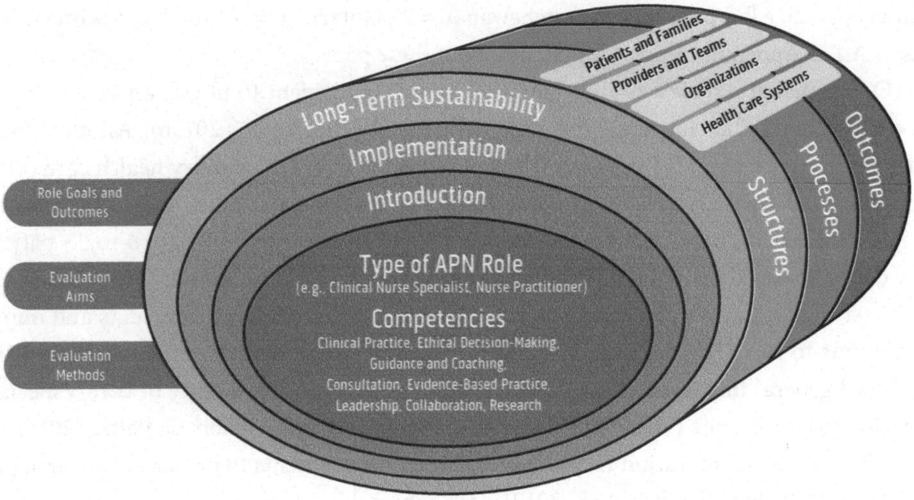

Source: Bryant-Lukosius, D., Spichiger, E., Martin, J., Stoll, H., Kellerhals, S. D., Fliedner, M., ... De Geest, S. (2016). Framework for evaluating the impact of advanced practice nursing roles. *Journal of Nursing Scholarship, 48*(2), 201–209. Reprinted with permission.

---

and *Canada*. Articles published after 2009 were included if they addressed research, quality improvement, or evaluation conducted in Canada. Literature reviews of any type and re-search protocols with a Canadian corresponding author were also included. The year 2009 was selected because research published in and prior to 2009 was already published in the 2010 special issue of the *Canadian Journal of Nursing Leadership* that focused on advanced practice nursing. Articles in this special issue continue to be some of the most downloaded articles in the journal.

The search for literature for this chapter was limited to two databases (Medline and CINAHL), did not use a comprehensive search strategy, and did not include a search of grey literature. Data were extracted from abstracts unless further clarification was needed from the full text. Notwithstanding these limitations, the review provides an information snapshot of the landscape of Canadian APN research that has an explicit focus on evaluating impacts or outcomes.

A total of 52 published papers were found with a focus on impact and/or outcomes of NP or CNS care in Canada: 16 were focused on NPs in primary care; 13 on NPs in acute care (includes in-patient, emergency, and ambulatory care); 10 on NPs in long-term care/home care; 12 on CNSs; and 2 included both CNSs and NPs. Data extracted included author name and province, purpose, method, and outcome/impact categorized as patient, provider, or system.

Nurse Practitioners in Primary Health Care

Of the 17 papers with a focus on primary care, 3 papers were systematic or scoping reviews of international studies. Two papers were regional in scope, one involved primary data collection in the four western provinces, and the other was a scoping review of research from Atlantic Canada. The remaining papers reported primary research conducted in British Columbia (n = 2), Alberta (n = 2), Saskatchewan (n = 2), Ontario (n = 5), and Nova Scotia (n = 1). Table A.1 in Appendix A provides details about these papers.

One systematic review found that NP care was equivalent to physician care in all but seven outcomes that favoured NP care (Martin-Misener et al., 2015b). Another found that the presence of an NP on a team decreased wait times for primary health care (PHC) appointments (Ansell, Crispo, Simard, & Bjerre, 2017) and another that NP panel size was dependent on patient characteristics and that on average, NPs saw 8 to 15 patients per day (Martin-Misener et al., 2016). Similarly, Curnew and Lukewich (2018) found that PHC settings with NPs and nurses had positive clinical outcomes for patients and improved access to care. Several papers reported primary research with patient outcomes that included general improvements in physiological health and the quality of care, especially for chronic conditions (Heale & Pilon, 2012; Hunter, Murphy, Babb, & Vallee, 2016). An NP-pharmacist collaboration resulted in specific improvements to prescribing of inappropriate medications (Fletcher et al., 2012). Two papers described high levels of patient satisfaction from care received through collaboration between an NP and physiotherapist to provide virtual services and improve access to physiotherapy services to a marginalized low-income population (Lovo, Harrison, O'Connell, Trask, & Bath, 2019; Oosman, Weber, Ogunson, & Bath, 2019).

Nurse Practitioners in Acute/Hospital Care

The 14 papers focused on NPs in acute care settings are outlined in Table A.2 in Appendix A. Five of these were literature reviews that were international in scope (Donald et al., 2015; Kilpatrick et al., 2015; Smigorowsky, Norris, McMurtry, & Tsuyuki, 2017; Smigorowsky, Sebastianski, & Norris, 2020; Spence, Ricci, & McCuaig, 2019); three were papers from Ontario (Hurlock-Chorostecki & Acorn, 2017; Nixon et al., 2020; Rietze, Heale, Hill, & Roles, 2016); British Columbia (Goldie, Prodan-Bhalla, & MacKay, 2012; Singh et al., 2019) and Alberta had two papers each (Li et al., 2017; Stahlke, Rawson, & Pituskin, 2017); Quebec (Kilpatrick et al., 2013) and Manitoba (Sawatzky, Christie, & Singal, 2013) each had one. Seven papers reported on quantitative studies, including two completed RCTs and one RCT protocol. Half of the remaining six were systematic reviews and half were qualitative papers. Comparing NP care to usual care (physician care) in acute care, two literature reviews found similar patient and health care system outcomes (Donald et al., 2015; Smigorowsky et al., 2020). Spence et al.'s (2019) review of NPs in surgical sites found NP care improved patient satisfaction, team communication, quality of and access to care, and decreased length of stay. Primary studies found patients with diabetes receiving NP care had improved glycemic control and quality of life (Li et al., 2017), patients with lymphoma had improved time to diagnosis (Nixon et al., 2020), and patients who were post-cardiac surgery had decreased symptoms and improved physical functioning (Sawatzky et al., 2013).

Nurse Practitioners in Long-Term/Home Care

The 10 papers focused on NPs in long-term care (n = 9) and home care (n =1) settings (Tung, Kaufmann, & Tanner, 2012) are outlined in Table A.3 in Appendix A. Five papers were international or national in scope; two were from Ontario; and there was one each from Quebec, Nova Scotia, and Saskatchewan. Among these, there was one systematic literature review (Donald et al., 2013); four quantitative papers (El-Masri, Omar, & Groh, 2015; Kaasalainen et al., 2016; Lacny et al., 2016; Tung et al., 2012); four qualitative papers (Carter et al., 2016; Kaasalainen et al., 2013; Ploeg et al., 2013; Sangster-Gormley et al., 2013); and one mixed-methods paper (Kilpatrick, Tchouaket, Jabbour, & Hains, 2020). Some of the benefits of advanced practice nurses identified in the systematic review included decreased rates of depression, urinary incontinence, pressure ulcers, and aggressive behaviours (Donald et al., 2013). Benefits of NP care for residents included reductions in pain (Kaasalainen et al., 2016), falls, restraint use, number of medications (Kilpatrick et al., 2020), and improved quality of care and informational and emotional support (Ploeg et al., 2013). Provider benefits of NP care included knowledge and skill development and capacity building (Kaasalainen et al., 2013; Sangster-Gormley et al., 2013). Some of the benefits to the health care system included reductions in emergency department transfers (El-Masri et al., 2015; Tung et al., 2012), improved access to care for residents (Carter et al., 2016), and cost-effectiveness (Lacny et al., 2016).

Clinical Nurse Specialists in Care Settings

There were 12 papers that focused on the outcomes of CNS care in in-patient, transitional, and outpatient settings. In-patient settings included cardiology, surgery, oncology, mental health, and palliative care. As shown in Table A.4 in Appendix A, five papers were international or national in scope, four were from Ontario, and three were from Quebec. Of these, there were four literature reviews (Bryant-Lukosius et al., 2015; Kilpatrick et al., 2015; Moore & McQuestion, 2012); three quantitative papers (Abela-Dimech, Johnston, & Strudwick, 2017; de Mestral et al., 2011; Kilpatrick et al., 2013); three quality-improvement papers (Fabbruzzo-Cota et al., 2016; Stilos & Daines, 2013; St-Louis & Brault, 2011); one qualitative paper (Desrochers, Donivan, Mehta, & Laizner, 2016); and one protocol paper (Jackson, Parkinson, Jackson, & Mantler, 2018).

Care provided by CNSs in transitional settings resulted in improved health outcomes for patients, for example, reduced mortality in post-cancer surgery patients, and improved treatment adherence and patient satisfaction in patients with health failure (Bryant-Lukosius et al., 2015). Provider benefits of CNS care included improved knowledge and skills as well as team communication (Kilpatrick et al., 2013). Health care system outcomes—such as length of stay, rehospitalization, and costs—were improved with CNS care in transitional care settings (Bryant-Lukosius et al., 2015) and in chronic disease management (Moore & McQuestion, 2012). Other examples of health care system outcomes of CNS care were reductions in hospital-acquired pressure ulcers (Fabbruzzo-Cota et al., 2016) and improvements in team referral processes (Stilos & Daines, 2013).

Conclusion

This chapter provides an overview of key historical and current contributions to the development of APN research and an evaluation of APN outcomes in Canada. This body of work includes a range of evidence-based knowledge products that have influenced APN development in Canada and internationally (Bryant-Lukosius & Martin-Misener, 2016). The APN frameworks have been impactful in guiding the introduction and implementation of new roles within Canada and around the world. Research chairs and organizations have trained and mentored APN scholars across Canada. APN research has informed the development of new roles and the conduct of practice analyses that have guided government policy as well as regulatory and educational policy documents.

Canadian literature published in the last decade demonstrates a breadth of research, evaluation, and quality-improvement approaches to examine APN outcomes and impact. Research has been performed in almost every province with authors who are from academic, policy, and practice environments. Our review is suggestive of an interesting trend toward examining outcomes of new approaches to health service delivery, sometimes in collaboration with a health care provider from another discipline such as a pharmacist or physiotherapist. Interprofessional teams that include APN roles are increasingly common, and more research is needed to determine the optimal size and composition of teams to meet the needs of specific populations.

Both NP and CNS research is occurring in a range of practice areas and commonly addresses patient and health care system outcomes. The Canadian CNS literature reflects the tripartite mandate of the CNS role with outcomes that focus on patients as well as providers and health care systems or organizations.

While research, quality improvement, and/or evaluation is being completed in almost all provinces across the country, more research and evaluation is needed to address the challenges and opportunities facing health care. Sustaining a path of continuous research and evaluation requires growth in workforce supply in three key areas: PhD-prepared researchers; APN clinicians engaged in research, evaluation, and APN policy; and administrative leaders who both conduct and support research, evaluation, and quality improvement. This is particularly important as provinces move toward becoming learning health care systems.

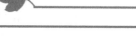

Critical Thinking Questions

1. What are the top three research priorities for improved integration of APN roles in Canada?
2. How has research contributed to the evolution of NP and CNS roles in Canada?

References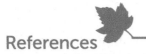

Abela-Dimech, F., Johnston, K., & Strudwick, G. (2017). Development and pilot implementation of a search protocol to improve patient safety on a psychiatric inpatient unit. *Clinical Nurse Specialist, 31*(2), 104–114. doi: 10.1097/NUR.0000000000000281

Ansell, D., Crispo, J. A. G., Simard, B., & Bjerre, L. M. (2017). Interventions to reduce wait times for primary care appointments: A systematic review. *BioMed Central (BMC) Health Services Research, 17*, 1–9. doi: 10.1186/s12913-017-2219-y

Boyko, J. A., Carter, N., & Bryant-Lukosius, D. (2016). Assessing the spread and uptake of a framework for introducing and evaluating advanced practice nursing roles. *World Views on Evidence-Based Nursing, 13*(4), 277–284. doi.org/10.1111/wvn.12160

Bryant-Lukosius, D., Carter, N., Kilpatrick, K., Martin-Misener, R., Donald, F., Kaasalainen, S., ... DiCenso, A. (2010). The clinical nurse specialist role in Canada. *Canadian Journal of Nursing Leadership, 23*(Special Edition), 140–166.

Bryant-Lukosius, D., Carter, N., Reid, K., Donald, F., Martin-Misener, R., Kilpatrick, K., ... DiCenso, A. (2015). The clinical effectiveness and cost-effectiveness of clinical nurse specialist-led hospital to home transitional care: A systematic review. *Journal of Evaluative Clinical Practice, 21*(5), 763–781. doi: 0.1111/jep.12401

Bryant-Lukosius, D., & Martin-Misener, R. (2016). *Advanced practice nursing: An essential component of country level human resources for health.* Policy paper for the International Council of Nurses. Retrieved from https://www.who.int/workforcealliance/knowledge/resources/ICN_PolicyBrief6AdvancedPracticeNursing.pdf

Bryant-Lukosius, D., Martin-Misener, R., Roussel, J., Carter, N., Kilpatrick, K., & Brousseau, L. (2017). Policy and the integration of advanced practice nursing roles in Canada: Are we making progress? In K. A. Goudreau & M. Smolenski (Eds.), *Health policy and advanced practice nursing, impact and implications* (2nd ed., pp. 357–374). New York, NY: Springer.

Bryant-Lukosius, D., Spichiger, E., Martin, J., Stoll, H., Degen Kellerhals, S., Fliedner, M., ... De Geest, S. (2016). Framework for evaluating the impact of advanced practice nursing roles. *Journal of Nursing Scholarship, 48*(2), 201–209.

Canadian Foundation for Healthcare Improvement (CFHI). (2018). Aligning outcomes and spending: Canadian experiences with value-based healthcare. Ottawa, ON: CFHI. Retrieved from https://www.cfhi-fcass.ca/sf-docs/default-source/documents/health-system-transformation/vbhc-executive-brief-e.pdf?sfvrsn=c884ab44_2

Canadian Institute for Health Information (CIHI). (2019). *Canada's health care provider data tables 2018.* Ottawa, ON: CIHI. Retrieved from https://www.cihi.ca/en/health-workforce

Canadian Nurse Practitioner Initiative (CNPI). (2006a). *Nurse practitioners: The time is now. A solution to improving access and reducing wait times in Canada.* Ottawa, ON: CNA. Retrieved from https://www.cna-aiic.ca/en/nursing-practice/the-practice-of-nursing/advanced-nursing-practice/nurse-practitioners/canadian-nurse-practitioner-initiative

CNPI. (2006b). *Implementation and evaluation toolkit for nurse practitioners in Canada.* Ottawa, ON: CNA. Retrieved from https://www.mycna.ca/~/media/nurseone/files/en/toolkit_implementation_evaluation_np_e.pdf

Canadian Nurses Association (CNA). (2014). *Pan-Canadian core competencies for the clinical nurse specialist.* Ottawa, ON: CNA. Retrieved from https://cna-aiic.ca/~/media/cna/files/en/clinical_nurse_specialists_convention_handout_e.pdf

CNA. (2019). *Advanced practice nursing: A pan-Canadian framework.* Ottawa, ON: CNA. Retrieved from https://www.cna-aiic.ca/en/nursing-practice/the-practice-of-nursing/advanced-nursing-practice

Carter, N., Sangster-Gormley, E., Ploeg, J., Martin-Misener, R., Donald, F., Wickson-Griffiths, A., … Schindel Martin, L. (2016). An assessment of how nurse practitioners create access to primary care in Canadian residential long-term care settings. *Canadian Journal of Nursing Leadership, 29*(2), 45–63. doi: 10.12927/cjnl.2016.24806

Chambers, L. W., & West, A. E. (1978). The St. John's randomized controlled trial of the family practice nurse: Health outcomes of patients. *International Journal of Epidemiology, 7*(2), 153–161.

Curnew, D. R., & Lukewich, J. (2018). Nursing within primary care settings in Atlantic Canada: A scoping review. *Sage Open,* 1–17. Retrieved from https://doi.org/10.1177/2158244018774379

de Mestral, C., Iqbal, S., Fong, N., LeBlanc, J., Fata, P., Razek, T., & Khwaja, K. (2011). Impact of a specialized multidisciplinary tracheostomy team on tracheostomy care in critically ill patients. *Canadian Journal of Surgery, 54*(3), 167–172. doi: 10.1503/cjs.043209

Desrochers, F., Donivan, E., Mehta, A., & Laizner, A. M. (2016). A psychosocial oncology program: Perceptions of the telephone-triage assessment. *Supportive Care in Cancer, 24*(7), 2937–2944.

DiCenso, A., Bryant-Lukosius, D., Martin-Misener, R., Donald, F., Abelson, J., Bourgeault, I., … Kioke, S. (2010). Factors enabling advanced practice nursing role integration in Canada. *Canadian Journal of Nursing Leadership, 23*(Special Edition), 211–238.

Donald, F., Kilpatrick, K., Reid, K., Carter, N., Bryant-Lukosius, D., Martin-Misener, R., … DiCenso, A. (2015). Hospital to community transitional care by nurse practitioners: A systematic review of cost-effectiveness. *International Journal of Nursing Studies, 52*(1), 436–451. doi: 0.1016/j.ijnurstu.2014.07.011

Donald, F., Kilpatrick, K., Reid, K., Carter, N., Martin-Misener, R., Bryant-Lukosius, D., … DiCenso, A. (2014). A systematic review of the cost-effectiveness of nurse practitioners and clinical nurse specialists: What is the quality of the evidence? *Nursing Research & Practice, 28*(3), 56–76. doi: 10.1155/2014/896587

Donald, F., Martin-Misener, R., Bryant-Lukosius, D., Kilpatrick, K., Kaasalainen, S., Kioke, S., … DiCenso, A. (2010). The primary healthcare nurse practitioner role in Canada. *Canadian Journal of Nursing Leadership, 23*(Special Edition), 88–113.

Donald, F., Martin-Misener, R., Carter, N., Donald, E. E., Kaasalainen, S., Wickson-Griffiths, A., … DiCenso, A. (2013). A systematic review of the effectiveness of advanced practice nurses in long-term care. *Journal of Advanced Nursing, 69*(10), 2148–2161. doi: 10.1111/jan.12140

Doran, D., Sidani, S., Keatings, M., & Doidge, D. (2002). An empirical test of the nursing role effectiveness model. *Journal of Advanced Nursing, 38*(1), 29–39.

El-Masri, M. M., Omar, A., & Groh, E. M. (2015). Evaluating the effectiveness of a nurse practitioner-led outreach program for long-term-care homes. *Canadian Journal of Nursing Research, 47*(3), 39–55.

Fabbruzzo-Cota, C., Frecea, M., Kozell, K., Pere, K., Thompson, T., Tjan, T. J., & Wong, A. (2016). A clinical nurse specialist-led interprofessional quality improvement project to reduce hospital-acquired pressure ulcers. *Clinical Nurse Specialist, 30*(2), 110–116. doi: 10.1097/NUR.0000000000000191

Fletcher, J., Hogg, W., Farrell, B., Woodend, K., Dahrouge, S., Lemelin, J., & Dalziel, W. (2012). Effect of nurse practitioner and pharmacist counseling on inappropriate medication use in family practice. *Canadian Family Physician, 58*(8), 862–868.

Goldie, C. L., Prodan-Bhalla, N., & MacKay, M. (2012). Nurse practitioners in postoperative cardiac surgery: Are they effective? *Canadian Journal of Cardiovascular Nursing, 22*(4), 8–15.

Heale, R., & Pilon, R. (2012). An exploration of patient satisfaction in a nurse practitioner-led clinic. *Nursing Leadership, 25*(3), 43–55.

Hunter, K. F., Murphy, R. S., Babb, M., & Vallee, C. (2016). Benefits and challenges faced by a nurse practitioner working in an interprofessional setting in rural Alberta. *Nursing Leadership, 29*(3), 61–70.

Hurlock-Chorostecki, C., & Acorn, M. (2017). Diffusing innovative roles within Ontario hospitals: Implementing the nurse practitioner as the most responsible provider. *Nursing Leadership, 30*(4), 60–66. doi: 10.12927/cjnl.2017.25448

Institute for Healthcare Improvement (IHI). (2019). *The triple aim.* Ottawa, ON: IHI. Retrieved from http://www.ihi.org

Irvine, D., Sidani, S., & Hall, L. M. (1998). Linking outcomes to nurses' roles in health care. *Nurse Economics, 16*(2), 58–64, 87.

Jackson, K. T., Parkinson, S., Jackson, B., & Mantler, T. (2018). Examining the impact of trauma-informed cognitive behavioral therapy on perinatal mental health outcomes among survivors of intimate partner violence (The PATH study): Protocol for a feasibility study. *Journal of Medical Internet Research (JMIR) Research Protocols, 7*(5), e134. doi: 10.2196/resprot.9820

Kaasalainen, S., Ploeg, J., McAiney, C., Schindel-Martin, L., Donald, L., Martin-Misener, R., … Sangster-Gormley, E. (2013). Role of the nurse practitioner in providing palliative care in long-term care homes. *International Journal of Palliative Nursing, 19*(10), 477–485.

Kaasalainen, S., Wickson-Griffiths, A., Akhtar-Danesh, N., Brazil, K., Donald, F., Martin-Misener, R., … Dolovich, L. (2016). The effectiveness of a nurse practitioner-led pain management team in long-term care: A mixed methods study. *International Journal of Nursing Studies, 62*, 156–167. doi: 10.1016/j.ijnurstu.2016.07.022

Kilpatrick, K., DiCenso, A., Bryant-Lukosius, D., Ritchie, J. A., Martin-Misener, R., & Carter, N. (2013). Practice patterns and perceived impact of clinical nurse specialist roles in Canada: Results of a national survey. *International Journal of Nursing Studies, 50*(11), 1524–1536. doi: 10.1016/j.ijnurstu.2013.03.005

Kilpatrick, K., Kaasalainen, S., Donald, F., Reid, K., Carter, N., Bryant-Lukosius, D., … DiCenso, A. (2014). The effectiveness and cost effectiveness of clinical nurse specialists in outpatient roles: A systematic review. *Journal of Evaluation in Clinical Practice, 20*(6), 1106–1123. doi: 10.1111/jep.12219

Kilpatrick, K., Reid, K., Carter, N., Donald, F., Bryant-Lukosius, D., Martin-Misener, R., … DiCenso, A. (2015). A systematic review of the cost effectiveness of clinical nurse specialists and nurse practitioners in inpatient roles. *Canadian Journal of Nursing Leadership, 28*(3), 56–76.

Kilpatrick, K., Tchouaket, É., Jabbour, M., & Hains, S. (2020). A mixed methods quality improvement study to implement nurse practitioner roles and improve care for residents in long-term care facilities. *BioMed Central (BMC) Nursing, 19*(6). doi: 10.1186/s12912-019-0395-2

Lacny, S., Zarrabi, M., Martin-Misener, R., Donald, F., Sketris, I., Murphy, A., DiCenso, A., & Marshall, D. A. (2016). Cost-effectiveness of a nurse practitioner-family physician model of care in a nursing home. *Journal of Advanced Nursing, 72*(9), 2138–2152.

Lamb, A., Martin-Misener, R., Bryant-Lukosius, D., & Latimer, M. (2018). Describing the leadership capabilities of advanced practice nurses using a qualitative descriptive study. *Nursing Open, 5*(3), 400–413. Retrieved from https://doi.org/10.1002/nop2.150

Li, S., Roschkov, S., Alkhodair, A., O'Neill, B. J., Chik, C. L., Tsuyuki, R. T., & Gyenes, G. T. (2017). The effect of nurse practitioner-led intervention in diabetes care for patients admitted to cardiology services. *Canadian Journal of Diabetes, 41*(1), 10–16. doi: 10.1016/j.jcjd.2016.06.008

Lopatino, E., Donald, F., DiCenso, A., Martin-Misener, R., Kilpatrick, K., Bryant-Lukosius, D., … Marshall, D. A. (2017). Economic evaluation of nurse practitioners and clinical nurse specialists: A methodological review. *Journal of International Studies in Nursing, 72*, 71–82.

Lovo, S., Harrison, L., O'Connell, M. E., Trask, C., & Bath, B. (2019). Experience of patients and practitioners with a team and technology approach to chronic back disorder management. *Journal of
Multidisciplinary Healthcare, 18*(12), 855–869. doi: 10.2147/JMDH.S208888

Marshall, D. A., Donald, F., Lacny, S., Reid, K., Bryant-Lukosius, D., Carter, N., … DiCenso, A. (2015).
Assessing the quality of economic evaluations of clinical nurse specialists and nurse practitioners:
A systematic review of cost-effectiveness. *NursingPlus Open, 1*, 11–17. Retrieved from https://doi.
org/10.1016/j.npls.2015.07.001

Martin-Misener, R., Donald, F., Wickson-Griffiths, A., Akhtar-Danesh, N., Ploeg, J., Brazil, K., …
Taniguchi, A. (2015a). A mixed methods study of the work patterns of full-time nurse practitioners
in Canadian nursing homes. *Journal of Clinical Nursing, 24*, 1327–1337. doi: 10.1111/jocn.12741

Martin-Misener, R., Harbman, P., Donald, F., Reid, K., Kilpatrick, K., Carter, N., … DiCenso, A.
(2015b). Cost-effectiveness of nurse practitioners in ambulatory care: Systematic review. *British
Medical Journal (BMJ) Open, 5*, e007167 doi: 10.1136/bmjopen-2014-007167

Martin-Misener, R., Kilpatrick, K., Donald, F., Bryant-Lukosius, D., Rayner, J., Valaitis, R., … Lamb,
A. (2016). Nurse practitioner caseload in primary health care: Scoping review. *International Journal
of Nursing Studies, 62*, 170–182.

Mitchell-DiCenso, A., Guyatt, G., Marrin, M., Goeree, R., Willan, A., Southwell, D., … Baumann,
A. (1996). A controlled trial of nurse practitioners in neonatal intensive care. *Pediatrics, 98*(6),
1143–1148.

Moore, J., & McQuestion, M. (2012). The clinical nurse specialist in chronic diseases. *Clinical Nurse
Specialist, 26*(3), 149–163. doi: 10.1097/NUR.0b013e3182503fa7

Nixon, S., Bezverbnaya, K., Maganti, M., Gullane, P., Reedijk, M., Kuruvilla, J., Prica, A., … Crump, M.
(2020). Evaluation of lymphadenopathy and suspected lymphoma in a lymphoma rapid diagnosis
clinic. *Journal of Clinical Oncology (JCO) Practice, 16*(1). doi: 10.1200/JOP.19.00202

Oosman, S., Weber, G., Ogunson, M., & Bath, B. (2019). Enhancing access to physical therapy services for people experiencing poverty and homelessness: The lighthouse pilot project. *Physiotherapy
Canada, 71*(2), 176–186. doi: 10.3138/ptc.2017-85.pc

Ploeg, J., Kaasalainen, S., McAiney, C., Martin-Misener, R., Donald, F., Wickson-Griffiths, A., …
Taniguchi, A. (2013). Resident and family perceptions of the nurse practitioner role in long term
care settings: A qualitative descriptive study. *BioMed Central (BMC) Nursing, 12*, 24. doi: 10.1186/1
0.1186/1472-6955-12-24

Porter, M. E. (2010). Value in healthcare. *The New England Journal of Medicine, 363*(27), 2477–2481.

Rietze, L., Heale, R., Hill, L., & Roles, S. (2016). Advance care planning in nurse practitioner practice:
A cross-sectional descriptive study. *Nursing Leadership, 29*(3), 106–119.

Sangster-Gormley, E., Carter, N., Donald, F., Martin-Misener, R., Ploeg, J., Kaasalainen, S., …
Wickson-Griffiths, A. (2013). A value added benefit of nurse practitioners in long-term care settings: Increased nursing staff's ability to care for residents. *Canadian Journal of Nursing Leadership,
26*(3), 24–37.

Sawatzky, J. A., Christie, S., & Singal, R. K. (2013). Exploring outcomes of a nurse practitioner-managed
cardiac surgery follow-up intervention: A randomized trial. *Journal of Advanced Nursing, 69*(9),
2076–2087. doi: 10.1111/jan.12075

Sidani, S., & Irvine, D. (1999). A conceptual framework for evaluating the nurse practitioner role in
acute care settings. *Journal of Advanced Nursing, 30*(1), 58–66.

Singh, S., Whitehurst, D. G., Funnell, L., Scott, V., MacDonald, V., Leung, P. M., … Feldman, F. (2019).
Breaking the cycle of recurrent fracture: Implementing the first fracture liaison service (FLS) in
British Columbia, Canada. *Archives Osteoporosis, 4*(1), 116. doi: 10.1007/s11657-019-0662-6

Smigorowsky, M. J., Norris, C. M., McMurtry, M. S., & Tsuyuki, R. T. (2017). Measuring the effect of nurse practitioner (NP)-led care on health-related quality of life in adult patients with atrial fibrillation: Study protocol for a randomized controlled trial. *Trials, 18*(1), 364. doi: 10.1186/s13063-017-2111-4

Smigorowsky, M. J., Sebastianski, M., & Norris, C. M. (2020). Outcomes of nurse practitioner-led care in patients with cardiovascular disease: A systematic review and meta-analysis. *Journal of Advanced Nursing, 76*(1), 81–95. doi: 10.1111/jan.14229

Spence, B. G., Ricci, J., & McCuaig, F. (2019). Nurse practitioners in orthopaedic surgical settings: A review of the literature. *Orthopedic Nursing, 38*(1), 17–24. doi: 10.1097/NOR.0000000000000514

Spitzer, W. O., Sackett, D. L., Sibley, J. C., Roberts, R. S., Gent, M., Kergin, D. J., ... Olynich, A. (1974). The Burlington randomized trial of the nurse practitioner. *New England Journal of Medicine, 290*(5), 251–256.

Stahlke, S., Rawson, K., & Pituskin, E. (2017). Patient perspectives on nurse practitioner care in oncology in Canada. *Journal of Nursing Scholarship, 49*(5), 487–494.

Stilos, K., & Daines, P. (2013). Exploring the leadership role of the clinical nurse specialist on an inpatient palliative care consulting team. *Nursing Leadership, 26*(1), 70–78.

St-Louis, L., & Brault, D. (2011). A clinical nurse specialist intervention to facilitate safe transfer from ICU. *Clinical Nurse Specialist, 25*(6), 321–326. doi: 10.1097/NUR.0b013e318233eaab

Tung, T. K., Kaufmann, J. A., & Tanner, E. (2012). The effect of nurse practitioner practice in home care on emergency department visits for homebound older adult patients: An exploratory pilot study. *Home Healthcare Nurse, 30*(6), 366–372. doi: 10.1097/NHH.0b013e318246dd53

Chapter 6

Competencies for the Clinical Nurse Specialist and Nurse Practitioner in Canada

Josette Roussel

JOSETTE ROUSSEL is an Executive Advisor at the Canadian Nurses Association, Ottawa, Ontario.

KEY TERMS

advanced practice nurses (APNs)
advanced practice nursing (APN)
APN competencies
clinical nurse specialist (CNS)
core competencies
framework
nurse practitioner (NP)

OBJECTIVES

1. Identify key elements from the literature on competency frameworks and their relation to APN.
2. Describe core competencies for APNs in Canada.
3. Describe the unique competencies for the CNS.
4. Describe the unique competencies for the NP.
5. Discuss overlapping competencies of the CNS and NP roles.

Introduction

This chapter describes the core competencies of all **advanced practice nurses (APNs)** as outlined in *Advanced Practice Nursing: A Pan-Canadian Framework* (Canadian Nurses Association [CNA], 2019) and focuses on the unique competencies of two **advanced practice nursing (APN)** roles in Canada: the **clinical nurse specialist (CNS)** and **nurse practitioner (NP)**. Key definitions of **APN competencies** and related concepts, as well as the overall CNA's APN **framework** of competencies for APNs in Canada, will be highlighted, and a description of the **core competencies** of APN will be provided that will serve as the basis for understanding the practice of CNSs and NPs in Canada.

Background

APN is a broad term referring to an advanced level of nursing practice that maximizes the graduate-level education of registered nurses (RNs) and NPs. All APNs have "in-depth nursing knowledge and expertise in complex decision-making to meet the health needs of individuals, families, groups, communities and populations" (CNA, 2019, p. 13). As such, NPs have graduate or postgraduate education with clinical experience and are able to autonomously diagnose, order, and interpret tests; prescribe medications; and perform specific procedures within their legislated scope of practice (CNA, 2016a). Likewise, CNSs are RNs with a graduate or doctorate degree in nursing, advanced nursing knowledge, and skills in making complex decisions. The CNS is an agent of change and has expertise in a clinical nursing specialty (CNA, 2016b).

The unique competencies for the NP were designed to facilitate the development of a national NP examination. As follow-up to the 2015 review of entry-level competencies for NPs, the Canadian Council for Registered Nurses Regulators (CCRNR) is exploring a new regulatory framework for the NP and is considering a national entry-level examination for all NPs in Canada (Stansfield, 2019). The unique competencies for the CNS were also developed to achieve greater clarity about this role in the Canadian health care landscape and to inform the development of standardized educational programs within Canada. There remains confusion about the differences between the role of the NP and the CNS. The unique competencies of these two APNs will be elaborated upon in order to provide clarity on the skills, knowledge, and judgment of nurses in these roles. As with other health care professional roles, there is an overlap of competencies between them.

Definition of Competencies

Competencies identify the range of functions, skills, knowledge, personal attributes, and behaviours needed to effectively perform a role within an organization (Lucia & Lepsinger, 1999). They are linked to a specific job and the related knowledge, skills, abilities, attitudes, and judgment required in order for a professional to become competent (Raymond, 2001). CNA (2005) defines competencies as the knowledge, skills, and abilities of a nurse to perform a specific action in a given practice situation. The International Council of Nurses (ICN) describes nurses' competence as the "effective application of a combination of knowledge, skill and judgement demonstrated by an individual in daily practice or job performance" (2009, p. 6). Competencies are highly relevant to today's health care context and are key enablers for nursing practice. Competencies are required whenever specific nursing roles are refined (CNA, 2000) in conjunction with the standards of nursing practice that nursing regulatory bodies develop to protect the public.

Competency Development

While the development of competencies is not new in nursing, it has become more relevant in recent years (Windsor, Douglas, & Harvey, 2012). A core competency is often linked to strategic, future-oriented, collective functions at the organizational level and therefore specifies the basic knowledge, attitudes, and skills needed to perform one's role as a health care professional (Moingeon & Edmondson, 1996; Prahalad & Hamel, 1990; Venes, 2013). The developmental process of a competency framework includes identifying a set of *core competencies* required for proficiency in a specific role or job (Chen & Naquin, 2005). Since the number and the level of competencies depend on the complexity of the role, developing competencies can take various forms. Some organizations define competencies in specific ways, such as in performance or behavioural indicators, while others develop competencies in more general terms (Chen & Naquin, 2005).

Defining competencies is important for the conceptualization and development of APN roles, specifically in the use of specialist competencies and nursing knowledge (ICN, 2008b). Doing so helps define and integrate APN roles and improve consensus on standards of care (Martin-Misener & Bryant-Lukosius, 2016).

Advanced Nursing Practice Competency Framework

In 2019, CNA revised and expanded the core competencies for APNs in its publication *Advanced Practice Nursing: A Pan-Canadian Framework*. The competencies in the framework were developed based on "an appropriate depth, breadth and range of nursing knowledge, theory and research, enhanced by clinical experience" (CNA, 2019, p. 29). The framework takes the approach that the blend of nurses' knowledge, skills, judgment, and personal attributes in a variety of environments specifically defines APN.

The core APN competencies in the 2019 framework, which build on competencies that were originally defined in a 2008 edition of the document, reflect APN role progression and new research. In addition to advanced clinical expertise requirements, these progressions include the promotion of leadership competencies and integration of research knowledge and skills; all have increasingly become core elements of APN education and role development (ICN, 2019). The 2019 CNA framework is used to develop educational curricula; outline concepts for research; shape government policy; and interpret APN to employers, the public, other health care workers, and policy-makers.

Core Competencies for Advanced Practice Nurses

An international review on APN frameworks found that competencies in research, leadership, knowledge brokering, and expert clinical judgment are common to many APN roles (Sastre-Fullana et al., 2014). Leadership roles in promoting evidence-based practice among clinical nurses are generally viewed as important.

In the revised 2019 framework, CNA included a new core competency category on education to describe the activities of APNs in this area. There is also expansion of the competencies in health system optimization. These core competencies are relevant to specialty practice and are exhibited by all APNs. The framework lists the competencies in six categories:

1. Direct comprehensive care competencies
2. Health system optimization
3. Education
4. Research
5. Leadership
6. Consultation and collaboration (CNA, 2019)

The framework also includes elements on how the APN role should be enacted. These elements are "effective and simultaneous interaction, blending and execution of knowledge, skills, judgment and personal attributes in a wide variety of practice environments that characterizes APN" (CNA, 2019, p. 29).

Direct Comprehensive Care

The advanced practice nurse provides comprehensive care to individual clients, communities, or populations. This is the cornerstone of APN and these competencies integrate extensive clinical experience with theory, research, and in-depth nursing and related knowledge (CNA, 2019). There remains discussion and debate on the interpretation of the direct comprehensive care competencies when introducing new APN roles. The nature of APN includes a high degree of autonomy in advance assessment, decision making, planning, development, and implementation of programs (Schober, 2017). In Hamric and Tracy (2019), the APN definition builds on and extends the understanding of APN proposed in previous editions. The definition states that clinical practice is a central competency of the APN role and informs other competencies. APN is also limited to roles that focus on clinical practice because nursing is a practice-oriented profession; interactions with clients are necessary to maintain and develop APN expertise.

Focusing on direct comprehensive care when discussing APN is not a value statement. Hamric and Tracy (2019) state that no value difference exists between nurses in non-APN roles and APN roles. Both are equally important to the overall growth and strengthening of nursing. As not all nurses with graduate education are practicing at the same level, the same holds true for all APNs. The key competencies exist to help clarify APN roles.

Health System Optimization

To demonstrate health system optimization, APNs contribute to the effective functioning of health systems through advocacy, the promotion of innovative client care, and the facilitation of equitable, client-centred health care (CNA, 2019). These competencies describe important contributions of APNs as we face challenges meeting complex population health care needs.

Education

The new educational competencies reflect APNs' commitment to professional growth and for upholding health and wellness learning for all other health care providers, students, clients, and families (CNA, 2019).

Research

Under the research competencies, APNs are committed to generating, synthesizing, critiquing, and applying research evidence. This remains an area that needs to be expanded as APNs have an essential research role to meet complex health care needs and create new evidence and practice guidelines (CNA, 2019).

Leadership

The leadership competencies of APNs describe the influence of the role in the organizations and communities they work in. APNs are innovative, improve care, promote the role, and are expected to be leaders (CNA, 2019). In a recent Canadian study, the authors state that it is important to clearly recognize APN leadership because nurses in these roles have an exceptional impact on patient, organization, and system outcomes (Lamb, Martin-Misener, Bryant-Lukosius, & Latimer, 2018).

Consultation and Collaboration

The consultation and collaboration competencies describe how APNs support teams, contribute to multilevel collaboration, and reduce the negative impacts of the determinants of health, which are important aspects of all nursing practice (CNA, 2019).

Nurse Practitioner Competencies

The revised entry-level NP competencies, outlined by CCRNR, are presented in four categories. These revised competencies include new elements such as cultural safety, the impact of power differentials in health service delivery with diverse populations, the increasing prevalence of concerns with mental health and addictions in Canada, and the recommendations of the Truth and Reconciliation Commission of Canada (CCRNR, 2016).

1. Client care
   A. Client relationship building and communication

    B. Assessment

    C. Diagnosis

    D. Management

    E. Collaboration, consultation, and referral

    F. Health promotion

2. Quality improvement and research

3. Leadership

4. Education

    A. Client, community, and health care team

    B. Continuing competence

    C. Professional roles and responsibilities

Within the categories, the descriptions outline the integrated knowledge, skills, judgments, and attributes required of an NP to practice safely and ethically in a designated role and setting, regardless of client populations or practice environments. The unique competencies for NPs are related to their additional "legislative authority, knowledge and skills to autonomously diagnose, order and interpret diagnostic tests, prescribe treatment (including drugs) and perform specific procedures (within their legislated scope of practice)" (CNA, 2019, p. 19). These core competencies were understood as building on those required of an RN. NPs are credentialed and expected to maintain hours of practice to keep their licence. There is more clarity on the role of the NP in health care as they have clear patient populations and provide increased access to care.

As NPs work in teams, it is important to decrease barriers to practice and permit them to work to the full potential of their competencies. As such, NP competencies include interprofessional collaboration, care coordination, coaching, and advanced clinical assessment skills; all are cornerstones of success (Bryant-Lukosius & DiCenso, 2004; Bryant-Lukosius, DiCenso, Browne, & Pinelli, 2004; DiCenso & Bryant-Lukosius, 2010).

Advanced clinical assessment skills are particularly important as they enable NPs to autonomously initiate treatment, identify changes in health status, and perform timely diagnoses to help patients avoid admission to emergency departments (Chavez, Dwyer, & Ramelet, 2017). NPs provide comprehensive care to clients of all ages using principles of health promotion and disease prevention; illness management; and supportive, curative, rehabilitative, and palliative care (CNA, 2016b). The NP's clinical approach is differentiated from that of a medical practitioner as they are grounded in professional nursing practice. The NP provides clinical care that incorporates professional nursing in psychological, social, and cultural factors that influence health and client care. NPs play an important role in improving access to primary care for vulnerable populations (Nelson et al., 2018).

There are many examples of NPs' clinical competencies in practice. For instance, they are particularly skilled at health education, which is a hallmark of nursing care and is the basis for many highly effective nursing interventions that support patient self-management of prevention practices. NPs are also well positioned to integrate mental health care and treatment in primary care (Creamer & Austin, 2017). The holistic approach to care and competencies by NPs addresses complex factors in mental illness. This specialty area is one in which NPs are committed to working with individuals who have a mental illness and who require more educational support to build more role competencies (Creamer & Austin, 2017).

Clinical Nurse Specialist Competencies

The CNS role involves analyzing, synthesizing, and applying nursing knowledge, theory, and research evidence to foster system-wide changes and advance nursing care and the profession as a whole (CNA, 2016b). The CNSs' expertise and competencies enable them to provide consultation on highly complex cases that will influence treatment (CNA, 2019). The unique competencies of the CNS therefore enable timely management and care of complex and vulnerable populations while providing education and support of the team and facilitating innovation in the health care system (Lewandowski & Adamle, 2009). Canadian researchers expressed the need for a pan-Canadian initiative to identify clear competencies for the CNS role (Bryant-Lukosius et al., 2010; Kilpatrick et al., 2011). To meet this need, the CNA Pan-Canadian Core Competencies for the Clinical Nurse Specialist serves as a framework "to reflect the diversity of specialty areas and practice environments in which CNSs work and to support evolution of the CNS role to meet the changing needs of patients and the Canadian health care system" (CNA, 2014, p. 1). The purpose of this CNS framework is to:

1. Promote clarity of the CNS role
2. Facilitate the understanding and highlight the importance of the CNS role for improving health and the delivery of health care services
3. Guide the development of CNS educational curricula and outcomes
4. Support CNSs in advancing their practice
5. Support employers who are implementing CNS roles in their organizations (CNA, 2014, p. 1)

These competencies are reflected in the following categories:

1. Clinical care competencies
2. Systems leadership competencies
3. Advancement of nursing practice competencies
4. Evaluation and research competencies

Adding to the confusion over the CNS role is the fact that they work in many distinct specialties, which can include, among others, pediatrics, oncology, and geriatrics. While all CNSs have a similar primary function to promote continuous improvement of patient outcomes and nursing care, the environments in which they operate vary considerably (CNA, 2016a). Thus, it was necessary for the CNS role competency framework to easily communicate common practice elements while allowing for this variation in practice environments.

In addition to the ability to provide consultation expertise, the CNS's specialty knowledge, skills, and abilities enable them to assist in the performance of specific treatments within their legislated scope of practice (CNA, 2019). The delineation of CNS practice helps to clarify their unique role. With their graduate-level education, CNSs are expert clinicians who provide direct clinical care, including health promotion, harm reduction, and management of disease and illness within a specialty practice. CNSs take a person-centred care approach

TABLE 6.1: Advanced Practice Nursing Core Competencies for the Clinical Nurse Specialist and Nurse Practitioner

Advanced Practice Nursing	
Clinical Nurse Specialist	**Nurse Practitioner**
Clinical Care Competencies: The CNS uses advanced and expert knowledge, skills, and abilities to develop, coordinate, and evaluate a collaborative plan of care for highly complex and unpredictable clinical situations with the focus on optimizing health and quality of life for the client. The CNS provides direct and indirect care based on his or her specialty knowledge, practice context, and specialty area.	Client Care: a. Client relationship building and communication b. Assessment c. Diagnosis d. Management e. Collaboration, consultation, and referral f. Health promotion The NP engages in the diagnostic process and develops differential diagnoses through identification, analysis, and interpretation of findings from a variety of sources.
Systems Leadership Competencies: The CNS leads change and influences clinical practice and political process within and across systems.	Leadership: The NP demonstrates leadership by using the nurse practitioner role to improve client care and facilitate system change.
Advancement of Nursing Practice Competencies: The CNS leads and fosters the development of individual regulated nurses and nursing practice.	Education: a. Client, community, and health care team b. Continuing competence c. Professional roles and responsibilities The NP integrates formal and informal education into practice.
Evaluation and Research Competencies: The CNS is a knowledge translator; searches for, critiques, interprets, synthesizes, uses, and disseminates evidence in clinical practice and for quality improvement and client safety initiatives. The CNS leads the development and evaluation of programs.	Quality Improvement and Research: The NP uses evidence-informed practice, seeks to optimize client care and health service delivery, and participates in research.

Source: Adapted from CNA. (2014). *Pan-Canadian core competencies for the clinical nurse specialist.* Ottawa, ON: CNA; CCRNR. (2016). *Entry-level competencies for nurse practitioners in Canada.* Beaverton, ON: CCRNR.

that emphasizes strengths and wellness over disease or deficit. CNSs influence nursing practice outcomes by leading and supporting nurses to provide scientifically grounded, evidence-based care. CNSs implement improvements in the health care delivery system (indirect care) and translate high-quality research evidence into clinical practice to improve clinical and fiscal outcomes (Fulton & Holly, 2018).

In oncology, for example, the CNS brings unique competencies to meet complex and varied patient needs. With their specialty knowledge of the cancer process and treatment options, the CNS coordinates activities for patients, uses advanced communication skills to support them and their carer(s) psychologically, and educates and promotes a healthy lifestyle to reduce the risk of recurrence. At the system level, the CNS leads the redesign of services to make them responsive to the patient's needs and supports local and national initiatives to promote awareness and prevention (Dempsey, Orr, Lane, & Scott, 2016).

Overlapping Advanced Practice Nursing Competencies

The need for greater role clarity has grown as health care has become more specialized and driven by outcomes. These changes spurred the development of the CNS and NP roles. As this process unfolded, however, some confusion arose about the distinct contribution of each role. This lack of clarity affects CNSs more than NPs. The NP role in primary care has been more prominent over the past decade and the NP title is protected in each province and territory. The lack of title recognition for CNSs, in contrast, has been a key reason for greater confusion about their role, as has a lack of consensus on entry-to-practice requirements (CNA, 2012, 2016a).

Collaboration between the CNS and NP is creating unique opportunities to bring comprehensive care to individuals and populations because their different roles are complementary. These unique competencies come together, for example, when the CNS provides expert nursing care for a population leading to the development of clinical care guidelines that promote the use of evidence, provide nurses with support and consultation, and facilitate system change. The NP's role in this scenario is more closely tied to their authority to write prescriptions, order and interpret tests, and perform procedures for the same population. The roles are shaped by health care needs and patient populations (Mohr & Coke, 2018).

Other overlapping competencies between CNSs and NPs include the fact that they are both autonomous and accountable at an advanced level of nursing practice and provide safe and competent care. They also both apply theories and diagnostic skills, drawing on their experiences in research, education, and leadership. Finally, they are required to maintain their distinct competencies related to clinical expertise through continuing professional development (ICN, 2019).

Conclusion

The pan-Canadian competencies for CNS and NP roles are contributing to role clarity, public awareness, and nurse mobility. The competencies are an important resource for many stakeholder groups such as nurses (RNs, CNSs, NPs), employers, educators, regulators, governments, and policy-makers. Several authors have suggested that nursing competency frameworks serve several diverse purposes (Black et al., 2008; ICN, 2003; Percival, 2004; Sastre-Fullana et al., 2014). As part of a framework for approving or recognizing nursing education programs in Canadian jurisdictions, competencies are used to describe what is expected of an entry-level graduate nurse to provide safe, competent, and ethical nursing care in a variety of practice settings. Competencies may also be used to develop practice standards; increase public and employer awareness of nurses' practice; facilitate the recognition of qualifications and skills required of internationally educated nurses; guide the development of definitions; clarify roles and responsibilities; facilitate the assessment of professional misconduct; and increase collaboration and communication (ICN, 2003; Percival, 2004).

Each set of competencies for nurses describes their unique and distinctive contributions to health care (ICN, 2008a, 2008b). Nursing competencies such as those in APN roles are consistent with the scope of practice and requirements of nursing as defined within the practice environment (ICN, 2008a, 2008b). The competencies for NPs and CNSs are progressive and build upon the competencies of the entry-level graduate nurse. NPs and CNSs have distinct and shared competencies leading to differences and similarities in how the two nursing roles are applied (DiCenso & Bryant-Lukosius, 2010). While the pan-Canadian framework for APNs establishes clarity on the NP and CNS roles, the individual core competencies serve as a foundation for NPs and CNSs, further delineating the differences and clarifying their contributions to the health care system.

In order to support CNSs and NPs in reaching their full potential, it is essential to continue to promote clarity of their practice and to identify how these APN roles contribute to the delivery of health care services. It is equally important to guide the development of educational curricula; support the implementation of advanced practice roles and levels of practice; offer guidance to employers, organizations, and health care systems; and promote appropriate governance in terms of policy, legislation, and credentialing (ICN, 2019). These elements will also ensure high-quality, accessible care to individuals and populations.

Critical Thinking Questions

1. Compare and contrast the CNS and NP roles in Canada.
2. Which competencies are common to the CNS and NP roles?
3. Why is it important to consider competencies when introducing these roles?
4. Where can CNS and NP roles make the most impact?

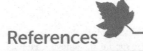

References

Black, J., Allen, D., Redfern, L., Muzio, L., Rushowick, B., Balaski, B., ... Round, B. (2008). Competencies in the context of entry-level registered nurse practice: A collaborative project in Canada. *International Nursing Review, 55*, 171–178.

Bryant-Lukosius, D., Carter, N., Kilpatrick, K., Martin-Misener, R., Donald, F., Kaasalainen, S., & DiCenso, A. (2010). The clinical nurse specialist role in Canada. *Nursing Leadership, 23*(Special Issue), 140–166. doi: 10.12927/cjnl.2010.22273

Bryant-Lukosius, D., & DiCenso, A. (2004). A framework for the introduction and evaluation of advanced practice roles. *Journal of Advanced Nursing, 48*(5), 530–540.

Bryant-Lukosius, D., DiCenso, A., Browne, G., & Pinelli, J. (2004). Advanced practice nursing roles: Development, implementation, and evaluation. *Journal of Advanced Nursing, 48*(5), 519–529.

Canadian Council of Registered Nurse Regulators (CCRNR). (2016). *Entry-level competencies for nurse practitioners in Canada.* Beaverton, ON: CCRNR.

Canadian Nurses Association (CNA). (2000). *A national framework for continuing competence programs for registered nurses.* Ottawa, ON: CNA.

CNA. (2005). *Canadian nurse practitioner core competency framework.* Ottawa, ON: CNA.

CNA. (2012). *Strengthening the role of the clinical nurse specialist in Canada.* Ottawa, ON: CNA.

CNA. (2014). *Pan-Canadian core competencies for the clinical nurse specialist.* Ottawa, ON: CNA.

CNA. (2016a). *Position statement: The clinical nurse specialist.* Ottawa, ON: CNA.

CNA. (2016b). *Position statement: The nurse practitioner.* Ottawa, ON: CNA.

CNA. (2019). *Advanced practice nursing: A pan-Canadian framework.* Ottawa, ON: CNA.

Chavez, K. S., Dwyer, A. A., & Ramelet, A.-S. (2017). International practice settings, interventions and outcomes of nurse practitioners in geriatric care: A scoping review. *International Journal of Nursing Studies, 78*, 61–75.

Chen, H.-C., & Naquin, S. S. (2005). *Development of competency-based assessment centers.* Retrieved from https://files.eric.ed.gov/fulltext/ED492404.pdf

Creamer, A.-M., & Austin, W. (2017). Canadian nurse practitioner core competencies identified: An opportunity to build mental health and illness skills and knowledge. *The Journal for Nurse Practitioners, 13*(5), e231–e236. Retrieved from https://doi.org/10.1016/j.nurpra.2016.12.017

Dempsey, L., Orr, S., Lane, S., & Scott, A. (2016). The clinical nurse specialist's role in head and neck cancer care: United Kingdom national multidisciplinary guidelines. *The Journal of Laryngology and Otology, 130*(S2), S212–S215. Retrieved from https://doi.org/10.1017/S0022215116000657

DiCenso, A., & Bryant-Lukosius, D. (2010). *Clinical nurse specialists and nurse practitioners in Canada: A decision support synthesis.* Ottawa, ON: CHSRF.

Fulton, J., & Holly, V. (2018). Characteristics of the CNS role and practice. Personal communication with Madrean Schober.

Hamric, A. B., & Tracy, M. F. (2019). A definition of advanced practice nursing. In M. F. Tracy & E. T. O'Grady (Eds.), *Advanced practice nursing: An integrative approach* (6th ed., pp. 61–79). St. Louis, MO: Elsevier.

International Council of Nurses (ICN). (2003). *An implementation model for the ICN framework of competencies for the generalist nurse.* Geneva, CH: ICN.

ICN. (2008a). *ICN regulation series: The scope of practice, standards and competencies of the advanced practice nurse.* Geneva, CH: ICN.

ICN. (2008b). *Nursing care continuum: Framework and competencies.* Geneva, CH: ICN.

ICN. (2009). *ICN regulation series: ICN framework of competencies for the nurse specialist.* Geneva, CH: ICN.

ICN. (2019). *Guidelines on advanced practice nursing.* Geneva, CH: ICN.

Kilpatrick, K., DiCenso, A., Bryant-Lukosius, D., Ritchie, J. A., Martin-Misener, R., & Carter, N. (2011). Practice patterns and perceived impact of clinical nurse specialist roles in Canada: Results of a national survey. *International Journal of Nursing Studies, 50*, 1524–1536.

Lamb, A., Martin-Misener, R., Bryant-Lukosius, D., & Latimer, M. (2018). Describing the leadership capabilities of advanced practice nurses using a qualitative descriptive study. *Nursing Open,* December, 400–413.

Lewandowski, W., & Adamle, E. (2009). Substantive areas of clinical nurse specialist practice: A comprehensive review of the literature. *Clinical Nurse Specialist, 23*(2), 73–90.

Lucia, A. D., & Lepsinger, R. (1999). *The art and science of competency models: Pinpointing critical success factors in organizations.* San Francisco, CA: Jossey-Bass/Pfeiffer.

Martin-Misener, R., & Bryant-Lukosius, D. (2016). Guest editors' reflections on progress in the development of advanced practice nursing in Canada. *Nursing Leadership, 29*(3), 6–13.

Mohr, L., & Coke, L. (2018). Distinguishing the clinical nurse specialist from other graduate nursing roles. *Clinical Nurse Specialist, 32*(3), 139–151.

Moingeon, B., & Edmondson, A. (1996). *Organizational learning and competitive advantage.* Thousand Oaks, CA: Sage.

Nelson, L. E., McMahon, J. M., Leblanc, N. M., Braksmajer, A., Crean, H. F., Smith, K., & Yue, Y. (2018). Advancing the case for nurse practitioner-based models to accelerate scale-up of HIV pre-exposure prophylaxis. *Journal of Clinical Nursing, 28,* 351–361.

Percival, E. (2004). *Common competencies for registered nurses in Western Pacific and South East Asian Region (WPSEAR).* Dickson, ACT: ANMAC.

Prahalad, C. K., & Hamel, G. (1990). The core competence of the corporation. *Harvard Business Review, 68*(3), 79–91. Retrieved from http://papers.ssrn.com/sol3/papers.cfm?abstract_id=1505251

Raymond, M. R. (2001). Job analysis and the specification of content for licensure and certification examinations. *Applied Measurement in Education, 14,* 369–415.

Sastre-Fullana, P., De Pedro-Gómez, J., Bennasar-Veny, M., Serrano-Gallardo, P., & Morales-Asencio, J. (2014). APN competency frameworks review. *International Nursing Review, 61,* 534–542.

Schober, M. (2017). *Strategic planning for advanced nursing practice.* New York, NY: Springer. doi: 10.1007/978-3-319-48526-3

Stansfield, K. (2019). *National nurse practitioner regulatory framework panel presentation during the Canadian Association of Schools in Nursing Graduate Studies Forum.* Ottawa, ON: CASN.

Venes, D. (Ed.). (2013). *Taber's cyclopedic medical dictionary* (22nd ed.). Philadelphia, PA: F. A. Davis.

Windsor, C., Douglas, C., & Harvey, T. (2012). Nursing and competencies: A natural fit. The politics of skill/competency formation in nursing. *Nursing Inquiry, 19,* 213–222. doi: 10.1111/j.1440-1800.2011.00549.x

Chapter 7

Understanding Regulatory, Legislative, and Credentialing Requirements in Canada

Lynn Miller

LYNN MILLER is a Strategy Policy Consultant at the Nova Scotia College of Nursing, Bedford, Nova Scotia. She is a nurse practitioner (NP)-Family/All Ages, an NP educator and maintains an NP practice in primary care and telemedicine.

KEY TERMS

competencies
continuing competence
legislation
regulation
self-regulation
standards

OBJECTIVES

1. Explore the evolution of advanced practice nursing (APN) legislation and regulation in Canada.
2. Explore the concepts of regulation and self-regulation in nursing and APN roles.
3. Examine the regulation of clinical nurse specialists and nurse practitioners.
4. Examine continued competence for APNs.
5. Explore the concepts of relational regulation and Right-touch regulation.

Introduction

Advanced practice nurses (APNs), as self-regulated nursing professionals, are subject to the same legislation that applies to all registered nurses (RNs), with additional legislation to define nurse practitioner (NP) scope of practice. Self-regulation is a privilege granted by government through legislation and grounded in the regulatory mandate of public protection. In this chapter, the various layers of professional regulation will be explored beginning with a definition of federal and provincial legislation. Regulation and self-regulation will then be examined as they apply to Canada's two APN roles: clinical nurse specialist (CNS) and nurse practitioner, including regulatory mechanisms such as competencies, scope of practice, standards, and continuing competence requirements. The chapter concludes with a look at Right-touch regulation; an approach that proactively manages risk and harm within the regulator's public protection mandate.

Federal and Provincial Legislation

Federal and provincial legislation form the outermost layer of professional regulation. Legislation, another term for a law or statute, is passed at the federal and provincial/territorial level to define the rights and responsibilities of government and citizens to govern individual and societal conduct, as well as to guide the delivery of services such as health care and justice. While acts are made at the broader federal or provincial government level, the responsibility for creating regulations is delegated to a ministry, department, or agency operating within that level of government (Canadian Nurses Association [CNA], 2019; Government of Canada, 2017). Regulations are used by governments and regulatory bodies to describe how acts are interpreted and operationalized (Balthazard, 2010; Morrison & Benton, 2010; Randall, 2000). Regulation of professions can either fall under a government ministry or department or be designated by legislation to a professional college or association. This is the process that enables self-regulation for the nursing profession.

What Is Self-Regulation?

Public protection is a basic principle of Canadian federal and provincial jurisprudence. For many professions in Canada, public protection is achieved through self-regulation, which is the authority granted to a profession to control processes such as education, admission, and licensure requirements, as well as standards and expectations for practice (Schiller, 2015). Governments grant this privilege based on the assumption that members of a profession have the knowledge and expertise to best make decisions about their practice in the public interest.

The privilege and responsibility of self-regulation are shared by the regulatory body and its registrants or members. Individuals must follow their professional standards and code of ethics, while the regulator is accountable to ensure that registrants/members practice in the public interest (Balthazard, 2010). While accomplished differently across jurisdictions, the primary role of nursing regulatory bodies in self-regulation includes promoting good practice, preventing poor practice, and intervening when practice is unacceptable (Nova Scotia College of Nursing [NSCN], 2019d). To achieve their mandate, regulators establish requirements for initial entry to practice, registration, and licensure; approve education programs based on competencies; develop standards of practice; provide continuing competence resources for their members; and develop professional conduct processes when practice concerns are identified (NSCN, 2019d; Randall, 2000).

Nursing Regulation in Canada: Then and Now

In the late 19th century, nursing was in its infancy as a profession, lacking consistent education requirements and unable to control who could call themselves a nurse. Two groups, the

American Society of Superintendents of Training Schools for Nurses of the United States and Canada formed in 1893 and the Associated Alumnae of the United States and Canada formed in 1896, began developing registration processes and standardizing education to advance the profession and make nursing accountable to the public (McIntyre & McDonald, 2010). The groups eventually separated due to political differences between the two countries, but efforts continued in Canada to produce a national approach to regulation. This marked the beginning of Canadian nursing regulation as provincial/territorial legislation gradually emerged and nursing regulatory bodies were created. Opposition to this movement came from many fronts in the early stages, including physicians and politicians, "who believed that their patients and constituents would be better served by an unregulated nursing marketplace [and] the fuss over legislation [would] put nurses in even greater danger of losing the womanly feelings of 'sympathy' and 'heart' so necessary … to proper nursing service" (K. MacPherson, as cited in Elliott, Rutty, & Villeneuve, 2013, p. 37). Provincial/territorial regulatory bodies and the year they were founded are shown in Figure 7.1. Some regulator names have changed as their governance models evolved or through amalgamation of territorial governments.

FIGURE 7.1: Provincial and Territorial Regulatory Bodies and Year Founded

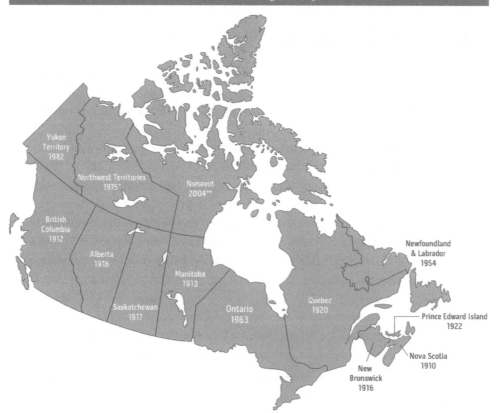

Notes: *Registered Nurses Association of Northwest Territories 1975–2004; **Registered Nurses Association of Northwest Territories and Nunavut after 2004

Source: Adapted from Elliott, J., Rutty, C., & Villeneuve, M. (2013). *Canadian Nurses Association: One hundred years of service.* Ottawa, ON: CNA.

Two Regulatory Models

There are currently two nursing regulatory bodies in place in Canada: the college model and the association model. Under the college model, the regulatory body's only legislated mandate and raison d'être is public protection through regulation of its members (Balthazard, 2018; College of Registered Nurses of Manitoba [CRNM], 2015b; NSCN, 2019b). Association regulators carry the dual role of regulation in the public interest along with a focus on their members through advocacy for the profession and contributing to public policy development (Balthazard, 2018; College and Association of Registered Nurses of Alberta [CARNA], 2015; Nurses Association of New Brunswick [NANB], 2015).

In the early part of the 21st century, some regulators moved away from the association model to adopt the college model, prompted by increased public and governmental scrutiny of existing self-regulation across all professions (Lahey, 2011). Those who support the college model argue that association regulators could find themselves in a conflict of interest if forced to choose between representing the profession and their members or protecting the public. Table 7.1 summarizes the current regulatory model in place in each jurisdiction and the enabling legislation.

TABLE 7.1: Regulators by Province and Enabling Legislation	
College of Registered Nurses of Newfoundland and Labrador (CRNNL)	Registered Nurses Act
College of Registered Nurses of Prince Edward Island (CRNPEI)	Nurses Act
Nova Scotia College of Nursing (NSCN)	Nursing Act
Nurses Association of New Brunswick (NANB)	Nurses Act
L'Ordre des infirmières et infirmiers du Québec (OIIQ)	Nurses Act
College of Nurses of Ontario (CNO)	Regulated Health Professions Act
College of Registered Nurses of Manitoba (CRNM)	Registered Nurses Act
Saskatchewan Association of Registered Nurses (SRNA)	Registered Nurses Act
College and Association of Registered Nurses of Alberta (CARNA)	Public Health Act/Health Professions Act
British Columbia College of Nursing Professionals (BCCNP)	Health Professions Act
Yukon Registered Nurses Association (YRNA)	Registered Nurses Profession Act
*Northwest Territories Registered Nurses Association (NWTRNA)/ **Registered Nurses Association of Northwest Territories and Nunavut (RNANT/NU)	*Nursing Profession Act/ **Nunavut Nursing Profession Act

Source: Adapted from Elliott, J., Rutty, C., & Villeneuve, M. (2013). *Canadian Nurses Association: One hundred years of service.* Ottawa, ON: CNA.

Recognizing the public protection mandate as their priority, Canada's 12 nursing regulators formed the Canadian Council of Registered Nurse Regulators (CCRNR) in 2011 to act as the national voice for nursing regulation in the public interest in Canada. The organization's priorities also assumed activities that were previously facilitated by CNA, including RN and NP licensure examinations and national regulatory frameworks (CCRNR, 2015a).

Understanding APN Regulation in Canada

APNs were not part of the health care landscape until the mid-20th century, although there are historical accounts of APNs working in both Newfoundland and Labrador and the Northwest Territories in the 1890s due to a lack of available physicians (Kaasalainen et al., 2010; see Chapter 1). The regulation of Canada's APN falls within the same legislative frameworks that regulate all nursing practice.

Clinical Nurse Specialists

Clinical nurse specialists are RNs with a graduate degree in nursing and clinical expertise in a specific client population. They use their knowledge, critical thinking, and leadership skills to manage complex client and system needs (McDonald, 2012). The CNS role falls within the legislated scope of RN practice and does not have additional regulation or title protection as is the case for NPs. This lack of title protection has been identified as a barrier to the sustainability of the CNS role (Bryant-Lukosius et al., 2010). To promote the CNS role, CNA developed the *Pan-Canadian Core Competencies for the Clinical Nurse Specialist* (CNA, 2014) to clarify the CNS role for clients, colleagues, employers, and government; however, at the regulatory level, CNSs are subject to the competencies and standards of practice for RNs established by their regulatory body.

Nurse Practitioners

Nurse practitioners are RNs with additional education and a legislated scope of practice that authorizes them to autonomously diagnose, order diagnostic tests, perform procedures, and prescribe pharmaceutical and non-pharmaceutical treatments for their clients. NPs also participate in the APN competencies of leadership, research, education, and program development. There are currently four streams of NP practice recognized across Canada—Family/All Ages or Primary Health Care, Pediatric, Adult, and Neonatal—although all streams are not recognized in every jurisdiction. In addition, while some regulators license NPs by their practice stream or specialty, others register and license NPs under a single category and regulate specialty practice through internal regulatory mechanisms. An important defining element of NP legislation is title protection. Similar to restrictions on use of the title RN, only those who have met the regulatory requirements for NP registration and/or licensure may use the title NP or one of the accepted variants, including RN(EC) in Ontario, RN(NP) in Saskatchewan, or RN(EP) in Manitoba (CNO, 2019; CRNM, 2015a; SRNA, 2017). Table 7.2 summarizes NPs by province and territory, and the year legislation was enacted authorizing NP practice.

TABLE 7.2: Nurse Practitioner Year of Initial Legislation by Province and Territory

British Columbia	2005
Alberta	1996
Saskatchewan	2003
Manitoba	2005
Ontario	1997
Quebec	2003
New Brunswick	2002
Nova Scotia	2002
Prince Edward Island	2006
Newfoundland and Labrador	1997
Northwest Territories, Nunavut	2004
Yukon	2009

Source: Adapted from Canadian Institute for Health Information (CIHI). (2006). *The regulation and supply of nurse practitioners in Canada: 2006 update*. Ottawa, ON: CIHI; Kaasalainen, S., Martin-Misener, R., Kilpatrick, K., Harbman, P., Bryant-Lukosius, D., Donald, F., ... DiCenso, A. (2010). A historical overview of the development of advanced practice nursing roles in Canada. *Nursing Leadership, 23*(Special Issue), 35–60.

The current approach to APN regulation in Canada is not without its challenges. McDonald, Herbert, and Thibeault (2006) blame this on "a patchwork of legislation and regulations governing all types of advanced practice nursing" (p. 176). Studies by Pulcini, Jelic, Gul, and Yuen Loke (2009) and Kleinpell et al. (2014) suggested that the variations in provincial/territorial legislation and regulation contribute to existing barriers to CNS and NP role implementation and scopes of practice. In addition, legislative changes at the federal level, while positive for APN role evolution, are often applied differently by provincial/territorial governments and nursing regulators, thus creating additional inconsistencies (Calnan & Fahey-Walsh, 2005). Recent examples include federal Medical Assistance in Dying (MAiD) and cannabis legislation, which were interpreted and enacted differently for NPs by both provincial/territorial governments and nursing regulators.

Regulatory Concepts

Nursing regulators rely on several key terms to define their structures and processes. While the definition of the terms may differ across jurisdictions, the intent is consistent across Canada, which is a critical requirement for mobility of professionals under the Canadian Free Trade Agreement (Internal Trade Secretariat, 2017).

Registration and Licensure

The term *registration* is used by some jurisdictions to encompass licensure and certification; however, it specifically defines the presence of a nurse's name on the regulatory body's membership list or register. Registration is considered the broadest and potentially weakest form of regulation (Balthazard, 2010; Randall, 2000). Licensure is considered more restrictive and not only defines the requirements for those who wish to practice nursing but also restricts this privilege to those who have an active licence (Balthazard, 2010). Criteria for registration and licensure may include successful completion of an education program approved by the regulator, successful completion of licensure examination(s) and jurisprudence examinations, proof of nursing practice (often measured by minimum number of practice hours), criminal record checks, and completion of continuing competency activities (Balthazard, 2010; CNO, 2018a; NSCN, 2019a).

In some jurisdictions—including Manitoba, New Brunswick, and Prince Edward Island—nurses may practice once their name appears on their regulatory body's register (Government of New Brunswick, 2002; Government of Prince Edward Island, 2019) while in others, registration alone does not grant a member the authority to practice nursing. In Nova Scotia, Saskatchewan, Newfoundland and Labrador, and Yukon, a nurse must be listed on the register in order to be granted a licence to practice (Government of Newfoundland and Labrador, 2013; Government of Nova Scotia, 2019; Government of Saskatchewan, 1988; Yukon Legislative Assembly, 2009). The terms *practice permit* or *certificate of registration* are used elsewhere, including Alberta, Ontario, the Northwest Territories, and Nunavut (Government of Alberta, 2013; Government of the Northwest Territories and Government of Nunavut, 2006; Government of Ontario, 1991), to denote the authority to practice in that province or territory.

Competencies

Competencies are statements describing the knowledge, skills, and judgment expected of a nurse in order to provide competent, safe, and ethical care to clients (Moghabghab, Tong, Hallaran, & Anderson, 2018). Competency statements serve many purposes, including guiding content for education programs and entry-to-practice examinations required for registration/licensure; acting as a framework for competence assessment; supporting self-reflection and direction for continuing competence activities; and informing government, employers, clients, and other stakeholders about the services the nurse is educated and competent to provide (CCRNR, 2015a, 2015b; CNA, 2010; CARNA, 2016; NSCN, 2019a).

In 2010, CNA released the *Canadian Nurse Practitioner Core Competency Framework*, an updated version of the original 2005 document that came from the Canadian Nurse Practitioner Initiative (CNA, 2010). Many regulators adapted or adopted this competency framework to develop and approve NP education programs and guide NP practice in their jurisdictions, with graduate education recognized as the preferred minimum requirement for entry-to-practice (Kaasalainen et al., 2010). In 2016, CCRNR released the report of a practice analysis completed to support the development of a national framework for NP licensure in Canada. One of the project's outputs was entry-level competencies for NPs, which have been adopted by nursing regulators across the country and have replaced the CNA document for regulatory purposes (CCRNR, 2016).

In 2014, CNA published the *Pan-Canadian Core Competencies for the Clinical Nurse Specialist*, which similarly outlines the expectations for CNS services across various practice settings. No matter their role, however, CNSs and NPs are expected to integrate registered nurse competencies with their own in providing client care (Black et al., 2008; NSCN, 2018).

Standards

Standards are authoritative statements that define the expected behaviours and professional and legal accountabilities for individual nursing practice. They guide practice and provide benchmarks for assessing provider performance in their interactions with clients and the public (NSCN, 2018). Once again, there are jurisdictional differences in the application of the term; with the British Columbia College of Nursing Professionals (BCCNP) referring to standards as limits and conditions (BCCNP, 2019b). Currently, CNS practice in Canada is measured against RN standards of practice, while NPs must adhere to these as well as their own standards of practice.

Scope of Practice

Scope of practice is a multi-layered, intricate relationship between the context of practice, nursing competencies, standards, and jurisdictional legislation and regulations. The scope of the profession delineates the outer limits of practice for nurses while remaining flexible so that the profession can evolve. Individual scope of practice is shaped by the needs of the nurse's client population, the practice setting, education, and regulatory and employer policies that permit or limit specific interventions (Schiller, 2015). Employers can further define, and even limit, scope of practice based on decisions about the type of client care services provided and who will provide them.

In addition to regulations and legislation, British Columbia, Alberta, and Ontario further define scope of practice for all nurses using controlled or restricted acts (CNO, 2018a; Schiller, 2015). This model identifies procedures or interventions that are considered high risk and require additional educational preparation before a nurse is authorized to perform them (Schiller, 2015).

Continuing Competence

Continuing competence has been described as a multi-dimensional and collaborative process that evolves over a nurse's career (Alexander, 2014; Brown & Elias, 2016; Takase, 2012). As a regulatory quality assurance mechanism, it is intended to demonstrate that nurses possess and maintain the necessary knowledge, skills, and judgment to provide safe client care (Morrison & Benton, 2010; NSCN, 2019a). Research into the value of continuing competence programs (CCP) is evolving; however, there is little evidence supporting the nature and quantity of CCP activities needed to demonstrate a nurse's competence (Brown & Elias, 2016; Takase, 2012).

Requirements for RNs vary across the country, but most include confirmation of practice hours, self-assessment of practice, identification of learning goals and a plan to achieve them, as well as a process to verify a registrant/member's program completion. Some regulators include activities such as a test on specific regulatory concepts or periodic multi-source feedback (MSF) from peers (Brown & Elias, 2016; CNO, 2018b). In most jurisdictions, CNSs and NPs complete the same CCP requirements as RNs, but in others—at present British Columbia, Ontario, and Nova Scotia—additional periodic activities are mandated, including MSF, clinic site visits, and/or objective structured clinical examinations (BCCNP, 2019a; CNO, 2018c).

Looking to the Future of APN Regulation

Relational Regulation and Right-Touch Regulation

Professional regulators are sometimes perceived negatively for their role in monitoring their members' activities, a perception that may have been reinforced for some RNs with the move by some regulators from an association model to a college model. In addition, regulation has traditionally taken a reactive approach to addressing performance that falls below expectations and standards set by regulatory bodies; however, this trend has come into question as consumers, governments, and other stakeholders are encouraged to question a profession's self-regulatory practices (Casey, 2008; Penney, Bayne, & Johansen, 2014). A new approach to self-regulation—called relational regulation—challenges regulators to find alternative ways to promote safe practice and improve the quality of care delivered other than imposing more stringent rules on health care providers (Cayton & Webb, 2014). By building relationships with their registrants/members and other stakeholders, regulators can still meet their mandate of public protection but also connect with their registrants/members collaboratively to meet the profession's mandate.

The BCCNP led the way in Canada for adoption of relational regulation, with Nova Scotia following shortly thereafter. Both BCCNP (2019c) and NSCN (2019c) share the principles upon which relational regulation is based, including the aforementioned relationship building, simplified communication that looks outward to serve the public rather than inward for the regulator, acceptance of mistakes and an approach to risk reduction that is collaborative and open, adoption of a *Right-touch* approach to regulation, and the use of principles to guide regulatory decisions.

Just culture is an element of the relational regulation philosophy. It acknowledges that errors happen for both human and system reasons, and the best way forward is not to attribute blame but instead look on errors as opportunities to learn and change. Just culture calls for changing priorities from provider-centric adherence to rules to focus more on avoiding harm while providing client care. This proactive rather than reactive approach challenges providers to base decisions on best evidence and collaboration with patients and other health care providers to support safe, quality care (Bayne, 2012).

Right-touch regulation uses evidence-informed strategies to assess risk and target resources more appropriately to manage it (Peterson & Fensling, 2011). The same evidence-informed decision making that CNSs and NPs use to deliver care can be employed by their regulatory bodies to proactively identify potential risks or problems before deciding on a solution (Bayne, 2012), which is the reverse of the current more reactive approach to professional regulation.

Conclusion

Advanced practice nurses have the privilege to self-regulate, but this is accompanied by an obligation to ground practice in legislative and regulatory boundaries. As advanced practice roles continue to evolve and be integrated into Canada's health care system, it is incumbent upon CNSs and NPs to be active participants in the regulatory process in order to fulfill their single and shared accountability for public protection. Groundbreaking approaches to regulation—including just culture, relational regulation, and Right-touch regulation—must be explored as mechanisms to support the evolution of APNs and the nursing profession as a whole.

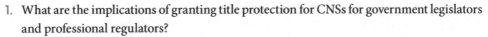

Critical Thinking Questions

1. What are the implications of granting title protection for CNSs for government legislators and professional regulators?
2. How does Right-touch regulation differ from the current model being used by your professional regulatory body? Can it be applied to health care providers who work in interprofessional or collaborative teams?
3. How do the principles of labour mobility outlined in the Canadian Free Trade Agreement impact movement of CNSs and NPs across jurisdictional boundaries?
4. What evidence supports the current continuing competence programs in meeting the regulatory mandate of public protection?

References

Alexander, M. (2014). Meeting the challenge of continued competence. Toronto, ON: HRPA. *Journal of Nursing Regulation, 5*(1), 3.

Balthazard, C. (2010). *What does it mean to be regulated?* Toronto, ON: HRPA. Retrieved from http://www.hrpa.ca/RegulationandHRDesignations/Documents/ProfessionalSelfRegulationandthe HumanResourcesManagementProfessioninOntarioAugust2008.pdf

Balthazard, C. (2018). *The differences between professional regulatory bodies and professional associations revisited.* Toronto, ON: HRPA. Retrieved from https://www.hrpa.ca/Documents/Regulation/ LinkedIn-Articles/75-Differences-between-regulatory-bodies-associations-revisited.pdf

Bayne, L. (2012). *Underlying philosophies and trends affecting professional regulation.* Vancouver, BC: CRNBC. Retrieved from https://www.nsrhpn.ca/wp-content/uploads/2014/08/philosophies-and-trends-affecting-regulation-2012.pdf

Black, J., Allen, D., Redfern, L., Muzio, I., Rushowicks, B., Balaski, B., … Round, B. (2008). Competencies in the context of entry-level registered nurse practice: A collaborative project in Canada. *International Nursing Review, 55*, 171–178.

British Columbia College of Nursing Professionals (BCCNP). (2019a). *Quality assurance and support: Nurse practitioners.* Vancouver, BC: BCCNP. Retrieved from https://www.bccnp.ca/PracticeSupport/RN_NP/QA/NP/Pages/Default.aspx

BCCNP. (2019b). *Scope of practice for nurse practitioners: Standards, limits and conditions.* Vancouver, BC: BCCNP. Retrieved from https://www.bccnp.ca/Standards/RN_NP/StandardResources/NP_ScopeofPractice.pdf

BCCNP. (2019c). *Strategic plan 2020–2023.* Vancouver, BC: BCCNP. Retrieved from https://www.bccnp.ca/bccnp/Documents/Strategic_plans/BCCNP_Strategic_Plan_2020-23.pdf#search=right%20touch%20regulation

Brown, S., & Elias, D. (2016). Creating a comprehensive, robust continuing competence program in Manitoba. *Journal of Nursing Regulation, 7*(2), 43–52.

Bryant-Lukosius, D., Carter, N., Kilpatrick, K., Martin-Misener, R., Donald, F., Kaasalainen, S., … DiCenso, A. (2010). The clinical nurse specialist role in Canada. *Advanced Practice Nursing, 23*(Special Issue December), 140–166.

Calnan, R., & Fahey-Walsh, J. (2005). *Practice consultation initial report.* Ottawa, ON: CNA.

Canadian Council of Registered Nurse Regulators (CCRNR). (2015a). *Competencies in the context of entry-level registered nurse practice.* Beaverton, ON: CCRNR. Retrieved from http://www.ccrnr.ca/entry-to-practice.html

CCRNR. (2015b). *Practice analysis study of nurse practitioners.* Beaverton, ON: CCRNR. Retrieved from http://www.ccrnr.ca/assets/ccrnr-practice-analysis-study-of-nurse-practitioners-report---final.pdf

CCRNR. (2016). *Entry-level competencies for nurse practitioners in Canada.* Beaverton, ON: CCRNR. Retrieved from https://cdn1.nscn.ca/sites/default/files/documents/resources/EntryLevelCompetenciesNP.pdf

Canadian Institute for Health Information (CIHI). (2006). *The regulation and supply of nurse practitioners in Canada: 2006 update.* Ottawa, ON: CIHI.

Canadian Nurses Association (CNA). (2010). *Canadian nurse practitioner core competency framework.* Ottawa, ON: CNA. Retrieved from http://www.cno.org/globalassets/for/rnec/pdf/competencyframework_en.pdf

CNA. (2014). *Pan-Canadian core competencies for the clinical nurse specialist.* Ottawa, ON: CNA.

CNA. (2019). *Regulation of RNs.* Ottawa, ON: CNA. Retrieved from https://www.cna-aiic.ca/en/nursing-practice/the-practice-of-nursing/regulation-of-rns

Casey, J. (2008). Key trends in professional regulation. *Fieldlaw, 5*, 1–3.

Cayton, H., & Webb, K. (2014). The benefits of a "right-touch" approach to health care regulation. *Journal of Health Services Research & Policy, 19*(4), 198–199. doi: 10.1177/1355819614546031

College and Association of Registered Nurses of Alberta (CARNA). (2015). *Together with RNs we protect the public.* Edmonton, AB: CARNA. Retrieved from http://www.nurses.ab.ca/content/carna/home/learn-about-carna.html

CARNA. (2016). *Entry-level competencies for nurse practitioners in Canada.* Edmonton, AB: CARNA. Retrieved from https://www.nurses.ab.ca/docs/default-source/document-library/standards/entry-level-competencies-for-nurse-practitioners-in-canada.pdf?sfvrsn=4fe67f33_12

College of Nurses of Ontario (CNO). (2018a). *Legislation and regulation RHPA: Scope of practice, controlled acts model.* Toronto, ON: CNO. Retrieved from http://www.cno.org/globalassets/docs/policy/41052_rhpascope.pdf

CNO. (2018b). *QA program.* Toronto, ON: CNO. Retrieved from https://www.cno.org/en/myqa/quality-assurance-page-2/

CNO. (2018c). *Registration requirements.* Toronto, ON: CNO. Retrieved from http://www.cno.org/en/become-a-nurse/new-applicants1/nurse-practitioner/registration-requirements-for-nps/

CNO. (2019). *Practice standard: Nurse practitioner.* Toronto, ON: CNO. Retrieved from http://www.cno.org/globalassets/docs/prac/41038_strdrnec.pdf

College of Registered Nurses of Manitoba (CRNM). (2015a). *What is an NP?* Winnipeg, MB: CRNM. Retrieved from http://www.crnm.mb.ca/aboutus-whatsanrnnp.php

CRNM. (2015b). *What we do.* Winnipeg, MB: CRNM. Retrieved from http://www.crnm.mb.ca/aboutus-whatwedo.php

Elliott, J., Rutty, C., & Villeneuve, M. (2013). *Canadian Nurses Association: One hundred years of service.* Ottawa, ON: CNA.

Government of Alberta. (2013). *Health Professions Act.* Edmonton, AB: Government of Alberta. Retrieved from http://www.qp.alberta.ca/1266.cfm?page=h07.cfm&leg_type=Acts&isbncln=9780779748136

Government of Canada. (2017). *Guide to making federal acts and regulations* (2nd ed.). Ottawa, ON: Government of Canada. Retrieved from https://www.canada.ca/en/privy-council/services/publications/guide-making-federal-acts-regulations.html

Government of New Brunswick. (2002). *An act respecting nurses and nurse practitioners.* Fredericton, NB: Government of New Brunswick. Retrieved from https://www.gnb.ca/legis/bill/editform-e.asp?ID=113&legi=54&num=4

Government of Newfoundland and Labrador. (2013). *Registered nurse regulations under the Registered Nurses Act.* St. John's, NL: Government of Newfoundland and Labrador. Retrieved from http://assembly.nl.ca/Legislation/sr/regulations/rc130066.htm

Government of the Northwest Territories and Government of Nunavut. (2006). *Nursing Profession Act.* Iqaluit, NU: Government of the Northwest Territories and Government of Nunavut. Retrieved from https://www.rnantnu.ca/documents/acts-legislation

Government of Nova Scotia. (2019). *Nursing Act.* Halifax, NS: Government of Nova Scotia.

Government of Ontario. (1991). *Nursing Act.* Toronto, ON: Government of Ontario. Retrieved from http://www.e-laws.gov.on.ca/html/statutes/english/elaws_statutes_91n32_e.htm

Government of Prince Edward Island. (2019). *Regulated Health Professions Act: Registered nurse regulations.* Charlottetown, PE: Government of Prince Edward Island. Retrieved from https://www.princeedwardisland.ca/sites/default/files/legislation/r10-1-9-regulated_health_professions_act_registered_nurses_regulations.pdf

Government of Saskatchewan. (1988). *The Registered Nurses Act.* Regina, SK: Government of Saskatchewan. Retrieved from http://www.qp.gov.sk.ca/documents/English/Statutes/Statutes/R12-2.pdf

Internal Trade Secretariat. (2017). *Canadian Free Trade Agreement.* Ottawa, ON: Government of Canada. Retrieved from https://www.cfta-alec.ca/wp-content/uploads/2017/06/CFTA-Consolidated-Text-Final-Print-Text-English.pdf

Kaasalainen, S., Martin-Misener, R., Kilpatrick, K., Harbman, P., Bryant-Lukosius, D., Donald, F., … DiCenso, A. (2010). A historical overview of the development of advanced practice nursing roles in Canada. *Nursing Leadership, 23*(Special Issue), 35–60.

Kleinpell, R., Scanlon, A., Hibbert, D., DeKeyser, F., East, L., Fraser, D., … Beauchesne, M. (2014). Addressing issues impacting advanced practice nursing worldwide. *The Online Journal of Nursing Issues, 19*(2). doi: 10.3912/OJIN.Vol19No02Man05

Lahey, W. (2011). Is self-regulation under threat? *Canadian Nurse, 107*(5), 7–8.

McDonald, D. (2012). *Who is the clinical nurse specialist?* Toronto, ON: CNO. Retrieved from https://www.canadian-nurse.com/en/articles/issues/2012/june-2012/who-is-the-clinical-nurse-specialist

McDonald, J. A., Herbert, R., & Thibeault, C. (2006). Advanced practice nursing: Unification through a common identity. *Journal of Professional Nursing, 23*(3), 172–179.

McIntyre, M., & McDonald, C. (2010). *Realities of Canadian nursing, professional, practice and power issues* (4th ed.). Philadelphia, PA: Wolters Kluwer.

Moghabghab, R., Tong, A., Hallaran, A., & Anderson, J. (2018). The difference between competency and competence: A regulatory perspective. *Journal of Nursing Regulation, 9*(2), 54–59.

Morrison, A., & Benton, D. C. (2010). Analyzing nursing regulation worldwide. *Journal of Nursing Regulation, 1*(1), 44–47.

Nova Scotia College of Nursing (NSCN). (2018). *Nurse practitioner standards of practice 2018.* Bedford, NS: NSCN. Retrieved from https://cdn1.nscn.ca/sites/default/files/documents/resources/NP-Standards-of-Practice.pdf

NSCN. (2019a). *Continuing competence program.* Bedford, NS: NSCN. Retrieved from https://www.nscn.ca/professional-practice/continuing-competence/continuing-competence-program

NSCN. (2019b). *Purpose, mission, vision and values.* Bedford, NS: NSCN. Retrieved from https://www.nscn.ca/explore-nscn/who-we-are/purpose-mission-vision-values

NSCN. (2019c). *Regulatory philosophies.* Bedford, NS: NSCN. Retrieved from https://www.nscn.ca/explore-nscn/who-we-are/regulatory-philosophies

NSCN. (2019d). *Self-regulation.* Bedford, NS: NSCN. Retrieved from https://www.nscn.ca/professional-practice/practice-support/practice-support-tools/self-regulation

Nurses Association of New Brunswick (NANB). (2015). *Mission, vision and public protection.* Fredericton, NB: NANB. Retrieved from http://www.nanb.nb.ca/index.php/about

Penney, C., Bayne, L., & Johansen, C. (2014). Developing a relational regulatory philosophy on a public protection mandate. *Journal of Nursing Regulation, 5*(3), 44–47.

Peterson, D., & Fensling, S. (2011). *Risk-based regulation: Good practice and lessons for the Victorian context.* Melbourne, AU: State Government of Victoria. Retrieved from http://www.energyandresources.vic.gov.au/about-us/publications/economics-and-policy-research/2011-publications/risk-based-regulation-good-practice-and-lessons-for-the-victorian-context

Pulcini, J., Jelic, M., Gul, R., & Yuen Loke, A. (2009). An international survey on advanced practice nursing education, practice and regulation. *Journal of Nursing Scholarship, 42*(1), 31–39.

Randall, G. E. (2000). *Understanding professional self-regulation.* Regina, SK: College of Paramedics of Saskatchewan. Retrieved from http://www.oavt.org/self_regulation/docs/about_selfreg_randall.pdf

Saskatchewan Registered Nurses Association (SRNA). (2017). *Registered nurse (nurse practitioner) practice standards.* Regina, SK: SRNA. Retrieved from https://www.srna.org/wp-content/uploads/2019/05/RNNPPracticeStandards2017.pdf

Schiller, C. J. (2015). Self-regulation of the nursing profession: Focus on four Canadian provinces. *Journal of Nursing Education and Practice, 5*(1), 95–106.

Takase, M. (2012). The relationship between the levels of nurses' competence and the length of their clinical experience: A tentative model for nursing competence development. *Journal of Clinical Nursing, 22*(9–10), 1400–1410.

Yukon Legislative Assembly. (2009). *Registered Nurses Profession Act.* Whitehorse, YT: Government of Yukon. Retrieved from http://www.gov.yk.ca/legislation/acts/renupr_c.pdf

Chapter 8

Advanced Practice Nursing Frameworks Utilized or Developed in Canada

Rosemary Wilson

ROSEMARY WILSON is Associate Professor at Queen's University, School of Nursing, Kingston, Ontario. She is also a nurse practitioner (NP)-Adult in chronic pain management at Kingston Health Sciences Centre, Kingston, Ontario.

KEY TERMS

advanced practice nursing
  (APN)
nursing frameworks

OBJECTIVES

1. Examine the development of advanced practice nursing (APN) frameworks in Canada.
2. Identify the APN frameworks most utilized in Canada.
3. Explore current trends and future development of APN frameworks.

Introduction

Nursing frameworks or models provide structure and guidance to clinical practice and are used by nursing educators to formulate curricula. This chapter will provide an overview of the development of **advanced practice nursing (APN)** frameworks and their use within Canada. Frameworks developed and advanced by Canadian researchers, professional bodies, and educators are highlighted chronologically, with earlier frameworks and models discussed first, followed by more recently developed conceptualizations.

The current definition of *advanced practice nursing* in Canada (Canadian Nurses Association [CNA], 2019) has emerged over time as APN roles have evolved, beginning with the national consensus work of the Canadian Nurse Practitioner Initiative (CNPI), which began in 2004. Embedded in the definition is the ability to use evidence and research to guide practice and influence policy.

Significance of Nursing Frameworks in Practice

Individual theoretical perspectives and world views of nurses continue to influence how nursing practice is conceived, implemented, and practiced (Jansen, 2010). Understanding the collective view of APN is important to the discipline of nursing. Not only must we be able to articulate what advanced practice is to those within the profession, it is also incumbent upon nursing to describe the nature of advanced practice to others. Conceptual frameworks and models assist in "conveying the reality of ANP through symbolic representation that often takes the form of words, pictures, or diagrams" (Chinn & Kramer, 2015, p. 159).

Advanced Practice Nursing Frameworks Utilized in Canada

Canadian nursing initially drew upon literature and research from other jurisdictions, most notably the United States (US), to shape APN curricula and roles in advanced practice. Four models are central to the development of APN in Canada: the Shuler Nurse Practitioner Practice Model, the National Organization of Nurse Practitioner Faculties (NONPF) domains of practice, Hamric's Model of Advanced Practice Nursing, and the Strong Model of Advanced Practice Nursing. Each is briefly discussed, with a synopsis of current use, including Canadian models of APN (see Table 8.1).

The Shuler Nurse Practitioner Practice Model

Salient nursing components of nurse practitioner (NP) practice are explicated in the model developed by Shuler and Davis (1993a). The authors intended to articulate a model that could be used by clinicians, as well as educators and researchers, to demonstrate how nursing and medicine are blended in practice. The nursing paradigm of person, health, nursing, and environment, as well as the nursing process, are clearly evident in the model. Preventive measures and health promotion activities also form key components of the model. Although Shuler 's model is lengthy and extensive, the authors provided an expanded explanation of its clinical application in an accompanying article shortly after the publication of the original article (Shuler & Davis, 1993b).

Despite its complexity, the practice model gained wide appeal and use in Canadian PHCNP programs since the 1990s and is the only APN framework to incorporate the competency of diagnosing, which makes it very specific to NP practice. While other models for the most part have replaced the Shuler model, references to the model are found in the current advanced health assessment curriculum in the Ontario Primary Health Care Nurse Practitioner (PHCNP) Program (2015).

Hamric's Model of Advanced Nursing Practice

In the first edition of *Advanced Nursing Practice: An Integrative Approach* edited by Hamric, Spross, and Hanson, published in 1996, the nature of APN is described using concentric circles to represent the characteristics of the model (Hamric, 1996). The model initially arose from Hamric's work with CNSs but evolved over time to be inclusive of all APN roles (Spross, 2014).

In the current model, primary criteria (i.e., graduate education, certification, and practice focused on patient/family) comprise the centre of the circle. The central competency of direct clinical practice encircles the primary criteria and surrounds the core competencies of leadership, collaboration, ethical decision making, guidance and coaching, consultation, and evidence-based practice (Spross, 2014). Graduate nursing education in Canada has utilized the work of Hamric extensively in classroom discourse on the nature of APN.

Strong Model of Advanced Practice Nursing

In the early 1990s at the Strong Memorial Hospital in Rochester, New York, APNs developed an organizational model to depict the five domains that characterized their advanced practice: direct comprehensive care, support of systems, education, research, and publication and scholarship (Ackerman, Norsen, Martin, Wiedrich, & Kiztman, 1996). The model is in a pentagonal shape with the patient at the centre, and the five domains each occupy a "slice" of the pentagon. Scholarship, collaboration, and empowerment are necessary threads that cross through the domains. Embedded in the model is the concept of the APN transitioning from novice to expert, depicted by shading of the pentagon (see Figure 8.1).

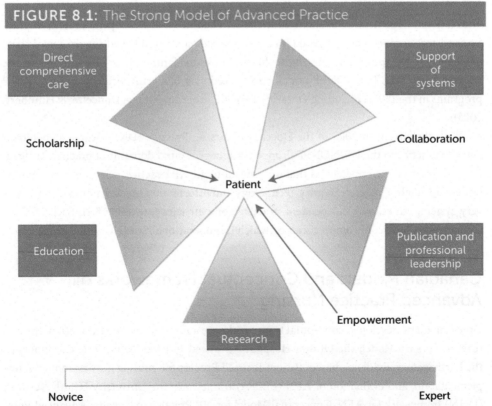

FIGURE 8.1: The Strong Model of Advanced Practice

Direct comprehensive care

Support of systems

Scholarship

Collaboration

Patient

Education

Publication and professional leadership

Empowerment

Research

Novice

Expert

Source: Adapted from Ackerman, M. H., Norsen, L., Martin, B., Wiedrich, J., & Kitzman, H. J. (1996). Development of a model of advanced practice. *American Journal of Critical Care,* 5(1), 68–73. Reprinted with permission.

In a pilot study (n = 18) that aimed to differentiate the roles of acute care nurse practitioners (ACNPs) from those of clinical nurse specialists (CNSs), Mick and Ackerman (2000) asked participants to self-rank individual expertise and relative importance of tasks with the five domains of the Strong Model. While the sample was small, clear differences in mean ranking scores were found between ACNP *and* CNS respondents, with CNSs self-ranking their expertise higher in all domains compared to ACNPs. Certain task aspects of direct clinical care were ranked higher among ACNPs than CNSs (i.e., history taking, initiating diagnostic tests, performing specialized procedures). The authors concluded from their pilot work that the Strong Model better described CNS practice than ACNP. It is critical to note, however, that not all the 12 participating ACNPs had formal NP education or had taken the ACNP certification examination when the survey was conducted.

Several tertiary hospitals in Canada adopted the Strong Model to guide APN in their institutions, including the Winnipeg Health Region and the Hospital for Sick Children (SickKids) in Toronto (LeGrow, Hubley, & McAllister, 2010). While the original Strong Model continues to guide practice in Winnipeg, modifications occurred in several Ontario institutions, and are discussed later in the chapter.

National Organization of Nurse Practitioner Faculties' Domains of Practice

The National Organization of Nurse Practitioner Faculties first developed domains of practice and core competencies in 1990 (2002a) and subsequently published supplemental competencies for NP specialties (2002b), including those for family nurse practitioners in the US (see Table 8.1). The NONPF documents served as a blueprint for developing PHCNP programs in the 1990s, including Ontario's PHCNP program (Cragg, Doucette, & Humbert, 2003).

With the advent in 2008 of the Doctor of Nursing Practice (DNP) degree as potential entry to practice in the US, NONPF dropped language around domains of practice. Instead, they outlined nine competencies that are central to all NP practice: scientific foundations, leadership, quality, practice inquiry, technology and information literacy, policy, health delivery system, ethics, and independent practice competencies (see Table 8.1). Each of these competencies have core competencies by which it is operationalized (NONPF, 2020).

Canadian Models and Conceptual Frameworks of Advanced Practice Nursing

Nine Canadian-developed conceptual frameworks are addressed in the next section: the Nature of Nursing Model; the Ottawa Hospital Advanced Practice Nurse Role Components; the Participatory, Evidence-based, Patient-focused Process for guiding the development, implementation, and evaluation of APN (PEPPA) framework; the University Health Network (UHN) framework for APN; Conceptual Model for NP Practice in Canada; Advanced Practice Nursing (APN) at SickKids; the Acute Care Nurse Practitioner Conceptual (ACNP) framework; the Saskatchewan Nursing Advanced Practice (SNAP) conceptual framework;

TABLE 8.1: Overview of APN Models Utilized or Developed in Canada

Model Name	Year	Country	Classification of Model	Key Elements
Shuler Nurse Practitioner Practice Model	1993	United States	Clinical practice model	• Person • Health • Nursing • NP role • Environment
Hamric's Model of Advanced Practice Nursing	1996	United States	Nature of advanced practice nursing	Primary criteria: • Central competency–practice • Core competencies • Critical environmental elements
The Strong Memorial Hospital Model of APN	1996	United States	Administrative or organizational	Five domains: 1. Direct comprehensive care 2. Support of systems 3. Education 4. Research 5. Publication and leadership
National Organization of Nurse Practitioner Faculties (NONPF): Family Nurse Practitioner (FNP) Competencies	2020	United States	Regulatory	NP competencies: • Scientific foundations • Leadership • Quality • Practice inquiry • Technology and information literacy • Policy • Health delivery system • Ethics • Independent practice

(Continued)

TABLE 8.1: Continued

Model Name	Year	Country	Classification of Model	Key Elements
The Nature of Nursing Model	2001	Canada	Differentiation between basic and advanced practice	• Theory • Pattern recognition • Practical knowledge • Practical wisdom • General to the particular
The Ottawa Hospital Advanced Practice Nurse Role Components	2001	Canada	Administrative or organizational	• Clinical practice • Consultation • Research • Education • Leadership/administration
Participatory, Evidence-based, Patient-focused Process for guiding the development, implementation, and evaluation of APN (PEPPA) Framework	2004	Canada	Role implementation and evaluation	Nine steps: 1. Define patient population and model of care 2. Identify stakeholders 3. Determine need for new model of care 4. Identify priority problems and goals to improve care 5. Define new model of care and APN role 6. Plan implementation 7. Initiate role implementation 8. Evaluate APN role and model of care 9. Determine future needs
University Health Network (UHN) Framework for APN	2004	Canada	Administrative or organizational	Core competencies: • Clinical practice • Leadership • Research • Change agent • Collaboration

Conceptual Model for NP Practice in Canada (CNPI)	2005	Canada	Nature of advanced practice nursing	• Vision of health • Client • Discipline • Context • Nurse practitioner • Inquiry/Evidence-based practice • Health care system • Greater society
Advanced Nursing Practice: A Pan-Canadian Framework	2019	Canada	Regulatory	• Definition and characteristics • Education • Roles • Regulation • Title protection • Scope of practice Competencies: • Direct comprehensive care • Optimizing health system • Educational • Research • Leadership • Consultation and collaboration Unique to CNS and NP: • Continuing competence • Professional liability protection • Strategies for successful implementation, integration, and sustainability • Evaluation

(Continued)

TABLE 8.1: Continued

Model Name	Year	Country	Classification of Model	Key Elements
APN Practice at SickKids	2010	Canada	Administrative or organizational	Five Domains: 1. Pediatric clinical practice 2. Research and scholarly activities 3. Interprofessional collaboration 4. Education and mentorship 5. Organizational and systems management
The Acute Care Nurse Practitioner Conceptual Framework	2012	Canada	Nature of advanced practice nursing	Process: • Boundary work • ACNP role enactment • Perceptions of team effectiveness Structure: • Patient level • ACNP level • Team level • Organization level • Health care system level Outcomes: • Quality • Safety • Cost • Team
The SNAP Conceptual Framework	2013	Canada	Administrative or organizational	Five domains: • Direct comprehensive care • Support of systems • Educative practice • Evidence-informed practice • Professional leadership

Source: Adapted from Spross, J. (2014). Conceptualizations of advanced practice nursing. In A. B. Hamric, C. M. Hanson, M. F. Tracy, & E. T. O'Grady (Eds.), *Advanced practice nursing: An integrative approach* (5th ed., p. 28). St. Louis, MO: Elsevier.

and the pan-Canadian APN framework (CNA, 2019). These Canadian practice frameworks and models have evolved from education, practice, and professional bodies, most notably, CNA.

The Nature of Nursing Model

In 2001, two nurse educators from Alberta, Kathleen Oberle and Marian Allen, explored the theoretical and philosophical literature in nursing to untangle confusion surrounding expert versus advanced practice, and to clarify the linkages between existing conceptual models and advanced practice. Their conceptualization of advanced practice articulates that an APN is first an expert practitioner, who has well-developed pattern recognition skills and practical knowledge (Oberle & Allen, 2001). What separates the APN from the expert practitioner, according to the authors, is the theoretical knowledge base of the APN gained from graduate education. The educational process, along with reflection, leads to transformation of practice. At the time of the Oberle and Allen (2001) publication, not all advanced practice educational programs in Canada were at the graduate level; their work propelled the debate and provided a theoretical basis for all APN preparation to be delivered through graduate educational programs.

The Ottawa Hospital Advanced Practice Nurse Role Components

A merger of three tertiary hospitals in 1998 was the impetus for clarification of APN in the new amalgamated entity, The Ottawa Hospital (TOH). Nursing leadership established a task force, and over a six-month period, a literature review was completed, focus groups were held, and input was sought from nurses, physicians, administration, and nursing faculty members from the University of Ottawa (De Grasse & Nicklin, 2001). The output was an ANP job description, an ANP framework, as well as assessment, implementation, and evaluation recommendations. Graduate education was considered to be "imperative" (De Grasse & Nicklin, 2001, p. 9). The role components within the framework include clinical practice, consultation, research, education, and leadership/administration. The model remains in use at The Ottawa Hospital with 10 APNs currently profiled on the hospital website (TOH, 2019).

PEPPA Framework

Classified as a role implementation and evaluation model, the PEPPA framework was developed by a CNS and APN researcher at McMaster University School of Nursing, Hamilton, Ontario (Bryant-Lukosius & DiCenso, 2004). The nine steps in the framework provide a logical template for engaging stakeholders in the process of designing, implementing, and evaluating an APN role within an agency or institution (see Figure 8.2).

Uptake of the PEPPA framework has been extensive; it is recognized as best practice for health care redesign, has been implemented in 16 countries, and has wide applicability across health systems (Bryant-Lukosius & Martin-Misener, 2015). The PEPPA framework has guided research investigations studying role implementation and evaluation in Canada (see Box 8.1).

FIGURE 8.2: The PEPPA Framework

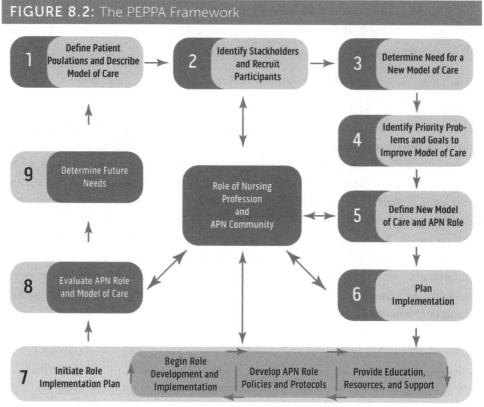

Source: Bryant-Lukosius, D., & DiCenso, A. (2004). A framework for the introduction and evaluation of advanced practice nursing roles. *Journal of Advanced Nursing, 48*(5), 530–540. Reprinted with permission.

BOX 8.1

Use of the PEPPA Framework in Studying Rural Nurse Practitioners

The PEPPA framework formed the conceptual framework for a 2004 study to define the role of rural nurse practitioners (NPs) in Nova Scotia. A mixed methods research design was employed using interviews and mailed questionnaires. Stakeholders were identified as per steps outlined in the PEPPA framework. Nine rural health board chairpersons were interviewed by telephone. The questionnaire was distributed to NPs, public health nurses, family practice nurses, and family physicians (n = 51). Findings demonstrated congruence between the health board chairpersons and the health care providers on the health care needs of rural Nova Scotians, the holistic nature of NP practice, and gaps in the current service model for primary health care. Further, the study identified a vision for NPs in rural communities, as well as the steps that required attention to optimize successful employment and integration of the NP role.

Source: Martin-Misener, R., Reilly, S. M., & Vollman, A. R. (2010). Defining the role of primary health care nurse practitioners in rural Nova Scotia. *Canadian Journal of Nursing Research, 42*(2), 30–47.

University Health Network Framework for Advanced Nursing Practice

Role ambiguity at the UHN sites in Toronto prompted a subcommittee of NPs to undertake a critical review of existing literature and to consult within the network in the early 2000s; the aim was to develop a comprehensive conceptual framework to promote role clarity (Miceviski et al., 2004). After reviewing four conceptual models for APN, including the Strong Model (Ackerman et al., 1996), the group decided to construct their own framework, the UHN Framework for Advanced Nursing Practice using components from several models (Miceviski et al., 2004).

Upon first glance, the UHN framework has visual features similar to the Strong Model. However, there are important distinctions. First, the model reads from left to right, starting with inputs into the central circle with five spokes, and ending with an arrow with outcomes, depicting the structure, process, and outcome elements of the framework. The inputs represent individual, organizational, professional, and societal variables that can affect APN practice; these could include such variables as patient acuity, educational preparation of the APN, entry to practice regulations, and societal values.

Advanced practice is conceptualized as having five core antecedents necessary for APN practice: advanced knowledge, scholarship, experience, communication, and compassion for others. The five antecedents make up the spokes or pillars of the central circle. Five APN competencies are identified as wedges between the five spokes and include clinical practice, leadership, research, change agent, and collaboration (Miceviski et al., 2004). These vary from the Strong Model domains in that education and support of systems are missing. Collaboration, which is a thread in the Strong Model, forms a competency in the UHN framework. The model also incorporates a systems approach, as the larger environment, with an interface of the following optimal characteristics, encompasses the inner circle: empowerment, autonomy, respect, inquiry, and advocacy. The output categories mirror those of the input: individual, organizational, professional, and societal. The authors infer that the model positions APNs at the point of care to engage in and contribute to clinical scholarship.

Conceptual Model for Nurse Practitioner Practice in Canada

In 2004, CNA launched the CNPI to develop a sustainable and integrated national framework to incorporate NPs into Canadian health care systems (CNPI, 2006). Health Canada provided funding for the project as part of a larger initiative of primary health care renewal in the country. One of the outputs of the two-year project was the development of a conceptual model for NP practice within the Canadian context (CNPI, 2006; see Figure 8.3).

The vision of health forms the inner circle of the model, surrounded by five "commonplaces," defined as the ordinary, everyday components that assist in conceptually organizing topics (Robinson Vollman & Martin-Misener, 2005). The commonplaces identified as central to nurse practitioner practice are client, from individual to communities; discipline, from narrow to broad; context, from micro- to multi-system; and nurse practitioner, from novice to expert, which signifies the fifth commonplace, time. These commonplace

FIGURE 8.3: Conceptual Model for Nurse Practitioner Practice in Canada

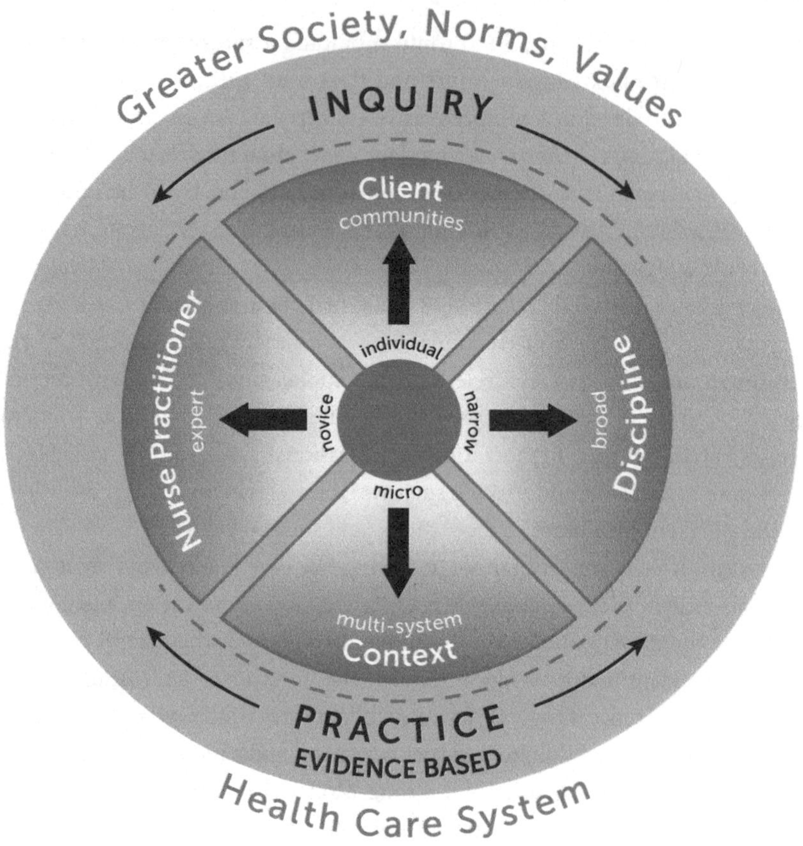

Source: Robinson Vollman, A., & Martin-Misener, R. (2005). A conceptual model for nurse practitioner practice. In Canadian Nurse Practitioner Initiative (2006), *Practice framework for nurse practitioners in Canada* (Appendix A) (pp. 1–13). Ottawa, ON: CNA. Reprinted with permission.

elements are encircled by evidence-based practice and inquiry, which make up the final ring around the model circle. Finally, the model is situated in the broader contexts of the health care system and the greater society, norms, and values. Despite the national exposure of the model in 2006, it is not widely represented in current literature or in NP educational program curricula.

Advanced Practice Nursing at SickKids

The tertiary children's hospital in Toronto, SickKids, has utilized the CNS role at their institution since the late 1960s (LeGrow et al., 2010). When the Strong Model was published, SickKids initially endorsed the model to guide their APN practice. Several years following the adoption of the Strong Model at SickKids, the APNs realized that inconsistency in its use was a problem. In analyzing the issues around the lack of uptake of the Strong Model, the APN Council concluded that they needed to develop a conceptual model that represented their vision, would guide APN practice, and address the unique aspects of their practice with ill children and their families.

To do this, they spent three months using innovative exercises and leadership techniques to capture the essence of the APN vision at SickKids. The effort was based on existing frameworks to invoke change and was deliberate in its approach. In the end, the APN Council achieved a vision to guide practice and fashioned a conceptual model with tenets rooted in the Strong Model (Ackerman et al., 1996). The framework has similar features to the UHN-FAPN model (Miceviski et al., 2004), but despite the attributes that appear comparable to those put forward at the UHN, the APN practice at SickKids model has decidedly different components (see Figure 8.4).

Rather than "inputs," the model begins at the left with acknowledgement of theories that are foundational elements. These include the Strong Model (Ackerman et al., 1996), the CNA APN standards and competencies, the Illness Belief Model (Wright, Watson, & Bell, 1996), and the Leadership Practice Model (Kouzes & Posner, 2002). The central circle, which is fashioned like the UHN-FAPN's model, has the child and family at the centre. Five small circles make spokes to the child and family and represent the SickKids APN core domains.

Interestingly, four of these domains are identical to the domains found in the Strong Model. The one Strong Model domain that is absent is leadership; in its place, the SickKids APN model identifies interprofessional collaboration as a key domain. Holistic care that encompasses the family is represented by the area between the spokes and depicts the context of communication, family-centred care, partnerships, human relationships, and collaboration. An encircling ring depicts the various settings, such as the home, community, hospital or ambulatory clinics, where holistic care is delivered by APNs. Like the UHN-FAPN model, an arrow leads to the right from the circle to outcomes. Unlike the UHN-FAPN model,

FIGURE 8.4: APN at SickKids

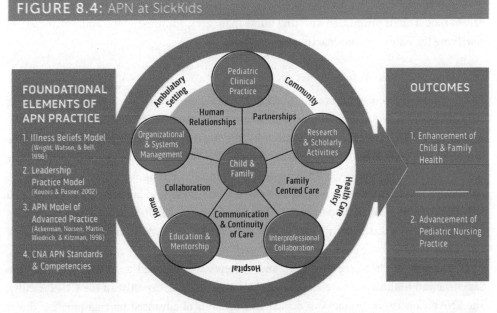

Source: LeGrow, K., Hubley, P., & McAllister, M. (2010). A conceptual framework for advanced practice nursing in a pediatric tertiary care setting: The SickKids' experience. *Nursing Leadership, 23*(2), 32–46. Reprinted with permission.

outcomes specific to child health and pediatric practice are expressed. A self-evaluation tool for the model is identified, but it does not provide a timeline for formal, planned evaluation of the model at SickKids (LeGrow et al., 2010).

The Acute Care Nurse Practitioner Conceptual Framework

A conceptualization of APN practice (Kilpatrick et al., 2012a) was developed from theoretical literature and a multiple-case study implemented in Quebec that explored role enactment by acute care NPs (ACNPs). In particular, the researchers investigated role boundaries, team processes with the enactment of ACNP roles, and the perception of effectiveness by team members (Kilpatrick et al., 2012a, 2012b).

Using cross-case analysis from the case-study findings, a new conceptual framework was constructed using identified process, structure, and outcome dimensions. In the centre, the three process dimensions of APN role enactment, boundary work, and team perception are shown with bivariate arrows, showing the interconnectedness of the processes. Concentric circles around the process dimensions depict how structure dimensions can restrict or expand the process dimensions. These elastic, concentric circles include patient, ACNP, team, organizational, and health care system-level structural dimensions that influence and affect the ability of the ACNP to carry out the role, to define boundaries, and to promote team effectiveness (Kilpatrick et al., 2012a, 2012b). Outcome dimensions are represented to the right of the concentric circles with quality, safety, cost, and team outcomes identified as key indicators of ACNP practice. The work addressed a gap in the understanding of the underlying processes and structures that occur with the introduction of an ACNP to the health care team (Kilpatrick et al., 2012a, 2012b). As the model is relatively new, further elucidation of ACNP team interaction and boundary work in other settings is important. The research-driven model holds promise in assisting nurse managers, administrators, and researchers in clarifying the nature of role enactment by ACNPs.

SNAP Conceptual Framework

Another reported conceptualization of APN was developed from the partnership, known as the Collaborative Nurse Practitioner Program (CNPP), between Saskatchewan Polytechnic School of Nursing, formerly SIAST, and the University of Regina (UR) Faculty of Nursing. Initially, the CNPP team looked at a number of APN models and frameworks to guide the CNPP's curriculum and program design. Identifying the Strong Model as a valid and reliable APN model, the team realized that the model's focus and language did not reflect a Saskatchewan nor Canadian context of APN. Therefore, the CNPP team adapted the Strong Model, and the Saskatchewan Nursing Advanced Practice (SNAP) Conceptual Framework was developed (Saskatchewan CNPPs, 2015; see Figure 8.5).

The Strong Model's core principles and concepts were aligned to fit the context of the Saskatchewan health system, reflect current literature, and the expertise of the CNPP faculty. The SNAP Conceptual Framework depicts five domains of advanced nursing practice: direct comprehensive care, support of systems, educative practice, evidence-informed practice, and professional leadership. Additionally, these concepts were mapped for consistency against

FIGURE 8.5: SNAP Conceptual Framework

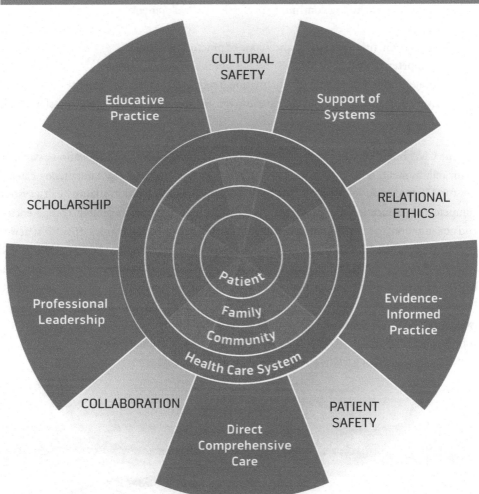

Source: Saskatchewan CNPPs. (2015). *Nurse practitioners—improving health care in communities.* Regina, SK: Saskatchewan Polytechnic and University of Regina. Reprinted with permission.

the core provincial RN(NP) competencies developed by the Saskatchewan Registered Nurses Association and the APN educational and practice competencies developed by the CNA.

In 2015, the SNAP Conceptual Framework was officially adopted as the conceptual framework to guide the CNPP's curricular and program design. The framework for advanced practice recognizes the expertise APN students bring to the program and reflects APN from both national and provincial competencies and practice standards.

Advanced Nursing Practice: A Pan-Canadian Framework

Building upon the work of the CNPI and the most recently identified Canadian APN competency framework, the CNA's pan-Canadian APN framework was refined from previous iterations, and includes strategies for successful APN role implementation, integration, and sustainability, as well as evaluation (CNA, 2019). The CNA presents the following framework elements:

- Definition and characteristics
- Education (including continuing professional development)
- Roles
- Regulation, title protection, and scope of practice
- Competencies (specific to CNS and NP roles)
- Strategies for successful implementation, integration, and sustainability
- Evaluation, including the Evaluation Framework Matrix (Bryant-Lukosius et al., 2016)

The CNA Board of Directors reiterated its endorsement of graduate education as a minimum requirement, and further refined the previous four overarching competency categories for APNs to include direct comprehensive care competencies; optimizing health system competencies; educational competencies; research competencies; leadership competencies; and consultation and collaboration competencies (CNA, 2019). The framework also renewed endorsement of the PEPPA framework with some additional resources (see Figure 8.2) and added a three-component conceptual framework for use in the implementation and evaluation of APN roles in acute care settings. The latter framework was adapted by Bryant-Lukosius et al. (2016) from the Nursing Role Effectiveness Model developed by Sidani in 1999 (see Figure 8.6). It is clear that the guidance provided by the national framework provides cohesion in the approach to APN definitions, roles, and educational preparation and remains central to ongoing discussions about APN practice in Canada.

FIGURE 8.6: Evaluation Framework Matrix—Key Concepts for Evaluating APN Roles

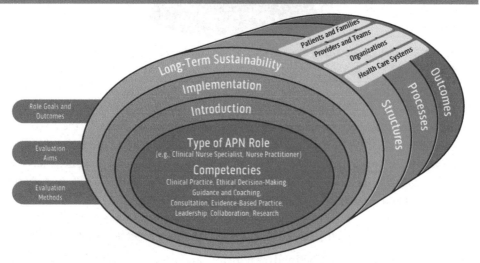

Source: Bryant-Lukosius, D., Spichiger, E., Martin, J., Stoll, H., Kellerhals, S. D., Fliedner, M., ... De Geest, S. (2016). Framework for evaluating the impact of advanced practice nursing roles. *Journal of Nursing Scholarship, 48*(2), 201–209. Reprinted with permission.

Conclusion

Within this sketch of APN conceptual models, several themes emerged. First, reliance on models from the US is decreasing as new Canadian models have emerged to address contextual nuances of our health care systems. Clearly, Hamric's Model of Advanced Nursing Practice (Hamric, 1996) continues to influence thinking surrounding the core elements of APN. Likewise, we can find the Strong Model (Ackerman et al., 1996) in use in Canadian acute care hospitals. However, the work of the CNPI in the early 2000s led to the development of a national competency framework that resulted in a better understanding of the nature of APN in Canada. Investigation of the impact of the original framework on the current state of APN practice (CNPI, 2016) and the refinement of the CNA's 2019 pan-Canadian framework clarifies some of the ambiguity surrounding the overlap and distinctions in CNS and NP roles and provides additional detail supporting professional development/continuing competency, research, leadership, role development, implementation, and evaluation.

Of the Canadian-developed frameworks presented, three are specific to NP practice, the remainder address APN generally, and it is important to note that four of the Canadian models were strongly influenced by the Strong Model. Of equal importance is the initiative of three tertiary hospitals to undertake conceptual development of APN role definitions and conceptualizations. Only one model clearly arose from research findings, while the PEPPA framework has been extensively used in research investigations (Boyko, Carter, & Bryant-Lukosius, 2016).

Despite the search to identify all APN conceptual models used or developed in Canada, it is quite possible that other models in use have not been reported in the literature. An inventory of APN framework utilization in practice settings was beyond the scope of this overview. Yet, with increased development of Canadian models since 2000, we need to grasp the extent of their use by APNs and how effective the models will prove to be in guiding role development and affecting APN sensitive outcomes. Continued inquiry into role implementation will help refine current APN frameworks and more clearly define the crucial elements that characterize the various advanced practice roles.

Critical Thinking Questions

1. What major driving forces in Canada led to the evolution of APN frameworks?
2. Compare and contrast the four Canadian models that were influenced by the Strong Model (i.e., UHN Framework for Advanced Practice Nursing, Advanced Practice Nursing at SickKids, the ACNP Conceptual Framework, and the SNAP Conceptual Framework). What contextual factors of the three settings might account for the different models?
3. How can APN models be used in nursing research? From your understanding of the models presented, which models could most easily be used to inform research?
4. How can the CNA's pan-Canadian framework influence the future landscape of APN practice in Canada?

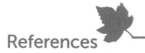

References

Ackerman, M. H., Norsen, L., Martin, B., Wiedrich, J., & Kitzman, H. J. (1996). Development of a model of advanced practice. *American Journal of Critical Care, 5*(1), 68–73.

Boyko, J. A., Carter, N., & Bryant-Lukosius, D. (2016). Assessing the spread and uptake of a framework for introducing and evaluating advanced practice nursing roles. *Worldviews on Evidence Based Nursing, 13*(4), 277–284. doi: 10.1111/wvn.12160

Bryant-Lukosius, D., & DiCenso, A. (2004). A framework for the introduction and evaluation of advanced practice nursing roles. *Journal of Advanced Nursing, 48*(5), 530–540.

Bryant-Lukosius, D., & Martin-Misener, R. (2015). *ICN policy brief. Advanced practice nursing: An essential component of country level human resources for health.* Geneva, CH: ICN. Retrieved from https://www.who.int/workforcealliance/knowledge/resources/ICN_PolicyBrief6AdvancedPractice Nursing.pdf

Bryant-Lukosius, D., Spichiger, E., Martin, J., Stoll, H., Kellerhals, S. D., Fliedner, M., ... De Geest, S. (2016). Framework for evaluating the impact of advanced practice nursing roles. *Journal of Nursing Scholarship, 48*(2), 201–209.

Canadian Nurse Practitioner Initiative (CNPI). (2006). *Nurse practitioners: The time is now.* Ottawa, ON: CNA.

CNPI. (2016). *The Canadian nurse practitioner initiative: A 10-year retrospective.* Ottawa, ON: CNA. Retrieved from https://www.cna-aiic.ca/-/media/cna/page-content/pdf-en/canadian-nurse-practitioner-initiative-a-10-year-retrospective.pdf

Canadian Nurses Association (CNA). (2019). *Advanced practice nursing: A pan-Canadian framework.* Ottawa, ON: CNA. Retrieved from https://www.cna-aiic.ca/-/media/cna/page-content/pdf-en/apn-a-pan-canadian-framework.pdf

Chinn, P. L., & Kramer, M. K. (2015). *Knowledge development in nursing: Theory and process* (9th ed.). St. Louis, MO: Elsevier Mosby.

Cragg, C. E., Doucette, S., & Humbert, J. (2003). Ten universities, one program: Successful collaboration to educate nurse practitioners. *Nurse Educator, 28*(5), 227–231.

De Grasse, C., & Nicklin, W. (2001). Advanced nursing practice: Old hat, new design. *Canadian Journal of Nursing Leadership, 14*(4), 7–12.

Hamric, A. B. (1996). A definition of advanced practice nursing. In A. B. Hamric, J. A. Spross, & C. M. Hanson (Eds.), *Advanced nursing practice: An integrative approach* (pp. 25–41). Philadelphia, PA: W. B. Saunders.

Jansen, M. P. (2010). Advanced practice within a nursing paradigm. In M. P. Jansen & M. Zwygart-Stauffacher (Eds.), *Advanced practice nursing: Core concepts for professional role development* (2nd ed., pp. 31–42). New York, NY: Springer.

Kilpatrick, K., Lavoie-Tremblay, M., Lamothe, L., Ritchie, J. A., & Doran, D. (2012a). Conceptual framework of acute care nurse practitioner role enactment, boundary work, and perceptions of team effectiveness. *Journal of Advanced Nursing, 69*(1), 205–217.

Kilpatrick, K., Lavoie-Tremblay, M., Ritchie, J. A., Lamothe, L., Doran, D., & Rochefort, C. (2012b). How are acute care nurse practitioners enacting their roles in healthcare teams? A descriptive multiple-case study. *International Journal of Nursing Studies, 49*(7), 850–862.

Kouzes, J. M., & Posner, B. Z. (2002). *The leadership challenge* (3rd ed.). San Francisco, CA: Wiley & Sons.

LeGrow, K., Hubley, P., & McAllister, M. (2010). A conceptual framework for advanced practice nursing in a pediatric tertiary care setting: The SickKids' experience. *Nursing Leadership, 23*(2), 32–46. doi: 10.12927/cjnl.2013.21831

Martin-Misener, R., Reilly, S. M., & Vollman, A. R. (2010). Defining the role of primary health care nurse practitioners in rural Nova Scotia. *Canadian Journal of Nursing Research, 42*(2), 30–47.

Miceviski, V., Korkola, L., Sakrssian, S., Mucahy, V., Shobbrook, C., Belford, L., & Kells, L. (2004). University Health Network framework for advanced nursing practice: Development of a comprehensive conceptual framework describing the multidimensional contributions of advanced practice nurses. *Nursing Leadership, 17*(3), 52–64. doi: 10.12927/cjnl.2004.16231

Mick, D. J., & Ackerman, M. H. (2000). Advanced practice nursing role delineation in acute and critical care: Application of the Strong model of advanced practice. *Heart & Lung, 29*(3), 210–221.

National Organization of Nurse Practitioner Faculties (NONPF). (2002a). *Domains and core competencies of nurse practitioner practice, 2002.* Washington, DC: NONPF.

NONPF. (2002b). *Nurse practitioner primary care competencies in specialty areas: Adult, family, gerontological, pediatric, and women's health.* Washington, DC: NONPF.

NONPF. (2020). *What are the NP core competencies?* Washington, DC: NONPF. Retrieved from https://www.nursepractitionerschools.com/faq/what-are-the-np-core-competencies/

Oberle, K., & Allen, M. (2001). The nature of advanced practice nursing. *Nursing Outlook, 49*(3), 148–153.

Ontario Primary Health Care Nurse Practitioner (PHCNP) Program. (2015). *Advanced health assessment and diagnosis (AHAD) I.* Toronto, ON: COUPN.

Robinson Vollman, A., & Martin-Misener, R. (2005). A conceptual model for nurse practitioner practice. In Canadian Nurse Practitioner Initiative (2006), *Practice framework for nurse practitioners in Canada* (Appendix A) (pp. 1–13). Ottawa, ON: CNA. Retrieved from www.npnow.ca/docs/tech-report/section3/05_PracticeFW_AppendixA.pdf

Saskatchewan Collaborative Nurse Practitioner Programs (CNPPs). (2015). *Nurse practitioners—Improving health care in communities.* Regina, SK: Saskatchewan Polytechnic and University of Regina. Retrieved from http://www.sasknursingdegree.ca/cnpp/vision-mission-values-and-the-snap-model/

Shuler, P. A., & Davis, J. E. (1993a). The Shuler Nurse Practitioner Practice model: A theoretical framework for nurse practitioner clinicians, educators, and researchers, part 1. *Journal of the American Academy of Nurse Practitioners, 5*(1), 11–18.

Shuler, P. A., & Davis, J. E. (1993b). The Shuler Nurse Practitioner Practice model: Clinical application, part 2. *Journal of the American Academy of Nurse Practitioners, 5*(2), 73–88.

Spross, J. (2014). Conceptualizations of advanced practice nursing. In A. B. Hamric, C. M. Hanson, M. F. Tracy, & E. T. O'Grady (Eds.), *Advanced practice nursing: An integrative approach* (5th ed., pp. 27–66). St. Louis, MO: Elsevier.

The Ottawa Hospital (TOH). (2019). *Advanced practice nurses.* Ottawa, ON: TOH. Retrieved from https://www.ottawahospital.on.ca/en/our-model-of-care/our-health-care-professional-team/nursing/advanced-practice-nurses/

Wright, L. M., Watson, W. L., & Bell, J. M. (1996). *Beliefs: The heart of healing in families and illness.* New York, NY: Basic Books.

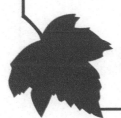

SECTION II

Social Determinants of Health and Advanced Practice Nursing

This section provides the reader with a broader examination of the traditional determinants of health such as social, economic, environmental, and behavioural elements affecting Indigenous, inner-city, rural and remote, LGBT2SQ, and migrant populations in Canada. Issues related to family and community, government policies, mental health and addiction, disease, homelessness and housing, racism, and youth that heavily influence these underserved populations are discussed. Additionally, contributions advanced practice nurses are making within the health care system for these populations are demonstrated in relation to health promotion, social inequality, and community health that influence their health and health care.

Chapter

9 Indigenous Populations

Mary Smith and Roger Pilon

MARY SMITH is currently an Assistant Professor at Queen's University, Kingston, Ontario, and has been a registered nurse since 1991. She completed the Ontario Primary Health Care Nurse Practitioner (PHCNP) Program in 2002 and has practiced in a variety of settings, including a remote First Nation community health centre, an Aging at Home program, and within a rural hospital's mental health care facility. Mary is a member of the Beausoleil First Nation community in Ontario and is passionate about fostering an understanding of Indigenous ways of being and knowing within nursing practice, research, education, and leadership.

ROGER PILON is an Associate Professor and Director at Laurentian University, School of Nursing, Assistant Professor at the Northern Ontario School of Medicine, and an NP-PHC in Sudbury, Ontario. His areas of research include Indigenous and francophone health, primary health care, and the integration of NPs into practice. Roger was one of the first primary health care nurse practitioners (PHCNPs) to be recognized in the province of Ontario in 1998. Since leaving full-time practice in 2008 to begin his academic career, Roger has maintained an active clinical practice in a local francophone community health centre and a First Nation community funded by the Aboriginal Healing and Wellness Strategy.

KEY TERMS

advanced practice nursing
(APN)
colonialism
Indigenous
primary health care (PHC)
reconciliation
social determinants of health
(SDH)

OBJECTIVES

1. Describe the relevance and interconnectedness between the social determinants of health (SDH) with primary health care (PHC) for advanced practice nursing (APN).
2. Define the meaning of *Indigenous Peoples*.
3. Interrelate concepts of reconciliation, colonialism, and cultural safety as associated with recent Canadian governmental inquiries and reports and their significance for APN.
4. Describe cultural safety in relation to power relationships and racism.
5. Exemplify health determinants in relation to APN domains of leadership, practice, education, and research.

Introduction

Within the realm of **advanced practice nursing (APN)**, both clinical nurse specialists (CNSs) and nurse practitioners (NPs) are making significant contributions to health care (Canadian Nurses Association [CNA], 2019). With educational training beyond that of the registered nurse, CNSs and NPs provide advanced knowledge, expertise, and leadership and are adept in disease prevention and health promotion. NPs specifically are regulated health providers involved in assessment, diagnosis, and treatment. Together, both CNSs and NPs are well positioned within the Canadian context to act upon the **social determinants of health (SDH)** and are guided through a holistic APN lens that links health and wellness with the socio-historical, political, economic, and cultural circumstances at play (Bourque Bearskin, 2011; CNA, 2019).

APN has its origins in outpost nursing in remote and isolated areas and in caring for Indigenous Peoples. These outpost nurses may have been involved in the legacy of the residential school system, which continues to shape health outcomes of Indigenous Peoples. In 2015, the Truth and Reconciliation Commission of Canada explicitly recognized the enduring trauma upon Indigenous Peoples and the necessity for all health care providers to learn their history. The history of health care involving Indigenous Peoples stems from a colonial structure. In 1876, the Medicine Chest clause, a Canadian government treaty provision, failed to provide equitable health care for Indigenous Peoples (McCallum, 2016). The Registered Nurses of Canadian Indian Ancestry, which has now become the Canadian Indigenous Nurses Association (CINA), sought to illuminate the ongoing health disparities that prevailed under the government's control of health resources through the Medical Services Branch (McCallum, 2016). Given the historical influence upon the health of Indigenous Peoples, **colonialism** and associated concepts, including cultural safety, will be prioritized and explained throughout this chapter as being highly significant to APN.

For consistency with the 2008 United Nations Declaration on the Rights of Indigenous Peoples (UNDRIP), the word *Indigenous* is applied throughout this chapter as the all-encompassing term inclusive of First Nations, Métis, and Inuit, while the term *Aboriginal* is still commonly used within government reports and statistics. It should be emphasized that First Nations, Métis, and Inuit are distinct peoples in terms of culture, language, and beliefs.

There are over 800 reserves and 600 Indigenous communities with greater than 70 languages across Canada (Statistics Canada, 2018). Indigenous Peoples' ability to speak an Indigenous language grew by 3.1% over the last 10 years, with Ojibway, Cree, and Inuktitut being the most frequently spoken Indigenous languages in Canada. The Indigenous population has grown by 42.5% since 2006 and is likely to exceed 2.5 million in the next two decades (see Figure 9.1; Statistics Canada, 2018). With a population of 1,673,785 as of 2016, this group is growing at a rate four times faster than the rest of the Canadian population. Life expectancy, including both on- and off-reserve Indigenous people, is 77.9 years compared to 82.9 years for the non-Indigenous population (Statistics Canada, 2015).

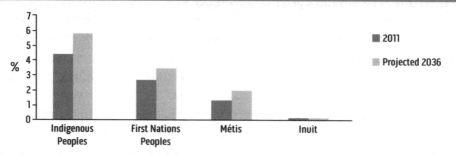

FIGURE 9.1: Population by Indigenous Identity as a Proportion of the Total Canadian Population, 2011 and 2036

Source: Statistics Canada. (2018). *First Nations people, Métis and Inuit in Canada: Diverse and growing populations.* Ottawa, ON: Statistics Canada. Retrieved from https://www.150.statcan.gc.ca/n1/pub/89-659-x/89-659-x2018001-eng.htm

A Lens for Advanced Practice Nursing

Determinants of Health

Primary health care (PHC) embraces comprehensive, principle-based population approaches across the lifespan. APN extends from PHC philosophy where human rights and social justice sustain accessible primary health care for all populations, particularly those disadvantaged by gender, ethnicity, or non-Western culture (CNA, 2015). While Mikkonen and Raphael (2010) describe the commonly known determinants of health, the First Nations Wholistic Policy and Planning model adds many more determinants as specific to Indigenous health (see Table 9.1). Additional determinants include colonialism, legal equity, lands, resources, language, and cultural identity (Indigenous Services Canada, 2018). For Indigenous populations globally, colonialism stands out as the root determinant from which all other determinants spiral (Allan, Smylie, Wellesley Institute, & Canadian Electronic Library, 2015). Furthermore, the World Health Organization (WHO) describes the health system as an intrinsic determinant of health (2010). The health care system calculates access to its resources through cost-driven policies influencing health care provision with vulnerable populations. All determinants of health are highly relevant to APN. For Indigenous communities across Canada, the socio-demographic determinants, including lack of housing and income, directly impact upon overall health and quality of life. APNs within nursing associations throughout Canada have been politically active. Through a leadership capacity, the CNA and the Registered Nurses Association of Ontario (RNAO) have lobbied government toward addressing socio-economic disparities that directly impact health status (CNA, 2015; RNAO, 2013).

Health Equity and Inequity

Health inequities remain a nationwide problem for Indigenous Peoples (Browne et al., 2016). Improvements through PHC can foster health overall with resulting reductions in wait times, emergency room visits, and better management of chronic diseases (Canadian Institutes of Health Research [CIHR], 2012; WHO, 2013). Health equity supports the best state of health

TABLE 9.1: Indigenous Determinants of Health

Indigenous Determinants of Health
• Community readiness
• Economic development
• Employment
• Environmental stewardship
• Gender
• Historical conditions and colonialism
• Housing
• Lands and resources
• Language, heritage, and strong cultural identity
• Legal and political equity
• Lifelong learning
• On and off reserve
• Racism and discrimination
• Self-determination and non-dominance
• Social services and supports
• Urban and rural

Source: Adapted from Assembly of First Nations. (2013). *First Nations wholistic policy and planning: A transitional discussion document on the social determinants of health.* Ottawa, ON: Public Health Agency of Canada. Retrieved from http://health.afn.ca/uploads/files/sdoh_afn.pdf

possible through the highest quality of care that is appropriate and consistent with the location and unique attributes of any given group of people (Varcoe, Wathen, Ford-Gilboe, Smye, & Browne, 2016).

APN is frequently involved in caring for groups with limited income who may live in urban, rural, or isolated communities. Moreover, throughout Canada, APN is making an impact upon health inequities through team-based, interprofessional PHC approaches within the communities where these health care providers choose to work. In Ontario, health care transformation includes new models of PHC, such as NP-Led Clinics, where NPs are primary health care providers in communities where primary health care is lacking. These NPs have emphasized that socio-economic circumstances are a priority and can have a negative impact on the care of chronic illnesses (Heale, James, Wenghofer, & Garceau, 2018). Archibald and Fraser (2013) further explain the capacity of NPs in addressing disparities at the individual or micro level also extends to the macro level, benefiting society as a whole. As consistent with the Canada Health Act, NPs have an important role in the provision of accessible health care.

Rethinking the SDH in relation to Indigenous Peoples' health in Canada involves understanding this complex history, which has not often been prioritized in APN education. Rather than focusing only on socially determined factors, all determinants, including economical and historical interfaces with past colonialist legacies that extend into the present, should be addressed (Greenwood, de Leeuw, Lindsay, & Reading, 2015). In the Interconnections Representation (see Figure 9.2), APN and associated domains of practice, leadership, research, and pedagogy are positioned as a sphere proximal to PHC where all interact to address the SDH and colonialist structures.

FIGURE 9.2: Interconnections Representation

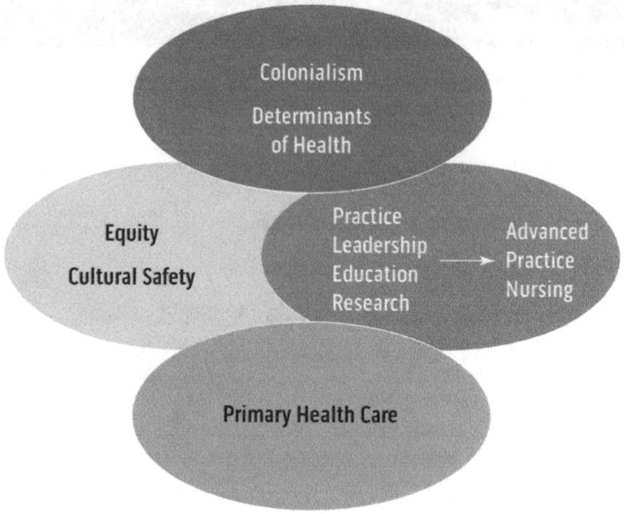

Source: Smith, M. (2019). Unpublished.

An SDH lens is necessary to understanding health inequities between Indigenous and non-Indigenous Peoples (Greenwood & de Leeuw, 2012). Identifying proximal, intermediate, and distal determinants is another way of recognizing what influences well-being (Reading & Wein, 2009). Proximal determinants include but are not limited to such areas as education, employment, and income that impact on mental, emotional, spiritual, and physical health. The intermediate determinants involve health systems, community structure, and organization and cultural permanence. They shape and influence the proximal determinants (Greenwood & de Leeuw, 2012; Reading & Wein, 2009). The distal determinants, which are broader, are the source of both proximal and intermediate determinants and encompass such elements as self-determination, colonialism, and racism (Greenwood & de Leeuw, 2012).

Colonialism: Legacies and Reconciliation

Although a full discussion of colonialism is beyond the scope of this chapter, a brief overview of critical features regarding colonialism and its impacts on the health and well-being of Indigenous Peoples in Canada will be discussed. Colonialism has been conceptualized in several ways. For example, Cote-Meek (2014) has suggested that colonization, which is the outcome of imperial ideology, is still ongoing today. Colonization should not be understood as a temporal concept that suggests colonialism no longer exists but rather as a way of critically explaining the ways in which colonialism has impacted Indigenous Peoples in the past and how it continues to do so today. Settler colonialism, as another distinctive type of colonialism, specifically encompasses Indigenous groups where settler society acquired dominance and authority.

Furthermore, structure is implicit within the concept of settler colonialism. An example is multiculturalism policies that become taken-for-granted ways that questionably have any helpful influence upon the relationship between settler and Indigenous Peoples. Reading (2015) further explains the universal consequences for all Indigenous Peoples globally arising from colonialism with ongoing intense changes to social, economic, and political structures. Disrupted access to water, food, and land as brought about by the Indian Act of 1876, the forced destruction of families through residential school systems, and the Sixties Scoop are but a few forces that culminated in disastrous repercussions that continue to be felt to this day (Reading, 2015).

Canada has been called on to be mindful of the recent Truth and Reconciliation Commission of Canada (TRC) with 94 Calls to Action. Reconciliation, as defined by the TRC, must involve respectful relationships with Indigenous Peoples. This requires learning and acknowledging the history of past harms, their causes, and ways to change. UNDRIP is addressed in Call to Action 43 by the TRC as the reconciliation framework to be fully implemented and adopted. It is also important to understand the TRC Call to Action 45, which specifically distinguishes the need to disclaim the Discovery Doctrine and apply UNDRIP. The Doctrine of Discovery originated in the 1400s, when lands were disposed and exploited regardless of the original dwellers (Assembly of First Nations, 2018). UNDRIP declares the rights of Indigenous Peoples globally, including free, prior and informed consent over resources and lands. Canada accepted it in 2016, but it has yet to pass its third reading to become law. The significance of land ownership cannot be understated in terms of its relationship to Indigenous health and well-being. Indigenous ways of being and knowing are intricately connected to the land, including hunting and fishing as a vital food source. The loss of land for Indigenous Peoples directly relates to catastrophic conditions and poor mental and physical health (Reading & Wein, 2009).

UNDRIP is also significant to the National Inquiry into Missing and Murdered Indigenous Women and Girls (MMIWG) with regard to furthering safety and security for Indigenous families and community. The final report included 231 Calls for Justice (National Inquiry into Missing and Murdered Indigenous Women and Girls, 2019). Both the TRC and MMIWG reports include recommendations for all health care sectors and emphasize the need for action toward education and practice, including but not limited to cultural safety training, anti-racism, and awareness of the history and ongoing legacies of colonialism. The aforesaid reports are essential to APN, which seeks to engage respectfully with Indigenous populations toward improving health outcomes.

Addressing SDH and Cultural Safety in Advanced Practice Nursing

Although there are a variety of conceptualizations to describe cultural relationships, cultural safety continues to resonate throughout the literature as an outcome that is on a learning continuum with cultural awareness and sensitivity, cultural competency, and cultural humility (First Nations Health Authority [FNHA], 2016). In summary, cultural awareness recognizes difference; cultural sensitivity acknowledges diversity; cultural competency involves health care practitioner skills and attitudes; and cultural humility requires self-reflection and lifelong learning (Allan, Smylie, Wellesley Institute, & Canadian Electronic Library, 2015; FNHA, 2016). As developed by Irihapeti Merenia Ramsden, a New Zealand Māori nurse, *cultural safety* has become a familiar term around the globe.

Cultural safety links with colonialism and the SDH in that it addresses power imbalances leading to disparities and poor health and well-being overall. Specifically, cultural safety is important in addressing racism (Allan, Smylie, Wellesley Institute, & Canadian Electronic Library, 2015). Racism and stereotypes within health care have and continue to jeopardize the well-being of Indigenous Peoples. Colonialism has cultivated varying forms of discrimination that may not always be immediately recognized; for example, Bourque Bearskin (2011) demonstrates experiences of racism toward Indigenous Peoples where cultural practices by families were denied within a critical care unit. In this example, the preoccupation with biomedical technical processes and procedures minimized the importance of cultural traditions. In times of critical illness and death, the denial of cultural practices for loved ones may further perpetuate traumatization (Bourque Bearskin, 2011). Furthermore, stigmatized perspectives held by advanced practitioners with diagnostic and prescriptive roles may lead to adverse outcomes where optimal treatments or diagnostic tests are delayed or withheld (Allan, Smylie, Wellesley Institute, & Canadian Electronic Library, 2015; Greenwood & de Leeuw, 2012).

Cultural Safety: Leadership, Practice, Education, and Research

In this section, previous discussions related to the SDH, colonialism, and reconciliation are integrated with specific APN practice. This discussion is framed from the perspective of interweaving APN leadership with practice, research, and education, reviewing where they intersect with the outcome of cultural safety, and specific systemic barriers will be highlighted.

Cultural safety is lifesaving and critical to APN. There are many tragic incidents reported throughout the media that demonstrate first-hand a pervasive lack of cultural safety within our health care system. A well-publicized case is that of Brian Sinclair, who at the age of 45 was discovered deceased in the emergency room 34 hours after he had arrived (Allan, Smylie, Wellesley Institute, & Canadian Electronic Library, 2015). The Jordan's Principle, in memory of Jordan River Anderson, was passed in 2007 to provide the necessary health care for Indigenous children regardless of jurisdictional boundaries. This principle, important to APN, represents Indigenous human rights issues in health care as Indigenous children have not always received equitable access to health care. As leaders in health care, APNs strive to advocate for and participate in activities building equity in health care. The 2016 CNA and CINA's joint statement on the government's announcement in support of Jordan's Principle specifically emphasizes the need to end jurisdictional disputes to fund health care that limit accessible health care for children. Through the domain of leadership, APNs play a key role in advocating for such essential policy changes.

Becoming attuned to the Non-Insured Health Benefit (NIHB) for First Nations Peoples is also relevant to APN. First Nations Peoples with status rely on NIHB to cover the costs of medications, treatments, therapies, and medical transportation. CNSs and NPs working with the First Nations population are required to be aware of which services are covered through NIHB. Moreover, many Indigenous persons who fall within the government categories of non-status First Nations and the Métis do not qualify to receive any support from NIHB (Allan, Smylie, Wellesley Institute, & Canadian Electronic Library, 2015). There are also regular changes to the services and medications that are covered through NIHB where many medications and services such as certain dental procedures are currently no longer covered. For First Nations children and their families living in often isolated communities, NIHB has declined critically vital medications, medical equipment, and therapies (Allan, Smylie, Wellesley Institute, & Canadian Electronic Library, 2015).

Indigenous Peoples may seek healing through the medicine wheel, including traditional medicines and smudging for experiences of trauma and pain (Bourque Bearskin, 2011). In traditional practices, sacred medicines—such as sage, sweetgrass, tobacco, and cedar—are used in ceremonies. These medicines may also be used in smudging. Smudging allows cleansing and a way to seek guidance from the Creator. The sacred medicines are ignited just enough to produce a smoke, which is fanned over an individual. While health care centres have differing policies about smudging, nurses need to know if there are spaces for smudging practices or traditional healers who can assist. Although the leadership in many health care centres are developing policies and safe, comfortable areas for private smudging, there continues to be ongoing challenges. Indigenous Peoples may feel ongoing trauma and may not want to participate in Canada's more traditional Western health care where there is disrespect for their Indigenous traditional ceremonies such as smudging (Allan, Smylie, Wellesley Institute, & Canadian Electronic Library, 2015). Person-centred care, where inequities in relationships are identified and balanced, is foundational for nursing and is consistent with cultural safety. Implicit within culturally safe practice are relational approaches that prioritize involvement of communities, families, and children as vital support systems (Bourque Bearskin, 2011). In this perspective, cultural safety is essential to nursing practice, education, and theory (Aboriginal Nurses Association of Canada [ANAC] & CNA, 2009).

Health care organizations are taking steps to further cultural safety. For example, the FNHA in British Columbia now has in place a declaration where individual health care practitioners and health regulators have signed their commitment to cultural safety and humility in practice. The commitment solidifies the mandate to further cultural humility and safety. This has been realized as a way forward toward a healthier system for all people. In addition, clinical leaders involved in policy development need to advocate for and engage Indigenous leaders and elders. Furthering the representation and engagement of Indigenous Peoples at all federal and provincial levels and within all sectors, including health care and education, remains a priority that requires a commitment to action by all administrators and leaders (FNHA, 2016).

Although there is evidence that cultural safety is becoming more well known within some health care educational programs, there are concerns that there remains a lack of cultural safety education in the majority of programs (Shah & Reeves, 2012). In British Columbia, the Provincial Health Services Authority (PHSA) has created the San'yas Indigenous Cultural Training program, which the British Columbia College of Nursing Professionals (BCCNP) has been advocating for all nurses to complete (BCCNP, 2019; PHSA in British Columbia, 2019). There is a need for faculty and students alike to address their own assumptions within the context of societal forces and egalitarian belief systems and for educators to engage students through classroom interactions and focused introspective dialogues (Browne, Smye, & Varcoe, 2005; McGibbon, Mulaudzi, Didham, Barton, & Sochan, 2014). The emphasis should be on addressing structural changes within curricula rather than including only more information to parts of already existing curricula.

The lack of cultural safety in education also relates to the prevailing under-representation of Indigenous nursing students and nurses throughout Canada. The Indigenous nursing workforce increased only slightly from 2.4% in 2011 to 3% in 2016 (CINA, 2016). In accordance with the TRC's Call to Action 23, APN educators are striving toward increasing the presence of Indigenous nurses. Decolonization and indigenization are approaches to address colonialism in health care and education. Furthermore, these concepts are necessary in supporting the increased presence of Indigenous health care providers. APN implies graduate prepared nurses are "advanced" and well versed in such concepts that connect colonialism and the lack of cultural safety to Indigenous non-participation in health care and education. Pete, Schneider, and O'Reilly (2013) bring light to the meanings behind indigenizing and decolonizing in relation to education and pedagogy. These concepts are described as interrelated whereas indigenizing concerns a holistic approach where Indigenous knowledge becomes the focal point that emphasizes relationships and addressing racism. Decolonizing involves reflecting upon the land or territory in which we work and live (Pete, Schneider, & O'Reilly, 2013). Decolonization further requires transforming the power imbalances within all sectors, including health, education, and research. Decolonization strategies identify covert racist systemic structures and dismantle taken-for-granted assumptions (McGibbon et al., 2014). In this respect, decolonization and indigenization are significant to addressing the SDH and cultural safety.

The necessity for cultural safety that stresses equitable relations through respectful consideration of historical, socio-political, and economic determinants is essential to furthering the representation of Indigenous students within the academy. Also important are flexible and relational approaches within APN education. Indigenous support networks within educational settings and distant learning opportunities where students may remain in home communities are strategies that may foster student recruitment and retention. As elders foster contextual wise practices, education that is inclusive of elders within APN education supports holistic contexts and participation by Indigenous Peoples (ANAC & CNA, 2009; Greenwood et al., 2015).

The principles of cultural safety are also significant to APN research. Cultural safety requires relationships with participants and communities where the methodology that guides the research is consistent with the world views of those being researched. This is different from the more traditional research project, which is primarily concerned with obtaining data whereupon project completion, the researcher(s) leaves the community, never to return again. Relationships with communities need to continue even long after the research is completed and research outcomes must benefit communities (Nelson & Wilson, 2018). Establishing trust is paramount to successful research. Indigenous ontologies and epistemologies or ways of being and knowing need to form the foundation for any research involving Indigenous Peoples.

Conclusion

This chapter has considered the SDH through a holistic APN lens seeking to further address the legacy of colonialism in conjunction with the environmental, physical, and social determinants that influence overall health and well-being. Health disparities are deeply linked with broader underlying factors, including the entrenched colonial, political, and social systems emanating from historical injustices. APN is uniquely positioned and challenged to demonstrate meaningful action in accordance with the recommendations as set forth by the TRC and MMIWG reports. Cultural safety as manifested through APN practice, education, leadership, and research is vital toward equity where harmful approaches are addressed and rectified. Through their expanded scope of practice, APN has great potential to further culturally safe care for all.

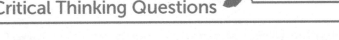

Critical Thinking Questions

1. Discuss ways APN may guide cultural safety through leadership, practice, education, and research.
2. Consider the difficulties described with regard to medical transportation and the services provided by NIHB. How could these difficulties be addressed? Are these micro-, meso-, or macro-level issues?
3. As a CNS or NP, you are asked to write a letter to advocate for a person in need of medical transportation through NIHB. Write a letter and discuss what you feel would be important to include about someone requiring transportation for chemotherapy treatments.
4. The manager of your unit asks you to take the lead toward enabling smudging within the facility. Consider how you might go about the development of a policy or protocol within your organization to facilitate traditional practices, including smudging.

References

Aboriginal Nurses Association of Canada (ANAC) & Canadian Nurses Association (CNA). (2009). *Cultural competency and cultural safety: Curriculum for Aboriginal Peoples.* Ottawa, ON: ANAC & CNA.

Allan, B., Smylie, J., Wellesley Institute, & Canadian Electronic Library (Firm). (2015). *First peoples, second class treatment: The role of racism in the health and well-being of Indigenous Peoples in Canada.* Toronto, ON: Wellesley Institute.

Archibald, M. M., & Fraser, K. (2013). The potential for nurse practitioners in health care reform. *Journal of Professional Nursing, 29*(5), 270–275. doi: 10.1016/j.profnurs.2012.10.002

Assembly of First Nations. (2013). *First Nations wholistic policy and planning: A transitional discussion document on the social determinants of health.* Ottawa, ON: Public Health Agency of Canada. Retrieved from http://health.afn.ca/uploads/files/sdoh_afn.pdf

Assembly of First Nations. (2018). *Dismantling the Doctrine of Discovery.* Retrieved from https://www.afn.ca/wp-content/uploads/2018/02/18-01-22-Dismantling-the-Doctrine-of-Discovery-EN.pdf

Bourque Bearskin, R. L. (2011). A critical lens on culture in nursing practice. *Nursing Ethics, 18*(4), 548–559.

British Columbia College of Nursing Professionals (BCCNP). (2019). *Cultural safety and humility.* Vancouver, BC: BCCNP. Retrieved from https://www.bccnp.ca/bccnp/cultural_safety/Pages/Default.aspx

Browne, A. J., Smye, V. L., & Varcoe, C. (2005). The relevance of postcolonial theoretical perspectives to research in Aboriginal health. *Canadian Journal of Nursing Research, 37*(4), 17–37.

Browne, A. J., Varcoe, C., Lavoie, J., Smye, V., Wong, S. T., Krause, M., … Fridkin, A. (2016). Enhancing health care equity with Indigenous populations: Evidence-based strategies from an ethnographic study. *BMC Health Services Research, 16,* 544. doi: 10.1186/s12913-016-1707-9

Canadian Indigenous Nurses Association (CINA). (2016). *Aboriginal nursing in Canada. ("Professional Occupations in Nursing" NOC 2016-301).* Ottawa, ON: CINA. Retrieved from https://nursing.usask.ca/documents/aboriginal/AboriginalRNWorkforceFactsheet.pdf

Canadian Institutes of Health Research (CIHR). (2012). *Health care in Canada, 2012: A focus on wait times.* Ottawa, ON: CIHR. Retrieved from https://secure.cihi.ca/free_products/HCIC2012-FullReport-ENweb.pdf

Canadian Nurses Association (CNA). (2015). *Position statement: Primary health care.* Ottawa, ON: CNA. Retrieved from https://www.cna-aiic.ca/~/media/cna/page-content/pdf-en/primary-health-care-position-statement.pdf

CNA. (2019). *Advanced practice nursing: A pan-Canadian framework.* Retrieved from https://www.cna-aiic.ca/-/media/cna/page-content/pdf-en/apn-a-pan-canadian-framework.pdf?la=en&hash=E1387634D492FD2B003964E3CD4188971305469E

CNA & CINA. (2016). *CNA and CINA's joint statement on the government's announcement in support of Jordan's Principle.* Ottawa, ON: CNA. Retrieved from https://www.cna-aiic.ca/en/news-room/news-releases/2016/cna-and-cinas-joint-statement-on-yesterdays-announcement-in-support-of-jordans-principle

Cote-Meek, S. (2014). *Colonized classrooms: Racism, trauma and resistance in post-secondary education.* Halifax, NS: Fernwood Publishing.

First Nations Health Authority (FNHA). (2016). *FNHA's policy statement on cultural safety and humility.* Vancouver, BC: FNHA. Retrieved from https://www.fnha.ca/Documents/FNHA-Policy-Statement-Cultural-Safety-and-Humility.pdf

Greenwood, M. L., & de Leeuw, S. N. (2012). Social determinants of health and the future well-being of Aboriginal children in Canada. *Paediatrics & Child Health, 17*(7), 381–384.

Greenwood, M., de Leeuw, S., Lindsay, N. M., & Reading, C. (2015). *Determinants of Indigenous Peoples' health in Canada: Beyond the social.* Toronto, ON: Canadian Scholars' Press.

Heale, R., James, S., Wenghofer, E., & Garceau, M. (2018). Nurse practitioner's perceptions of the impact of the nurse practitioner-led clinic model on the quality of care of complex patients. *Primary Health Care Research & Development, 19*(6), 553–560. doi: 10.1017/S1463423617000913

Indigenous Services Canada. (2018). *Preventing and managing chronic disease in First Nations communities: A guidance framework.* Ottawa, ON: Government of Canada. Retrieved from http://publications.gc.ca/collections/collection_2018/aanc-inac/H34-313-1-2017-eng.pdf

McCallum, M. J. L. (2016). The Indigenous nurses who decolonized health care. *Briarpatch, 45*(6), 30–35.

McGibbon, E., Mulaudzi, F. M., Didham, P., Barton, S., & Sochan, A. (2014). Toward decolonizing nursing: The colonization of nursing and strategies for increasing the counter-narrative. *Nursing Inquiry, 21*(3), 179–191. doi: 10.1111/nin.12042

Mikkonen, J., & Raphael, D. (2010). *Social determinants of health: The Canadian facts.* Toronto, ON: York University School of Health Policy and Management.

National Inquiry into Missing and Murdered Indigenous Women and Girls (Canada), Depository Services Program (Canada), & Canada Privy Council Office. (2019). *Reclaiming power and place: Final report of the national inquiry into missing and murdered indigenous women and girls.* Ottawa, ON: Privy Council Office. Retrieved from http://publications.gc.ca/collections/collection_2019/bcp-pco/CP32-163-2-3-2019-eng.pdf

Nelson, S., & Wilson, K. (2018). Understanding barriers to health care access through cultural safety and ethical space: Indigenous People's experiences in Prince George, Canada. *Social Science & Medicine, 218*, 21–27. doi: 10.1016/j.socscimed.2018.09.017

Pete, S., Schneider, B., & O'Reilly, K. (2013). Decolonizing our practice—Indigenizing our teaching. *First Nations Perspectives, 5*(1), 99–115.

Provincial Health Services Authority (PHSA) in British Columbia. (2019). *San'yas Indigenous cultural safety training.* Victoria, BC: PHSA in British Columbia. Retrieved from http://www.sanyas.ca/home

Reading, C. (2015). Structural determinants of Aboriginal peoples' health. In M. Greenwood, S. de Leeuw, N. M. Lindsay, & C. Reading (Eds.), *Determinants of Indigenous Peoples' health in Canada: Beyond the Social* (pp. 3–15). Toronto, ON: Canadian Scholars' Press.

Reading, C. L., & Wein, F. (2009). *Health inequalities and social determinants of Aboriginal Peoples' health.* Prince George, BC: NCCAH. Retrieved from https://www.ccnsa-nccah.ca/docs/determinants/RPT-HealthInequalities-Reading-Wien-EN.pdf

Registered Nurses' Association of Ontario (RNAO). (2013). *Fairer societies for better health equity.* Toronto, ON: RNAO. Retrieved from https://rnao.ca/sites/rnao-ca/files/Fairer_Societies_for_Better_Health_Equity_july_2013.pdf

Shah, C. P., & Reeves, A. (2012). Increasing Aboriginal cultural safety among health care practitioners. *Canadian Journal of Public Health, 103*(5), e397.

Statistics Canada. (2015). *Projections of the Aboriginal populations, Canada.* Ottawa, ON: Statistics Canada. Retrieved from https://www150.statcan.gc.ca/n1/pub/89-645-x/89-645-x2010001-eng.htm

Statistics Canada. (2018). *First Nations people, Métis and Inuit in Canada: Diverse and growing populations.* Ottawa, ON: Statistics Canada. Retrieved from https://www150.statcan.gc.ca/n1/pub/89-659-x/89-659-x2018001-eng.htm

Truth and Reconciliation Commission of Canada. (2015). *Calls to action.* Winnipeg, MB: Truth and Reconciliation Commission of Canada. Retrieved from http://trc.ca/assets/pdf/Calls_to_Action_English2.pdf

United Nations (UN). (2008). *United Nations declaration on the rights of Indigenous Peoples.* New York, NY: UN. Retrieved from https://www.un.org/esa/socdev/unpfii/documents/DRIPS_en.pdf

Varcoe, C. M., Wathen, C. N., Ford-Gilboe, M., Smye, V., & Browne, A. (2016). *VEGA briefing note on trauma- and violence-informed care.* Ottawa, ON: CIHR. Retrieved from https://vegaproject.mcmaster.ca/docs/default-source/pdf/briefing-note-trauma-and-violence-informed-care.pdf?sfvrsn=e9e58971_0

World Health Organization (WHO). (2010). *A conceptual framework for action on the social determinants of health. Social determinants of health discussion paper 2 (policy and practice).* Geneva, CH: WHO. Retrieved from https://www.who.int/sdhconference/resources/ConceptualframeworkforactiononSDH_eng.pdf

WHO. (2013). *Closing the health equity gap: Policy options and opportunities for action.* Geneva, CH: WHO. Retrieved from https://apps.who.int/iris/bitstream/handle/10665/78335/9789241505178_eng.pdf;jsessionid=4A631141B895A40A5C0F5FB8F0D6F9AF?sequence=1

Chapter 10

Inner-City Populations

Jennifer Beaveridge, Michelle Carter, and Angela Russolillo

JENNIFER BEAVERIDGE is a family nurse practitioner (NP), Regional Department Head and Director of Nurse Practitioners with Vancouver Coastal Health in North Vancouver, British Columbia. She has practiced in primary health care for 15 years with vulnerable and marginalized inner-city populations. Jennifer has a specialty practice with substance use disorder, HIV, hepatitis C, and gendering-affirming care. Jennifer is the Clinical Lead and Adjunct Professor for the family nurse practitioner program at the University of Northern British Columbia, Prince George, British Columbia, and Adjunct Professor at the University of British Columbia School of Nursing, Vancouver, British Columbia. She is a consultant for the BCCNP, including the NP licensing examinations and the NP quality assurance program.

MICHELLE CARTER is a clinical nurse specialist (CNS) in Psychiatry at St. Paul's Hospital, Vancouver, British Columbia. Her focus is on the development, implementation, and evaluation of evidence-based psychiatric care practices. In an effort to impact system-wide changes, she is often involved in the creation of interdisciplinary guidelines, care processes, education, quality improvement, and research. Michelle is also an Adjunct Professor at the University of British Columbia School of Nursing, Vancouver, British Columbia, and guest lectures on topics related to psychiatry and nursing leadership.

ANGELA RUSSOLILLO is a Practice Consultant with Providence Health Care, Vancouver, British Columbia. She has over a decade of nursing experience in both acute and community mental health. Currently, she works with local, regional, and provincial stakeholders to ensure policy and practice standards promote the provision of safe and ethical patient care. In addition to her clinical practice–oriented work, Angela's research focuses on health services use among people who are substance dependent, mentally ill, and who experience additional sources of hardship such as involvement with the criminal justice system or homelessness.

KEY TERMS

advanced practice nurses
  (APNs)
inner-city populations
social determinants of health
trauma-informed practice
urban health penalty

OBJECTIVES

1. Recognize, screen, and identify the factors that influence health and social outcomes for inner-city populations.
2. Identify the strategies, approaches, and frameworks that shape how advanced practice nurses (APNs) care for individuals with complex health challenges.
3. Understand the role of APNs working with inner-city populations.

Introduction

In the 21st century, cities play a dominant role in the day-to-day lives of individuals around the globe. Nearly 55% of the world's population resides in urban areas and this number is only expected to increase over the next three decades (United Nations [UN], 2018). Rapid population growth and urbanization are among the leading global trends that may have a significant impact on individual and population-level health (World Health Organization [WHO], 2010). Health and disease in urban populations have been the subject of considerable popular and scientific literature. Historically, perspectives on cities were that their size and density, combined with unplanned growth, result in exposures that produce excess morbidity and mortality (Vlahov, Galea, Gibble, & Freundeberg, 2005). Contemporary arguments associate cities with more favourable outcomes and advantages suggesting that urban living provides greater opportunities for wealth, social cohesion, access to health services, and reductions in health problems (Eckert & Kohler, 2014; Leon, 2008; Vlahov, Galea, & Freudenberg, 2005). Nevertheless, inner-city environments continue to threaten public health, including the rise of homelessness, mental illness, availability of illicit drugs, and the spread of infectious diseases along with other environmental risks, for example, pollution (Gruebner et al., 2017; Wasylenki, 2001). The purpose of this chapter is to provide an overview of the social, political, and economic factors associated with inner-city health and provide both practice and policy-level approaches to intervene and improve the health of individuals.

Inner-City Health in Canada

The health of **inner-city populations** has emerged as a central concern across Canada and represents both social and geographical constructs and social containers (Murphy, Fafard, & O'Campo, 2012) where many of the most harmful health inequities become evident (Vlahov, Boufford, Pearson, & Norris, 2010). A significant number of social, political, and economic disparities converge within cities (i.e., poverty, homelessness, food insecurity, racism) and create barriers to healthy and sustainable communities. There is little dispute that housing and health are inextricably linked. A number of Canadian cities struggle to provide adequate housing and to ensure that priority is given to the most vulnerable and marginalized members of society. People experiencing homelessness have shorter-than-average life expectancies (Hwang, Wilkins, Tjepkema, O'Campo, & Dunn, 2009), and their lives are threatened with morbidity rates that are dramatically higher than people living in secure housing (Aldridge et al., 2018; Fazel, Geddes, & Kushel, 2014). Homelessness and other risk factors (i.e., illicit drugs, food insecurity, pollution) are overrepresented in urban areas and require attention from health professionals because the inner-city environment influences all aspects of health across the lifespan.

Despite enormous advances in health and social programming, urban health inequalities continue to persist and the question of when and why actions are (or are not) taken is vital. Now more than ever there is an urgency to uncover the connections between health and inner cities, and **advanced practice nurses (APNs)** can play a key role in health care delivery with this population. Canadians over the past decade have witnessed numerous consequences resulting from the convergence of health and urban living. These issues range from the declaration of a public health emergency in 2016 in response to unprecedented mortality from opioids (Belzak & Halverson, 2018) to unparalleled damage resulting from global warming and a failure to acknowledge the human impact on climate change (Karl & Trenberth, 2003). Considerable pressure has been placed on the heads of government and policy-makers to intervene in a meaningful way to end these complex health issues. Unfortunately, policy action is often gradual and protracted, failing to provide timely solutions to evolving issues. In order to expedite action, it is essential to involve health professionals in preventing and reducing population-level health impacts, as well as providing primary health care needs associated with city and urban environments. We all live, work, and play in cities worldwide and need to advocate for the health and well-being of our communities.

Advanced Practice Nursing and Inner-City Populations

Both clinical nurse specialists (CNSs) and nurse practitioners (NPs), as APNs, play key roles in addressing the health care inequities in vulnerable inner-city populations, as well as increasing access to public and primary health care. Since its inception, the NP role has been addressing health care inequities in vulnerable and marginalized populations. NPs work to address health care disparities for inner-city populations at both the population and patient-specific levels through policy and direct patient care. The role of the NP includes diagnosing, treating, and managing acute, chronic, and complex health conditions. NPs bring expert knowledge, including a skill set that employs complex decision making, as well as the knowledge to address and identify population health care trends and create strategies to address the social determinants of health, health promotion, illness, and injury prevention (Canadian Nurses Association [CNA], 2010; International Council of Nurses [ICN], 2008).

NPs can be the most responsible provider (MRP) and are often the primary health care providers in inner-city settings. Across Canada, the scope of the NP role has grown over time, with the most recent changes to include prescribing controlled drugs and substances, opioid agonist therapies, and the ability to treat both human immunodeficiency virus (HIV) and hepatitis C. NPs can be flexible in where they deliver health care, including in-office or clinic, house calls, outreach services, and telehealth services.

The NP role, which combines the core values of nursing and medical knowledge, truly shines when working with both the social and medical complexities that are often disproportionately represented in inner-city populations. A study in Ontario identified 35% of family physician offices worked with unemployed populations compared to two-thirds of NPs working in community health centres, where more than 30% of clients were homeless, and over 50% of NPs were working in NP-Led Clinics (Koren, Mian, & Rukholm, 2010).

The CNS is uniquely positioned to analyze, synthesize, and apply research evidence to foster system-wide changes and APN. Drawing on their knowledge of research processes and methodologies, CNSs can not only develop critical research questions but can also translate findings into evidence-informed care (Bryant-Lukosius et al., 2010). In the context of urban health, there are several important concepts that have yet to be explored. For example, few studies have investigated the characteristics of urban contexts in relation to health or the ways in which these characteristics might be modifiable (Galea & Vlahov, 2005). Such findings have the potential to inform public policies that impact the social determinants of health, as well as clinical interventions that directly improve health care outcomes. As knowledge translators, CNSs can further integrate evidence into practice through the development of innovative care programs, clinical protocols, and nursing standards (Bryant-Lukosius et al., 2010).

Social Determinants of Health

The social determinants of health refer to the economic and social factors that impact health. These include access to care, gender, genetics, race and culture, employment, childhood experiences, social supports, physical living environments, health behaviours, literacy and education, as well as social status and income (Government of Canada, 2019; WHO, 2019). The WHO (2019) suggests that health is determined by one's circumstances and environment. Although many social determinants of health impact inner cities, the following are of relevance to APNs: housing, access to health and social services, and childhood development. The social determinants of health not only contribute to health care outcomes but also have a major impact on health expenditure. Inner-city populations often lack equitable access to the social determinants of health, resulting in poorer health care outcomes (Wasylenki, 2001). Addressing the social determinants can solve health inequities and improve individual and population health for inner cities.

Housing

On average, over 30,000 Canadians are homeless each night, with 2.3 million (8% of the population older than 15 years old) identifying that they have experienced homelessness at some time in their life (Rodrigue, 2016). In 2016, Statistics Canada released a study that identified contributing factors to homelessness as adverse childhood experiences, including physical and emotional abuse, disability, Indigenous identity, immigration, victims of crime, and those with weaker social networks (Rodrigue, 2016). The inner city has an above-average unemployment rate, workers making lower pay, people with disabilities who are living in poverty, and poor living and housing conditions (Wasylenki, 2001). It is imperative that APNs are aware of the populations most vulnerable to homelessness.

Those who are homeless or precariously housed have an increased risk of morbidity and mortality due to the social and health impacts of homelessness. Compared to those who have permanent housing, there is a substantial increase in mortality among those who are younger (Fazel, Geddes, & Kushel, 2014). The causes of the disproportionate mortality result from infectious diseases such as tuberculosis and HIV, chronic illnesses such as heart disease, substance-use disorders, suicides, injuries that are unintentional, overdose and poisoning, as well as homicides (Fazel, Geddes, & Kushel, 2014). Hwang and Burns (2014) identify six key health interventions that need to be targeted in order to address homelessness: (1) primary health care, (2) mental health care, (3) substance-use services, (4) medical respite programs, (5) homeless youth, and (6) supportive housing.

A systematic review conducted on housing interventions studies between 1887 and 2007 that were aimed at improving health care outcomes identified three main areas that can be addressed by housing: warmth, respiratory, and mental health conditions that have shown statistically significant outcomes (Thomson, Thomas, Sellstrom, & Petticrew, 2009). More recently Curl and Kearns (2015) identified that improvement and access to housing is more of a curative approach to health care outcomes than a prevention strategy. Although there is still evidence lacking on the benefits of health care outcomes from prevention, the evidence is clear that adequate housing can have a curative impact on health.

Access to Health Care and Social Services

Canada has over 4.8 million people who identify as being unattached and not receiving regular primary health care services (Statistics Canada, 2017). Ensuring equitable access to quality health care services is an important step in addressing health care disparities associated with social and economic status. Access to health care can be operationally defined as the actual use of health care services and any factors that may facilitate or impede service use (Andersen, Rice, & Kominski, 2001). This perspective encourages consideration of not only service availability but also variables that affect service uptake.

There is evidence suggesting that access to health care is not equitable across Canada. That is, those with higher socio-economic status have increased access for nearly every available health care service, while those from disadvantaged social groups are less likely to receive appropriate health care when required (Canadian Medical Association [CMA], 2013). A study in Ontario identified that those living in more influential, higher economic neighbourhoods had 45% shorter waiting times for coronary angiograms and a 23% higher rate of receiving the coronary angiogram (Alter, Naylor, Austin, & Tu, 1999). In the case of low-income urban areas, individuals are more likely to report difficulty securing appointments, less monitoring of chronic health conditions, and more hospitalizations for conditions that could be treated in primary health care (Bierman et al., 2010; CMA, 2013). Barriers to access in inner-city settings include lack of information about sources of care, concerns related to child care, perceived complexity around health care system organization, as well as challenges related to transportation and communication (House et al., 2000; Kalich, Heinemann, & Ghahari, 2015; Loignon et al., 2015a, 2015b).

Even when inner-city patients can find appropriate health care, the access to health care services may still be impeded and have barriers. Language difficulties, low health literacy, cultural differences, and discrimination by health care workers pose potential barriers to full patient engagement (Bierman et al., 2010). In working toward health care equity, we must look beyond service availability and consider individual characteristics (i.e., cultural beliefs, availability of child care, ability to pay for services/medications not covered by provincial plans), system factors (i.e., lack of primary health care provider, length of procedural wait-lists, attitudes of health care workers), and barriers that affect access to health care in inner cities (CMA, 2013).

Childhood Development

The development of a child is impacted by several factors, including their living environment, social supports, access to health care and prevention services, and adverse childhood experiences. Adverse childhood experiences (ACEs) include physical and emotional abuse, and household dysfunction experienced between the ages of 0–17 years (Brown et al., 2010; Felitti et al., 1998). The impact of ACEs has been well researched and has proven to have a significant impact on health care outcomes in adulthood. The higher the number of adverse experiences, the greater the risk of developing a chronic illness and disability later in life (Brown et al., 2010; Felitti et al., 1998).

Through increasing access to primary health care and public health services, children at risk can be identified earlier. APNs can screen for ACEs and identify at-risk children. The ACE screening tool is a simple questionnaire that APNs can utilize. It includes 10 questions related to an individual's exposure to adverse events in childhood, including verbal, emotional, and sexual abuse, as well as having divorced parents and living with someone with a mental health or substance abuse issue (Felitti et al., 1998). The questionnaire generates a score; the higher the score, the greater the likelihood of the individual experiencing poorer health care outcomes and inequities with the social determinants of health. The Centers for Disease Control and Prevention (CDC) states that one in six people screened will have more than four ACEs (CDC, 2019). Preventing ACEs health care outcomes could, for example, lead to the prevention of over 21 million cases of depression (CDC, 2019).

Overall, APNs are pivotal in addressing health inequities. Medicine focused on prevention through behaviour modification for groups that are at higher risk of poor health care outcomes; however, a paradigm shift is required to move from individual blame to addressing the environments impacting individuals. This could be achieved by creating equitable access to resources and support in order to address health care outcomes (Andermann, 2016). All health care providers require knowledge in the social determinants of health in order to truly impact health at an individual and population level.

Approaches to Inner-City Health Care

Many individuals living within an inner-city experience an **urban health penalty** due to high concentrations of poverty, unemployment, and exposure to unhealthy environments (Wasylenki, 2001). Since poor health tends to emerge from complex interactions between socio-economic factors, environment, and biology, multi-faceted strategies that extend beyond the traditional medical model are needed to improve individuals' health status. In this section, we discuss key approaches to inner-city health care at the patient, practice, and policy levels.

Philosophical Approaches

Improving inner-city health care equity and outcomes requires an underlying focus on patient-centred care. This philosophy takes into account the unique needs, values, and preferences of the individual and seeks to empower patients as experts in their own care (Mead & Bower, 2000). In practical terms, patient-centred care encourages clinicians to partner with patients in the co-design and delivery of individualized treatment that is both meaningful and realistic (Santana et al., 2018).

Patient-centred care is foundational to a number of important practice frameworks. In aiming to recognize and account for power imbalances and experiences of marginalization, **trauma-informed practice** has emerged as a particularly useful framework across urban health care settings. Trauma-informed practice is grounded in an understanding of, and responsiveness to, the pervasive and long-term impact of trauma on physical and mental health (Hopper, Bassuk, & Olivet, 2010). To provide health care that is trauma-informed, the entire system (i.e., environment, team, policies) must reflect an understanding of trauma in ways that promote recovery and avoid retraumatization (British Columbia Provincial Mental Health and Substance Use Planning Council, 2013). Although trauma-informed practice can be adapted to support specific clinical contexts, four core principles have been identified: trauma awareness; safety and trustworthiness; choice, control, and collaboration; and strengths and skill building (see Figure 10.1; Purkey, Patel, & Phillips, 2018). Implementation of these principles requires thoughtful review of multiple operational domains, including staff training, physical environment, care procedures, and program evaluation (British Columbia Provincial Mental Health and Substance Use Planning Council, 2013).

Harm reduction presents another critical approach to urban health as highlighted by the opioid crisis. Broadly defined, harm reduction refers to evidence-based, patient-centred interventions that aim to reduce the health and social harms of substance use without necessarily requiring abstinence (Hawk et al., 2017). Health care professionals who engage in harm reduction empower individuals with choice around health behaviours in order to enhance the knowledge and skills required to live safer and healthier lives (British Columbia Ministry of Health, 2005). Safe injection sites, needle exchange programs, overdose prevention sites, and opioid agonist therapy are examples of harm reduction strategies currently used in Canada.

FIGURE 10.1: Core Principles of Trauma-Informed Practice

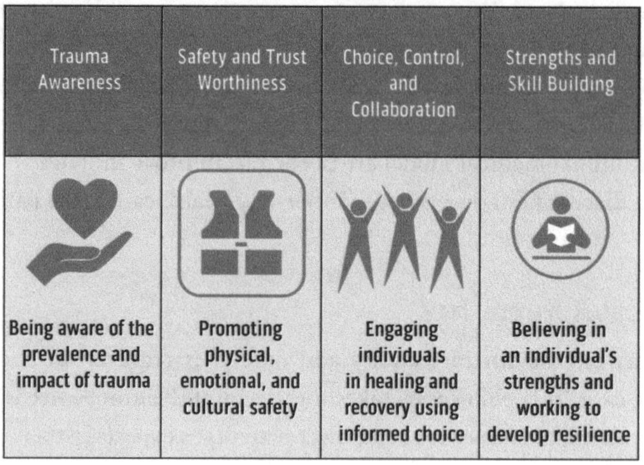

Trauma Awareness	Safety and Trust Worthiness	Choice, Control, and Collaboration	Strengths and Skill Building
Being aware of the prevalence and impact of trauma	Promoting physical, emotional, and cultural safety	Engaging individuals in healing and recovery using informed choice	Believing in an individual's strengths and working to develop resilience

Source: Adapted by Carter, M. (2020).

Patient Level

Building on the concept of patient-centred care, there is growing evidence to suggest that the quality of patient-provider relationships is crucial to effective treatment and improved health care outcomes, especially in vulnerable populations. Central to the development of strong therapeutic relationships is the clinician's ability to demonstrate "social competence" and adapt their practice to the social conditions of the person seeking health care (Loignon et al., 2015a, 2015b). At the patient level, this can take the form of assessing psychosocial challenges and facilitating access to support services (Andermann, 2016).

Assessing Psychosocial Challenges

Health care professionals working in inner-city communities should consider biomedical morbidity in the context of unique, and often complex, psychosocial circumstances. Along with clinical red flags and patient cues, there are several evidence-based tools to support the assessment of prevalent urban health such as unemployment and food insecurity and factors that can impede care such as low health literacy (Andermann, 2016). Of note, sensitive inquiry is significant in and of itself, that is, perceived provider compassion is positively correlated with both patient engagement and quality of health care (Goodrich & Cornwell, 2008).

Connecting Patients to Appropriate Resources

Once a social assessment has been made, providers can connect patients with key resources within and beyond the health care system. From medical specialists and housing organizations to school support and employment agencies, clinicians need to be familiar with the full range of health care and social programs available in their community or work closely with team members who have this expertise. Health care professionals can further assist individuals by advocating for, and facilitating access to, government benefits that may reduce social or economic strain, for example, low-cost daycare (Andermann, 2016).

Practice Level

Beyond patient-provider interactions, practice level interventions are important in improving inner-city health. The challenge in identifying practice strategies that broadly apply to inner-city communities lies in the scope of research conducted to date, which has largely focused on interventions aimed at specific patient populations (i.e., individuals who are homeless) or diseases (i.e., HIV). Reflecting a small sample of current evidence, Table 10.1

TABLE 10.1: Examples of Evidence-Informed Inner-City Interventions

Intervention Category	Key Points	Source(s)
Access to care	• Isolated and hard-to-reach patients benefit from integrated and proactive approaches to care delivery (i.e., assertive outreach, patient tracking, case managers). • Patient navigators—individuals who work with patients to help understand and manoeuvre through complex care systems—improve timely access to health services for vulnerable populations.	Freund, 2011; Hwang & Burns, 2014
Housing support	• Provision of housing (i.e., Housing First model) improves a range of health and social outcomes (i.e., increased housing tenure) for homeless populations, particularly among those experiencing mental illness and substance use disorders.	Hwang & Burns, 2014
Substance use care	• Methadone and buprenorphine, two forms of opioid replacement therapy, are effective for treating opioid dependency; however, methadone is more effective at retaining people in treatment. Supervised injectable opioid agonist therapy might be indicated for people refractory to standard treatment. • Supervised injection sites, where health care professionals provide harm reduction supplies and supervise drug consumption, reduce overdose deaths, ambulance call-outs, public injecting, and needle sharing.	British Columbia Centre on Substance Use & British Columbia Ministry of Health, 2017; Potier, Laprévote, Dubois-Arber, Cottencin, & Rolland, 2014
Infectious disease care	• Targeted screening in primary care, use of dried blood spot testing, and outreach improve uptake of hepatitis C virus testing. • HIV risk reduction interventions, including screening programs, psychosocial interventions (i.e., cognitive behavioural therapy), and opioid replacement therapy increase HIV testing uptake and decrease high-risk sexual and injecting behaviours.	Jones et al., 2013; Underhill, Dumont, & Operario, 2014

highlights empirical findings related to a few select social and health domains. The table is not exhaustive but instead provides practical examples of interventions that might apply to a variety of inner-city practice settings.

Policy Level

From a public health perspective, inner-city health policies should address social, economic, and health care inequities, while reflecting a systems approach, where interactions, both synergistic and antagonistic, between urban environment and individual well-being are carefully considered. While the scope of inner-city health care policy is expansive, most policies fall into one of three broad categories: improving physical environment; improving social environment; and improving access to quality health care services (Freudenberg, Galea, & Vlahov, 2006). Many policies operate directly within inner-city communities to improve living conditions, while others target higher levels of social organization to bring about new health care resources and services. Examples of Canadian policies that could potentially impact inner-city health include social assistance initiatives (i.e., the National Child Benefit) and criminal sentencing reform (Canadian Institute of Health Information [CIHI], 2006, 2008; Cook & Roesch, 2012).

Conclusion

Although the social determinants of health are not a new concept, they continue to contribute to health care and social inequities in inner-city populations. The intersections of poverty, unemployment, homelessness, and access to care play a critical role in the health of inner-city populations. APNs play an important role in addressing the barriers to health care services and reducing the inequities experienced by individuals and populations living in Canadian inner cities. From primary health care to policy and research, APNs influence health care outcomes across the lifespan. It's essential to further understand the relationship between the social determinants of health and the health of inner-city populations. Informed decision making alongside advocacy are fundamental to addressing the unique and often complex health care challenges facing individuals and communities within our cities.

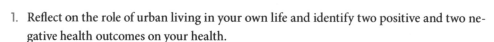

Critical Thinking Questions

1. Reflect on the role of urban living in your own life and identify two positive and two negative health outcomes on your health.
2. Explain the urban health penalty and its influence on contemporary health care and public policy.
3. Identify two research questions or quality improvement ideas that will improve health care for individuals impacted by homelessness, poverty, or addiction.

4. How does health care differ between rural and urban environments? As an APN, how would you describe your role in promoting health for individuals residing within large cities? What challenges might you encounter?
5. Design a health care intervention strategy targeted at reducing morbidity and mortality for homeless individuals.
6. What key impacts can APNs have on population health and addressing health care inequities with inner-city populations?

References

Aldridge, R., Story, A., Hwang, S., Nordentoft, M., Luchenski, S., Hartwell, G., ... Hayward, A. (2018). Morbidity and mortality in homeless individuals, prisoners, sex workers, and individuals with substance use disorders in high-income countries: A systematic review and meta-analysis. *The Lancet, 391*, 241–250.

Alter, D., Naylor, C., Austin, P., & Tu, J. (1999). Effects of socioeconomic status on access to invasive cardiac procedures and on mortality after acute myocardial infarction. *New England Journal of Medicine, 341*, 1359–1367. doi: 10.1056/NEJM199910283411806

Andermann, A. (2016). Taking action on the social determinants of health in clinical practice: A framework for health professionals. *Canadian Medical Association Journal, 188*(17–18), E474–E483. doi: 10.1503/cmaj.160177

Andersen, R. M., Rice, T. H., & Kominski, G. F. (2001). *Changing the U.S. health care system: Key issues in health services, policy, and management.* San Francisco, CA: Jossey-Bass.

Belzak, L., & Halverson, J. (2018). The opioid crisis in Canada: A national perspective [La crise des opioïdes au Canada : Une perspective nationale]. *Health Promotion and Chronic Disease Prevention in Canada: Research, Policy and Practice, 38*(6), 224–233. doi: 10.24095/hpcdp.38.6.02

Bierman, A. S., Johns, A., Hyndman, B., Mitchell, C., Degani, N., Shack, R. R., ... Parlette, V. (2010). *Ontario women's health equity report: Social determinants of health & populations at risk: Chapter 12.* Toronto, ON: ICES. Retrieved from http://www.powerstudy.ca/wp-content/uploads/downloads/2012/10/Chapter12-SDOHandPopsatRisk.pdf

British Columbia Centre on Substance Use & British Columbia Ministry of Health. (2017). *A guideline for the clinical management of opioid use disorder.* Victoria, BC: Government of British Columbia. Retrieved from https://www.bccsu.ca/wp-content/uploads/2017/06/BC-OUD-Guidelines_June2017.pdf

British Columbia Ministry of Health. (2005). *Harm reduction: A British Columbia community guide.* Victoria, BC: Government of British Columbia. Retrieved from https://www.health.gov.bc.ca/library/publications/year/2005/hrcommunityguide.pdf

British Columbia Provincial Mental Health and Substance Use Planning Council. (2013). *The trauma-informed practice guide.* Victoria, BC: Government of British Columbia. Retrieved from http://www.llbc.leg.bc.ca/public/pubdocs/bcdocs2017_2/682595/2013_tip-guide.pdf

Brown, D. W., Anda, R. F., Felitti, V. J., Edwards, V. J., Malarcher, A. M., Croft, J. B., & Giles, W. H. (2010). Adverse childhood experiences are associated with the risk of lung cancer: A prospective cohort study. *BioMed Central (BMC) Public Health, 10*(20), 1–12. doi: 10.1186/1471-2458-10-20

Bryant-Lukosius, D., Carter, N., Kilpatrick, K., Martin-Misener, R., Donald, F., Kaasalainen, S., ... DiCenso, A. (2010). The clinical nurse specialist role in Canada. *Nursing Leadership, 23*(Special Edition), 140–166.

Canadian Institute of Health Information (CIHI). (2006). *Improving the health of Canadians: An introduction to health in urban places.* Ottawa, ON: CIHI. Retrieved from https://secure.cihi.ca/free_products/PH_Full_Report_English.pdf

CIHI. (2008). *Reducing gaps in health: A focus on socio-economic status in urban Canada.* Ottawa, ON: CIHI. Retrieved from https://healthofficerscouncil.net/wp-content/uploads/2012/12/urban-health-officers-reducing_gaps_in_health_report_en_081009.pdf

Canadian Medical Association (CMA). (2013). *Ensuring equitable access to health care: Strategies for governments, planners and the medical profession.* Ottawa, ON: CMA. Retrieved from https://policybase.cma.ca/en/permalink/policy11062

Canadian Nurses Association (CNA). (2010). *Canadian nurse practitioner core competency framework.* Ottawa, ON: CNA. Retrieved from http://www.cno.org/globalassets/for/rnec/pdf/competencyframework_en.pdf

Centers for Disease Control and Prevention (CDC). (2019). *Preventing adverse childhood experiences.* Atlanta, GA: CDC. Retrieved from https://www.cdc.gov/violenceprevention/childabuseandneglect/aces/fastfact.html?CDC_AA_refVal=https%3A%2F%2Fwww.cdc.gov%2Fviolenceprevention%2Fchildabuseandneglect%2Facestudy%2Faboutace.html

Cook, A. N., & Roesch, R. (2012). "Tough on crime" reforms: What psychology has to say about the recent and proposed justice policy in Canada. *Canadian Psychology, 53*(3), 217.

Curl, A., & Kearns, A. (2015). Can housing improvements cure or prevent the onset of health conditions over time in deprived areas? *BioMed Central (BMC) Public Health, 15,* 1191. doi: 10.1186/s12889-015-2524-5

Eckert, S., & Kohler, S. (2014). Urbanization and health in developing countries: A systematic review. *World Health & Population, 15*(1), 7–20. doi: 10.12927/whp.2014.23722

Fazel, S., Geddes, J., & Kushel, M. (2014). The health of homeless people in high-income countries: Descriptive epidemiology, health consequences, and clinical and policy recommendations. *The Lancet, 384,* 1529–1540.

Felitti, V. J., Anda, R. F., Nordenberg, D., Williamson, D. F., Spitz, A. M., Edwards, V., ... Marks, J. (1998). Relationship of childhood abuse and household dysfunction to many of the leading causes of death in adults: The Adverse Childhood Experiences (ACE) study. *American Journal of Preventive Medicine, 14*(4), 245–258.

Freudenberg, N., Galea, S., & Vlahov, D. (2006). *Cities and the health of the public.* Nashville, TN: Vanderbilt University Press.

Freund, K. M. (2011). Patient navigation: The promise to reduce health disparities. *Journal of General Internal Medicine, 26*(2), 110–112.

Galea, S., & Vlahov, D. (2005). Urban health: Evidence, challenges, and directions. *Annual Review of Public Health, 26,* 341–365.

Goodrich, J., & Cornwell, J. (2008). *Seeing the person in the patient: The point of care review paper.* London, UK: The King's Fund. Retrieved from https://www.kingsfund.org.uk/sites/default/files/Seeing-the-person-in-the-patient-The-Point-of-Care-review-paper-Goodrich-Cornwell-Kings-Fund-December-2008.pdf

Government of Canada. (2019). *Social determinants of health and health inequalities.* Ottawa, ON: Government of Canada. Retrieved from https://www.canada.ca/en/public-health/services/health-promotion/population-health/what-determines-health.html

Gruebner, O., Rapp, M., Adli, M., Kluge, U., Galea, S., & Heinz, A. (2017). Cities and mental health. *Deutsches Arzteblatt International, 114*(8), 121–127.

Hawk, M., Coulter, R. W., Egan, J. E., Fisk, S., Friedman, M. R., Tula, M., & Kinsky, S. (2017). Harm reduction principles for healthcare settings. *Harm Reduction Journal, 14*(1), Article 70. https://doi.org/10.1186/s12954-017-0196-4

Hopper, E. K., Bassuk, E. L., & Olivet, J. (2010). Shelter from the storm: Trauma-informed care in homelessness services settings. *The Open Health Services and Policy Journal, 3*(1), 80–100.

House, J. S., Lepkowski, J. M., Williams, D. R., Mero, R. P., Lantz, P. M., Robert, S. A., & Chen, J. (2000). Excess mortality among urban residents: How much, for whom, and why? *American Journal of Public Health, 90*(12), 1898.

Hwang, S., Wilkins, R., Tjepkema, M., O'Campo, P., & Dunn, J. (2009). Mortality among residents of shelters, rooming houses, and hotels in Canada: 11-year follow-up study. *British Medical Journal, 339*(7729), 1068–1070.

Hwang, S. W., & Burns, T. (2014). Health interventions for people who are homeless. *The Lancet, 384*(9953), 1541–1547.

International Council of Nurses (ICN). (2008). *The scope of practice, standards and competencies of the advanced practice nurse.* Geneva, CH: ICN.

Jones, L., Bates, G., McCoy, E., Beynon, C., McVeigh, J., & Bellis, M. A. (2013). Effectiveness of interventions to increase hepatitis C testing uptake among high-risk groups: A systematic review. *The European Journal of Public Health, 24*(5), 781–788.

Kalich, A., Heinemann, L., & Ghahari, S. (2015). A scoping review of immigrant experience of health care access barriers in Canada. *Journal of Immigrant and Minority Health, 18*(3), 697–709.

Karl, T., & Trenberth, K. (2003). Modern global climate change. *Science, 302*(5651), 1719–1723.

Koren, I., Mian, O., & Rukholm, E. (2010). Integration of nurse practitioners into Ontario's primary health care system: Variations across practice settings. *Canadian Journal of Nursing Research, 42*(2), 48–69.

Leon, D. (2008). Cities, urbanization and health. *International Journal of Epidemiology, 37*(1), 4–8.

Loignon, C., Fortin, M., Bedos, C., Barbeau, D., Boudreault-Fournier, A., Gottin, T., … Haggerty, J. L. (2015a). Providing care to vulnerable populations: A qualitative study among GPs working in deprived areas in Montreal, Canada. *Family Practice, 32*(2), 232–236.

Loignon, C., Hudon, C., Goulet, É., Boyer, S., De Laat, M., Fournier, N., … Bush, P. (2015b). Perceived barriers to healthcare for persons living in poverty in Quebec, Canada: The EQUIhealThY project. *International Journal for Equity in Health, 14*(1), 4. doi: 10.1186/s12939-015-0135-5

Mead, N., & Bower, P. (2000). Patient-centredness: A conceptual framework and review of the empirical literature. *Social Science & Medicine, 51*(7), 1087–1110.

Murphy, K., Fafard, P., & O'Campo, P. (2012). Introduction-knowledge translation and urban health equity: Advancing the agenda. *Journal of Urban Health, 89*(6), 875–880.

Potier, C., Laprévote, V., Dubois-Arber, F., Cottencin, O., & Rolland, B. (2014). Supervised injection services: What has been demonstrated? A systematic literature review. *Drug and Alcohol Dependence, 145*, 48–68.

Purkey, E., Patel, R., & Phillips, S. P. (2018). Trauma-informed care: Better care for everyone. *Canadian Family Physician, 64*(3), 170–172.

Rodrigue, S. (2016). *Insights on Canadian society: Hidden homelessness in Canada.* Ottawa, ON: Statistics Canada. Retrieved from https://www150.statcan.gc.ca/n1/pub/75-006-x/2016001/article/14678-eng.htm

Santana, M. J., Manalili, K., Jolley, R. J., Zelinsky, S., Quan, H., & Lu, M. (2018). How to practice person-centred care: A conceptual framework. *Health Expectations, 21*(2), 429–440.

Statistics Canada. (2017). *Primary health care providers, 2016*. Ottawa, ON: Statistics Canada. Retrieved from https://www150.statcan.gc.ca/n1/pub/82-625-x/2017001/article/54863-eng.htm

Thomson, H., Thomas, S., Sellstrom, E., & Petticrew, M. (2009). The health impacts of housing improvement: A systematic review of intervention studies from 1887 to 2007. *American Journal of Public Health, 99*(3), 681–692. doi: 10.2105/AJPH.2008.143909

Underhill, K., Dumont, D., & Operario, D. (2014). HIV prevention for adults with criminal justice involvement: A systematic review of HIV risk-reduction interventions in incarceration and community settings. *American Journal of Public Health, 104*(11), e27–e53.

United Nations (UN). (2018). *World urbanization prospects*. New York, NY: UN. Retrieved from https://population.un.org/wup/Publications/Files/WUP2018-Report.pdf

Vlahov, D., Boufford, J. I., Pearson, C. E., & Norris, L. (Eds.). (2010). *Urban health: Global perspectives*. Indianapolis, IN: John Wiley & Sons.

Vlahov, D., Galea, S., & Freudenberg, N. (2005). The urban health "advantage." *Journal of Urban Health: Bulletin of the New York Academy of Medicine, 82*(1), 1–4.

Vlahov, D., Galea, S., Gibble, E., & Freudenberg, N. (2005). Perspectives on urban conditions and population health. *Cadernos De Saúde Pública, 21*(3), 949–957.

Wasylenki, D. (2001). Inner-city health. *Canadian Medical Association Journal, 164*(2), 214–215.

World Health Organization (WHO). (2010). Urbanization and health. *Bulletin of the World Health Organization, 88*(4), 241–320. Retrieved from https://www.who.int/bulletin/volumes/88/4/10-010410/en/

WHO. (2019). *The determinants of health*. Geneva, CH: WHO. Retrieved from https://www.who.int/hia/evidence/doh/en/

Chapter 11

Rural and Remote Populations

Mary Ellen Labrecque, Janet Luimes, and Brenda Mishak

MARY ELLEN LABRECQUE is an RN(NP) and Assistant Professor and Director, Nurse Practitioner Program in the College of Nursing at the University of Saskatchewan, Saskatoon, Saskatchewan. Her professional nursing practice experience includes acute, community, industrial, and tertiary care in urban, rural, and northern communities as an RN, CNS, and NP.

JANET LUIMES is an RN(NP) and Assistant Professor, Academic Programming in the College of Nursing at the University of Saskatchewan, Saskatoon, Saskatchewan. She has worked in a variety of professional settings, including acute care, telehealth, family practice, nursing education, and program planning and evaluation, in Ontario, Saskatchewan, and Alberta.

BRENDA MISHAK is an Assistant Professor in the College of Nursing at the University of Saskatchewan, Saskatoon, Saskatchewan. She has spent her professional career in primary health care in rural and northern communities as a public health nurse, nurse practitioner, and nursing administration.

KEY TERMS

advanced practice nurses (APNs)
advanced practice nursing (APN)
remoteness index (RI)
rural

OBJECTIVES

1. Define *rural* and describe rural populations in Canada.
2. Discuss the social determinants of health related to rural people, communities, and health care services.
3. Explore opportunities and challenges in rural practice.
4. Identify a "view to the future" of advanced practice nursing in rural settings.

Introduction

From a historical perspective, nurses can be credited with establishing health care services in **rural** and remote Canada (Kaasalainen et al., 2010). From the earliest federal and provincial records on the delivery of rural health care services, nurses are identified as providing care to people in the smallest and most remote communities in our country. With the development of the first community nursing positions, both in rural outposts and hospitals, nurses have been referred to as the "unsung heroes" (Waldram, Herring, & Young, 1995) who functioned in expanded **advanced practice nursing (APN)** roles, focused on meeting the needs of the populations served, and consistently advocated on issues related to the social determinants of health.

For all **advanced practice nurses (APNs)** providing care in geographically rural and remote communities, they need the ability to understand the context of health care services from the perspective of social determinants of health in order to address illness prevention and health promotion for rural populations. Living in a rural or remote setting in Canada places populations at a disadvantage predominantly in relation to access to health care, perspectives on confidentiality, and the limited use of technology to enhance rural health services.

This chapter will assist APNs in appreciating the interconnected elements of rural and remote geography as a social determinant of health.

Defining *Rural*

There is no definitive definition that has been used to describe or inform the concept of *rural* in Canada. *Rural* has been defined for statistical purposes by population divisions as a community with a population of less than 1,000, or in health research using a Statistics Canada definition of *rural and small town* (du Plessis, Beshiri, Bollman, & Clemenson, 2001) as "communities with a core population of less than 10,000 people, where less than 50% of the employed population commutes to larger urban centers for work" (MacLeod et al., 2017, p. 3). While there are multiple definitions of *rural*, Reimer and Bollman (2010) identify that there are two commonalities in most efforts to define *rural*: geographical locations with low population density and lengthy distances to higher population densities.

Literature on the concept of *rural* identifies that objectivity and subjectivity are associated with the term (Kulig & Williams, 2011). Research describing the meaning of *rural* has explored the perspectives of people in rural communities, health care providers, and health researchers. Understandably, the differing perspectives are as varied as the geographical and population diversity that spans the country. In general, people who live in rural areas have been reported to describe *rural* in terms of their relationships in and with the community, land, and location. Health care providers tend to focus on availability of health services resources, and health researchers and policy-makers on the intersection of living rural and health.

From a Canadian nursing perspective, registered nurses (RNs) and nurse practitioners (NPs) who participated in a national study on practice in rural and remote Canada were asked to define *rural* (Kulig et al., 2008). Results of the thematic analysis indicated that nurses who work in rural settings described their practice by the characteristics and geographical area of their communities, health care resources, and rural nursing practice. Community characteristics most often depicted differences between rural and urban economy, transportation, and availability of retail stores. Responses also defined *rural communities* in terms of strong, positive, and supportive interpersonal relationships. Geographical descriptions provided by these rural nurses were synonymous with definitions in the literature about population density and distance from urban centres. One unique characteristic was the inclusion of rural as including living on small islands, often not considered in rural descriptions in Canada, and the additional challenges in accessing health care services.

Access to health care resources were also described by the nurse participants in a similar manner to reports on limitations of rural health services (Kulig et al., 2008): communities at a distance from large urban centres; scarce resources for diagnostic, emergency, and specialty services; and dependence on medical evacuation by airplane or poorly maintained rural roads. In creating a descriptive definition of *rural*, these nurses focused on practice differences and suggested that increased autonomy and responsibility were an inherent part of being a first-line rural health care provider. Additionally, the literature supports the rural nurses in defining their practice by the type of skills they needed to develop, such as how to communicate patient presentations over the telephone when attempting to access support from specialists and emergency services at a distance to their communities (i.e., physician consultation by phone). Combined with the common practice of providing care to family, friends, and neighbours, one of the many elements that can contribute to professional ethical dilemmas and personal challenges is the provision of care to a rural population (Kulig et al., 2008), and descriptions of rural nursing practice support rural and urban differences and how entry-level competencies are enacted.

A newer approach to exploring geography in relation to health is the Remoteness Index (RI; Alasia, Bédard, Bélanger, Guimond, & Penney, 2017). Developed by Statistics Canada researchers, census subdivisions were designated as having levels of remoteness that respond to distance from population centres over 1,000 and the population of the community. The index is a scale that can also be sectioned into categories for population and designation as rural, remote, and urban. Researchers used the RI to investigate the relationship between causes of mortality and the distance of rural communities to larger centres (Subedi, Greenberg, & Roshanafshar, 2019). Findings from this study suggested that remoteness of a community is positively associated with increasing rates of preventable and treatable mortality (i.e., ischemic heart disease, breast and colorectal cancers) and decreased access to facilities and resources to provide health care services to address causes of mortality. Most often, distance to services, or increasing RI, was an important link in causes of mortality.

These definitions and indexes of rural and remote are important aspects of rural that need to be considered by APNs. In working within small rural communities, it is important that APNs understand the history and context of the origins and health care services management of their community; develop a network of interprofessional colleagues and resources for consultation and referral; maintain a list of regional resources; and collaborate with community members to explore their perception on services that align with local cultural beliefs on health and illness.

Rural Populations

Numerous studies have identified that rural populations have access to fewer health care resources and have a health status lower than urban populations (Aalhus, Oke, & Fumerton, 2018; Pong, DesMeules, & Lagace, 2009). Health care financial resources are commonly designated based on population size and the need to locate specialized diagnostic services in urban centres. It is well known that the number of health care resources and services are incrementally associated with increased health status. Presumably, decentralizing health care resources and services would increase the accessibility for rural people and improve their health status. Considering that the population of rural people has a large involvement in economic and agricultural resource development in Canada (Canadian Rural Revitalization Foundation [CRRF], 2015), ideally an investment in the health of rural people can also be seen as an investment in rural industry and food production, which is important to the overall health of the country.

Analysis of the Canadian population statistics identifies that approximately 81% of the population resides in urban settings (Piecher, 2019), in relative proximity to the Canadian–United States border. The remaining 19% of the population are spread over the large expanse of land across all provinces and territories. The CRRF (2015) documents an example of the rural nature of Canada in the description of Saskatchewan as having the most rural roads per person of any region, nationally and internationally, in the world (Stewart, 2006). This network of rural roads provides avenues for rural people to access larger centres for health care services and emergency transportation. However, access to emergency care involves time and travel over long distances, which can negatively impact health outcomes. In the province of Saskatchewan, the benefit of a large network of rural highways also provides a level of risk, as the province has high rates of collisions and fatalities on rural roadways (Saskatchewan Government Insurance, 2019).

Rural populations are as culturally diverse as the expansive Canadian geography. The most recent immigration statistics indicate that in rural areas there is an increasing immigrant and newcomer population (Carter, Morrish, & Amoyaw, 2008). Although immigrant populations are considering rural and remote communities in Canada as potential locations for residing, a scoping review by Patel, Dean, Edge, Wilson, and Ghassemi (2019) suggests that living rural for immigrant populations involved social determinants of health (i.e., cultural services, employment, and social inclusion) that differ in degree of influence in comparison to other rural residents.

Social Determinants of Health and Rural Populations

The World Health Organization (WHO; 2020) has stated the social determinants of health are the conditions in which people are born, grow, live, work, and age as well as the systems and forces that shape daily life. Systems and forces include economics, social policy, social norms, and politics (WHO, 2020). Raphael (2016), a prominent Canadian author and expert on the social determinants of health, provides high-quality evidence to support the social determinants as having a greater influence on health and incidence of illness than traditional biomedical and behavioural risk factors. According to Raphael (2016), the social determinants of health must meet four criteria: (1) be important to the health of Canadians, (2) be understandable to Canadians, (3) have clear policy relevance to Canadian decision makers and citizens, and (4) be especially timely and relevant. He identifies the following 16 social determinants of health: "Indigenous ancestry, disability, early life, education, employment and working conditions, food security, gender, geography, health care services, housing, im-migrant status, income and its distribution, race, social safety net, social exclusion[/inclusion], and unemployment and employment security" (2016, p. 11).

The social determinants of health are primary drivers of health care inequalities, including differences in health status seen between rural and urban communities. Rural communities generally experience poorer health outcomes than urban communities, making them a vulnerable or an at-risk population (Aalhus et al., 2018; Pong et al., 2009). Rural Canadians are more likely to live in poorer socio-economic conditions, have lower education, exhibit less healthy behaviours (for example, higher smoking rates), and have higher overall mortality rates than urban residents (Aalhus et al., 2018; DesMeules & Pong, 2006; Pong et al., 2009, 2011). Additional health disparities for rural residents include potential for fewer social, educational, and employment opportunities; less choices and access to healthy food options; and increased vulnerability to chronic disease such as cancer, cardiovascular disease, respiratory disease, and mental health and substance abuse disorders (Aalhus et al., 2018; Pong et al., 2009). DesMeules et al. (2011) report rural residents have increased mortality rates from circulatory disease, injury, and suicide when compared to urban populations. More rural and remote residents self-report poor or fair for their health status, activity limitations, and living with disabilities (Pong et al., 2011).

There are unique challenges to delivery of health care in rural and remote communities. Many of these challenges relate to poor access due to isolated geographical locations and low population densities. Limited availability of health care providers, hospitals, primary care clinics, and public transportation all negatively impact timely access to health care for acute, chronic, and preventative care visits. Limited laboratory, diagnostic imaging, counselling, physiotherapy, home care, and other services, all of which could be recommended to optimize patient care, can further result in delayed detection and treatment of disease compromising health outcomes (Mattos et al., 2019).

Rural residents have identified lack of access to public transportation and the need to travel longer distances as a barrier to health care and their social supports (Mattos et al., 2019; Pong et al., 2011). Connecting with community and family has been identified as an important part of quality of life for rural residents (Mattos et al., 2019). However, this benefit of forming close community ties is changing as more rural youth migrate to urban centres (i.e., an increase in the need for reliable transportation and the ability to travel; Patel et al., 2019) and rural public transportation options deteriorate (i.e., bus services). Without transportation options, there is inherit risk of social isolation imposed by rural geography.

Some of the notable concerns for rural women involve travel to access urban childbirth facilities (Health Canada, 2017). Historical provincial and federal health services policies on transportation assistance to hospitals for childbirth have been less than beneficial for women and their families. Recent changes to these policies, supporting the provision of fathers or a family member/friend to accompany pregnant women, have been long overdue. For rural mothers, limited rural childbirth options impact the entire rural family unit, when mothers leave the community and families need to arrange alternate care during their absence. As most women are encouraged to travel to an urban community at 38 weeks of gestation, family units can be disrupted for a few weeks prior to confinement. Although this has been the normal pathway to childbirth for rural women and families, it is strikingly different than the experiences of urban women and families. Other differences include access to specialty obstetrical services for women with health challenges in pregnancy (i.e., gestational diabetes, pre-eclampsia, and developmental concerns). If health challenges present in pregnancy, the financial implications for families increase with additional travel to urban appointments or a prolonged hospital admission. Such additional financial strains on rural families can cloud the excitement that commonly surrounds the birth of a child.

Residents of urban and rural communities show marked differences in their access to and use of health services. For instance, hospitalization rates rise with increasing degree of rurality, but average lengths of hospital stays decrease. Pong et al. (2011) identified that greater proportions of rural residents reported receiving care in emergency departments or outpatient clinics. The use of emergency services is influenced by many factors, including culture, education, finances, and public policy.

When examining culture, it is also important to consider that rural communities often have a higher proportion of Indigenous Peoples who experience significant health disparities when compared to non-Indigenous people (Pong et al., 2011). Indigenous Peoples experience higher rates of infant and child mortality; maternal morbidity and mortality; preventable chronic diseases; interpersonal violence, homicide, and suicide; and shortened life expectancy (National Collaborating Centre for Aboriginal Health [NCCAH], 2013). The health inequities experienced by Indigenous Peoples are rooted in a history of colonization and the social determinants of health.

Health Care in Rural Communities

Barriers and facilitators of rural APNs are like urban concerns where physician, government policies, and public support are the primary drivers and roadblocks to optimal ANP integration (Alden-Bugden, 2019). However, rural APNs also face unique barriers related to limited resource availability: they are often required to do more with less, managing the health care needs of entire communities with limited access to nearby diagnostic services or specialist consultants.

As identified by Kulig et al. (2008), other unique challenges for health care providers in rural communities commonly include the provision of care for people they know (i.e., friends and neighbours) because they are one of few providers in the community. Consequently, resulting professional ethical dilemmas may ensue. For example, a patient may visit the off-duty NP's home seeking medical attention or ask about medical test results when they run into a provider at a public venue such as the community arena. Privacy and confidentiality also present unique challenges in rural settings due to the closeness of the communities, overlapping roles of community members, and the fact that residents are often aware of the intimate details of their neighbours' lives (Werth, Hastings, & Riding-Malon, 2010). For instance, a community member may notice their neighbour's vehicle in the health clinic parking lot and inquire if their neighbour is having health difficulties. When caring for vulnerable

populations, such as those with mental health, addictions, LGBTQ2, or end-of-life care, special consideration for privacy and confidentiality is paramount. A breach in confidentiality
or privacy for such patients not only threatens their future utilization of health services but
may negatively impact their health status.

There has been little research done in the area of ethical considerations when providing
care in rural communities. Roberts, Battaglia, and Epstein (1999) reported the following factors intensified ethical dilemmas for health care providers in rural settings: overlapping relationships; conflicting roles; altered therapeutic boundaries between caregivers, patients, and
families; challenges in preserving patient confidentiality; heightened cultural dimensions of
mental health care; limited resources; and greater stresses experienced by rural caregivers.
The Canadian Nurses Association's Code of Ethics for Registered Nurses (2017) provides useful guidance for all RNs and NPs on navigating ethical dilemmas, including privacy, confidentiality, boundaries, and resource availability. It is also important for providers to be aware
of legal and regulatory parameters, and how these interact with the Code of Ethics.

Entry-Level Rural Competencies for Advanced Practice Nursing

The scope of practice for rural APNs differs significantly from urban practice. In key national
studies on rural nursing practice in Canada (MacLeod et al., 2004, 2017; MacLeod, Kulig,
& Stewart, 2019), researchers reported that rural nurses described their practice as crossing
multiple clinical areas within the context of a day of work. These included teaching crutch
walking to managing labour and delivery to caring for acutely ill patients requiring medical
evacuation to a trauma centre (MacLeod et al., 2019). One of the challenges for APN education programs has been the preparation of nurses for practice in rural communities. Health
care educational programs often have an urban-centric approach to content and delivery
of education. Many of the students who enrol in NP programs obtain work in large urban
centres. The challenge for educators is not to overlook a focus on rural practice and the effect
of diversity in federal, provincial, and regional governmental involvement in health care organizations, policies, and settings where APNs are employed.

There are few nursing or APN education programs in Canada that include an emphasis on rural practice (Zimmer et al., 2014). Within the diversity of NP education programs,
students may not have the opportunity to experience a rural clinical setting. The delivery
of education focused on the application of competencies for positions in resource-scarce
rural geographical locations is important to prepare NPs for rural practice settings. The
rural health services workforce has embraced NPs as essential members of health care teams.
Although integration of NPs into rural health care systems differs across provincial boundaries, the limited health human resources available in rural communities can be suggested as
benefiting from increased access to acute and primary health care with the expansion in the
scope of practice of NPs.

Knowledge gained through APN educational programs about evidence-informed assessment, diagnosis, and management of common medical conditions often does not consider

the limited resources available in rural health care facilities. Therefore, the application of clinical knowledge in the provision of care for patients in a rural community is not operationalized in the same manner as when providing care in urban settings. For example, patients seen in a remote area clinic for a chronic condition may need the lifestyle education and support provided by the NP versus referral to an urban chronic disease management program. In rural acute care settings, management of acute complications of chronic illnesses may lead to patient transfers, by road or air, to larger centres to access diagnostic procedures unavailable in rural communities. The process for patient transfers, or the method of collaboration for patient transfers, differs depending on the geographical and policy barriers (i.e., crossing provincial boundaries) that may hinder access to resources in large urban settings.

The entry-level competencies for APNs have limited focus on disaster nursing as an element of education for rural or urban practice (Canadian Council Registered Nurse Regulators [CCRNR], 2012). As the numbers of natural disasters are increasing (Mehrabi et al., 2019; Wahlstrom & Guha-Sapir, 2015), nurses in Canada need to understand their role in disaster planning, preparedness, operations, and review. Natural disasters—such as forest fires, storm floods, droughts, earthquakes, and extreme temperatures—have become more common. However, there are few APN programs that reportedly include information about disaster planning and operations (Kulig et al., 2017).

For rural APNs, education and participation in disaster preparedness and planning should be an integral aspect of nursing employment. The International Council of Nurses (ICN) has recently updated nursing competencies on disaster nursing (2019). The document identifies that nurses provide essential services in interprofessional teams when responding to disasters. In developing competencies for disasters, nursing professional associations need to support the integration of knowledge about disaster response and ensure that nurses can obtain training and ongoing refresher courses with mock disaster events to ensure they are open to taking leadership opportunities.

To date, there have been few Canadian studies on disaster nursing, but Kulig et al. (2017) explored rural nurses' experiences with disasters. They identified that few NPs reported assisting with a disaster event, and participation in disaster events was linked to length of time practicing in rural settings, distance from a major centre, and engagement in their community. Importantly, the experience of involvement in disaster events was not found to be supported with debriefing, which may affect their mental health and well-being given their connection to the community and potentially witnessing the effects of the disaster on family and friends.

The Future of Rural Advanced Practice Nursing

Telehealth has the potential to bridge geographical barriers to accessing health care services, benefiting health outcomes, and reducing expenditures (Jong, Mendez, & Jong, 2019). The words *telehealth, telemedicine, telenursing,* and *e-health* are often used interchangeably. According to the WHO, telehealth is used to connect patients to health care providers over geographical distances. Utilizing telehealth facilitates assessment, diagnosis, and development of treatment plans in patient care without the need for patient travel to providers or specialists. Telehealth also facilitates rural research, continuing education, and interprofessional care (WHO, 2016).

Telehealth has been effectively implemented in various rural and remote locations in Canada with success in reducing acute medical transfers (Canadian Agency for Drugs and Technologies in Health [CADTH], 2016; Mendez, Jong, Keays-White, & Turner, 2013), facilitating access to chronic disease specialists (CADTH, 2016; Jong & Kraishi, 2004), providing mental health services (Jong, 2004), providing oversight of advanced life support (Jong, 2010), facilitating point-of-care ultrasound (Jong et al., 2019), and facilitating access to allied health professions such as dieticians, speech language pathology, and physiotherapy (Jong et al., 2019).

Patients have reported positive experiences with the use of telehealth, including more timely access to health care, decreased burden of travel and related expenses, as well as enhanced social support by being able to stay closer to home (Jong et al., 2019; Nasser & Chen, 2014). Rural health care providers also benefit from telehealth through the collaborative support offered and opportunities for continuing education. However, telehealth continues to be underutilized (Jong et al., 2019; Nasser & Chen, 2014). With advancing technology, limitations such as unreliable or unavailable broad bandwidth are no longer the primary barrier to utilization of telehealth. Rather, practitioner reluctance and unfamiliarity with telehealth equipment, associated costs of the technology, and limitations in remuneration for providers using this technology are likely inhibiting realizing the full potential telehealth can offer rural and remote communities (Bradford, Caffery, & Smith, 2016) and APNs to reduce barriers to care. It will be interesting to reflect on the experience of coronavirus disease 2019 (COVID-19) and the long-term implementation of this advancing technology.

Conclusion

Throughout this chapter, information was presented to assist APNs in appreciating the interconnected elements of rural geography as a social determinant of health. People living in rural communities in Canada have lower health status than urban populations, and APNs in rural settings need to make themselves aware of the health challenges in the local rural populations where they are employed. For APNs, providing care in geographically rural communities encompasses building an understanding of the historical context of access to health care services, perspectives on confidentiality, and advancing the use of technology to find potential avenues to enhance the health of the population through health promotion and prevention strategies.

Critical Thinking Questions

1. How does geography affect NP practice in rural settings?
2. Rural communities are culturally diverse. How would cultural diversity of communities influence how care is delivered in rural settings?
3. What are the differences between primary care and acute care NP practice in urban and rural settings?

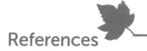

References

Aalhus, M., Oke, B., & Fumerton, R. (2018). *The social determinants of health of resource extraction and development in rural and northern communities: A summary of impacts and promising practices for assessment and monitoring.* British Columbia Observatory Population & Public Health and BC Centre for Disease Control. Retrieved from https://www.northernhealth.ca/sites/northern_health/files/services/office-health-resource-development/documents/impacts-promising-practices-assessment-monitoring.pdf

Alasia, A., Bédard, F., Bélanger, J., Guimond, E., & Penney, C. (2017). *Measuring remoteness and accessibility: A set of indices for Canadian communities.* Ottawa, ON: Statistics Canada. Retrieved from https://www150.statcan.gc.ca/n1/pub/18-001-x/18-001-x2017002-eng.htm

Alden-Bugden, D. (2019). The role and scope of the NP in Canada. *The Nurse Practitioner, 44*(9), 8–10.

Bradford, N. K., Caffery, L. J., & Smith, A. C. (2016). Telehealth services in rural and remote Australia: A systematic review of models of care and factors influencing success and sustainability. *Rural Remote Health, 16*(4), 3808.

Canadian Agency for Drugs and Technologies in Health (CADTH). (2016). *Telehealth: Summary of evidence.* Ottawa, ON: CADTH. Retrieved from https://www.cadth.ca/sites/default/files/pdf/telehealth_bundle.pdf

Canadian Council of Registered Nurse Regulators (CCRNR). (2012). *Competencies in the context of entry-level registered nurse practice.* Beaverton, ON: CCRNR. Retrieved from http://www.ccrnr.ca/assets/jcp_rn_competencies_2012_edition.pdf

Canadian Nurses Association (CNA). (2017). *Code of ethics for registered nurses.* Ottawa, ON: CNA.

Canadian Rural Revitalization Foundation (CRRF). (2015). *State of rural Canada: 2015.* Retrieved from http://sorc.crrf.ca/

Carter, T., Morrish, M., & Amoyaw, B. (2008). Attracting immigrants to smaller urban and rural communities: Lessons learned from the Manitoba Provincial Nominee Program. *Journal of International Migration and Integration, 9*, 161–183.

DesMeules, M., & Pong, R. (2006). *How healthy are rural Canadians? An assessment of their health status and health determinants.* Canadian Institute for Health Information and Public Health Agency of Canada. Retrieved from https://secure.cihi.ca/free_products/rural_canadians_2006_report_e.pdf

DesMeules, M., Pong, R., Read Guernsey, J., Wang, F., Luo, W., & Dressler, M. P. (2011). Rural health status and determinants in Canada. In J. C. Kulig & A. M. Williams (Eds.), *Rural health status and determinants in Canada* (pp. 23–46). Vancouver, BC: UBC Press.

du Plessis, V., Beshiri, R., Bollman, R. D., & Clemenson, H. (2001). Definitions of rural. *Rural and Small Town Canada Bulletin, 3*(30), 1–17. Catalogue no. 21-006-XIE. Ottawa, ON: Statistics Canada.

Health Canada. (2017). *Medical transportation benefits information.* Ottawa, ON: Government of Canada. Retrieved from https://www.canada.ca/en/health-canada/services/first-nations-inuit-health/noninsured-health-benefits/benefits-information/medical-transportation-benefits-information-first-nations-inuit-health.html

International Council of Nurses (ICN). (2019). *Core competencies in disaster nursing: Version 2.0.* Geneva, CH: ICN.

Jong, M. (2004). Managing suicides via videoconferencing in a remote northern community in Canada. *International Journal of Circumpolar Health, 63*(4), 422–428.

Jong, M. (2010). Resuscitation by video in northern communities. *International Journal of Circumpolar Health, 69*(5), 519–527.

Jong, M., & Kraishi, M. (2004). A comparative study on the utility of telehealth in the provision of rheumatology services to rural and northern communities. *International Journal of Circumpolar Health, 53*(4), 415–421.

Jong, M., Mendez, I., & Jong, R. (2019). Enhancing access to care in northern rural communities via telehealth. *International Journal of Circumpolar Health, 78*(2), 1554174. doi: 10.1080/22423982.2018.1554174

Kaasalainen, S., Martin-Misener, R., Kilpatrick, K., Harbman, P., Bryant-Lukosius, D., Donald, F., … DiCenso, A. (2010). A historical overview of the development of advanced practice nursing roles in Canada. *Nursing Leadership, 23*(Special Issue), 35–60.

Kulig, J., Penz, K., Karunanayake, C., MacLeod, M., Jahner, S., & Andrews, M. (2017). Experiences of rural and remote nurses assisting with disasters. *Australian Emergency Nursing Journal, 20*(2), 98–106.

Kulig, J. C., Andrews, M. E., Stewart, N. J., Pitblado, R., MacLeod, M. L. P., Bentham, D., … Smith, B. (2008). How do registered nurses define rurality? *Australian Journal of Rural Health, 16*(1), 28–32. doi.org/10.1111/j.1440-1584.2007.00947.x

Kulig, J. C., & Williams, A. M. (Eds.) (2011). *Health in rural Canada.* Vancouver, BC: UBC Press.

MacLeod, M., Kulig, J., & Stewart, N. (May, 2019). Lessons on twenty years of research on nursing practice in rural and remote Canada. *Canadian Nurse.* Retrieved from https://www.canadian-nurse.com

MacLeod, M. L. P., Kulig, J. C., Stewart, N. J., Pitblado, J. R., & Knock, M. (2004). The nature of nursing practice in rural and remote Canada. *Canadian Nurse, 100*(6), 27–31.

MacLeod, M. L. P., Stewart, N. J., Kulig, J. C., Anguish, P., Andrews, M. E., Banner, D., … Zimmer, L. (2017). Nurses who work in rural and remote communities in Canada: A national survey. *Human Resources for Health, 15*(34). doi: 10.1186/s12960-017-0209-0

Mattos, M. K., Burke, L. E., Baernholdt, M., Hu, L., Nilsen, M. L., & Lingler, J. H. (2019). Perceived social determinants of health among older, rural-dwelling adults with early-stage cognitive impairment. *Dementia, 18*(3), 920–935. https://doi.org/10.1177/1471301217694250

Mehrabi, Z., Donner, S. D., Rios, P., Guha-Sapir, D., Rowhani, P., Kandlikar, M., & Ramankutty, N. (2019). Can we sustain success in reducing deaths to extreme weather in a hotter world? *World Development Perspectives, 14.* http://dx.doi.org/10.14288/1.0378870

Mendez, I., Jong, M., Keays-White, D., & Turner, G. (2013). The use of remote presence for health care delivery in a northern Inuit community: A feasibility study. *International Journal of Circumpolar Health, 72.* doi: 10.3402/ijch.v72i0.21112

Nasser, A., & Chen, N. (2014). Telehealth in rural Canada. Successes and challenges. *University of Western Ontario Medical Journal, 83*(1), 49–50. Retrieved from http://www.uwomj.com/wp-content/uploads/2014/10/v82no1_16.pdf

National Collaborating Centre for Aboriginal Health (NCCAH). (2013). *An overview of Aboriginal health in Canada.* Ottawa, ON: Public Health Agency of Canada. Retrieved from https://www.ccn-sa-nccah.ca/docs/context/FS-OverviewAbororiginalHealth-EN.pdf

Patel, A., Dean, J., Edge, S., Wilson, K., & Ghassemi, E. (2019). Double burden of rural migration in Canada? Considering the social determinants of health related to immigrant settlement outside the cosmopolis. *International Journal of Environmental Research and Public Health, 16*(5), E678. doi: 10.3390/ijerph16050678

Piecher, H. (2019). *The urbanization of Canada 2018.* London, UK: Statista. Retrieved from https://www.statista.com/statistics/271208/urbanization-in-canada/#statisticContainer

Pong, R., DesMeules, M., & Lagace, C. (2009). Rural-urban disparities in health: How does Canada fare and how does Canada compare with Australia? *Australian Journal of Rural Health, 17*(1), 25–64.

Pong, R. W., DesMeules, M., Heng, D., Lagace, C., Guernsey, J. R., Kazanjian, A., ... Luo, W. (2011). Patterns of health services utilization in rural Canada. *Chronic Diseases and Injuries in Canada, 31*(Supplement 1), 1–36.

Raphael, D. (2016). *Social determinants of health: Canadian perspectives* (3rd ed.). Toronto, ON: Canadian Scholars' Press.

Reimer, B., & Bollman, R. D. (2010). Understanding rural Canada: Implications for rural development policy and rural planning policy. In D. Douglas (Ed.), *Rural planning and development in Canada* (pp. 10–52). Toronto, ON: Nelson Education.

Roberts, L. W., Battaglia, J., & Epstein, R. S. (1999). Frontier ethics: Mental health care needs and ethical dilemmas in rural communities. *Psychiatric Services, 50*(4), 497–503. doi: 10.1176/ps.50.4.497

Saskatchewan Government Insurance. (2019). *2018 Saskatchewan traffic collisions report.* Regina, SK: Saskatchewan.ca.

Stewart, I. (2006). "Municipal road network." In *Encyclopedia of Saskatchewan.* Regina, SK: Canadian Rural Revitalization Foundation.

Subedi, R., Greenberg, T. L., & Roshanafshar, S. (2019). Does geography matter in mortality? An analysis of potentially avoidable mortality by remoteness index in Canada. *Health Report, 30*(5), 3–15. doi: 10.25318/82-003-x201900500001-eng

Wahlstrom, M., & Guha-Sapir, D. (2015). *The human cost of weather related disasters, 1995–2015.* Geneva, CH: Centre for Research on the Epidemiology of Disasters.

Waldram, J. B., Herring, A., & Young, T. K. (1995). *Aboriginal health in Canada.* Toronto, ON: Oxford University Press.

Werth, J. L., Hastings, S. L., & Riding-Malon, R. (2010). Ethical challenges in practicing in rural areas. *Journal of Clinical Psychology, 66*(5), 537–548. https://doi.org/10.1002/jclp.20681

World Health Organization (WHO). (2016). *Global diffusion of ehealth: Making universal health coverage achievable.* Geneva, CH: WHO.

WHO. (2020). *Social determinants of health.* Geneva, CH: WHO. Retrieved from https://www.who.int/social_determinants/sdh_definition/en/

Zimmer, L. V., Banner, D., Aldiabat, K., Keeler, G., Kleptetar, A., Ouellette, H., ... MacLeod, M. (2014). Nursing education for rural and northern practice in Canada. *Journal of Nursing Education and Practice, 4*(8), 162–172. doi: 10.5430/jnep.v4n8p162

Chapter

12

LGBT2SQ Populations

Erin Ziegler

ERIN ZIEGLER is a nurse practitioner (NP)-PHC and Assistant Professor in the Daphne Cockwell School of Nursing at Ryerson University, Toronto, Ontario. Erin's clinical practice is focused on providing primary care to LGBT2SQ individuals. Her research focuses on the delivery of primary care to LGBT2SQ individuals, advanced nursing practices, and education. She is a team member with the Canadian Centre for Advanced Practice Nursing Research at McMaster University, Hamilton, Ontario.

KEY TERMS

gender identity
LGBT2SQ
sexual orientation

OBJECTIVES

1. Discuss and differentiate between the concepts of gender and sexuality.
2. Explore personal values and beliefs and examine the advanced practice nurse's role in working with LGBT2SQ individuals.
3. Understand advanced practice nursing and nurse practitioner roles in caring for LGBT2SQ individuals.

Introduction

The umbrella term **LGBT2SQ** (lesbian, gay, bisexual, transgender, two-spirit, and queer) includes a broad range of identities related to gender and sexuality. Advanced practice nurses (APNs) may encounter LGBT2SQ individuals in all areas of health care. In order to provide competent and culturally sensitive care to this population, it is important for APNs to understand the unique health care needs of this vulnerable and marginalized population.

Although grouped together as a community, it is important to note the distinct differences between one's sexuality and/or **gender identity**. An individual's sexual identity is referred to as their **sexual orientation**, the gender to which they are attracted. Sexual orientation can be heterosexual, homosexual, or bisexual. Those attracted to individuals of the opposite sex identify as heterosexual, whereas those attracted to individuals of the same sex may identify as homosexual. Women who are sexually attracted to women may use the term *lesbian* to describe their sexual orientation, and men who are sexually attracted to men may use the term *gay*. Individuals who are attracted to both men and women may use the term *bisexual*. *Queer* is often used as an all-encompassing term for individuals who do not identify as heterosexual.

Sex and *gender* are often used interchangeably yet are two very different terms. *Sex* refers to an individual's chromosomes (XX or XY) and their genitalia. *Gender* refers to the social classifications of male or female. Gender identity is one's sense of self as male or female and can be classified as cisgender or transgender. When an individual's gender identity aligns with their sex assigned at birth, they are cisgender. Transgender individuals have an incongruence in their gender identity and the sex assigned at birth. A transgender female is an individual who was born male, identifies as female, and may use female pronouns (LGBT Health Program, 2015). *Two-spirit* is a term that includes a range of sexual and gender identities and is used by some Indigenous Peoples. The term may refer to Indigenous individuals who embody both female and male spirits or who identify as lesbian, gay, bisexual, or queer (National Collaborating Centre for Aboriginal Health, 2016).

Statistics Canada (2015) reported that 1.7% of Canadians between the ages of 18 and 59 identified as gay or lesbian, whereas 1.3% of Canadians in the same age group identified as bisexual. Canadian censuses currently collect gender data only as male or female, excluding the transgender population (Davidson, 2015; Statistics Canada, 2016). The most recent estimate is that there are approximately 200,000 transgender adults in Canada (Giblon & Bauer, 2017). There are no Canadian statistics on the number of Indigenous individuals who identify as two-spirit.

Barrier to Accessing Health Care

Advanced practice nurses should be informed about health disparities that affect the LGBT2SQ population, including discrimination, prejudice, stigma, heterosexism, and homophobic environments (Institute of Medicine, 2011; Rutherford, McIntyre, Daley, & Ross, 2012). A history of discrimination, negative past experiences with health care services, and fear of disclosing their sexuality or gender identity to health care practitioners are common barriers to health care access experienced by this population. Two-spirit individuals experience higher levels of stigma when compared to other LGBTQ communities in Canada (Brotman, Ryan, Jalbert, & Rowe, 2002). Fear of victimization or refusal of services have also been expressed as a concern when accessing health care services. Up to 17% of transgender individuals have reported experiencing refusal of medical care because of their gender identity or expression (Grant et al., 2010).

In health care settings, homophobia, a negative feeling toward those who identify as homosexual, or heterosexism, the assumption that everyone is heterosexual, are barriers to care (Dorsen, 2012) and may contribute to the fear of discrimination experienced by this population. Disclosing one's sexuality or gender identity, or choosing not to, is a key decision that LGBT2SQ individuals often need to make with each new health care encounter, and the decision is often based on previous experience. Disclosure or non-disclosure can impact the experience with the health care practitioner and the quality of care. Non-disclosure can result in individuals not receiving optimal health care, including misdiagnosis or delays in medical treatment (Polonijo & Hollister, 2011). Individuals who chose to disclose to their health care practitioner have reported improved communication, comfort, satisfaction, and increased likelihood of obtaining health services (Steele, Tinmouth, & Lu, 2006).

In addition to the potential for discrimination, the presence of heterosexism from a health care practitioner may impact care delivery and services provided. Assuming all individuals are heterosexual can create a barrier within the client-practitioner relationship. An example of a hetero-normative assumption is that all sexually active women require contraception. During a clinical encounter, the advanced practice nurse taking the health history, including asking a general question about sexuality, finds that a female client responds affirmatively, indicating she is sexually active. In follow-up, the advanced practice nurse asks about the use of contraception, assuming the woman is in a sexual relationship with a male partner. If this female is engaged in a same-sex relationship, she now must decide if she wants to disclose her sexuality to the advanced practice nurse and explain why she does not need contraception. The purpose for asking about sexual activity is for the advanced practice nurse to accurately understand potential risks to the client. Asking the question about sexual activity in a non-assumptive way—such as "Are you sexually active with men, women, or both?"—would create an opportunity for the client to discuss their sexuality in a non-judgmental and safe environment.

Transgender individuals often experience additional barriers when accessing health care, specifically around the medical aspects of transition, such as hormone therapy and surgeries. Access to a practitioner who is knowledgeable about transgender health care has been identified as a major barrier in this population (Cruz, 2014; Gardner & Safer, 2013; Heinz & MacFarlane, 2013; Roberts & Fantz, 2014). Limited transgender-specific content in health education programs is the main contributor to this barrier (Alegria, 2011; Roberts & Fantz, 2014). Those individuals who do have access to a health care provider may experience further barriers in accessing coverage for cross-sex hormones and gender-affirming surgery. Under Canada's universal health system, health care delivery and insurance are mandated at a provincial level. Cross-sex hormone therapy is covered under some provincial benefits or by private insurance (Rotondi et al., 2013). Gender-affirming surgery is necessary for many transgender individuals and is covered in Canada with special provincial specific applications and approval requirements. Gender-affirming surgeries may include mastectomy, hysterectomy, metoidioplasty, phalloplasty, orchiectomy, and vaginoplasty. The long application process, surgery-specific criteria such as 12 months of hormone use, referral to another practitioner for secondary assessment, combined with another waiting list to see the surgeon and have the surgery, further contribute to the barriers and delays in accessing care by the transgender population.

Health of LGBT2SQ Individuals

While there are no LGBT2SQ-specific diseases, there are risk factors and risk behaviours that increase the rate of certain diseases in the LGBT2SQ population. Discrimination and stigma have been factors in high rates of mental health issues, suicide, and substance use disorders in the LGBT2SQ population (Institute of Medicine, 2011). Compared to their heterosexual counterparts, lesbian, gay, and bisexual adults are two times more likely to experience a mental health condition, such as depression or anxiety (Medley, Lipari, & Bose, 2016). Risk of suicidal thoughts and behaviours is also elevated (Haas et al., 2011), with a two times greater risk of suicide attempts (King et al., 2008). Rates of depression, anxiety, and suicide have been reported even higher in the transgender population (Institute of Medicine, 2011; Roller, Sedlak, & Draucker, 2015). A large study of transgender individuals in Ontario found that 35% had seriously considered suicide and 11% attempted suicide in the previous year (Bauer, Scheim, Pyne, Travers, & Hammond, 2015).

Substance use, such as tobacco, alcohol, and recreational drugs, is higher in the LGBT2SQ population. For some individuals, substance use has been used as a coping mechanism to deal with stigma and discrimination (Makadon, Mayer, Potter, & Goldhammer, 2015). Research has found that lesbian and bisexual women have higher rates of alcohol use and dependence (Green & Feinstein, 2012), and gay and bisexual men have higher use of recreational drugs such as marijuana and stimulants (Stall et al., 2001). Lesbian, gay, and bisexual individuals use tobacco up to two times more than heterosexual individuals (Conron, Mimiaga, & Landers, 2010; McElroy, Everett, & Zaniletti, 2011). Increased discrimination encountered by transgender individuals may be a factor in the further higher rates of drug and alcohol use, especially in transgender women. Studies have found that transgender women report higher use of drug injection, alcohol, and marijuana (Herbst et al., 2008).

The health care needs of the LGBT2SQ population are similar to those of the general population in terms of illness, chronic disease, and preventative care; however, it is important to remember that there may be resistance or barriers to access health care services for this population. Furthermore, as previously discussed, there are some increased risk factors associated with the LGBT2SQ population. Sedentary lifestyles and poor diet have contributed to high rates of obesity in lesbian women, increasing their risk of type 2 diabetes, coronary artery disease, stroke, and breast cancer (Boehmer, Bowen, & Bauer, 2007; Bowen, Balsam, & Ender, 2008). Higher rates of body dissatisfaction may be present in gay men, increasing their risk of eating disorders (Yean et al., 2013).

To "screen what you have" is an easy rule to remember when discussing health promotion and preventative screening for cervical, breast, and prostate cancer with this population, especially transgender individuals. A transgender male may have a cervix and therefore require Papanicolaou (Pap) testing, according to current screening guidelines. Studies have demonstrated that lesbian women are screened less for cervical cancer than the general population due to a perceived lower risk of human papilloma virus infection; however, there is no difference in the risk (Marrazzo, Koutsky, Kiviat, Kuypers & Stine, 2003; Tracy, Schluterman, & Greenberg, 2013).

Sexual health is an important aspect to health care for every individual regardless of their gender or sexual orientation. Prevention of sexually transmitted infections (STIs) and family planning should be discussed with everyone regardless of their sexuality and/or gender identity. It is important to remember that it is behaviour and not activity that increases the risk of STIs. Discussing safe sex practices and having open, safe spaces for talking about sexual activity is important for the LGBT2SQ population. Screening for STIs is important in all individuals engaged in sexual activity, and LGBT2SQ individuals may be at higher risk for some STIs. The Government of Canada's (2019) *Canadian Guidelines on Sexually Transmitted Infections* recommended annual screening for chlamydia, gonorrhea, syphilis, and human immunodeficiency virus (HIV) for all gay and bisexual men who have sex with men or transgender individuals. Individuals who have multiple or anonymous partners or who have unprotected sex under the influence of drugs or alcohol should be screened every three to five months. Women should be screened according to sexual history and risk factors. Further prevention against HIV with the use of PrEP (pre-exposure prophylaxis) therapy may be warranted in men who have sex with men, including gay, bisexual, and transgender women due to the higher risk of HIV exposure. PrEP is a prevention strategy using prophylaxis antiviral medications to reduce the risk of HIV infection in high-risk individuals (Tan et al., 2017) and an important aspect of harm reduction and health promotion for this population.

Many LGBT2SQ individuals have or want to have children. Pregnancy, surrogacy, or adoption are options that can be explored. APNs should learn to counsel patients appropriately and refer them to services if needed. Contraception should be part of the discussions around healthy sexual activities. It is important to avoid making assumptions about the need for contraception in this population. Lesbian and bisexual women may have sex with men and many transgender men still have reproductive organs, therefore contraception needs should be explored on an individual basis. It is important to counsel transgender men that testosterone therapy is not a reliable form of contraception.

Providing Safe and Inclusive Health Care

Advanced practice nurses can play a key role in creating safe environments for LGBT2SQ individuals that promote equity, inclusivity, and improve health care access by assessing their workplace to ensure that health care services and programs are inclusive of the needs of LBGT2SQ individuals, including clients and staff. Everyone, regardless of their sexuality and/or gender identity, should be able to see that their identity is acknowledged and welcomed within any organization (Registered Nurses Association of Ontario [RNAO], 2007). Displaying safe space signs; using appropriate forms, assessment tools, and educational materials; and having gender-neutral washrooms are important in providing inclusive and nondiscriminatory health care (Ard & Makadon, 2012; Coren, Coren, Pagliaro, & Weiss, 2011; Mayer et al., 2008). It is also important to be aware of community resources and organizations that are safe for clients, such as where a transgender female can go for a mammogram.

Advocating for safe and inclusive health care services in your organization and community is a key role for APNs.

As APNs, a key aspect of providing affirming clinical encounters is to ensure that you are not making any assumptions about an individual's gender or sexuality. Take a minute to evaluate your beliefs. Do you have any moral, ethical, or religious beliefs that could impact the care you provide to the LGBT2SQ population? Have you made hetero-normative assumptions in your clinical practice? Have you identified any limitations in your knowledge or skill in caring for this population? Self-reflection and being aware of one's own personal biases and assumptions can help to improve the care you provide to this population.

Being non-judgmental and open is important when taking a social and/or sexual health history from LGBT2SQ clients. Developing an approach to history taking that is inclusive, asking the same questions of all clients, and normalizing the approach will help to ensure an open conversation. Set the stage by saying, "I am going to ask you some questions about your sexual health and gender identity. I ask everyone these questions because it is important for your overall health." When meeting a new client, ask about preferred name and pronouns. Asking "Do you have sex with men, women, or both?" can be used to start the conversation about sexual orientation and activity. Asking about the 5 Ps (partners, practices, past STI history, protection, and pregnancy plans) is an effective way to assess sexual risk (National LGBT Health Education Center, 2015).

Conclusion

Advanced practice nurses play an important role in the provision of health care services for the LGBT2SQ population. Through advanced knowledge and skill, APNs can advocate for improved access to health care and ensure that services are inclusive and safe. The advanced roles and scopes of practice of APNs have situated them in key positions in the delivery of health care services for LGBT2SQ individuals.

Critical Thinking Questions

1. How can APNs advocate and be allies for LGBT2SQ individuals and their health care needs?
2. Explore your own sexuality and gender. How comfortable are you with your own identity?
3. How comfortable are you with those who have an identity that differs from yours?
4. Think about your current workplace. Would it be considered a safe space?
5. What is your workplace doing to be inclusive of LGBT2SQ individuals and where should changes be made?

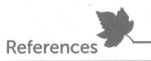

References

Alegria, C. (2011). Transgender identity and health care: Implications for psychosocial and physical evaluation. *Journal of the American Academy of Nurse Practitioners, 23*(4), 175–182.

Ard, K., & Makadon, H. (2012). *Improving the health care of lesbian, gay, bisexual and transgender (LGBT) people: Understanding and eliminating health disparities.* Boston, MA: Fenway Institute. Retrieved from https://www.lgbthealtheducation.org/publication/improving-the-health-care-of-lesbian-gay-bisexual-and-transgender-lgbt-people-understanding-and-eliminating-health-disparities/

Bauer, G., Scheim, A., Pyne, J., Travers, R., & Hammond, R. (2015). Intervenable factors associated with suicide risk in transgender persons: A respondent driven sampling study in Ontario, Canada. *BioMed Central (BMC) Public Health, 15*(525). doi: 10.1186/s12889-015-1867-2

Boehmer, U., Bowen, D., & Bauer, G. (2007). Overweight and obesity in sexual-minority women: Evidence from population-based data. *American Journal of Public Health, 97*(6), 1134–1140.

Bowen, D., Balsam, K., & Ender, S. (2008). A review of obesity issues in sexual minority women. *Obesity, 16*(2), 221–228.

Brotman, S., Ryan, B., Jalbert, Y., & Rowe, B. (2002). Reclaiming space-regaining health: The health care experiences of two-spirit people in Canada. *Journal of Gay & Lesbian Social Services, 14*(1), 67–87.

Conron, K., Mimiaga, M., & Landers, S. (2010). A population-based study of sexual orientation identity and gender difference in adult health. *American Journal of Public Health, 100*(10), 1953–1960.

Coren, J., Coren, C., Pagliaro, S., & Weiss, L. (2011). Assessing your office for care of lesbian, gay, bisexual, and transgender patients. *The Health Care Manager, 30*(1), 66–70.

Cruz, T. M. (2014). Assessing access to care for transgender and gender nonconforming people: A consideration of diversity in combating discrimination. *Social Science & Medicine, 110*, 65–73. http://dx.doi.org/10.1016/j.socscimed.2014.03.032

Davidson, T. (2015). A review of transgender health in Canada. *University of Ottawa Journal of Medicine, 5*(2), 40–45.

Dorsen, C. (2012). An integrative review of nurse attitudes towards lesbian, gay, bisexual and transgender patients. *Canadian Journal of Nursing Resreach, 44*(3), 18–43.

Gardner, I., & Safer, J. (2013). Progress on the road to better medical care for transgender patients. *Current Opinion in Endocrinology, Diabetes & Obesity, 20*(6), 553–558. http://dx.doi.org/10.1097/01

Giblon, R., & Bauer, G. (2017). Health care availability, quality, and unmet need: A comparison of transgender and cisgender residents in Ontario, Canada. *BMC Health Services Research, 17*(283). doi: 10.1186/s12913-017-2226-z

Government of Canada. (2019). *Canadian guidelines on sexually transmitted infections.* Ottawa, ON: Public Health Agency of Canada. Retrieved from https://www.canada.ca/en/public-health/services/infectious-diseases/sexual-health-sexually-transmitted-infections/canadian-guidelines.html

Grant, J., Mottet, L., Tanis, J., Harrison, J., Herman, J., & Keisling, M. (2010). *National transgender discrimination survey report on health and health care.* Washington, DC: National Center for Transgender Equality and National Gay and Lesbian Task Force.

Green, K., & Feinstein, B. (2012). Substance use in lesbian, gay and bisexual populations: An update on empirical research and implications for treatment. *Psychology of Addictive Behaviours, 26*(2), 265–278.

Haas, A., Eliason, M., Mays, V., Mathy, R., Cochran, S., D'Augelli, A., ... Clayton, P. (2011). Suicide and suicide risk in lesbian, gay, bisexual and transgender populations: Review and recommendations. *Journal of Homosexuality, 58*(1), 10–51.

Heinz, M., & MacFarlane, D. (2013). Island lives: A trans community needs assessment for Vancouver Island. *SAGE Open, 3*(3). doi: 10.1177/2158244013503836

Herbst, J., Jacobs, E., Finlayson, T., McKleroy, V., Neumann, M., Crepaz, N., & HIV/AIDS Prevention Research Synthesis Team. (2008). Estimating HIV prevalence and risk behaviors of transgender persons in the United States: A systematic review. *AIDS & Behavior, 12*(1), 1–17.

Institute of Medicine. (2011). *The health of lesbian, gay, bisexual, and transgender people: Building a foundation for better understanding.* Washington, DC: National Academies Press.

King, M., Semlyen, J., See Tai, S., Killaspy, H., Osborn, D., Popelyuk, D., & Nazareth, I. (2008). A systematic review of mental disorder, suicide, and deliberate self harm in lesbian, gay and bisexual people. *BioMed Central (BMC) Psychiatry, 8*(70), 1–17.

LGBT Health Program. (2015). *Guidelines and protocols for hormone therapy and primary health care for trans clients.* Toronto, ON: Sherbourne Health Centre.

Makadon, H., Mayer, K., Potter, J., & Goldhammer, H. (2015). *The Fenway guide to lesbian, gay, bisexual and transgender health* (2nd ed.). Philadelphia, PA: Sheridan Books.

Marrazzo, J., Koutsky, L., Kiviat, N., Kuypers, J., & Stine, K. (2003). Papanicolaou test screening and prevalence of genital human papillomavirus among women who have sex with women. *American Journal of Public Health, 91*(6), 947–952.

Mayer, K., Bradford, J., Makadon, H., Stall, R., Goldhammer, H., & Landers, S. (2008). Sexual and gender minority health: What we know and what needs to be done. *American Journal of Public Health, 98*(6), 989–995.

McElroy, J., Everett, K., & Zaniletti, I. (2011). An examination of smoking behavior and opinions about smoke-free environments in a large sample of sexual and gender minority community members. *Nicotine & Tobacco Research, 13*(6), 440–448.

Medley, G., Lipair, R., & Bose, J. (2016). *Sexual orientation and estimates of adult substance use and mental health: Results from the 2015 national survey on drug use and health.* Rockville, ML: SAMHSA. Retrieved from https://www.samhsa.gov/data/sites/default/files/NSDUH-SexualOrientation-2015/NSDUH-SexualOrientation-2015/NSDUH-SexualOrientation-2015.htm

National Collaborating Centre for Aboriginal Health. (2016). *An introduction to the health of two-spirit people: Historical, contemporary and emergent issues.* Ottawa, ON: NCCIH. Retrieved from https://www.nccih.ca/docs/emerging/RPT-HealthTwoSpirit-Hunt-EN.pdf

National LGBT Health Education Center. (2015). *Taking routine histories of sexual health: A system-wide approach for health centers.* Boston, MA: Fenway Institute. Retrieved from https://www.lgbthealtheducation.org/wp-content/uploads/COM-827-sexual-history_toolkit_2015.pdf

Polonijo, A., & Hollister, B. (2011). Normalcy, boundaries, and heterosexism: An exploration of online lesbian health queries. *Journal of Gay & Lesbian Social Services, 23*(2), 165–187.

Registered Nurses Association of Ontario (RNAO). (2007). *Position statement: Respecting sexual orientation and gender identity.* Toronto, ON: RNAO. Retrieved from https://rnao.ca/policy/position-statements/sexual-orientation-gender-identity

Roberts, T., & Fantz, C. (2014). Barriers to quality health care for the transgender population. *Clinical Biochemistry, 47*(10–11), 983–987.

Roller, C. G., Sedlak, C., & Draucker, C. B. (2015). Navigating the system: How transgender individuals engage in health care services. *Journal of Nursing Scholarship, 47*(5), 417–424. http://dx.doi.
org/10.1111/jnu.12160

Rotondi, N. K., Bauer, G. R., Scanlon, K., Kaay, M., Travers, R., & Travers, A. (2013). Nonprescribed
hormone use and self-performed surgeries: "Do-it-yourself" transitions in transgender communities in Ontario, Canada. *American Journal of Public Health, 103*(10), 1830–1836. http://dx.doi.
org/10.2105/AJPH.2013.301348

Rutherford, K., McIntyre, J., Daley, A., & Ross, L. (2012). Development of expertise in mental health
service provisions for lesbian, gay, bisexual and transgender communities. *Medical Education, 46*,
903–913. doi: 10.1111/j.1365-2923.2012.04272.x

Stall, R., Paul, J., Greenwood, G., Pollack, L., Bein, E., Crosby, G., … Catania, J. (2001). Alcohol use,
drug use and alcohol-related problems among men who have sex with men: The urban men's health
study. *Addictions, 96*(11), 1589–1601.

Statistics Canada. (2015). *Canadian community health survey.* Ottawa, ON: Statistics Canada. Retrieved from http://www23.statcan.gc.ca/imdb/p2SV.pl?Function=getSurvey&SDDS=3226

Statistics Canada. (2016). *Canadian demographics at a glance.* Ottawa, ON: Statistics Canada. Retrieved from http://www.statcan.gc.ca/pub/91-003-x/91-003-x2014001-eng.pdf

Steele, L., Tinmouth, J. M., & Lu, A. (2006). Regular health care use by lesbians: A path analysis of
predictive factors. *Family Practice, 23*(6), 631–636.

Tan, D., Hull, M., Yoong, D., Tremblay, C., O'Bryne, P., Thoman, R., … and the Biomedical HIV Prevention Working Group of the CIHR Canadian HIV Trials Network. (2017). Canadian guidelines
on HIV pre-exposure prophylaxis and nonoccupational exposure prophylaxis. *Canadian Medical
Association Journal, 189*, E1448–E1458.

Tracy, J., Schluterman, N., & Greenberg, D. (2013). Understanding cervical cancer screening among
lesbians: A national survey. *BMC Public Health, 13*, 442.

Yean, C., Benau, E., Dakanalis, A., Hormes, J., Perone, J., & Timko, C. (2013). The relationship of sex
and sexual orientation to self-esteem, body shape satisfaction, and eating disorder symptomato-
logy. *Frontiers in Psychology, 4*, 887.

Chapter 13

Refugee and Migrant Populations

Vanessa Wright and Shannon Sweeney

VANESSA WRIGHT is a nurse practitioner (NP)-PHC at Crossroads Clinic in Women's College Hospital, Toronto, Ontario, where she provides comprehensive medical services to newly arrived refugees. She has worked across a variety of community health centres (CHCs) in Toronto and provided PHC and emergency nursing care in medically underserviced First Nations communities in northern Ontario. Vanessa's work as an emergency nurse at Mount Sinai Hospital in Toronto, Ontario, led her to become the nursing lead for the Toronto Addis Ababa Academic Collaboration Emergency Medicine Team, where she supported the educational partnership between Addis Ababa University and the University of Toronto. Her other professional experiences include working as a field nurse for Doctors Without Borders in South Africa, South Sudan, Zambia, India, in HIV, malnutrition, gender-based violence, and reproductive health projects. She sits on the health advisory council for the Canadian Centre for Victims of Torture, acts as an expert presenter for The Centre for Addiction and Mental Health's (CAMH's) Immigrant and Refugee Mental Health course, and is an association member with Doctors Without Borders.

SHANNON SWEENEY has worked as a nurse practitioner (NP)-PHC at numerous community health centres across the Greater Toronto Area. She has provided holistic primary health care to refugees, new immigrants, and marginalized families across a variety of communities. She is particularly passionate about refugee women's health issues and supporting breastfeeding mothers. Shannon has been involved in developing a diabetes program and a women's health and prenatal care program for a refugee clinic in Toronto's east end. Her goal is to spread awareness about the unique health issues faced by newly arrived refugees and immigrants in Canada. Shannon sat on the perinatal committee at Fairview Community Health, was the women and children's outreach program coordinator at Scarborough Centre for Healthy Communities, and has participated in multiple outreach and community-based primary health care initiatives throughout her years as an NP-PHC.

<table>
</table>

KEY TERMS	OBJECTIVES

KEY TERMS

advanced practice nurses
   (APNs)
advocacy
migrants
migration
refugees
resettlement
social determinants of health

OBJECTIVES

1. Distinguish how the physical and social conditions of the migratory process impact short- and long-term health outcomes for refugees in their post-migration settlement in Canada.
2. Appreciate key concepts of health assessment for newly arrived refugees and migrants as supported by evidenced-based clinical guidelines.
3. Gain insight into aspects of advocacy and culturally sensitive care that the advanced practice nurse is well suited to provide refugee and migrant populations.

Introduction

Approximately 286,000 newcomers resettle in Canada each year, and about 10% of them are refugees (Minister for Immigration, Refugees and Citizenship Canada, 2018). There are many reasons, voluntary or involuntary, that a person may have left their country; however, in the case of those who are vulnerable and marginalized, the boundaries between forced and voluntary migration are often blurred (Van Hear, 2011). The unique health considerations of newcomers are influenced by their country of origin as well as post-migratory stressors, including limited access to health care, poor living conditions, and elevated poverty (Schulpen, 1996; Sanmartin & Ross, 2006). This chapter will examine health concerns specific to refugees and migrants through the social determinants of health, which directly influence their overall health and well-being within the Canadian context.

Defining Refugee and Migrant Groups

Refugee

A refugee is a person who has been forced to leave their country based on a well-founded fear of persecution on the basis of race, religion, sexual orientation, political opinion, or membership in a particular social group; and whose state cannot or will not protect them from their persecution. Accordingly, refugees are individuals whose claims of persecution are recognized by the state in which they have sought sanctuary under the signatory of the United Nations Convention Relating to the Status of Refugees (United Nations General Assembly, 1951).

Asylum Seeker

An asylum seeker is a person who has left their country of origin and crossed an international border. They have formally applied for and are awaiting recognition as a refugee. An asylum seeker's case has not yet been decided as they must demonstrate they are fleeing persecution.

Resettled Refugee

A resettled refugee is a person who has been officially recognized as a refugee and offered permanent residency in the country where their application was successful.

Internally Displaced Person

An internally displaced person is a person who is forcibly displaced from their home for many of the same reasons as refugees; however, they have not crossed an internationally recognized border and are displaced within their own countries.

Migrant

A migrant is a person who crosses an international border but does not meet the Geneva Convention's definition of a refugee. This term is used broadly, as are reasons a person might migrate voluntarily or involuntarily, for example, fleeing natural disasters, starvation, and extreme poverty (United Nations High Commissioner for Refugees [UNHCR], 1977, 2014).

Refugee Resettlement Pathways in the Canadian Context

Refugee resettlement in Canada takes place in two distinct pathways. One, refugees can make a claim for asylum at a border crossing upon arrival in Canada or shortly thereafter. The second involves acceptance of a refugee's claim before arrival, wherein their resettlement is initiated from abroad and they arrive with permanent residency status. Individuals who apply for refugee status upon arrival in Canada are referred to as refugee claimants. Refugee claimants must present their claim for asylum before the Immigration and Refugee Board of Canada. During the time it takes for their claim to be heard and determined, refugee claimants may be eligible for social assistance (Immigration, Refugees and Citizenship Canada [IRCC], 2017). In addition, refugee claimants can also apply to IRCC for a work permit during this time.

Of those who arrive in Canada as resettled and with permanent residency status, approximately one-half arrive as government-assisted refugees (GARs). GARs' financial and settlement support is provided by federal funding and government-funded agencies within their first year. The other half arrive as privately sponsored refugees (PSRs). PSRs are sponsored by community groups, non-governmental organizations, faith groups, or private citizens, who carry the financial, settlement, and social support responsibility for the PSR(s) up to one year. Lastly, a smaller proportion of refugees are resettled through the Blended Visa Office-Referred program, which was created in 2013 and denotes financial support as shared by both the government and private groups (Citizenship and Immigration Canada [CIC], 2015a).

Social Determinants of Refugee and Migrant Health

It is widely accepted that the health and wellness of individuals and populations are directly influenced by the social conditions of their lives (Commission on Social Determinants of Health, 2008). Raphael, Bryant, and Curry-Stevens (2004) list 14 factors that are strong predictors of poor health outcomes in terms of physical and mental health and social affliction: (1) Indigenous ancestry, (2) disability, (3) early life, (4) education, (5) employment and working conditions, (6) food security, (7) gender, (8) health care services, (9) housing, (10) income distribution, (11) race, (12) social safety net, (13) social exclusion, and (14) unemployment and employment security. In examining these 14 factors, it becomes clear that those with greater access to resources have improved health outcomes as a result of the political and social structures that create inequities within and between populations (Irwin & Scali, 2010). Herein, the social determinants of health are embedded in the structural factors that are formative to one's health and social equity, including material conditions, social relationships, and health-related behaviours (Brunner & Marmot, 2005).

The extent to which one's social determinants of health are affected by their social, political, and material conditions pre-migration has been well documented, particularly surrounding exposure to trauma, poor living conditions, and inadequate health care (Steel, Dunlavy, Harding, & Töres, 2017). Recent studies suggest that as migration becomes an integral part of socialization, it is imperative to understand how both social and structural determinants of health affect one's well-being (Mentis, 2016). A multitude of pre-migration stressors can affect one's health, including inadequate food, shelter, health care access, lack of safety, and family and community disruption. For the purposes of this chapter, however, migrant groups and their resettlement in Canada will be examined through the material, structural, and social post-migration factors that strongly influence them. Herein, we recognize that chronic stress after arriving in the host country is associated with poorer quality of life and health (Steel et al., 2017).

Post-Migration Impact on Health

Finances

Economic insecurity is a widespread and common concern among the refugee population in Canada. Financial support varies across provinces and is comparable to funds provided by government social assistance, with housing supplements available under certain circumstances (CIC, 2015a, 2015b). In a study performed by DeVoretz, Pivnenko, and Beiser (2004), economic performance by the average refugee was evaluated as relatively strong for those who were able to attain employment, yet economic poverty to this day is an endemic and growing problem for refugees. Furthermore, DeVoretz et al. found that income level for refugees on social assistance did not change seven years after initial evaluation. Both refugee service providers and refugees themselves note that the level of government social assistance is hardly enough to cover the cost of basic living needs for both singles and large families (Korn, Coric, & Hynie, 2014). Poverty levels are greatly influenced by local economic milieu, employment opportunities, navigation within the settlement sector, and access to financial services, which can vary widely from city to city (Korn et al., 2014). Perhaps one of the most common and disheartening experiences refugees face is the struggle to find Canadian employment because of professional bodies and employers' lack of acceptance of foreign credentials, language-related barriers, and lack of prior Canadian work experience. The inability to secure suitable work compels many migrants to take up low-skilled, precarious work to survive. Therefore, markers of economic hardship appear to be one of the most—if not the most—important health determinants for refugee well-being (Salami et al., 2017).

Housing

Refugees often encounter great difficulty sourcing safe and affordable housing upon arrival. They encounter many of the same barriers navigating housing networks as other low-income immigrants; however, they have the added emotional stress of being displaced from their homeland, often under traumatic experiences, and family separation. Among the various cities and communities refugees arrive in, they may find themselves segregated into low-income neighbourhoods, particularly with challenging housing conditions (Murdie, 2008). Evidence from Toronto indicates that refugee claimants have a much more difficult pathway to secure housing than do sponsored refugees (Murdie, 2008). In addition, poor-quality housing has been associated with mental and physical health outcomes, including increased prevalence of chronic diseases such as chronic respiratory infections; infectious diseases such as tuberculosis; and silent environmental harms, including lead poisoning (Hood, 2005). A large national study conducted out of Montreal, Vancouver, and Toronto found that a high proportion of refugees, compared to other newcomers, spent time in temporary housing (shelters, with friends, with acquaintances or strangers), exemplifying the precariousness and safety concerns for this under-housed population (Hiebert, 2011). This holds true for most refugee claimants who, upon arrival, will often make contact with settlement agencies and connect with an urban shelter, where they will live while they search for affordable housing. Sourcing adequate housing is particularly difficult for large refugee families and for those with disabilities, where larger apartments or homes are typically not affordable or available (Korn et al., 2014).

Education

Refugees experience lower rates of access to post-secondary education in Canada than other newcomers, despite the priority many refugee youth place on education (Ferede, 2010). Loss or non-recognition of previous educational documents, linguistic limitations, or fears of entering the school system at an advanced age are some of the systemic barriers refugee youth may face to furthering their education. The educational pathway of refugee youth is frequently disrupted during their forced migration and compounded by their felt need to provide immediate income for their family living in the same vicinity or to send income abroad (Shakya et al., 2010). This lack of access to higher education contributes to limited social and economic advancement, allowing many refugees to experience unemployment, underemployment, and lower incomes compared to other newcomers (DeVoretz et al., 2004).

Social Exclusion

Recognizing various post-migratory conditions that affect health and mental health of refugee and migrant populations would not be complete without reviewing the impact of social conditions for newcomers, specifically forms of social exclusion. Social exclusion for newcomer groups is often embedded through the post-migration trajectory and significantly influenced by linguistic barriers as well as barriers to social service and system navigation. These barriers exclude refugees from accessing needed services, community integration, and opportunities (Korn et al., 2014). The repercussions of social exclusion can be particularly felt for those who have migrated without family members and whose social support needs may not be fully met (Korn et al., 2014). The "healthy immigrant effect" chronicles the detrimental health impact of social exclusion on the newcomer, a phenomenon in which the immigrant arrives in Canada healthier than the average Canadian, and then shows declines in perceived and observed measures of health over time (de Maio & Kemp, 2010).

Refugee Health Care and Unique Considerations

It is common for refugees to prioritize meeting basic resettlement needs such as housing, food, and income for themselves and their families upon arrival rather than seeking access to health care. Unfortunately, when access to health care is neglected, the structural and material influences that impact one's health, particularly in the refugee population, take greater significance (Asgary & Segar, 2011). However, when attempting to access health care in Canada, immigrants and refugees report barriers that include navigating structural and system complexities and health insurance (Korn et al., 2014). Of note, linguistic and cultural communication difficulties are the most frequently cited barrier to receiving health care in newcomer populations (Pottie, Ng, Spitzer, Mohammed, & Glazier, 2008). For these reasons, this population typically has less access to health care and presents with unique health issues that require careful consideration by those working in the health care sector (Pottie et al., 2011).

Health Care Coverage for Refugees in Canada

Interim Federal Health Program (IFHP) is the federal health insurance for resettled refugees, refugee claimants, protected persons, and victims of human trafficking. Those who are granted refugee status prior to arrival (GARs and PSRs) are provided with provincial health insurance upon arrival in Canada, in addition to health insurance provided by IFHP to cover medication costs and supplemental services during their first year of resettlement (IRCC, 2017). Refugee claimants are provided with IFHP for both medical services (similar to provincial coverage) and supplemental coverage. Misconceptions abound regarding IFHP and coverage options for individuals presenting with this form of documentation. In 2012, Campbell, Klei, Hodges, Fisman, and Kitto (2012) conducted research with a variety of migrants across Toronto and found many commented on the two-tier health care system in place: one that would accept Ontario Health Insurance Plan (OHIP), and those that would accept IFHP. It is imperative to dispel such myths and create greater access to health care services for those with IFHP. To do so, health care providers across Canada simply need to register at Medavie Blue Cross to become a provider and obtain a corresponding provider number (https:// docs.medaviebc.ca/providers/forms/providerifhpregistrationformtermsandconditions.pdf).

Guidelines for Immigrant and Refugee Care

The study of health equity reflects the value of social justice and exposes the causes of health disparities as rooted in social structures (Reutter & Kushner, 2010). The profession of nursing, proposed by Reutter and Kushner (2010), aligns directly with social justice and health equity constructs from the profession's historical and philosophical roots. In that regard, nurses at the forefront of community and acute care are well poised to assess, educate, and communicate health inequities and interventions that could improve health care. Numerous health care bodies have developed guidelines for health care providers caring for refugee patients. The 2011 Canadian Collaboration for Immigrant and Refugee Health's (CCIRH) "Evidenced-Based Clinical Guidelines for Immigrant and Refugees" provide an evidenced-based practical approach for the care of newcomers (Pottie et al., 2011). In addition, an online checklist for migrants from specific regions has been adapted from the guidelines (http://www.ccirhken.ca) and a series of short podcasts have been created (http://www.cochrane.org/evidence/podcasts?title=&body_value=Immigrant+health). Also of value, the Canadian Pediatric Society has developed evidenced-based guidelines, clinical and advocacy tools, and training materials for health care providers that focus on newcomer child health: Caring for Kids New to Canada (http://www.kidsnewtocanada.ca).

The Immigration Medical Examination

The immigration medical examination (IME) is a cursory health examination conducted by a designated Immigration and Citizenship Canada physician. It is for all refugees and is intended to screen for the burden of illness and some communicable diseases; however, it does not provide a comprehensive clinical examination for refugees (Gushulak, Pottie, Roberts, Torres, & DesMeules, 2011). The examination consists of a basic history, physical examination, HIV and syphilis testing for those over 15 years of age, a chest image for those over 11 years of age, and urinalysis for those over five years of age. For refugee claimants, the IME is conducted in Canada soon after one's refugee claim is made. For GARs and PSRs, the IME is generally performed within the year before their arrival in Canada.

Considerations for Medical History Taking with Refugee Patients

For patients with limited English proficiency, the use of a trained interpreter is recommended to allow for safe, high-quality, efficient health care. Using a relative for interpretation entails the risk that important information may not be relayed due to limitations in language ability, cultural barriers, and social ties to the next of kin (Hadziabic & Hjelm, 2013). This is particularly true for youth and children, where interpretation has weighted responsibility and can disrupt family roles and dynamics (Hilliard, 2018).

Creating a rapport with the refugee patient and recognizing the time it may take to gather a comprehensive history is critical. In this regard, it may take several visits to elicit various aspects of a patient's health status and history. Often within the first appointment, the patient's immediate health concerns are addressed, ensuring that the patient feels safe and comfortable. It is important that health care confidentiality be explained to the patient, and that information shared within the appointment is kept within the domain and not shared with immigration, potentially affecting their refugee status.

Obtaining a migration history (including country of birth and all countries visited during migration) is essential to understanding health risk and exposure within each country. In addition, a thorough family history can provide valuable information on existing social stressors and supports, as well as hereditary diseases. This question also opens a gateway to noting available familial supports the patient may have in their host country or abroad. A social history, including educational level and employment history in their country of origin, is informative, as is exploring a patient's current living situation and economic means. This information will also likely be helpful when creating care plans for these patients and when linking with various language, employment, educational, and social services within Canada. Lastly, within a review of systems, the health care provider may find inquiring about appetite and sleep as a non-intrusive way to explore the patient's mental health. Reasons why the refugee patient has fled their country of origin may be disclosed to the health care provider within their series of appointments; however, it is recommended that this be done on the patient's own terms without probing.

Opportunities for health education and system navigation within the first series of appointments with the refugee patient are important to recognize and address. Areas to explore include health insurance (IFHP, OHIP); differences between acute and primary care; specialist referrals; use of emergency services, walk-in clinics, pharmacies, and social assistance. In addition, there may be an increase in unwanted pregnancies during the period soon after migration (Pottie et al., 2011). For female refugee patients of child-bearing years, sensitively exploring contraceptive needs early in the migration process and connecting them with the desired intervention can help allay some of these concerns. Additional preventative health screening includes a review of immunization history and administration of a full primary series according to age bracket and federal and provincial vaccination policies (Public Health Agency of Canada [PHAC], 2018). Immunization records from one's country of origin may be utilized when considered accurate, therefore avoiding the duplication of vaccinations.

Considerations for Conducting Physical Examinations with Refugee Patients

Connecting refugees to primary care early in their migration trajectory is of utmost importance to address the multitude of significant and complex health needs this population often presents with (Robertshaw, Dhesi, & Jones, 2017; Stagg, Jones, Bickler, & Abubaker, 2012). Most refugees originate from low- and middle-income countries; therefore, there is a higher prevalence of pre-existing infectious diseases such as tuberculosis, HIV, and hepatitis B compared with host populations (Pottie et al., 2011). In addition, the risk of contracting infectious diseases due to insufficient vaccine coverage is important to recognize (Clark & Mytton, 2007). Migrant populations also suffer from non-communicable diseases, including hypertension, diabetes, chronic respiratory diseases, to name a few, which may be under-managed and exacerbated when they arrive in their host country (Amara & Aljunid, 2014).

It is also important to recognize the high rates of sexual and gender-based violence refugees are exposed to, increasing their risk of acquiring sexually transmitted infections, as well as additional physical and psychological sequelae (Keygnaert, Vettenburg, & Temmerman, 2012). In many instances, female refugees have never undergone screening for cervical cancer (Pottie et al., 2011). A gynecological examination is important to conduct; however, it is often not appropriate on an initial assessment unless urgently indicated. Over time, with development of patient-provider rapport, tailored patient education, and professional interpreters, the uptake of cervical cancer screening and gynecological examinations may improve (Wiedmeyer, Lofters, & Rashid, 2012).

Table 13.1 outlines specific elements to include when initially conducting a physical examination on a refugee patient and corresponding rationale. For further recommended investigations in refugee health assessments, including preventative health and infectious disease screening for adults, please refer to http://www.ccirhken.ca and CCIRH guidelines (Pottie et al., 2011); and for children, Canadian Pediatric Society's Caring for Kids New to Canada website (http://www.kidsnewtocanada.ca).

TABLE 13.1: Components of Initial Physical Assessment of Refugee Patients

Physical Examination	Rationale
Vital signs, including blood pressure and body mass index	Refugees (as well as other immigrant groups) often gain weight after arrival in Canada due to changes in access and type of food and levels of physical activity (McDonald & Kennedy, 2005)
Screening and/or referral for eye examination	Unrecognized visual loss in not uncommon in refugees (Pottie et al., 2011)
Screening and referral for dental examination	There are high rates of dental caries among refugees, and early intervention is beneficial (Pottie et al., 2011)
Cardiovascular examination	May yield undiagnosed congenital or rheumatic heart disease
Respiratory examination	Identification of respiratory diseases such as tuberculosis
Abdominal examination	Identification of enlarged liver, spleen
Lymph node examination	Abnormalities can identify hematologic, malignant, or infectious disease
Integumentary examination	Clubbing of digits may indicate congenital heart disease, chronic lung infections, cirrhosis of the liver, or whipworm infections (Rutherford, 2013) Dermatologic examination may yield an opportunity to document physical signs of previous violence or torture

Source: Adapted by Wright & Sweeney (2019).

Addressing Mental Health Concerns in Refugee Patients

A further concern for refugee populations is the burden of mental health they experience. Violence experienced in their countries of origin, including sexual abuse and torture, are reported, which may lead to psychological and physical trauma (Fazel, Wheeler, & Danesh, 2015). Pre-migration traumas are compounded by post-migration stressors, including loss of social networks, financial insecurity, lack of housing, and cross-cultural stress while integrating into countries of settlement (Miller, Worthington, Muzurovic, Tipping, & Goldman, 2002). Health care providers working with this population should be aware of the high rates of depression and post-traumatic stress disorder (PTSD), where approximately 9% of adult refugees suffer from PTSD, which is approximately 10 times the amount in the age-matched American population (Fazel et al., 2015). Such conditions may present as somatic symptoms such as changes in sleep, appetite, concentration, and energy, particularly in children and youth.

Despite the overwhelming hardships many refugees have traversed, the majority do not suffer from severe mental health issues and corresponding sequalae. There are many points along a refugee's settlement into their host country that can be particularly stressful, including the refugee determination process itself. With appropriate supports and a strong therapeutic alliance between the patient and health care provider, it has been demonstrated that many mental health symptoms resolve once the refugee determination process is complete, often without medical treatment. Guidelines recommend screening for depression only in the presence of integrated systems that can provide appropriate follow-up (Pottie et al., 2011). In addition, screening for exposure to trauma is not advised as it may cause more harm than benefit (Pottie et al., 2011). Those with significant health concerns may benefit from seeking additional support and management through specialized mental health services, including psychiatry and centres for victims of trauma.

Documentation Requests for Refugee Hearings

Refugee claimants will have a hearing before the Immigration and Refugee Board of Canada to present their case. The time it takes for this hearing to occur from when a refugee claim is made varies from province to province; however, it appears the average length of time is approximately 18 months. Some refugee claimants may request a letter of documentation to support their medical health for their hearing. These letters can document physical scars and mental health sequalae that may have resulted from pre-migration injury and trauma. These documentation letters can be very valuable from a documentation perspective when discussed with the refugee claimant's lawyer. In addition, concerns over poor memory, concentration, and mental health fragility are noteworthy if they may affect the refugee claimant's ability to respond to questioning during their hearing. When writing letters for refugee hearings, it is important to remain objective, refrain from commenting on the credibility of the claim itself, and focus the documentation on medical issues noted in the clinical setting.

Migrant Farm Worker Health Care

Migrant agricultural workers have been coming to Canada since 1996 under the Seasonal Agricultural Worker Program (SAWP), a federal initiative based on reciprocal contracts with Commonwealth Caribbean countries and Mexico. SAWP is part of the Temporary Foreign Worker (TFW) program, which allows migrant workers to enter Canada through three streams: SAWP, Canada Caregiver Program, and International Mobility Program (Pysklywec, McLaughlin, Tew, & Haines, 2011). Approximately 310,000 TFWs entered Canada in 2015, and this number has been growing annually (Preibisch & Hennebry, 2011; Statistics Canada, 2018). Of this, about 40,000 migrant agricultural workers are employed through the SAWP and come from the United States, Mexico, and the Caribbean (McLaughlin, 2010; Orkin, Lay, McLaughlin, Schwandt, & Cole, 2014; Pysklywec et al., 2011). The majority of migrant agricultural workers are employed in Ontario, Quebec, British Columbia, and Alberta and can stay in Canada for up to eight months of the year, where many return annually (Pysklywec et al., 2011).

Migrant agricultural workers represent a particularly vulnerable subset of migrants who come to Canada for temporary employment; however, there is limited research regarding the health of this population. Prior to arrival, they undergo health screening in the form of an immigration physical, which includes a physical examination, urine and blood testing (HIV, syphilis), and chest radiography (Orkin et al., 2014). As a result of selection bias and screening, most migrant agricultural workers are in good health when they first arrive (Preibisch & Hennebry, 2011). Migrant agricultural workers qualify for medical coverage during their stay; however, coverage is subject to provincial variability and often relies on the employer to facilitate health care access (Pysklywec et al., 2011).

Common health concerns for this population are related to the temporary nature of their employment and include demanding and potentially dangerous working conditions, overcrowded living conditions, and the emotional stress of prolonged family separation (Cajax & Cohen, 2019; Pysklywec et al., 2011). Workers experience a variety of occupational health issues, in addition to the existing chronic health concerns they may already possess, including repetitive lifting, bending, exposure to extreme weather conditions, and pesticides. Barriers to accessing health services are compounded by lack of English proficiency, lack of health literacy and education, job insecurity, limited access to transportation, and extended working hours (Cajax & Cohen, 2019; Preibisch & Hennebry, 2011; Pysklywec et al., 2011).

Although there is limited research on this highly vulnerable population, and more longitudinal Canadian studies are needed, most communities who employ migrant agricultural workers across Canada have formed support networks and community groups. Such groups have often developed informally and serve as major assets in assisting with translation, coordinating various services, and linking migrant agricultural workers to the community. Several web-based resources have been developed to provide additional information regarding the health and occupational risks of migrant works (see Additional Resources at the end of chapter). Clinicians, health promoters, and allied health providers may find these resources helpful in the development and provision of innovative health care access when working with this population.

Advocacy for Migrant Health Populations

Advanced practice nurses (APNs) are uniquely positioned across Canada within primary and acute care settings to advocate and advance newcomer health. The profound health systems knowledge nurses possess is integral to address, access, and leverage the optimally integrated care that newcomers often require. The workings of this coveted knowledge base can be seen in nurses working at the bedside, in public health departments, community clinics, and in long-term care homes, among many other practice settings. Within these domains, nurses are poised to build trusting relationships, establish integrated referral pathways, and continue to build organizational networks based on cultural understanding.

At an individual, family, organizational, or community level, APNs have a recognized role to advance and assist individuals, families, and colleagues in navigating health and social support systems to better address social determinants of health (Yanicki, Kushner, & Reutter, 2015). Recognizing the multitude of post-migratory stressors—including language barriers, unemployment, financial strain, access to housing, and social isolation—is vital for the health of newcomers. The opportunity for nurses to act as advocates and assist individuals or families in health navigation cannot be done in isolation, but with knowledge of local resources and social networks. Community resources focusing on education, employment, financial assistance, and recreation can be particularly valuable referral pathways to establish in advancing the health of newcomers.

From an organizational perspective, many avenues of advocacy can present and be addressed when caring for newcomers. As previously mentioned, within Canada, linguistic barriers are cited as the main obstacle to health care services for immigrant populations, particularly newcomers (Pottie et al., 2011; Toronto Public Health, 2011). Language barriers can result in misdiagnosis, medication errors, and hospital admissions and readmissions (Laher, Sultana, Aery, & Kumar, 2018). Using a trained interpreter has shown that patients have a higher satisfaction with care provision, improved information recall, improved physical functioning, and higher likelihood of obtaining preventative health care (Laher et al., 2018). As our country's linguistic diversity continues to grow, it is imperative that health care providers and institutions consider how language needs are addressed and managed across a range of health care settings.

Additionally, creating organizational partnerships with community and government organizations offers channels for community mobilization, networking shared resources, and collaborative initiatives. This can be achieved through formal and informal partnerships with settlement organizations, public health departments, mental health service organizations, interpretation agencies, legal aid, shelters, and community housing groups. The landscape and demographic of the newcomer population can change rapidly from city to city, depending on immigration policy, service provision, access to employment, and housing. Intersectoral partnerships can bridge many gaps in service provision for newcomers and create the reflexivity that is often needed depending on local service provision and migration volumes.

Lastly, in addition to recognizing strategies for long-term engagement, and mobilization of broader support networks, the implementation of cultural competency training within institutions and organizations can help improve health outcomes by navigating communication barriers and cultural differences (Ingram, 2012).

To effectively provide care to the diverse populations we serve across Canada, health care providers must be aware of and sensitive to our own cultural background and that of our patients. The Process of Cultural Competence in the Delivery of Healthcare Services Model (Campinha-Bacote, 1999) was created for nurses; however, it has been used across health professions as an approach toward cultural competence and reflection. The model is based on the notion that all encounters are cultural encounters and there is a direct relationship between health care professionals' knowledge of cultural competence and positive patient health outcomes (Ingram, 2012). Campinha-Bacote's model includes five constructs representing the pneumonic ASKED:

- Cultural **A**wareness: Self-examination of one's own biases, stereotypes, prejudices
- Cultural **S**kills: Collect culturally relevant data regarding the patient's presenting problem and conduct culturally sensitive physical examination
- Cultural **K**nowledge: Seeking and obtaining a sound educational base regarding culturally and ethnically diverse groups
- Cultural **E**ncounters: Process of interacting with patients from diverse backgrounds to validate, refine, and modify existing values, beliefs, and practices
- Cultural **D**esire: Motivation of the health care provider to want to engage in the process of becoming culturally competent

Conclusion

Refugees face unique pre-migratory social and material conditions that strongly influence their post-migration settlement and integration. It is vital to recognize structural factors rooted in poverty and exclusion that can perpetuate poor health outcomes for newcomer groups within our societies. Delivery of health care to newcomer populations is a growing and advancing field where service models are being developed and integrated within existing structures. In that regard, APNs are extremely well suited across the Canadian health care system to create channels of clinical, political, material, and social advocacy to advance the health and well-being of refugee and migrant groups.

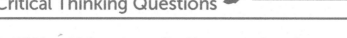

Critical Thinking Questions

1. Which social determinant of health appears to have the most significant impact on the health of refugees in Canada?
2. Use the "Evidence-Based Clinical Guidelines for Immigrants and Refugees" found at www.ccrihken.ca along with Table 13.1 to determine what laboratory screening and physical examination components should be included during the initial visit for a 38-year-old female refugee claimant who has newly arrived from the Democratic Republic of Congo.

3. Describe opportunities for advocacy at the individual, systems, and public policy levels that APNs are uniquely positioned to provide, promote, and enhance well-being among refugees.

Additional Resources

1. The International Organization for Migration (IOM): https://health.iom.int
    Frameworks can be viewed to gain perspective of how the social determinants of health impact migrant health
2. United Nations High Commissioner for Refugees (UNHCR): https://www.unhcr.org/aboutus.html
    Information that details the accounts of forced migration around the globe, including international policy, statistics of migration patterns/trends, evaluation of program and policy implementation
3. The 2011 Canadian Collaboration for Immigrant and Refugee Health (CCIRH): "Evidenced Based Clinic Guidelines for Immigrant and Refugees," published in the *Canadian Medical Association Journal*: http://www.cmaj.ca/content/183/12/E824
4. Caring for Kids New to Canada: http://www.kidsnewtocanada.ca
    Information related to caring for newcomer child and youth populations, created by the Canadian Pediatric Society
5. The Refugee Mental Health Project, offered through the Centre for Addiction and Mental Health: https://www.porticonetwork.ca/web/rmph
    Offers online courses, webinars, and community of practice for health care and settlement workers focusing on refugee mental health
6. Interim Federal Health Program (IFHP), federal health care coverage for refugees offered through Medavie Blue Cross
    For coverage details: https://docs.medaviebc.ca/providers/guides_info/IFHP-Information-Handbook-for-Health-care-Professionals-April-1-2016.pdf;
    How to sign up as a provider: https://www.canada.ca/en/immigration-refugees-citizenship/services/refugees/help-within-canada/health-care/professionals.html
7. Migrant Worker Health Canada: www.migrantworkerhealth.ca
    An evidence-based educational initiative that aims to facilitate collaborative strategies to increase health care access for migrant workers, with contacts and resources to assist health care professionals

References

Amara, A. H., & Aljunid, S. M. (2014). Noncommunicable diseases among urban refugees and asylum-seekers in developing countries: A neglected health care need. *Global Health, 10*(24). doi: 10.1186/1744-8603-10-2

Asgary, R., & Segar, N. (2011). Barriers to health care access among refugee seekers. *Journal of Health Care for the Poor and Underserved, 22*(2), 506–522. https://doi.org/10.1353/hpu.2011.0047

Brunner, E., & Marmot, M. (2005). Social organization, stress and health. In M. Marmot & R. Wilkinson (Eds.), *Social determinants of health* (pp. 17–43). Oxford, UK: Oxford University Press.

Cajax, C. S., & Cohen, A. (2019). "I will not leave my body here": Migrant farmworkers' health and safety amidst a climate of coercion. *International Journal of Environmental Research and Public Health, 16*(5). Retrieved from https://www.ncbi.nlm.nih.gov/pmc/articles/PMC6695666/

Campbell, R. M., Klei, A. G., Hodges, B. D., Fisman, D., & Kitto, S. (2012). A comparison of health access between permanent residents, undocumented immigrants and refugee claimants in Toronto, Canada. *Journal of Immigrant and Minority Health, 16*(1), 165–176. doi: 10.1007/s10903-012-9740

Campinha-Bacote, J. (1999). A model and instrument for addressing cultural competence in health care. *Journal of Nursing Education, 38*(5), 203–207. Retrieved from https://www.healio.com/nursing/journals/jne

Citizenship and Immigration Canada (CIC). (2015a). *In Canada processing of convention refugees abroad and members of the humanitarian protected persons abroad class-Part 2 [Resettlement Assistance Program (RAP)].* Ottawa, ON: CIC. Retrieved from https://www.canada.ca/content/dam/ircc/migration/ircc/english/resources/manuals/ip/ip03-part2-eng.pdf

CIC. (2015b). *Privately sponsored refugee resettlement in Canada.* Ottawa, ON: CIC. Retrieved from https://www.canada.ca/content/dam/ircc/migration/ircc/english/pdf/pub/psr_eng.pdf

Clark, R. C., & Mytton, J. (2007). Estimating infectious disease in UK asylum seekers and refugees: A systematic review of prevalence studies. *Journal of Public Health, 29,* 420–428. doi: 10.1093/pubmed/fdm063

Commission on Social Determinants of Health. (2008). *Closing the gap in a generation: Health equity through social action on the social determinants of health.* Geneva, CH: WHO. Retrieved from https://www.who.int/social_determinants/final_report/csdh_finalreport_2008.pdf

de Maio, F. G., & Kemp, E. (2010). The deterioration of health status among immigrants to Canada. *Global Public Health, 5*(5), 462–478. http://doi.org/10.1080/17441690902942480

DeVoretz, D., Pivnenko, S., & Beiser, M. (2004). *The economic experience of refugees in Canada.* Bonn, DE: IZA. Retrieved from http://repec.iza.org/dp1088.pdf

Fazel, M., Wheeler, J., & Danesh, J. (2015). Prevalence of serious mental disorder in 7000 refugees resettled into western countries: A systematic review. *Lancet, 365*(9467), 1309–1314. http://doi.org/10.1016/S0140-6736(05)61027-6

Ferede, M. K. (2010). Structural factors associated with higher education access for first generation refugees in Canada: An agenda for research. *Refuge, 27*(2), 79–88. Retrieved from https://refuge.journals.yorku.ca/index.php/refuge

Gushulak, B. D., Pottie, K., Roberts, J. H., Torres, S., & DesMeules, M. (2011). Migration and health in Canada: Health in a global village. *Canadian Medical Association Journal, 183*(12), 952–958. http://doi.org/10.1503/cmaj.090287

Hadziabic, E., & Hjelm, K. (2013). Working with interpreters: Practical advice for use of an interpreter in healthcare. *International Journal of Evidence Based Health Care, 11,* 69–76. doi: 10.1111/1744-1609.12005

Hiebert, D. (2011). Immigrants and refugees in housing markets of Montreal, Toronto and Vancouver, 2011. *Canadian Journal of Urban Research, 26*(2), 52–78.

Hilliard, R. (2018). *Caring for kids new to Canada: Using interpreters in the health care settings.* Ottawa, ON: CPS. Retrieved from http://www.kidsnewtocanada.ca/care/interpreters

Hood, E. (2005). Dwelling disparities: How poor housing leads to poor health. *Environmental Health Perspectives, 113*(5), 310–317. doi: 10.1289/ehp.113-a310

Immigration, Refugees and Citizenship Canada (IRCC). (2017). How Canada's refugee system works. Ottawa, ON: Government of Canada. Retrieved from https://www.canada.ca.en/immigration-refugees-citizenship/services/refugees/canada-role.html

Ingram, R. R. (2012). Using Campinha-Bacote's process of cultural competence model to examine the relationship between health literacy and cultural competence. *Journal of Advanced Nursing, 68*(3), 695–704. doi: 10.1111/j.1365-2648.2011.05822.x

Irwin, A., & Scali, E. (2010). *Action on the social determinants of health: Learning from previous experiences. Social Determinants of Health Discussion Paper 1.* Geneva, CH: WHO. Retrieved from https://www.who.int/social_determinants/corner/SDHDP1.pdf

Keygnaert, I., Vettenburg, N., & Temmerman, M. (2012). Hidden violence is silent rape: Sexual and gender-based violence in refugees, asylum seekers and undocumented migrants in Belgium and the Netherlands. *Culture Health and Sexuality, 14*(5), 505–520. doi: 10.1080/13691058.2012.671961

Korn, A., Coric, K., & Hynie, M. (2014). Working with vulnerable populations: Best practices, innovation and impact. *Canadian Diversity, 11*(1), 106–109.

Laher, N., Sultana, A., Aery, A., & Kumar, N. (2018). *Access to language interpretation services and impact on clinical and patient outcomes: A scoping review.* Toronto, ON: Wellesley Institute. Retrieved from https://www.wellesleyinstitute.com/wp-content/uploads/2018/04/Language-Interpretation-Services-Scoping-Review.pdf

McDonald, J. T., & Kennedy, S. (2005). Is migration to Canada associated with unhealthy weight gain? Overweight and obesity among Canada's immigrants. *Social Science and Medicine, 61*(12), 2469–2481. http://doi.org.10.1016/j.socsimed.2005.05.004

McLaughlin, J. (2010). Determinants of health of migrant farm workers in Canada. *Health Policy Research Bulletin, 17*, 30–32. Retrieved from http://scholars.wlu.ca/cgi/viewcontent.cgi?article=1002&context=brantford_hs

Mentis, A.-F. A. (2016). Child migration: From social determinants of health to the development agenda and beyond. *Medicine, Conflict and Survival, 32*(3), 221–227. http://doi.org/10.1080/13623699.2016.1258806

Miller, K. E., Worthington, G. J., Muzurovic, J., Tipping, J., & Goldman, A. (2002). Bosnian refugees and the stressors of exile: A narrative study. *American Journal of Orthopsychiatry, 72*, 341–354. doi: 10.1037/0002-9432.72.3.341

Minister for Immigration, Refugees and Citizenship Canada. (2018). *Annual report to Parliament on immigration, 2018.* Ottawa, ON: Government of Canada. Retrieved from https://www.canada.ca/en/immigration-refugees-citizenship/corporate/publications-manuals/annual-report-parliament-immigration-2018/report.html

Murdie, R. A. (2008). Pathways to housing: The experiences of sponsored refugees and refugee claimants in accessing permanent housing in Toronto. *Journal of International Migration and Integration, 9*(1), 81–101. doi: 10.1007/s12134-008-0045-0

Orkin, A. M., Lay, M., McLaughlin, J., Schwandt, M., & Cole, D. (2014). Medical repatriation of migrant farm workers in Ontario: A descriptive analysis. *Canadian Medical Association Journal, 2*(3), E192–E198. Retrieved from https://www.ncbi.nlm.nih.gov/pmc/articles/PMC4183168

Pottie, K., Greenaway, C., Feightner, J., Welch, V., Swinkles, H., Rashid, M., … Tugwell, P. (2011). Evidence-based clinical guidelines for immigrants and refugees. *Canadian Medical Association Journal, 183*(12), 824–925. https://doi.org/10.1503/cmaj.090313

Pottie, K., Ng, E., Spitzer, D., Mohammed, A., & Glazier, R. (2008). Language proficiency, gender and self-reported health: An analysis of the first two waves of the longitudinal survey of immigrants to Canada. *Canadian Journal of Public Health, 99*(6), 505–510. Retrieved from https://www.jstor.org/stable/41995162

Preibisch, K., & Hennebry, J. (2011). Temporary migration, chronic effects: The health of international migrant workers in Canada. *Canadian Medical Association Journal, 183*(9), 1033–1088. doi: 10.1503/cmaj.090736

Public Health Agency of Canada (PHAC). (2018). *Provincial and territorial immunization information: Immunization schedules by province and territory.* Ottawa, ON: Government of Canada. Retrieved from https://www.canada.ca/en/public-health/services/provincial-territorial-immunization-information.html

Pysklywec, M., McLaughlin, J., Tew, M., & Haines, T. (2011). Doctors within borders: Meeting healthcare needs of migrant farm workers in Canada. *Canadian Medical Association Journal, 183*(9), 1039–1042. doi: 10.1503/cmaj.091404

Raphael, D., Bryant, T., & Curry-Stevens, A. (2004). Toronto health charter outlines future health policy directions for Canada and elsewhere. *Health Promotion International, 19*(2), 269–273. doi: 10.1093/heapro/dah214

Reutter, L., & Kushner, K. E. (2010). Health equity through action of the social determinants of health: Taking up the challenge in nursing. *Nursing Inquiry, 17*(3), 269–280. Retrieved from http://www.nbpeipublichealth.ca/uploads/8/1/6/0/81605148/reutter-2010-nursinginquiry-healthequitythroughactiononthesdoh-takingupthechallengeinnursing.pdf

Robertshaw, L., Dhesi, S., & Jones, L. L. (2017). Challenges and facilitators for health professionals providing primary healthcare for refugees and asylum seekers in high income countries: A systemic review and thematic synthesis of qualitative research. *British Medical Journal Open, 7.* doi: 10.1136/bmjopen-2017-015981

Rutherford, J. D. (2013). Digital clubbing. *Circulation, 127,* 1997–1999. Retrieved from http://doi.org/10.1161/CIRCULATIONHA.112.000163

Salami, B., Yaskina, M., Hegadoren, K., Diaz, E., Merhali, S., Rammohan, A., & Ben-Shlomo, Y. (2017). Migration and social determinants of mental health: Results from the Canadian health measures survey. *Canadian Journal of Public Health, 108*(4), 362–367. doi: 10.17269/CJPH.108.6105

Sanmartin, C., & Ross, N. (2006). Experiencing difficulties accessing first-contact health services in Canada. *Health Policy, 1,* 103–119. Retrieved from https://www.ncbi.nlm.nih.gov/pmc/articles/PMC2585333/

Schulpen, T. (1996). Migration and child health: The Dutch experience. *European Journal of Pediatrics, 155,* 351–356.

Shakya, Y., Yogendra, B., Gurgue, S., Hynie, M., Akbari, A., Malik, M., ... Alley, S. (2010). Aspirations for higher education among newcomer refugee youth in Toronto: Expectations, challenges and strategies. *Refuge, 27*(2), 65–78. Retrieved from https://refuge.journals.yorku.ca/index.php/refuge/article/view/34723

Stagg, H. R., Jones, J., Bickler, G., & Abubaker, I. (2012). Poor uptake of primary healthcare registration among reentrants to the UK: A retrospective cohort study. *British Medical Journal Open, 2,* e001453. doi: 10.1136/bmjopen-2012-001453

Statistics Canada. (2018). How temporary were Canada's temporary foreign workers? Ottawa, ON: Statistics Canada. Retrieved from https://www150.statcan.gc.ca/n1/daily-quotidien/180129/dq180129b-eng.htm

Steel, J. L., Dunlavy, A. C., Harding, C. E., & Töres, T. (2017). The psychological consequences of pre-emigration trauma and post-migration stress in refugees and immigrants from Africa. *Journal of Immigrant and Minority Health, 19*(3), 523–532. doi: 10.1007/s10903-106-0478-z

Toronto Public Health. (2011). *The global city: Newcomer health in Toronto.* Toronto, ON: City of Toronto. Retrieved from https://www.toronto.ca/legdocs/mmis/2011/hl/bgrd/backgroundfile-42361.pdf

United Nations General Assembly. (1951). *Convention relating to the status of refugees.* United Nations treaty series. Geneva, CH: United Nations. Retrieved from https://treaties.un.org/pages/ViewDetailsII.aspx?src=TREATY&mtdsg_no=V-2&chapter=5&Temp=mtdsg2&clang=_en

United Nations High Commissioner for Refugees (UNHCR). (1977). *Note on non-refoulement, EC/SCP/2.* Geneva, CH: UNHCR. Retrieved from https://www.unhcr.org/excom/scip/3ae68ccd10/note-non-refoulement-submitted-high-commissioner.html

UNHCR. (2014). *Protecting refugees and the role of the UNHCR.* Geneva, CH: UNHCR. Retrieved from https://www.unhcr.org/about-us/background/509a836e9/protecting-refugees-role-unhcr.html

Van Hear, N. (2011). *Mixed migration: Policy changes.* Oxford, UK: The Migration Observatory. Retrieved from https://migrationobservatory.ox.ac.uk/resources/primers/mixed-migration-policy-challenges/

Wiedmeyer, M., Lofters, A., & Rashid, M. (2012). Cervical cancer screening among vulnerable women. *Canadian Family Physician, 58*(9), 521–526. Retrieved from https://www.cfp.ca/content/cfp/58/9/e521.full.pdf

Yanicki, S. M., Kushner, K. E., & Reutter, L. (2015). Social inclusion/exclusion as matters of social (in)justice: A call for nursing action. *Nursing Inquiry, 22*(2), 121–123. doi: 10.1111/nin.12076

SECTION III

Advanced Practice Nursing Role Competencies in Canada: A Case Study Approach

This section applies the Canadian Nurses Association's advanced practice nursing (APN) pan-Canadian framework competencies. Using a case study approach, the reader will see how each competency is operationalized by a clinical nurse specialist and nurse practitioner to demonstrate how both APN roles approach the competency in practice. In this section, there may appear to be repetition between the chapters and subchapters, but as a whole section, each competency discussion demonstrates consistency in practice approaches between advanced practice nurses and further informs and substantiates the competency discussion.

Chapter

14A

Direct Comprehensive Care Competencies

Clinical Nurse Specialist

Laurie Clune

LAURIE CLUNE is a registered nurse with experience as a clinical consultant in the community. Currently she is an Associate Professor in the Faculty of Nursing and Vice Chair, Research Ethics Board, at the University of Regina, Regina, Saskatchewan.

KEY TERMS

advanced practice nurses (APNs)
clinical nurse specialist (CNS)
direct comprehensive care competencies

OBJECTIVES

1. Describe how the CNS enacts direct comprehensive care competencies in practice.
2. Discuss the importance of the CNS comprehensive care competencies in Canada's complex health care environment.
3. Explore the application of the CNS role in practice.

Introduction

Advanced practice nurses (APNs), including the **clinical nurse specialist (CNS)** and nurse practitioner (NP), play a central role in enhancing and coordinating the care of complex clients and reshaping the health care system thus improving the quality of care. Several competencies required by APNs are identified in the pan-Canadian APN framework (Canadian Nurses Association [CNA], 2019). The first direct comprehensive care competency is exemplified by a nurse having graduate education and clinical expertise in a specialized area of nursing. As well, this competency is demonstrated by a CNS's clinical leadership in the application of current nursing knowledge, theory, research, and practice skills in the clinical setting to improve health care and education for patients, families, health care professionals, and the community.

This chapter will examine the **direct comprehensive care competencies** as they apply to the CNS role, focusing on the areas of graduate education, leading the team, advancing nursing practice, and enhancing health care. A case study will be utilized to illustrate the application of the competencies in practice.

Direct Comprehensive Care

The CNS is a registered nurse with graduate education and in-depth knowledge in a selected area of clinical practice. The knowledge and skills of a CNS position them to lead the inter-professional team, advance practice, and enhance health care.

Graduate Education

The CNS's advanced academic preparation builds upon baccalaureate-level nursing competencies to create a deeper knowledge base and enhanced practice skills (Baer & Weinstein, 2013). Coursework in health policy, research, health care system management, nursing education, and administration prepares the CNS for a key role in advancing nursing practice and directing comprehensive health care (Canadian Association of Schools of Nursing [CASN], 2015). Graduate education supports the CNS in developing a comprehensive and substantive understanding of nursing knowledge, theory, and research. A more critical awareness of the complex challenges faced in the health care system emerges. The CNS develops abilities to conduct a systematic inquiry of research, analyze existing scholarship, and critically appraise evidence so that new practice interventions can be developed, applied, and evaluated in the practice setting. Through graduate education, the CNS develops in-depth knowledge of nursing and the health care system, which is utilized in the practice setting to enhance and direct the care of patients (CASN, 2016).

Leading the Team

The knowledge gained through graduate education positions the CNS as a leader in directing comprehensive health care. As a member of an interprofessional health care team, the CNS acts as a role model, mentor, and advocate for enhancements to the quality of health care for patients, families, communities, and specific populations (Anderson, Champ, Vimy, Delure, & Watson, 2016; Bryant-Lukosius et al., 2015a).

Cook, McIntyre, Recoche, and Lee (2019) found members of the interprofessional health care team describe the CNS as a leader in the health care team because they act as a key contact, communicator, and coordinator of patient care; support and advocate for the patient care and nursing practice; have expert knowledge, which is shared with patients and team members through education; possess advanced health assessment skills, which result in referrals and symptom/side effect management. Therefore, the CNS leads the team to ensure safety, quality of care, and positive health outcomes.

Advancing Practice

The clinical role of the CNS revolves primarily around directing the care of complex or difficult patient or nursing situations. The CNS strategizes to improve and resolve challenging situations by drawing on their in-depth knowledge of nursing and other relevant sciences (CASN, 2016; CNA, 2019). Integral to this facilitation and resolution, the CNS assesses, develops, or contributes to the plans to enhance clinical care by providing information and/or education throughout the illness trajectory of the patient. The level of direct clinical involvement a CNS has with the client—whether it be nursing staff, other health care professionals, community care workers, or even the patient as client—may vary given the circumstances.

The CNS as a clinician is integrally involved in work with health care providers to assess, plan, implement, and evaluate care of patients/clients because of the increasing acuity and complexity of health care delivery. Many CNSs in clinical situations facilitate and coordinate the care of complex patient/clients' situations during their hospital stays and upon discharge home or to other health care facilities. This coordination of care role assumed by CNSs has resulted in fewer readmissions of certain populations of patients (Barber, 2016; Bryant-Lukosius et al., 2010, 2015a, 2015b).

The CNS utilizes proficiency in the nursing process, communication strategies, collaboration techniques, and knowledge of the workings of partnerships and relationships to prepare for management of complex situations. However, evaluation, assessment and professional accountability, awareness of the availability of information or resources, along with current advanced nursing knowledge, assist the CNS to better understand and resolve issues related to clinical situations. The goal of the CNS is to gather as much information from the team, patient, or family concerning a situation, issue, or presenting problem.

Enhancing Care

The development of procedures, techniques, and protocols for nurses and health care team members is another aspect of the CNS's role in directing comprehensive care. As the CNS works directly in the clinical setting with staff, their ability to guide and shape practice through mentorship and education is facilitated. The CNS may mentor staff by directly providing care or monitoring the practice of staff. The CNS is aware of the educational and support needs of patients, families, and staff because of their level of practice involvement. This can result in the CNS facilitating change by reviewing current practice trends; creating a study; developing new policies, procedures, and protocols; booking equipment; holding in-services; working individually with staff; and creating informal and formal learning opportunities. The CNS's provision of education and guidance to nurses, the interprofessional health care team, and patients and their families have a direct impact on making positive changes toward enhancing the comprehensiveness of care.

Working directly with patients and staff allows the CNS to examine issues and trends that emerge in the practice setting for specific subgroups of patients. For example, a patient who lived in a rural area may not have access to the same services available in urban areas (Honey & Wright, 2018; Loughery & Woodgate, 2015). In these situations, nurses require up-to-date and accurate knowledge to guide their work with these patient groups. Hence, the CNS plays a central role in sharing new knowledge and instituting new protocols that direct care.

The following case study illustrates how the CNS directs comprehensive care competencies with a complex patient living in a rural setting. The scenario demonstrates how the CNS has an impact not only for the specific patient and their care but also for health care team education, patient satisfaction, and future patients.

CASE STUDY

The Story of Jose

Source of Consultation: The pre-operative RN, a member of the surgical oncology interprofessional health care team, asked the CNS to meet with a patient named Jose.

Reason for Consultation: Jose is a 58-year-old, divorced male diagnosed with colon cancer and scheduled for surgery. He lives in a rural part of the province and has come to the hospital (500 km away) to have his first meeting with the surgeon, pre-operative testing, and attend the pre-operative clinic program. Jose has come alone to the clinic. While he has a fiancée and daughter, he has not told them the details of his illness and surgery.

Team Members Involved in Collaboration: Twice weekly, the surgical oncology interprofessional health team of a tertiary urban hospital meets to discuss current patients, issues, and concerns. The team—composed of a surgeon, oncologist, radiologist, charge nurse, pre-operative clinic nurse, CNS, NP, physiotherapist, pharmacist, occupational therapist, and social worker—identifies patients who may require the services of specific team members, like the CNS.

Clinical
Past medical history: Jose does not like going to the doctor. He has not had a
   wellness physical examination in over 20 years. A fecal immunochemical test (FIT)
   kit was mailed to Jose by the provincial cancer agency. The kit is sent to residents
   who are between the ages of 50–74, have a valid health card, and no previous
   diagnosis of colorectal cancer. Jose completed the test and mailed the kit in for
   analysis. A week later, Jose's family physician called to tell him the test results
   were abnormal. He travelled to the hospital for a colonoscopy. The results showed
   cancerous cells. Jose was then referred to a surgeon and is scheduled for surgery
   in one week.
No past surgeries, hospital admissions, or allergies
No family history of cancer
The Pre-Operative questionnaire completed by Jose indicates:
Social support: Lisa (fiancée) and Anna (daughter)
Education: Completed college education and has a diploma in business management
Occupation: Manager for a supermarket
Finances: Financially stable
Benefits: Comprehensive health insurance plan

Housing: Four-bedroom ranch-style bungalow; stairs to basement only

Address: Rural village, 500 km from hospital; no cancer care services in the rural area

Health care provider: Family physician

Approximate travel costs to come to hospital (fuel, hotel, meals, parking): $300 per night

Assessment: Elena, the team's CNS, asked Jose to come to her office for a meeting on the first day of his pre-operative clinic visit. Elena has created a welcoming environment for discussions with oncology patients by having comfortable chairs and soft lighting. A "Do not disturb" sign was placed on the door so that there would be no interruptions. The conversation began with Elena asking, "I understand you have come a long way to the hospital today. How long does it take to get here?" Over the course of an hour, Elena assessed Jose's physical, informational, emotional, psychological, social, spiritual, and practical needs.

Findings: Subjective

Jose loves his rural community and does not like coming to the city for medical appointments. "I just want to get back to normal at home," said Jose. He voiced concern about his family members and has not told his fiancée Lisa about his diagnosis or the exact reason for his surgery. When asked why, he said, "I don't want to worry her." As well, having Lisa coming to the hospital "would be too expensive" due to the travel costs associated with taking time off work, driving to the city, staying at a hotel, and purchasing food. Anna is Jose's 21-year-old daughter. She is away at university and does not know of her father's health issues. Jose said, "I want her to focus on her studies. She doesn't need to worry about me."

Findings: Objective

Jose is medically stable, willing to discuss his needs, wants to protect his family, and is experiencing some potential financial stress and burden with coming to the hospital for health care and treatment. Cancer care services are not available in the area where Jose lives.

Problem Identification: Jose's social support system (Lisa and Anna) is currently not available to him and unaware of the diagnosis, treatment, and discharge care requirements. Attending appointments at the city hospital are difficult and costly for the patient. There is a lack of cancer supports in Jose's home community, which may hinder his recovery.

Impression: Jose requires support in sharing the news of his illness and treatment with his social support system. While he is currently financially stable, extended stays and the requirement to return to the city for follow-up may be costly. Strategies for Jose to receive emotional support in his community need to be investigated.

Plan and Interventions: Encourage Jose to share his medical information with his family. The CNS or social worker can be available to help facilitate this discussion.

Online support and meeting services with hospital health care professionals for the patient can be established to minimize the necessity to come to hospital, but still provide ongoing support. If a visit to hospital is required, cluster appointments and tests can be arranged. Establish a preferred hospital rate for Jose and his family at hotels closest to the hospital and in the cafeteria. Make a referral to the oncology social worker, who can provide additional support to Jose and his family as required.

Evaluation: The number of visits Jose makes to the hospital are decreased from what is outlined in the care pathway. Instead, some visits and consultations will occur online with some follow-up appointments done virtually. Jose's family physician performs the physical health assessment under the guidance of the surgeon. Jose meets with health care team members by telephone weekly and his family feel supported throughout the illness trajectory. Jose and his family utilize the preferred rates of stay in the local hotel and hospital cafeteria.

Education
Recommendations/Interventions for Patient and Nursing Staff: Elena sends an email to the oncology program's medical and nursing staff, secretary, and volunteers to remind them of the preferred rates at local hotels, the parking arcade, and hospital cafeteria for patients who travel more than 100 km to hospital. She reinforces this when interacting with these individuals over the next two weeks.

    During the next interprofessional health care team rounds, Elena proposes setting up a virtual hotline that rural patients can use to call the hospital, and that staff can use to call patients living in rural settings.

Ongoing Care of the Client in the Practice Setting: Elena speaks to the ambulatory care oncology nurses and secretary about clustering rural patients' appointments.

In-Services for Interprofessional Health Care Team: Elena is a member of the organizing committee for the next hospital oncology education day. At a meeting of the committee she suggests that the focus of the day is on the experiences of rural patients with complex health needs, and how to improve their care.

Researcher
Patient-Centred and Evidence-Informed: To establish therapeutic communication with Jose, Elena created a meeting environment that was comfortable for him and free of interruptions (Baer & Weinstein, 2013). During the initial assessment interview, Elena used Fitch's supportive care framework (2008) to assess Jose's physical, emotional, practical, informational, spiritual, social, and psychological needs.

Outcomes Measurement of Clients with Similar Complex Health Care Issues: A retrospective chart review was conducted for patients who live in rural areas and travel more than 100 km to the hospital to examine patient outcomes. A satisfaction survey was developed to examine the experiences of rural oncology patients (Honey & Wright, 2018; Watson, Vimy, Anderson, Champ, & Delure, 2016).

Discussion

The case study illustrates how the CNS's involvement in directing comprehensive health care can have a positive outcome for the care of a client with complex care issues.

Graduate Education

Graduate education exposes the CNS to the nursing literature, which assists them in developing advanced ways of assessing and treating a patient. In the CNS-patient interview, evidence-informed interventions are used to enhance therapeutic communication. Traditionally, communication between the nurse and patient occurs in an examination room, hallway, or at the bedside. In these medical places, nurse-patient discussions are often superficial and limited (Amoah et al., 2019; Baer & Weinstein, 2013). First, a patient's condition may limit their ability to engage in communication. As well, most patients are acutely aware of the demands placed on a nurse when providing care to multiple patients. Nurse interruptions are frequently a reason patients do not share information with nurses (Amoah et al., 2019). In many cases, nurses control and limit conversations to specific close-ended questions about the patient's condition or treatment such as "On a scale of 1–10, what is your pain like?" to which a patient is expected to respond with brief, quantifiable answers. Nurses also communicate with patients when providing education.

The oncology research literature describes strategies to enhance therapeutic communication (Baer & Weinstein, 2017; Barber, 2016; Bryant-Lukosius et al., 2015b; Fitch, 2008; Forshaw, Hall, Boyes, Carey, & Martin, 2017; Loughery & Woodgate, 2015, 2019). By speaking to the patient pre-operatively, factors such as pain, which may limit the interaction, are minimized. In this case, the CNS decorated her office space to foster therapeutic communication, using furniture and lighting, and a door sign to minimize interruptions (Baer & Weinstein, 2013, 2017). The use of Fitch's (2008) seminal supportive care framework to guide conversation topics demonstrates a CNS using advanced communication techniques to facilitate good communication.

Leading the Team

By seeking out the assistance of the CNS for a complex client like Jose, the pre-operative RN, a member of the surgical oncology interprofessional health care team, illustrated the leadership role a CNS has on the team. The RN, recognizing that the client presented unique challenges, such as living a long distance from the hospital and not telling his family about his diagnosis, utilized the clinical expertise of the CNS to assist in care planning. The CNS, taking a leadership role in the interprofessional health care team's education, is another example of advanced practice.

Advancing Practice

Educating the interprofessional health care team on the health care needs of a rural patient like Jose demonstrates the CNS advancing practice. Rural patients have needs that are distinct due to geography and limited access to health care services (Butow et al., 2012; Honey & Wright, 2018; Loughery & Woodgate, 2019; Watson et al., 2016). Informally, by talking to nurses and staff about the unique needs of rural patients, new ways of thinking about every-day issues and traditional practices can lead to improved health care outcomes. Formally, by making the rural patient experience the focus of an educational day, the CNS is leading the team and advancing practice to enhance the care of this subpopulation of patients.

Enhancing Care

By implementing strategies to ease the financial burden, such as discounted hotel and food rates, clustering appointments, meeting virtually with the patient, etc., the CNS is taking active steps to enhance care, not only for Jose, but also for any future rural patients. Seeking feedback on the experiences of rural patients is a way of evaluating the effectiveness of the interventions and seeking alternatives to enhance care from the patients' standpoint.

Conclusion

The CNS is a clinical leader who is responsible for direct comprehensive care competencies. The way the CNS utilizes nursing knowledge and advanced practice skills to enhance the quality of patient care, particularly for those with complex needs, demonstrates the actualization of this competency. Supporting the education of interprofessional health care team members and facilitating the adoption of new practice innovations demonstrates how the CNS is a leader. Evaluating the effectiveness of enhanced care strategies illustrates the CNS's graduate education and clinical expertise in a specialized area of nursing. The CNS's understanding and use of current nursing knowledge, theory, research, and practice skills in the clinical setting are utilized to enhance care and education for patients, families, health care professionals, and the community.

Critical Thinking Questions

1. Describe ways in which a CNS can influence patient and organizational outcomes.
2. Explain ways in which a CNS can demonstrate leadership in the interprofessional health care team.
3. Identify other ways a CNS can utilize theory and research-informed sources to contribute to or enhance everyday nursing practices.

References

Amoah, V. M. K., Anokye, R., Boakye, D. S., Acheampong, E., Budu-Ainooson, A., Okyere, E., ... Afriyie, J. O. (2019). A qualitative assessment of perceived barriers to effective therapeutic communication among nurses and patients. *BioMed Central (BMC) Nursing, 11*(4). Retrieved from https://bmcnurs.biomedcentral.com/articles/10.1186/s12912-019-0328-0

Anderson, J., Champ, S., Vimy, K., DeIure, A., & Watson, L. (2016). Developing a provincial cancer patient navigation program utilizing a quality improvement approach; Part one: Designing and implementing. *Canadian Oncology Nursing Journal, 26*(4), 122–128. doi: 10.5737/23688076262122128

Baer, L., & Weinstein, E. (2013). Improving oncology nurses' communication skills for difficult conversations outcome. *Clinical Journal of Oncology Nursing, 17*(3), E45–E51.

Baer, L., & Weinstein, E. (2017). Communication skills for difficult conversations. *Clinical Journal of Oncology Nursing, 17*(3), 45–51. doi: 10.1188/13.CJON.E45-E51

Barber, C. (2016). Role of care co-ordinators in cancer clinical nurse specialist teams. *Cancer Nursing Practice, 15*(3), 31–36. doi: 10.7748/cnp.15.3.31.s25

Bryant-Lukosius, D., Carter, N., Kilpatrick, K., Martin-Misener, R., Donald, F., Kaasalainen, S., … DiCenso, A. (2010). The clinical nurse specialist role in Canada. *Nursing Leadership, 23*(Special Edition), 140–166.

Bryant-Lukosius, D., Carter, N., Reid, K., Donald, F., Martin-Misener, R., Kilpatrick, K., … DiCenso, A. (2015a). The clinical effectiveness and cost-effectiveness of clinical nurse specialist-led hospital to home transitional care: A systematic review. *Journal of Evaluation in Clinical Practice, 21*(5), 763–781.

Bryant-Lukosius, D., Cosby, R., Earle, C., Bakker, D., Fitzgerald, B., Burkoski, V., & Green, E. F. (2015b). Effective use of advanced practice nursing roles in cancer control: Results of a systematic review. *Cancer Nursing, 38*(4S), 0–134.

Butow, P. N., Phillips, F., Schweder, J., White, K., Underhill, C., & Goldstein, D. (2012). Psychosocial well-being and supportive care needs of cancer patients living in urban and rural/regional areas: A systematic review. *Supportive Care in Cancer, 20*(1), 1–22.

Canadian Association of Schools of Nursing (CASN). (2015). *Nursing practice in master's education.* Ottawa, ON: CASN. Retrieved from http://www.casn.ca/wp-content/uploads/2014/10/Nursing-Practice-in-Masters-paper.pdf

CASN. (2016). *Position statement on masters level of nursing.* Ottawa, ON: CASN.

Canadian Nurses Association (CNA). (2019). *Advanced practice nursing: A pan-Canadian framework.* Ottawa, ON: CNA. Retrieved from https://www.cna-aiic.ca/-/media/cna/page-content/pdf-en/advanced-practice-nursing-framework-en.pdf

Cook, O., McIntyre, M., Recoche, K., & Lee, S. (2019). "Our nurse is the glue for our team"—Multidisciplinary team members' experiences and perceptions of the gynaecological oncology specialist nurse role. *European Journal of Oncology Nursing, 41*, 7–15. doi: 10.1016/j.ejon.2019.05.004

Fitch, M. I. (2008). Supportive care framework. *Canadian Oncology Nursing Journal, 18*(1), 6–24.

Forshaw, K., Hall, A. E., Boyes, A. W., Carey, M. L., & Martin, J. (2017). Patients' experiences of preparation for radiation therapy: A qualitative study. *Oncology Nursing Forum, 44*(1), E1–E9. doi: 10.1188/17.ONF.E1-E9

Honey, M., & Wright, J. (2018). Nurses developing confidence and competence in telehealth: Results of a descriptive qualitative study. *Contemporary Nurse, 54*(4–5), 472–482. doi: 10.1080/10376178.2018.1530945

Loughery, J., & Woodgate, R. L. (2015). Supportive care needs of rural individuals living with cancer: A literature review. *Canadian Oncology Nursing Journal, 25*(2), 157–178.

Loughery, J., & Woodgate, R. (2019). Supportive care experiences of rural women living with breast cancer: An interpretive descriptive qualitative study. *Canadian Oncology Nursing Journal, 29*(3), 170–176.

Watson, L. C., Vimy, K., Anderson, J., Champ, S., & DeIure, A. (2016). Developing a provincial cancer patient navigation program utilizing a quality improvement approach; Part three: Evaluation and outcomes. *Canadian Oncology Nursing Journal, 26*(3), 186–193.

Chapter

14B

Direct Comprehensive Care Competencies

Nurse Practitioner

Monakshi (Mona) Sawhney

MONAKSHI (MONA) SAWHNEY is a nurse practitioner (NP)-Adult with a specialty practice in acute pain management at North York General Hospital, Toronto, Ontario, and chronic pain management at Kingston Health Sciences Centre, Kingston, Ontario. She is also an Assistant Professor at Queen's University, School of Nursing, and Department of Anesthesia and Perioperative Medicine, Kingston, Ontario.

KEY TERMS

clinical competencies
direct comprehensive care

OBJECTIVES

1. Compare and contrast the pan-Canadian advanced practice nursing (APN) direct comprehensive care competencies with practice standards developed by provincial regulatory nursing bodies.
2. Explore the application of the nurse practitioner clinical role in practice.

Introduction

Advanced practice nurses (APNs) provide health care services to individuals, families, communities, and at the population health level in a variety of practice settings (Canadian Nurses Association [CNA], 2019). The **direct comprehensive care** competencies or **clinical competencies** in advanced practice are characterized by the provision of clinical care that is grounded in specialty nursing knowledge in the nursing profession. Nurse practitioners (NPs) enact the APN clinical competencies through the application of theoretical, research-based, and experiential concepts that guide complex nursing assessments, decision making, and intervention strategies. Additionally, NPs have the legislative authority to utilize their knowledge and skills to autonomously diagnose, order diagnostic tests, prescribe treatments (including medications), and perform specified procedures (CNA, 2019). Therefore, NPs practice according to legislation (both federal and provincial/territorial), professional and ethical standards, and relevant policies (CNA, 2010). This chapter will explore the direct comprehensive care competencies for the NP role. A case study by a hospital-based NP will be utilized to demonstrate application of the NP clinical competencies.

Direct Comprehensive Care

In both primary health care and acute care settings, NPs spend the majority of their time involved in direct patient care (Donald et al., 2014; Heale, Dahrouge, Johnston, & Tranmer, 2018; Keenan, Mutterback, Velthuizen, Pantalone, & Gossack-Keenan, 2018; Martin-Misner et al., 2019). The clinical role of the NP is built on and extends the APN direct comprehensive care competencies outlined by the CNA. These competencies include advanced assessment and intervention strategies; evidence-informed decision making; assessment or measurement of outcomes; minimization of adverse events; identification of key determinates of health and population-level trends that have health implications; illness prevention and health promotion; and dissemination of knowledge (CNA, 2019). For an NP to effectively enact their role as a clinician, they must utilize all of the APN competencies (optimizing health systems, education, research, leadership, consultation, and collaboration) in their clinical practice.

NPs lead care by using their expanded scope of practice to conduct autonomous assessments and make diagnoses and treatment decisions. When making treatment decisions, NPs utilize an evidence-informed approach that includes the latest research, patient preferences, and available resources (DiCenso, Ciliska, & Guyatt, 2005). The NP clinical role improves team functioning, and interprofessional collaboration, team dynamics, quality of care, and professionalism (Heale, James, Wenghofer, & Garceau, 2018; Hurlock-Chorostecki et al., 2016). In addition, NPs disseminate knowledge through teaching, coaching, and mentoring other members of the interprofessional team (Kilpatrick et al., 2019).

Regardless of the clinical practice setting, NPs optimize outcomes for patients and families through collaboration and consultation with other health care providers (Kilpatrick et al., 2019). This is a key factor in the prevention and management of patient-related adverse events. NPs help guide decision making and use a patient- and family-centred approach when providing care. Other NP-related outcomes include patient education, health promotion, illness prevention, and improved pain management (Acorn, 2015; Goldie, Prodan-Bhalla, & Mackay, 2012; Heale, Wenghofer, James, & Garceau, 2018; Kilpatrick et al., 2019).

CASE STUDY

The Story of Miguel

Chief Complaint: Miguel is a 58-year-old male who underwent a bowel resection one day earlier for colon cancer. To manage his post-operative pain, he is receiving epidural ropivacaine 0.2% and hydromorphone 0.04 mg/mL at a rate of 3mL/hr. He is also receiving acetaminophen 1,000 mg orally q 6h for pain. His epidural catheter is placed at the T9/T10 dermatome. Overnight he had very little pain (1 or 2/10); however, this morning he describes having severe pain 8/10 in his abdomen (the area of his surgery). He is on the Enhanced Recovery After Surgery (ERAS) protocol, so he is started on a regular diet this morning, but reports feeling very nauseated due to pain. He has not been out of bed since surgery. Yasmin, the NP-Adult for the Acute Pain Service, has been called by the RN caring for Miguel to assess him.

History of Present Illness: Miguel underwent his routine colon screening (fecal immunochemical test [FIT]) and due to abnormal results, underwent a colonoscopy. A suspicious lesion was identified, biopsied, and reported positive for cancerous cells. Thus, he underwent a colon resection yesterday.

Past Medical History: BMI = 27, hypertension

Social History: Miguel has been divorced for many years, has one daughter (age 21 years). He is currently engaged to be married (to Lisa). He completed college education and has a diploma in business management. He currently works as a manager for a supermarket in a rural area of the province, is financially stable, and has good benefits from his employer. He does not wish to disclose information about his cancer to his family members as he does not want to burden them.

Family History: No history of cancer

Physical Examination
Afebrile
Cardiac: BP 128/72, heart rate 102 (normal sinus rhythm)
Respiratory: RR 14, O_2 saturation 99% with 2L/minute oxygen via nasal prongs; normal breath sounds bilaterally, but it is painful to take a deep breath
Gastrointestinal: No bowel sounds; reports feeling nauseated, no vomiting
Urinary: Urinary catheter in place, draining yellow-coloured urine 50mL/hr
Integumentary: Skin intact; surgical incision is covered with a dry dressing. Epidural catheter site on the patient's back is dry and intact.
Neurological: Oriented to person, place, time; motor strength: upper extremities are 5/5 strength; lower extremities 5/5 plantar and dorsi flexion of feet, bending and straightening of knees, 3/5 hip flexors (straight leg raise against resistance) due to pain in abdomen; sensation: decreased sensation to cold T10 to T12
Pain: 8/10 in abdomen at rest and when taking a deep breath
Psycho-emotional: Anxious and focused on the pain
All other systems within normal limits
Relevant Diagnostic Tests:
Hgb = 113, WBCs = 13.0×10^9/L
Electrolytes and creatinine within normal limits

INR = 1.1; prothrombin time (PT) = 11 seconds; partial thromboplastin time (PTT) = 35 seconds

Allergies: None

Medications: Bisoprolol 5 mg po daily, Acetaminophen 1,000 mg po q6h, Daltaparin 5,000 IU sc, epidural ropivacaine and hydromorphone at 3 mL/hr

Plan: After assessing Miguel, Yasmin decides to test the effectiveness of the epidural to see if the epidural catheter is still in place to provide analgesia; the Daltaparin is held until after it is determined to maintain or remove the epidural. The epidural is tested with Lidocaine 1% total of 5 mL, vital signs, sensory and motor function, and pain are monitored for the next hour. Miguel's pain decreased to 4/10, pulse = 72/min, BP = 110/60, sensation is decreased between T9 to T12, he has normal motor function in the upper and lower extremities with strength in legs and feet 5/5. Yasmin orders an increase in the epidural rate to 6 mL/hour to help maintain effective analgesia, and continues to monitor over the day; the Daltaparin is also restarted. An NSAID is not prescribed as Yasmin is aware of research findings that indicate NSAIDs may contribute to anastomosis leaks in patients who undergo colorectal surgery (Fjederholt et al., 2018; Huang, Tang, & Young, 2018; Kverneng et al., 2017). Yasmin also provides education to Miguel and his family regarding pain assessment and management and learns that Miguel is very concerned about ongoing pain if the cancer is not "cured." Miguel asks Yasmin if they can collaborate with his primary health care provider, an NP, regarding his post-operative pain when he is ready for discharge home.

Yasmin documents and communicates the outcome of the assessment and intervention to the interprofessional team (including the RN, physiotherapist, pharmacist, CNS on the in-patient surgical unit, surgeon, and anaesthesiologist). On post-operative day 2, Miguel is walking, eating, and his pain is well controlled. Anticoagulation bloodwork is monitored, his INR remains at 1.1, and his epidural catheter is removed at the end of day 2 and he is transitioned to oral hydromorphone 2 mg po prn for pain, in addition to acetaminophen. An NSAID is not prescribed, and Miguel is informed to avoid NSAIDs for the next 6 weeks. On post-operative day 3, prior to Miguel's discharge home, Yasmin contacts his primary health care NP and discusses his post-operative pain, discharge pain plan, and prescriptions.

Discussion

An analysis of Miguel's case study illustrates that the NP, Yasmin, demonstrated many of the APN and NP competencies (CNA, 2010, 2019). She provided care that was grounded in a nursing role with the aim of supporting Miguel through the experience of colon surgery and pain management to attain/regain optimal function enhanced by specialty knowledge relevant to anaesthesia and pain management. An advanced assessment and intervention strategies that were appropriate for Miguel's condition were provided. Additionally, the practice demonstrated the delivery of evidence-informed care, with integration data from multiple sources (Miguel, the RN, and evidence-informed research).

Yasmin provided education and anticipated and prevented adverse events by monitoring patient outcome and bloodwork. For example, she monitored Miguel's response to treatment and monitored bloodwork to ensure safe discontinuation of his epidural (Sawhney, Chambers, & Hysi, 2018). She communicated with the patient and other team members in resolving issues by finding a solution that would meet his unique needs, while balancing the need for system efficiency. Yasmin engaged other members of the interprofessional team, including the RN staff, CNS, physiotherapy, surgeon, and primary health care provider, to facilitate communication about his needs and experience.

Conclusion

NPs' care decisions are based on an analysis of health information obtained through utilization of APN competencies and obtaining additional information through the NP clinical competencies of advanced health assessment, diagnostic reasoning, and therapeutic planning. An NP's clinical practice is rooted in advanced nursing competencies that provide the foundation for the values, knowledge, and theories of professional nursing practice, and the utilization of expanded skills and scope that are grounded in patient- and family-centred care and collaborative relationships. All of this incorporates health promotion, illness and injury prevention, rehabilitative, curative, supportive, and palliative care (CNA, 2019). Legislation has been passed in all jurisdictions in Canada that broadens the full scope of practice for NPs with the intention of increasing access to care for patients, increasing interprofessional collaboration, and maintaining safety (CNA, 2019).

It is the advanced nursing roots of the NP that differentiates the NP role from other, medical-based roles that share similar scopes of practice. It is important that NPs themselves understand and can clearly articulate that it is the synergy of the APN and NP clinical competencies—the advanced nursing knowledge, coupled with the expanded scope of practice—that distinguishes the NP role from other similar roles.

Critical Thinking Questions

1. How do the NP and CNS roles differ in terms of clinical accountability?
2. Which of the NP clinical competencies would be the most challenging to initiate? Why?
3. What supports are available to an NP to implement or develop clinical competencies?

References

Acorn, M. (2015). Nurse practitioners as most responsible provider: Impact on care for seniors admitted to an Ontario hospital. *International Journal of Nursing & Clinical Practices, 2*, 1–11.

Canadian Nurses Association (CNA). (2010). *Canadian nurse practitioner core competency framework.* Ottawa, ON: CNA. Retrieved from https://www.cna-aiic.ca/~/media/cna/files/en/competency_framework_2010_e.pdf

CNA. (2019). *Advanced practice nursing: A pan-Canadian framework.* Ottawa, ON: CNA. Retrieved from https://cna-aiic.ca/-/media/cna/page-content/pdf-en/apn-a-pan-canadian-framework.pdf

DiCenso, A., Ciliska, D. K., & Guyatt, G. (2005). Introduction to evidence-based nursing. In A. Di-Censo, G. Guyatt, & D. K. Ciliska (Eds.), *Evidenced-based nursing: A guide to clinical practice* (pp. 20–43). St. Louis, MO: Elsevier/Mosby.

Donald, F., Kilpatrick, K., Reid, K., Carter, N., Martin-Misener, R., Bryant-Lukosius, D., … DiCenso, A. (2014). A systematic review of the cost-effectiveness of nurse practitioners and clinical nurse specialists: What is the quality of the evidence? *Nursing Research and Practice, 2014.* http://dx.doi.org/10.1155/2014/896587

Fjederholt, K. T., Okholm, C., Svendsen, L. B., Achiam, M., Kirkegard, J., & Mortensen, F. V. (2018). Ketorolac and other NSAIDs increase the risk of anastomotic leakage after surgery for GEJ cancers: A cohort study of 557 patients. *Journal of Gastrointestinal Surgery, 22,* 587–594.

Goldie, C. L., Prodan-Bhalla, N., & Mackay, M. (2012). Nurse practitioners in postoperative cardiac surgery: Are they effective? *Canadian Journal of Cardiovascular Nursing, 22*(4), 8–15.

Heale, R., Dahrouge, S., Johnston, S., & Tranmer, J. (2018). Characteristics of nurse practitioner practice in family health teams in Ontario, Canada. *Policy, Politics, & Nursing Practice, 19*(3–4), 72–81.

Heale, R., James, S., Wenghofer, E., & Garceau, M. L. (2018). Nurse practitioner's perceptions of the impact of the nurse practitioner-led clinic model on the quality of care of complex patients. *Primary Health Care Research & Development, 19,* 553–560.

Heale, R., Wenghofer, E., James, S., & Garceau, M. L. (2018). Quality of care for patients with diabetes and multimorbidity registered at nurse practitioner-led clinics. *Canadian Journal of Nursing Research, 50*(1), 20–27.

Huang, Y., Tang, S. R., & Young, C. J. (2018). Nonsteroidal anti-inflammatory drugs and anastomotic dehiscence after colorectal surgery: A meta-analysis. *Australian and New Zealand (ANZ) Journal of Surgery, 88,* 959–965.

Hurlock-Chorostecki, C., van Soren, M., MacMillan, K., Sidani, S., Donald, F., & Reeves, S. (2016). A qualitative study of nurse practitioner promotion of interprofessional care across institutional settings: Perspectives from different healthcare professionals. *International Journal of Nursing Sciences, 3,* 3–10.

Keenan, A. M., Mutterback, E. E., Velthuizen, K. M., Pantalone, M. E., & Gossack-Keenan, K. L. (2018). Perceptions of the effectiveness of advanced practice nurses on a neurosurgery unit in a Canadian tertiary care centre: A pre-and-post implementation design. *International Journal of Nursing Sciences, 5,* 138–143. doi: 10.1016/j.ijnss.2018.03.008

Kilpatrick, K., Jabbour, M., Tchouaket, E., Acorn, M., Donald, F., & Hains, S. (2019). Implementing primary healthcare nurse practitioners in long-term care teams: A qualitative descriptive study. *Journal of Advanced Nursing, 75,* 1306–1315.

Kverneng, D., Hultberg, E., Angenete, M., Lydrup, L., Rutegard, J., Matthiessen, P., & Rutegard, M. (2017). Nonsteroidal anti-inflammatory drugs and the risk of anastomotic leakage after anterior resection for rectal cancer. *European Journal of Surgical Oncology, 43*(10), 1908–1914.

Martin-Misener, R., Wong, S. T., Johnston, S., Blackman, S., Scott, C., Hogg, W., … Wuite, S. (2019). Regional variation in primary care improvement strategies and policy: Case studies that consider qualitative contextual data for performance measurement in three Canadian provinces. *British Medical Journal Open, 9*(10), e029622. doi: 10.1136/bmjopen-2019-029622

Sawhney, M., Chambers, S., & Hysi, F. (2018). Removing epidural catheters in surgical patients: Guidance for nurses. *Nursing2018, 48*(12), 47–49.

Chapter

15A

Optimizing Health System Competencies

Clinical Nurse Specialist

Ken McDonald

KEN MCDONALD is a clinical nurse specialist (CNS) in mental health and substance abuse with the Fraser Health Authority, Vancouver, British Columbia. He is currently the RN/CNS councillor of the Nurses and Nurse Practitioners of British Columbia (NNPBC), the province's professional nursing organization.

KEY TERMS

advanced practice nurses (APNs)
clinical nurse specialists (CNSs)
competency
optimizing

OBJECTIVES

1. Discuss the optimizing health system competency.
2. Explore the clinical nurse specialist role in optimizing the health system.
3. Discuss skills and decision-making skills required to support optimizing the health system.

Introduction

Clinical nurse specialists (CNSs), as **advanced practice nurses (APNs)**, are often presented with opportunities to improve the functioning of or **optimizing** the health care system within their organization. This is a particularly influential activity because of the nature of systems, which will be discussed in more detail later in this chapter, that allows for this work to impact diverse parts of the practice environment and create change for many people. Commensurate with this potential for such a far-reaching impact is the benefit of understanding the complexity of this work and having a diverse set of knowledge and skills to support safe and effective system optimization. This chapter will provide background information about topics such as general systems theory and some of the important skills that are not uniquely nursing, a case study, and discussion demonstrating optimizing a health system project to better understand the strengths and opportunities for improvement of a health system.

Optimizing Health System Competency

This competency is a new addition to the Canadian Nurses Association's pan-Canadian APN framework (Canadian Nurses Association [CNA], 2019). It is defined as "contributing to the effective functioning of health systems through advocacy, promoting innovative client care and facilitating equitable, client-centred health care" (CNA, 2019, p. 30). General systems theory describes a system as "multiple, interdependent parts that collectively form more than the sum of their parts" (Suter et al., 2013, p. 58). This holistic interdependency results in two key systems features: they are not understandable by investigating the parts in isolation; and a change in a part results in changes in another part of the system (Cordon, 2013). A system can be part of a large socio-cultural phenomena such as how power is distributed, or smaller and less complex such as the components that contribute to a single medication being administered. A system can be both the individual pieces and total culmination of these pieces.

Lewandowski and Adamle's (2009) literature review related to APN confirmed facilitating change and innovation is a significant activity of CNS work. Similarly, a 2009 survey study of 505 CNSs indicated that CNSs are often involved in system-wide planning and innovation to achieve desirable organizational outcomes (Baldwin, Clark, Fulton, & Mayo, 2009).

Optimization often requires diverse knowledge and abilities, many of which are not uniquely nursing. Some broad categories are financial analysis, business communication, project management, quality or process improvement, and change management techniques. Specific examples from the literature are LEAN (a process improvement approach to reduce waste), SIX SIGMA (a process improvement approach to reduce errors), and Prosci ADKAR (a change management model; Gocsik & Barton, 2014; Patton, Lim, Ramlow, & White, 2015; Spruce & Butler, 2017). Health system optimization is often complex and can therefore require equally diverse skills and abilities.

The CNS is well situated to assist in the development and implementation of educational programs in order to optimize the management and performance of nursing practices, lead nursing research initiatives, improve patient outcomes, and lead health care teams. In this capacity, the CNS drives the structuring and optimization of health care organizations (Henderson, 2004).

The CNS is also positioned to optimize the nursing process, improve the quality of nursing care, and drive the development of specialty nursing (Lampe, Geddie, Aguirre, & Sole, 2013). The value of the CNS in primary health care and home care has been described more clearly in the US versus Canadian literature. The contributions of CNS tertiary care prevention, nursing service, and follow-up care for patients with chronic conditions, such as cardiovascular disease, diabetes, osteoporosis, and chronic pain, have been well established (Tian et al., 2014).

BreatheWELL at Home, a Fraser Health program in British Columbia, established a multi-sector partnership designated to assist clients to gain more control over their chronic obstructive pulmonary disease (COPD) and decrease tertiary care admissions. Led by CNSs, a patient-centred approach allowed clients to establish their own goals to manage symptoms and exacerbations through support, coaching, and education through home visits and telehealth. The results showed a 28% reduction in emergency room visits, 35% reduction in admissions, and a 16% reduction in hospital stay for those who were admitted (Fraser & Park, 2013). As well, the CNS reported that nurses expressed higher job satisfaction in assisting clients to better understand their COPD, which resulted in increased confidence in self-management and improved health. Similarly, a review by the Ontario Ministry of Health and Long-Term Care (MOHLTC) demonstrated that a CNS-led interprofessional approach to wound care was effective in reducing healing times by eight weeks, and treatment costs by approximately $18,000 per person (Browne, Birch & Thabane, 2012).

Kilpatrick, Tchouaket, Carter, Bryant-Lukosius, and DiCenso (2016) completed a survey of 445 CNSs and reported on the facilitators and barriers to APNs participating in organizational leadership work. One of the key implications to the study was in identifying structures and processes that influence the CNS role. In turn, these may inform approaches used by providers and decision makers that optimize the CNS role across health care settings and support the delivery of high-quality care.

With a rapidly aging population, along with associated alterations in health across the disease spectrum and management, the CNS will increasingly occupy a principal role in secondary prevention (McClelland, McCoy, & Burson, 2013). The emergence of patient-centred home care designed to improve access, coordination, quality, satisfaction, and comprehensive health care provides the CNS with a key role in implementing changes at multiple levels of the health care system (Fagerstrom, 2009).

The knowledge related to how CNSs optimize the health system is growing, but there is still a lot to learn. Even where there have been attempts to further this line of inquiry, the results can still be somewhat incomplete. Key unanswered questions include the optimal skill development path; what and who benefits most from CNS role participation; and the overall impact of the CNS role itself.

CASE STUDY

The Story of Duante

Duante is a clinical nurse specialist for the mental health and substance use services of a large health organization responsible for the region's full continuum of client care, including acute, outpatient, subacute, tertiary, and community services. As the only CNS for the region, most of his work focuses on opportunities that will help multiple sites and services. Duante enjoys the diversity this offers and the opportunities to improve such a large and complex set of systems that affect the lives of many people.

Recently, Duante was invited to a meeting with one of the service's senior administrative leaders. The provincial coroner had launched an inquest to investigate a cluster of suicide deaths in one of the communities within the region. The coroner issued a recommendation for the organization to complete an internal review of its suicide prevention processes and make necessary improvements to reduce the chance of future deaths. Duante was assigned the task of completing this work. Duante started with a plan to examine the current system for suicide assessment and intervention. This led to discovering that a key part of the system, an intervention called suicide safety planning, was being offered in less than 10% of appropriate cases.

A comprehensive review of suicide prevention literature was conducted that examined best practices and existing suicide prevention protocols. As well, the organization's suicide death reports were examined, and Duante dialogued with internal clinical staff and colleagues in other organizations. The analysis uncovered this was related to inefficiencies in documentation, safety planning health records management, and poor staff awareness and training for safety planning. Duante engaged with clients and other members of the health care team to resolve these barriers and advocate within the system.

With this information, Duante proposed possible solutions and set forth to collaborate with stakeholders from the related supporting systems. To speed up documentation, a piloted standardized safety plan form was created, and plans proceeded to integrate it into the various health records systems, making it available to partnering services/agencies. Duante also developed an online self-learning staff education module to support awareness and safety planning skills, which reduced education costs. These system improvements were launched over a one-year period ensuring the health care team understood these changes and used them effectively.

The result was very positive. Twelve months after its launch, chart audits indicated safety planning was being used in over 70% of appropriate cases, which was a significant increase from the baseline measurement. Staff training records showed that most staff had completed the online course and post-learning assessment surveys and were consistently positive. Health record improvements and the ability to share the document with external services had other stakeholders requesting copies of the materials for their own adoption. As a result of these system changes, there was a drop in suicide deaths in the at-risk community that had experienced the initial cluster of deaths that started this process in motion.

Discussion

In the case study, the CNS, Duante, was able to increase the use of an important suicide prevention intervention, which has reduced the number of deaths by suicide. Although one area was initially targeted, other communities benefited, leading to an optimization for this sector of the health system. An essential step in system optimization is to effectively identify gaps in the system and develop the strategies to produce the desired change. Duante was particularly aware that misidentifying an opportunity could result in the wrong solutions, wasting resources, and enabling continued suboptimal functioning. He utilized several experts in implementing the new processes, which included an online learning content developer in the education department, an electronic medical records database designer with the information management systems services, and a manager and privacy expert with the health records management department.

Duante frequently had to advocate for clients during the planning and implementation processes. As health organizations have many competing priorities, even very useful initiatives can be postponed or cancelled. He frequently communicated the importance of the suicide prevention optimization work to maintain its presence on the organization's leadership work plan and keep supporting team members focused and participating in the changes. He provided the senior leadership committee with regular updates about his progress and frequently reminded them about the tragedy of suicide deaths and the coroner's involvement. Through these actions, Duante advocated to keep the suicide prevention system optimization work at the forefront of the agenda and prevent it from being sidelined.

A potential barrier was met during implementation. The local telephone crisis line service was one of the necessary improvements voiced by clients and family members. However, due to confidentiality concerns, the health records and privacy departments generally did not allow this practice. Duante persuaded the leaders of these departments to approve an exception by presenting the evidence and representing clients' expressed needs. With their agreement, Duante was able to include design features and processes that facilitated sharing the safety plan with whomever the client chose. This improvement was possible only due to Duante's advocacy within the system.

In implementing the improvements to the organization's suicide prevention safety program, Duante communicated the changes to formal authorities and key informal stakeholders, as well as to all clinical staff. Implementation was continually monitored through ongoing data collection, acknowledging success stories, as well as providing coaching and feedback where it was needed. For this initiative, implementation was considered complete after one year.

Conclusion

CNSs are knowledgeable APNs who are well positioned within the health care system to support client care and positive outcomes in many ways, including health system optimization. The interconnected nature and potentially large size of many health care systems can make this complex and challenging. To effectively accomplish this work, the CNS must employ a variety of skills and draw on their expertise and networks. How CNSs can be involved in health system optimization continues to grow; however, there are still many unanswered questions. This competency is important because it offers the opportunity to impact health care organizations, the people who work within them, and the clients they serve, which can have impacts on communities provincially, federally, and globally. By using skills such as gap analysis, planning, client and team member engagement, advocacy, resource allocation, and implementation, the CNS is more likely to demonstrate successful outcomes. Health system optimization initiatives can be challenging and rewarding. To enhance effectiveness in this area, additional research by APNs, including CNSs, will be required. This might possibly require the development of an equally broader skill set and abilities that are not uniquely nursing but which place the CNS in an optimal role for this undertaking.

Critical Thinking Questions

1. The health care system is large, and there are many opportunities for system optimization. How would you describe the role of the CNS in identifying if a health system optimization project is needed in your workplace?
2. How would you communicate your ideas to your organization's leaders and/or stakeholders to engage them in optimizing a health system?
3. What skills align with your current strengths? What skills would you like to explore and develop further?

References

Baldwin, K. M., Clark, A., Fulton, J., & Mayo, A. (2009). National validation of the NACNS clinical nurse specialist competencies. *Journal of Nursing Scholarship, 41*(2), 193–201.

Browne, G., Birch, S., & Thabane, L. (2012). *Better care: An analysis of nursing and healthcare outcomes.* Ottawa, ON: CHSRF/CNA. Retrieved from http://archives.enap.ca/bibliotheques/2013/06/030429355.pdf

Canadian Nurses Association (CNA). (2019). *Advanced practice nursing: A pan-Canadian framework.* Ottawa, ON: CNA. Retrieved from https://www.cna-aiic.ca/-/media/cna/page-content/pdf-en/apn-a-pan-canadian-framework.pdf

Cordon, C. (2013). System theories: An overview of various system theories and its application in healthcare. *American Journal of Systems Science, 2*(1), 13–22.

Fagerstrom, L. (2009). Developing the scope of practice and education for advanced practice nurses in Finland. *International Nursing Review, 56,* 269–272.

Fraser, J., & Park, G. (2013). *BreatheWELL at home: Access and leadership in COPD self-management.* PowerPoint presentation for the Home Care Knowledge Network Better Care for People Living with Chronic Disease Webinar Series. Retrieved from http://www.cdnhomecare.ca/media.php?mid=3276

Gocsik, T., & Barton, A. (2014). Performance improvement methods to optimize clinical workflow, a practical approach. *Clinical Nurse Specialist, 28*(4), 197–200.

Henderson, S. (2004). The role of the clinical nurse specialist in medical surgical nursing. *Medical-Surgical Nursing, 13,* 38–41.

Kilpatrick, K., Tchouaket, A., Carter, N., Bryant-Lukosius, D., & DiCenso, A. (2016). Structural and process factors that influence clinical nurse specialist role implementation. *Clinical Nurse Specialist, 30*(2), 89–100.

Lampe, J. S., Geddie, P. I., Aguirre, L., & Sole, M. L. (2013). Finding the right fit: Implementation of a structured interviewing process for clinical nurse specialists. *Advanced Critical Care, 24,* 194–202.

Lewandowski, W., & Adamle, K. (2009). Substantive areas of clinical nurse specialist practice, a comprehensive review of the literature. *Clinical Nurse Specialist, 23*(2), 73–90.

McClelland, M., McCoy, M. A., & Burson, R. (2013). Clinical nurse specialists: Then, now, and the future of the profession. *Clinical Nurse Specialist, 27,* 96–102.

Patton, C., Lim, K., Ramlow, L., & White, K. (2015). Increasing efficiency in evaluation of chronic cough: A multidisciplinary, collaborative approach. *Quality Management in Health Care, 24*(4), 177–182.

Spruce, K., & Butler, C. (2017). Enhancing outcomes for outpatient percutaneous coronary intervention. *Clinical Nurse Specialist, 31*(6), 319–328.

Suter, E., Goldman, J., Martimianakis, T., Chatalalsingh, C., DeMatteo, D. J., & Reeves, S. (2013). The use of systems and organizational theories in the interprofessional field: Findings from a scoping review. *Journal of Interprofessional Care, 27,* 57–64.

Tian, X., Lian, J.-X., Ma, L., Wang, Y., Cao, H., & Song, G.-M. (2014). Current status of clinical nurse specialists and the demands of osteoporosis specialized nurses in mainland China. *International Journal of Nursing Sciences, 1*(3), 306–313.

Chapter

15B

Optimizing Health System Competencies

Nurse Practitioner

Paul Tylliros

PAUL TYLLIROS is a nurse practitioner (NP)-PHC working in northwestern Ontario with an Indigenous health access organization. He has been a nurse practitioner since 2012 and a registered nurse since 2004. Paul has experience working with various federally and provincially funded health care organizations in Ontario and Manitoba since 2004.

KEY TERMS

advanced practice nursing (APN) competencies
health care settings
optimize health system

OBJECTIVES

1. Discuss the importance of the nurse practitioner (NP) role in optimizing health systems in today's complex health care environment.
2. Explore the NP role in relation to optimizing health systems.
3. Discuss potential outcomes for patients, families, and communities when NPs optimize health systems.

Introduction

The current landscape of health care delivery in Canada includes multi-faceted approaches within primary, secondary, and tertiary **health care settings**. Optimization of the nurse practitioner (NP) role within these diverse health care settings requires recognition and support for the full scope of NP practice and competencies from multiple levels of government and community stakeholders. The NP should be able to integrate diversity and creativity in their approach and delivery of health care to meet the many unique health care demands across these sectors (Bryant-Lukosius & Martin-Misener, 2015). The expected result would be that clients and communities would have the opportunity for enhanced continuity and sustainability of access to health care and improved client care outcomes (Bryant-Lukosius & Martin-Misener, 2015).

The NP is well situated to lead or participate in initiatives that **optimize health system** sectors for the benefit of improved access, especially in remote, isolated, and rural settings, and especially for Indigenous Peoples in northern Canada. The Canadian Nurses Association's (CNA) **advanced practice nursing (APN) competencies** illustrate the full capacity to function in diverse health care environments. Nevertheless, several aspects of health care delivery and the surrounding policy, legislation, geographical, and physical limitations can complicate the ability to implement and sustain the optimization of such health systems (Bryant-Lukosius & Martin-Misener, 2015; CNA, 2019).

The importance of the role of the NP is supported by evidence that demonstrates NPs can have an impact in optimizing health systems using a broad range of interventions from direct client care management, streamlining care delivery, and coordination of services to advocating and creating health care policy (DiCenso & Bryant-Lukosius, 2010; Little & Reichert, 2018).

Optimizing Health System Competency

In the CNA's 2019 pan-Canadian APN competencies, optimizing health system refers to the ability of APNs to make contributions that improve efficiencies in health systems functioning through advocacy, promoting innovative client care, and facilitating equitable, client-centred health care (CNA, 2019).

The NP's optimization of the health system competency contributes to the processes within health care systems via creative client care solutions, promoting health care access, advocating for equitable health services, and is geared toward increasing client-centred health care. Furthermore, essential to the delivery and execution of health care services, NPs exercising the optimizing health system competency engage clients and communities, health teams, and existing health delivery mechanisms in promoting health care access and resolving and mitigating the challenges to access and sustainability of health delivery (CNA, 2019).

Through active participation, NPs seeks to understand the unique knowledge base of the population and communities they serve to optimize the best approach to delivering health care. For example, Indigenous communities have unique traditions and practices that factor in their definition and values of health and wellness. These include a traditional system of knowing and being that provides a different framework from which the NP practices when obtaining individual health information. Therefore, using and implementing creative health care assessment strategies would be an appropriate demonstration of optimizing the unique health care system in assessing and meeting the health care demands of this population (Bryant-Lukosius & Martin-Misener, 2015; CNA, 2019; de Witt & Ploeg, 2005; World Health Organization [WHO], 2016).

The NP's role is fundamental in building strategies and influencing government and health policy with their advanced practice knowledge and judgment. Nurse practitioners are significantly positioned to address legislation and political agendas that either challenge or

TABLE 15B.1: Optimizing Health System Competencies

- Engage clients and other team members in resolving issues at the health system level
- Generate and incorporate new nursing knowledge to develop standards of care, practice guidelines, care protocols, programs, and policies
- Advocate for clients in relation to care, the health system and policy decisions that broadly affect health (e.g., determinants of health), and quality of life
- Understand and integrate the principles of resource allocation and cost effectiveness in organizational and health system-level decision-making
- Contribute to system-level change through policy and guideline development and effective use of resources
- Participate in strategic planning for their health care service, department, or facility
- Contribute to, consult, or collaborate with other health care personnel on recruitment and retention activities
- Implement improvements in health care, including delivery structures and processes
- Understand legislative and socio-political issues that influence health policy and use this knowledge to build strategies to improve health, health care access, and healthy public policy
- Identify gaps in the health system and develop strategies to facilitate and manage change
- Advocate for changes in health policy by participating on regional, provincial/territorial, and federal committees that influence decision-making

Source: CNA. (2019). *Advanced practice nursing: A pan-Canadian framework.* Ottawa, ON: CNA. Retrieved from https://www.cna-aiic.ca/-/media/cna/page-content/pdf-en/apn-a-pan-canadian-framework.pdf

facilitate health care access. Historical data are clear in demonstrating NPs have been uniquely positioned with knowledge and expertise to provide access to care for remote northern Canadian communities, namely Indigenous communities (CNA, 2019). Armed with this evidence, NPs can and do advance health care outcomes surrounding all chronic disease management. Also, NPs promote public health initiatives, identify gaps in health care systems, and offer solutions to empower and manage change and client satisfaction over other health care providers (CNA, 2010, 2019).

Lastly, by optimizing health systems, NPs reduce barriers to access to health care, improve wait times, and lessen the burden on the health care system. This is achieved by providing access for clients with early diagnosis, interventions, management of acute and chronic health conditions, and offering educational wellness solutions with continuity of care (Hurlock-Chorostecki & McCallum, 2016). Table 15b.1 describes the competency, Optimizing Health System, which is one of eight core competencies for APN practice (CNA, 2019).

Limitations exist for the NP in executing full scope of practice and optimization of health systems, such as insufficient comprehensive team-based funding models that support the NP role. Many regions of Canada do not have a primary health care (PHC) provider/family physician and would benefit from the implementation of the NP role (Bryant-Lukosius & Martin-Misener, 2015; Little & Reichert, 2018).

CASE STUDY

The Story of Thomas

Thomas, an NP living in a small northwestern Ontario community of approximately 15,000 people, is employed by an Indigenous health access centre funded by both provincial and federal agencies. This is a new role for Thomas and his mandate is to provide and coordinate health care services to this community and 12 neighbouring remote Indigenous communities situated approximately 75 km from the nearest town and tertiary health care centre.

The health care service agreement identifies the provision of primary health care services to all ages and to collaborate with existing health and administration personnel in each of the communities, including the chief and council leadership.

One of these communities has been without health care access for 12 weeks due to the lack of available health care providers in the region. The population is approximately 150 people, with individuals' ages ranging from 18 to 45 years. Prior to this, the community's health care services had been infrequently available due to the limited primary health care resources available and geographical barriers.

Thomas finds this an exciting opportunity to practice utilizing his knowledge, skill, and abilities in a capacity not practiced in before. After careful consideration, meetings with his agency, and a review of his service delivery expectations, it is determined that he will provide outreach health care services one day per week initially to establish access to health care for these Indigenous communities.

For Thomas to provide health care services, he will first need to identify the stakeholders and leaders in the communities. Thomas initiates meetings and introductions to the councillors, chief, and elders of the communities. Further, he creates a working relationship with the community health director and administration to identify the immediate health care gaps that need to be addressed first. The feedback of health care needs includes a lack of chronic disease management, particularly for clients with diabetes and cardiovascular disease, child immunization, and women's health screening.

Thomas has been an NP for six years and has gained valuable and insightful perspectives and experiences in community health capacity building in order to ascertain how he will optimize and provide health care services to these remote communities.

After only four short months, community members and leaders report they are happy with how Thomas has optimized health care services in the communities that is evidenced by improved continuity of care, coordination of health care services with physician collaboration, public health nursing, community health representatives, community health nurses, laboratory services, and medication dispensing and distribution. Thomas has been involved in implementing health programs for chronic diseases, men's and women's health, cancer screening, and child and infant health programs. Due to his efforts, the communities have also seen an increase in health care access and collaboration with physicians and specialists from the nearest tertiary care centre benefiting the overall health of the communities served.

Discussion

In the case, Thomas illustrates through his role as an NP several strategies to optimize health system competency. Various elements of his practice and collaboration were essential to benefit individuals and the community accessing health care. Thomas recognized the importance of his participation in optimizing the health systems within his community. These included but were not limited to advocating for clients, improving quality of patient care, increasing comprehensiveness of care, understanding resource allocation and effectiveness within the health system, increasing patients' subjective experiences, and most significantly, increasing access to health care (Little & Reichert, 2018).

Although NPs have been utilized across Canada, including in remote and rural outposts and health centres since the 1970s, the shortage of primary care providers, access, and lengthy wait times are still apparent (de Witt & Ploeg, 2005; Little & Reichert, 2018). Therefore, an NP such as Thomas is well situated in rural northwestern Ontario to address first-hand the complexities and challenges faced by many northern Canadian communities. Furthermore, associated with the shortage of health care providers is the lack of interprofessional collaboration with physician specialists, nurses, and administration required to facilitate health care delivery in remote/rural communities. Such interprofessional collaboration was achieved by Thomas's efforts in coordinating the implementation and utilization of health programs, laboratory services, urgent medical transportation services, and establishing a physician partnership if physician consultation was required (Little & Reichert, 2018).

Once Thomas understood the multiplicity of collaboration required, he further explored the fundamental processes necessary to sustain these services. He explored the evidence and sought assistance internally and externally of his professional group to determine if there was a comprehensive team-based funding model that would support the NP role in increasing access to PHC. The gaps and challenges are evident with many northern communities facing limited access to a primary care provider or infrequent physician availability. These communities would greatly benefit from the implementation of NPs (Little & Reichert, 2018).

Government legislation and policies continue to restrict some NPs in rural settings such as Ontario. Although the NP has provincial authority and legislation to prescribe and manage controlled substances, the NP continues to be restricted in ordering CT/MRI and specific laboratory testing to investigate symptoms and cause of illness in some provinces. Policies and current legislation that inform the scope of NP practice can either assist or detract from the NP's ability to pursue further diagnostic investigations, which has an impact on the ability to optimize health systems and facilitate client care and treatment (Little & Reichert, 2018).

With increasing supportive evidence, health authorities recognize the potential cost savings to the health system from utilizing and engaging NPs in rural and remote communities. This is further supported by initiatives to increase and integrate the NP along with appropriate technology into the primary health care system, including the expansion of NP-Led Clinics in Ontario (Wilson & Mattison, 2018).

Thomas's example applied current evidence into his role of providing health care services to these remote communities. He recommended the optimization of various sectors that make up the continuity of care within this practice environment, the use of interprofessional collaboration, the use of electronic medical records technology, and utilizing the full scope of NP practice (Wilson & Mattison, 2018).

Although many questions arose in terms of role clarity and scope of practice, Thomas was purposefully instrumental in introducing his role, allowing opportunities for role clarity with clients, community members, and leadership. Thomas took the initiative to hold meetings and in-services about his role and practice in the community. This further promoted the role of the NP and increased the understanding of NP education, skill, and competencies (CNA, 2014).

Unfortunately, incorporating physicians into the health care rotation with remote communities was not a favourable option for visiting physicians. Physicians are normally perceived as better utilized within urban, community, and hospital/urgent care settings. The evidence supports this as NPs are well received in remote communities and have been utilized in remote and northern Canadian communities since the 1970s (de Witt & Ploeg, 2005; DiCenso & Bryant-Lukosius, 2010).

Key learning opportunities for Thomas included adapting to the unique practice environment, assessing the current challenges and successes while building on community strengths. NPs are well situated to achieve improved health status and outcomes, thus optimizing on community capacity in areas requiring modification such as transportation, client discharge, and follow-up appointments. Therefore, NPs can be adaptive and flexible to a variety of populations, and health system needs, combined with the lack of providers in northern communities, have facilitated the acceptance and addition of the NP role in northern health care systems (DiCenso & Bryant-Lukosius, 2010).

Nurse practitioners utilize expert knowledge and abilities to optimize their role in improving health and health care system outcomes. Remote nursing stations are established in communities with small populations that often have higher than normal health care demands placed on the health care provider. However, the NP is well positioned to practice in these small communities as they are not reliant on the volume of health care, but rather the access of health care (Wilson & Mattison, 2018).

Thomas, through self reflection, acknowledges the profound impact he was having in utilizing his knowledge, skill, and expertise in delivering health care services. He also recognized that this remains a satisfying and fulfilling career and practice opportunity in a challenging health care setting. He was able to identify, through his experience, how the effectiveness of NPs can be paramount in the remote communities where he is located. Thomas has acquired expert knowledge in optimizing several aspects of the health care process and systems to promote access to care. As a result, he was recognized as a leader and a key facilitator among his peers and communities. During this time, he gained critical insight and foresight with the health care delivery processes and systems where he continues to work with remote Indigenous communities in an effort to reduce the disparity between health care needs and achieved health care outcomes.

Conclusion

Moving forward with purposeful initiatives, identifying gaps in the health care system, advocating for change, and participating in strategic planning are fundamental for the NP. As the NP engages in these activities to optimize health systems, they are, in effect, enacting competencies as defined by the CNA (2010, 2014, 2016, 2019).

Furthermore, NPs participate by advocating for access to care and the legislation and organizational policies that impact clients' right to care and the resulting health outcomes. Nurse practitioners are also well situated in identifying key factors affecting health, such as the determinants of health and quality of life indicators for rural and remote communities.

The integration of NPs into the northern health care system has been an important human resource strategy for optimizing access to primary health care services and has facilitated significant acceptance in addressing the shortage of providers in Canada's northern communities. As a result, NPs have demonstrated adaptive and flexible approaches in meeting the health care demands of a variety of populations (DiCenso & Bryant-Lukosius, 2010).

Lastly, findings are consistent across studies identifying APNs that NPs are effective and safe health care practitioners who can positively influence the individual, provider, and health system outcomes (Little & Reichert, 2018).

Critical Thinking Questions

1. What benefits and challenges do you foresee as NPs continue to optimize health systems?
2. Which aspects of the CNA optimizing health system competency did Thomas utilize and execute?
3. What future considerations exist for NPs in optimizing health systems? What areas of health care would be most beneficial as the next steps?
4. Are there any opportunities in your organization or health care practice setting to expand health services or change the way you optimize health systems?

References

Bryant-Lukosius, D., & Martin-Misener, M. (2015). *ICN policy brief. Advanced practice nursing: An essential component of country level human resources for health.* Geneva, CH: ICN. Retrieved from http://fhs.mcmaster.ca/ccapnr/documents/ICNPolicyBrief6AdvancedPracticeNursing.pdf

Canadian Nurses Association (CNA). (2010). *Canadian nurse practitioner core competency framework.* Ottawa, ON: CNA. Retrieved from http://www.cno.org/globalassets/for/rnec/pdf/competencyframework_en.pdf

CNA. (2014). *Optimizing the role of nurses in primary health care: Final report.* Ottawa, ON: CNA. Retrieved from https://cna-aiic.ca/~/media/cna/page-content/pdf-en/optimizing-the-role-of-nurses-in-primary-care-in-canada.pdf

CNA. (2016). *Position statement: Nurse practitioner.* Ottawa, ON: CNA. Retrieved from https://www. cna-aiic.ca/-/media/cna/page-content/pdf-en/the-nurse-practitioner-position-statement_2016.pdf

CNA. (2019). *Advanced practice nursing: A pan-Canadian framework.* Ottawa, ON: CNA. Retrieved from https://www.cna-aiic.ca/-/media/cna/page-content/pdf-en/apn-a-pan-canadian-framework.pdf

de Witt, L., & Ploeg, J. (2005). Critical analysis of the evolution of a Canadian nurse practitioner role. *Canadian Journal of Nursing Research, 37*(4), 116–137.

DiCenso, A., & Bryant-Lukosius, D. (2010). *Clinical nurse specialists and nurse practitioners in Canada: A decision support synthesis.* Ottawa, ON: CHFI. Retrieved from https://www.cfhi-fcass.ca/Search-ResultsNews/10-06-01/b9cb9576-6140-4954-aa57-2b81c1350936.aspx

Hurlock-Chorostecki, C., & McCallum, J. (2016). Nurse practitioner role, values in hospital: New strategies for hospital leaders. *Nursing Leadership, 29*(3), 82–92.

Little, L., & Reichert, C. (2018). *Fulfilling nurse practitioners' untapped potential in Canada's health care system: Results from the CFNU pan-Canadian nurse practitioner retention & recruitment study.* Ottawa, ON: CFNU. Retrieved from https://nursesunions.ca/wp-content/uploads/2018/06/CFNU_UntappedPotential-Final-EN.pdf

Wilson, M. G., & Mattison, C. A. (2018). *Rapid synthesis: Enhancing health system integration of nurse practitioners in Ontario.* Hamilton, ON: McMaster University Health Forum. Retrieved from https://macsphere.mcmaster.ca/bitstream/11375/23852/1/Enhancing%20Health%20System%20Integration%20of%20Nurse%20Practitioners%20in%20Ontario.pdf

World Health Organization (WHO). (2016). *Indigenous populations.* Geneva, CH: WHO.

Chapter 16A

Educational Competencies

Clinical Nurse Specialist

Line Beaudet and Steve Gagné

LINE BEAUDET is an advanced practice nurse in neurosciences and Principal Scientist at the Centre de recherche du Centre hospitalier de l'Université de Montréal (CRCHUM), Montreal, Quebec. She is an Associate Professor at the Faculty of Nursing, Université de Montréal, Montreal, Quebec.

STEVE GAGNÉ is an advanced practice nurse in critical care and Associate Scientist at the Centre de recherche du Centre hospitalier de l'Université de Montréal (CRCHUM), Montreal, Quebec. He is an Associate Clinical Nurse Specialist at the Faculty of Nursing, Université de Montréal, Montreal, Quebec.

KEY TERMS

clinical nurse specialist (CNS)
coaching
education
mentoring
preceptorship

OBJECTIVES

1. Appraise the core educational competencies of the clinical nurse specialist (CNS).
2. Discuss how these competencies can develop throughout the professional career of the CNS.
3. Identify the impact of these competencies on the different spheres of influence of the CNS (patients and families, providers and teams, organization, health care system, and society).

Introduction

The increasing complexity of health care, the emergence of new practices, and the evolution of health knowledge are all elements that call on the educational competencies of the **clinical nurse specialist (CNS)**. These include **education, mentoring, preceptorship,** and **coaching.** Educational competencies are based on the clinical expertise of the CNS in their specialized area of nursing, as well as on caring, academic, and personalized support skills developed during graduate education and throughout their career in broader health care environments

(O'Grady & Johnson, 2019). Although distinct, these competencies are at the heart of the CNS's advanced practice and promote the engagement of patients, families, caregivers, and interdisciplinary teams in their specific learning activities (Canadian Nurses Association [CNA], 2019; O'Grady & Johnson, 2019).

This chapter defines the core educational competencies of the CNS. It discusses how the CNS can develop these competencies during a professional career. Finally, based on a case study, it highlights the impacts of educational competencies on the various spheres of influence of the CNS such as patients and families, providers and teams, the organization, the health care system, and society.

Educational Competencies of the Clinical Nurse Specialist

Several relational approaches emerge from the literature related to the core educational competencies of the CNS, particularly education, mentoring, preceptorship, and coaching. Although they share common elements, various aspects distinguish them, for example, their purpose, their duration, as well as their process and the focus of the interaction (O'Grady & Johnson, 2019).

Patient and Family Education

The CNS draws on extensive disciplinary and empirical knowledge, as well as evidence-informed educational strategies, and is recognized as an expert in patient, family, and public education (Morin, 2018). This is illustrated by the CNS's ability to grasp the complex health situations that are encountered, the particularities of the environment, as well as the diversity of patient and family needs, concerns, and preferences in order to adjust their teaching and educational strategies (O'Grady & Johnson, 2019). More specifically, patient and family education encompass informational and interactive learning activities, delivered as needed over several weeks, in individual, group, or telehealth formats (Tessier, 2012). The CNS's educational mission is founded on sustainability and aims to make information accessible at the local, national, and international levels, as well as to empower and promote the health of the population served (Winnipeg Regional Health Authority [WRHA], 2012).

This competency includes educational approaches that foster individual and family well-being and quality of life such as health education, therapeutic education, motivational interviewing, providing role models, peer support, problem-solving, demonstration and training, as well as family system, psycho-educational, and behavioural approaches (Bonnin & Palicot, 2001; Morin, 2018; Tessier, 2012). The education provided by the CNS assists patients and their families in making difficult decisions and life choices and fosters the development of confidence in managing the impact of concomitant acute and chronic physical and mental health issues (Morin, 2018; O'Grady & Johnson, 2019).

Staff and Interdisciplinary Team Education

With recognized expertise in clinical practice, knowledge of adult education, and evidence-informed outcomes in their area of nursing specialization, the CNS contributes to the education and professional development of caregivers and the interprofessional health care team (Jokiniemi, 2014; Mathieu, Bell, Ramelet, & Morin, 2016). Education for caregivers and the interprofessional health care team includes pedagogical activities, both informal and formal, whether face-to-face, online, or in writing (WRHA, 2012). For example, the CNS initiates and supports the conceptualization, delivery, and evaluation of training, educational activities, and residency programs for health care providers, students, and managers based on an analysis of their learning needs (Jokiniemi, 2014; WRHA, 2012). The CNS is responsible for the development, integration, and use of clinical pathways, new technologies, and best practice guidelines within the organization (Chick, Negley, Sievers, & Tammel, 2012; Gurzick & Kesten, 2010; Mohr & Coke, 2018). Many CNSs with a university affiliation are also accountable for the supervision or the direction of APN students (Mathieu et al., 2016).

The CNS education competency is rooted in a co-development approach with the caregivers and the interprofessional health care team (O'Grady & Johnson, 2019). It includes diversified educational strategies, including reflective practice, knowledge mapping, concept mapping, series mapping, high-fidelity simulation, role modelling, demonstration, journal clubs, quality of care audits, and joint monitoring of clinical and administrative performance indicators (Chick et al., 2012). In short, this competency of the CNS promotes the development and transfer of knowledge, the continuous optimization of practice, and greater involvement of staff nurses in resolving organizational challenges and issues within the ever-changing health care system (CNA, 2019; Mathieu et al., 2016; Mohr & Coke, 2018).

Mentoring, Preceptorship, and Coaching

Inspired by a humanist model of nursing and a partnership perspective with patients, families, caregivers, interprofessional health care teams, and undergraduate and graduate students, the CNS draws on other educational competencies, such as mentoring, preceptorship, and coaching (CNA, 2019; O'Grady & Johnson, 2019).

Mentoring is defined by Meier (2013) as "a nurturing process in which a more skilled or more experienced person, serving as a role model, teaches, sponsors, encourages, counsels, and befriends a less-skilled or less-experienced person for the purpose of promoting the latter's professional and/or personal development" (p. 343). Mentoring involves the establishment and long-term maintenance of a trusting, voluntary, and mutual relationship between mentor and mentee (Meier, 2013). Mentoring by a CNS aims to increase the mentee's level of satisfaction and self-confidence, as well as passing on humanist values and knowledge, particularly at the empirical, experiential, ethical, and political levels (Mijares & Bond, 2013).

The second competency, preceptorship, constitutes an "educational process embedded in a dynamic nursing environment where expert nurses guide nurses or nursing students through structured hands-on clinical experiences to hone their skills and socialize them to the profession and/or specific clinical settings" (Ward & McComb, 2017, p. e878). Unlike mentoring, preceptorship is not a voluntary commitment between tutor and preceptor. It is limited in time and oriented to the integration of concrete skills and the attainment of specific objectives (Meier, 2013).

As for coaching, this competency corresponds to a "skilled, purposeful, results-oriented, and structured relationship-centered interaction with clients for the purpose of promoting achievement of client goals" (O'Grady & Johnson, 2019, p. 184). The clients, whether a patient and his family coping with multiple chronic illnesses or health professionals facing a new or complex situation, are able to articulate their goals and take ownership of their choices as well as the changes they are making (O'Grady & Johnson, 2019). The CNS's coaching is like a catalyst that assists clients to clarify their expectations, specify the nature of their solutions, anticipate and take up challenges, and lastly, fine-tune the approach undertaken to achieve the goals set (Ervin, 2005; O'Grady & Johnson, 2019).

In summary, mentoring, preceptorship, and coaching are complementary educational competencies the CNS can draw on in their roles of teaching and supporting the transition experiences of patients, families, caregivers, interprofessional health care teams, and students. Each of these competencies contributes to meeting the specific learning needs of clients and health professionals and to the development and integration of evidence-based knowledge.

Developing Lifelong Educational Competencies

In order to develop the breadth of educational competencies needed and the confidence to apply their abilities, the CNS must engage in continuous professional development throughout their career (CNA, 2019). There are several learning approaches available (CNA, 2019; WRHA, 2012):

- Complete and maintain certification in their area of specialization
- Stay abreast of developments in their field of practice and in adult education by creating and maintaining their own awareness program
- Join a mentoring program with an experienced CNS within their organization
- Participate in a co-development group and community of practice dedicated to APNs
- Engage in national associations of APNs, and patient and family advocacy
- Obtain and maintain an APN affiliation with a faculty of nursing
- Collaborate closely with dynamic interprofessional health care teams and experienced researchers
- Publish articles and design written and online educational materials
- Assume responsibility for committees, workshops, webinars, podcasts, and conferences at the academic, clinical, scientific, and policy levels
- Conduct an annual evaluation of their professional development as a CNS within a competency framework
- Seek and receive feedback from peers and supervisors on professional development, and develop an action plan based on learning objectives to be achieved

CASE STUDY

The Story of Alinta

Alinta is a CNS in the emergency department (ED) of a university hospital. At a monthly meeting with the head nurse and the department manager, they review the profiles of newly recruited nurses, as well as the number of positions to be filled to complete their team. The retention rate is around 70%. The novice nurses state that there is a significant gap between the theoretical concepts covered in undergraduate nursing education and the clinical reality of the tertiary care hospital centre. The complexity of the clients is making the ED an unattractive environment for new graduates. The management team proposes reviewing the orientation process for novice nurses in the ED. In order to resolve the situation, Alinta proposes implementing a residency program in the ED. She explains that, based on results elsewhere, such a program would permit, among other things, the acquisition of skills in assessing the physical and mental condition of clients in various complex health situations. In addition, the residency program would be based on best practices identified in the critical care and adult learner literature. The CNS knows that this type of professional inquiry is essential to ensure optimal quality of care and safe health care delivery in the ED.

In order to develop a relevant course curriculum for the novice nursing team in the ED, Alinta consults with the faculty who provides critical care training at the university affiliated with the hospital centre. She reviews the course outlines and the activities carried out in the skills laboratory to obtain an accurate picture of a new graduate starting a career in the ED. For a CNS, it is important to build on prior learning to foster a continuum of learning. This statement is one of the premises of the competency-based approach. Based on the concepts and theoretical ideas presented in the undergraduate nursing program, the CNS can design a structured education plan for hiring that is part of a professionalization process that will meet the needs and expectations of nursing staff, as well as fulfill the mission of the ED and the organization.

For Alinta, the objectives pursued by the residency program stem from the competencies listed by the Canadian Nurses Association related to the ED specialty, and from the professional associations of the specialty. The content of the education days must also meet the standards of nursing practice published by the National Emergency Nurses Affiliation and the Emergency Nurses Association. To ensure compliance, Alinta ensures that the curriculum and the student learning objectives for the various education days of the residency program are consistent with the professional aspirations presented by the various North American emergency care associations. Depending on the objectives pursued, the CNS will utilize a variety of educational strategies that allow for the development of a nurse's clinical judgment and clinical leadership in order to meet the competency indicators of a nurse working in the ED.

The residency program needs to consider different components in health sciences pedagogy and promote the educational principles of the adult learner. Alinta includes a variety of teaching strategies to stimulate learning and promote their integration into practice using presentations, hands-on demonstrations, clinical observation, video viewing, concept mapping, high-fidelity simulation, peer-to-peer case study analysis, and preceptorship. Although Alinta is responsible for creating and designing the residency program, she surrounds herself with experienced clinical nurses in the ED and a nurse educator to design and fine-tune the content, as well as to deliver the educational aspects of the residency program. Collaboration with a team of experienced nurse clinicians will facilitate discussions and foster the clinical reasoning and critical thinking skills required of novice nurses.

Discussion

In the case study, Alinta demonstrates a desire to develop the knowledge and competencies appropriate to the ED specialization and to prepare novice nurses to better develop in the clinical setting. To consolidate their clinical judgment, Alinta opted to create a residency program. This initiative is consistent with recommendations from the Institute of Medicine (2011) that a residency program can facilitate the role transition of nurse caregivers. In addition, the results of several studies (Casse, 2019; Goode, Reid Ponte, & Sullivan Havens, 2016; Meyer Bratt, 2013) highlight the benefits of such a curriculum for novice health professionals in different spheres of influence.

Sphere of Influence: Individual/Family

The structure of a nursing residency program is a way of encouraging novice nurses to ground their clinical practice on evidence-informed outcomes (Barnett, Minnick, & Norman, 2014). As part of the education activities, novice nurses can ask themselves questions about current practices related to best practices. In helping to develop this type of educational initiative aimed at health care personnel, the CNS contribution encompasses improving patient and family satisfaction with health care, better management of the health care episode that will optimize length of stay, and early detection of complications that may arise for the patient (Micevski et al., 2004).

Sphere of Influence: Professionals

By sharing knowledge and clinical expertise with interprofessional health care teams, the CNS contributes to the development of the practice of health care in their institution. In this case, Alinta's vision of initiating a residency program permits novice nurses to reduce the gap between theoretical concepts and clinical reality. The main objective is to facilitate the role transition of novice nurses (Boyer, Valdez-Delgado, Huss, Barker, & Mann-Salinas, 2017; Goode et al., 2016). By favouring pedagogical strategies that allow these nurses to participate actively in their learning, the CNS contributes to the integration of nursing and speciality knowledge (Meyer Bratt, 2013). The CNS participates in developing the clinical leadership of the novice nurse, as well as their competencies and professional confidence in order to provide quality care (Goode et al., 2016). In seeking the collaboration of experienced nurse clinicians and nurse educators in a preceptorship program, the CNS promotes the development of a culture of support and learning among nurses (Meyer Bratt, 2013).

Sphere of Influence: Organization

With recruitment and retention continuing to be challenges for health care organizations, the CNS can help to maintain the nursing workforce. As some 13% of nurses leave the profession within the first year of their careers and 37% consider changing jobs (Rosseter, 2014), initiatives by a CNS, in conjunction with the management and education team and other partners of the health care organization, can contribute to the stabilization of the nursing workforce. The implementation of a residency program has a direct impact on the organization's human resources. This program for novice nurses reduces the turnover rate of new graduates, while increasing job satisfaction and personnel retention (Chant & Westendorf, 2019; Eckerson, 2018). Also, the human resources department can use this type of initiative as a promotional tool for recruitment at job fairs (Pillai, Manister, Coppolo, Ducey, & McManus-Penzero, 2018).

Sphere of Influence: Health Care System and Society

The practice of integrating a residency program into a novice nurse's career path has been in existence for over 40 years (Pillai et al., 2018). This type of on-the-job continuing education has been part of the American recommendations for health care facilities since its introduction (Institute of Medicine, 2011). The creation of a residency program is an example of how an innovative CNS's idea can influence the health care system. For institutions, this type of CNS project is essential for developing the competencies of novice nurses and providing them with appropriate clinical support. In this way, the CNS contributes to maintaining access to health care in an efficient and optimal manner.

Conclusion

The literature affirms that CNSs' educational competencies facilitate the provision of knowledge and new practices to clients, professionals, organizations, and the health care system. To do this, the CNS can rely on proven clinical, pedagogical, and scientific competencies, particularly education, mentoring, preceptorship, and coaching. These considerable assets enable the CNS to draw on a variety of strategies in adult education. The CNS is encouraged to develop educational competencies throughout their professional career and to mobilize internal and external resources. In this way, the CNS can pass on the benefits of their expertise to the various parties involved by acting as a role model for new generations of nurses.

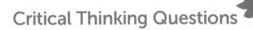

Critical Thinking Questions

1. An innovative treatment was recently approved by Health Canada. As a CNS, you are responsible for developing a webinar for patients and caregivers in your area of specialization. How would you do this?
2. New legislation passed by parliament will transform nursing and interprofessional practice in your province and organization. What educational strategies should the CNS focus on and why?
3. The integration of patient/family partners is increasingly valued from the beginning of the development of any educational program and throughout the different phases of the process. How can their integration influence the results of an educational program for clients, professionals, the organization, and the health care system?

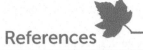

References

Barnett, J. S., Minnick, A. F., & Norman, L. D. (2014). A description of U.S. post-graduation nurse residency programs. *Nursing Outlook, 62*, 174–184.

Bonnin, F., & Palicot, A. M. (2001). L'éducation pour la santé: un service au public, un enjeu de la modernisation du système de santé. Proposition du réseau des comités d'éducation pour la santé [Health education: A service to the public, an issue in the modernization of the health system. Proposal from the network of health education committees]. *Santé publique, 3*(13), 287–294.

Boyer, S. A., Valdez-Delgado, K. K., Huss, J. L., Barker, A. J., & Mann-Salinas, E. A. (2017). Impact of nurse residency program on transition to specialty practice. *Journal of Nurses in Professional Development, 33*(5), 220–227.

Canadian Nurses Association (CNA). (2019). *Advanced practice nursing: A pan-Canadian framework.* Ottawa, ON: CNA. Retrieved from https://www.cna-aiic.ca/-/media/cna/page-content/pdf-en/advanced-practice-nursing-framework-en.pdf

Casse, K. (2019). ED opportunities for new graduates: Implementing an emergency nurse residency program. *Nursing Management, 50*(4), 36–41.

Chant, K. J., & Westendorf, D. S. (2019). Nurse residency programs: Key components for sustainability. *Journal for Nurses in Professional Development, 35*(4), 185–192.

Chick, K., Negley, K., Sievers, B., & Tammel, K. (2012). Enhancing patient education through clinical nurse specialist collaboration. *Clinical Nurse Specialist, 26*(6), 317–322.

Eckerson, C. M. (2018). The impact of nurse residency program in United States on improving retention and satisfaction of new nurse hires: An evidence-based literature review. *Nurse Education Today, 71*, 84–90.

Ervin, N. E. (2005). Clinical coaching: A strategy for enhancing evidence-based nursing practice. *Clinical Nurse Specialist, 19*(6), 296–301.

Goode, C. J., Reid Ponte, P., & Sullivan Havens, D. (2016). Residency for transition into practice: An essential requirement for new graduates from basic RN programs. *The Journal of Nursing Administration, 46*(2), 82–86.

Gurzick, M., & Kesten, K. S. (2010). The impact of clinical nurse specialists on clinical pathways in the application of evidence-based practice. *Journal of Professional Nursing, 26*(1), 42–48.

Institute of Medicine. (2011). *The future of nursing: Leading change, advancing health.* Washington, DC: The National Academies Press. Retrieved from https://www.ic4n.org/wp-content/uploads/2018/03/The-Future-of-Nursing-Report-2010.pdf

Jokiniemi, K. (2014). *Clinical nurse specialist in Finnish health care* (Doctoral thesis, University of Eastern Finland). Dissertations in Health Sciences, Number 249. Retrieved from https://core.ac.uk/download/pdf/32427141.pdf

Mathieu, L., Bell, L., Ramelet, A. S., & Morin, D. (2016). Les compétences de leadership pour la pratique infirmière avancée : Proposition d'un modèle de développement pour la formation infirmière et la pratique clinique [Leadership skills for advanced nursing practice: Proposal of a development model for nursing education and clinical practice]. *Revue francophone internationale de recherche infirmière.* doi: 10.1016/j.refiri.2016.04.003

Meier, S. R. (2013). Concept analysis of mentoring. *Advances in Neonatal Care, 13*(5), 341–345.

Meyer Bratt, M. (2013). Nurse residency program: Best practices for optimizing organizational success. *Journal for Nurses in Professional Development, 29*(3), 102–110.

Micevski, V., Korkola, L., Sarkissian, S., Mulcahy, V., Shobbrook, C., Belford, L., & Kells, L. (2004). University Health Network framework for advanced nursing practice: Development of a comprehensive conceptual framework describing the multidimensional contributions of advanced practice nurses. *Nursing Leadership, 17*(3), 52–64.

Mijares, L., & Bond, M. L. (2013). Mentoring: A concept analysis. *The Journal of Theory Construction & Testing, 17*(1), 23–28.

Mohr, L. D., & Coke, L. A. (2018). Distinguishing the clinical nurse specialist from other graduate nursing roles. *Clinical Nurse Specialist, 32*(3), 139–151.

Morin, D. (2018). *La pratique infirmière avancée : Vers un consensus au sein de la francophonie* [Advanced nursing practice: Toward a consensus within the Francophonie]. Montreal, QC: Secrétariat international des infirmières et infirmiers de l'espace francophone (SIDIIEF).

O'Grady, E., & Johnson, J. E. (2019). Guidance and coaching. In M. F. Tracy & E. T. O'Grady (Eds.), *Hamric and Hanson's advanced practice nursing: An integrative approach* (pp. 180–202). St. Louis, MO: Elsevier.

Pillai, S., Manister, N. N., Coppolo, M. T., Ducey, M. S., & McManus-Penzero, J. (2018). Evaluation of a nurse residency program. *Journal for Nurses in Professional Development, 34*(6), E23–E28.

Rosseter, R. J. (2014). *Nursing shortage fact sheet.* Washington, DC: American Association of Colleges of Nursing. Retrieved from https://www.lwtech.edu/about/foundation/raisebsnup/docs/nursing-shortage-fact-sheet.pdf

Tessier, S. (2012). *Les éducations en santé : Éducation pour la santé, éducation thérapeutique, éducation à porter soins et secours* [Health education: Health education, therapeutic education, education in providing care and aid]. Paris, FR: Maloine.

Ward, A. E., & McComb, S. A. (2017). Formalising the precepting process: A concept analysis of preceptorship. *Journal of Clinical Nursing, 27*, e873–e881.

Winnipeg Regional Health Authority (WRHA). (2012). *A guide to successful integration of a clinical nurse specialist.* Winnipeg, MB: WRHA. Retrieved from https://www.wrha.mb.ca/extranet/nursing/files/CNS-Toolkit.pdf

Chapter

16B

Educational Competencies

Nurse Practitioner

Françoise (Frankie) Verville

FRANÇOISE VERVILLE is the Program Head and Professor for the Collaborative Nurse Practitioner Program at Saskatchewan Polytechnic, School of Nursing, and Graduate Adjunct Professor, Faculty of Nursing, University of Regina, both in Regina, Saskatchewan. She is a nurse practitioner (NP)-Family/All Ages who, in addition to her teaching and administrative responsibilities, has been involved in advocating for the NP role and profession as an executive member of the Saskatchewan Association of Nurse Practitioners. Françoise maintains a clinical practice in both rural and urban communities.

KEY TERMS

educational competencies
interprofessional education
(IPE)
preceptorship

OBJECTIVES

1. Explore the advanced practice nursing educational competencies from the perspective of the nurse practitioner (NP) role.
2. Examine the preceptor role as it relates to NP students.
3. Demonstrate the application of advanced practice nursing educational role competencies.

Introduction

The Canadian Nurses Association's (CNA) advanced practice nursing (APN) pan-Canadian framework (2019) articulated competencies that highlight the role of nurse practitioners (NPs) in the area of education. These competencies are broad concepts that describe what advanced practice nurses (APNs) who are in the clinical nurse specialist (CNS) and NP roles must demonstrate in their practice to improve the health of the clients and populations they serve (CNA, 2019; Melnyk, Gallagher-Ford, Long, & Fineout-Overholt, 2014).

Additionally, regulatory bodies across Canada have integrated **educational competencies** in their documents that describe entry to practice requirements of NPs (Canadian Council of Registered Nurse Regulators [CCRNR], 2015; College of Nurses of Ontario [CNO], 2018;

Saskatchewan Registered Nurses Association [SRNA], 2017). These regulatory standards describe what a competent NP graduate must demonstrate in practice as it pertains to education. Nursing regulatory bodies provide examples of how these competencies can be operationalized and continuously developed in the practice setting.

Information related to these competencies, which provides NP students the opportunity to integrate theoretical and practical knowledge into the practice setting under the direction of their clinical preceptors, is scaffolded throughout graduate NP education. In practice, NPs enact these competencies by developing and deepening personal knowledge in their area of practice, teaching and mentoring the broader interprofessional team, precepting NP students, and influencing change at the organizational level. A key component related to the application of these competencies is the need for practicing NPs to support and mentor students within the profession in the development of their knowledge, skills, and abilities, which are all critical elements to a successful transition into the role (CNA, 2019).

This chapter will focus on the CNA's educational competencies described in the framework for the NP role and how they support the learning needs of clients, interprofessional health care teams, as well as students.

Educational Competencies

Advanced practice nursing educational competencies address three broad areas: (1) the client (individual, family, or community), (2) the health care team (intra- and interprofessional), and (3) APN students (CNA, 2019). Furthermore, acquisition of knowledge related to these competencies is not in a silo but rather requires an understanding of the other APN competencies, which include direct clinical practice, research, leadership, consultation, and collaboration. Unfortunately, NPs can find it difficult to enact educational competencies due to certain organizational factors and limited resources. Table 16b.1 describes the APN educational competencies.

TABLE 16B.1: Advanced Practice Nursing Educational Competencies

- Develop educational programs and/or identify resources to address the priority learning needs of clients, communities, and health care team members
- Disseminate evidence-informed knowledge to clients, communities, and health care team members through formal and informal mechanisms
- Create opportunities that enhance and contribute to interprofessional collaboration in order to improve client care
- Create relationships (i.e., cross appointments) with academic organizations to develop new knowledge and improve knowledge translation
- Build capacity within the organization that advocates for, contributes to, and supports ongoing learning within a collaborative practice
- Ensure preceptorship and mentorship are integrated into the practice setting to build capacity and facilitate the development of a robust NP workforce

---

Source: Adapted from CNA. (2019). *Advanced practice nursing: A pan-Canadian framework.* Ottawa, ON: CNA. Retrieved from https://cna-aiic.ca/-/media/cna/page-content/pdf-en/apn-a-pan-canadian-framework.pdf

Client Education

NPs provide direct client care to a variety of populations. In addition to providing direct clinical care, they also work with clients to identify goals of care and provide education to improve client self-efficacy, a key component to achieving these goals (Archiopoli et al., 2016; Hessler et al., 2019). Self-efficacy is an important theoretical concept and is believed to affect all aspects of human behaviour, including health. This construct, initially developed as part of social learning theory by Albert Bandura, relates to an individual's perception of their capacity to achieve their goals (Archiopoli et al., 2016). Self-efficacy is influenced by both internal and external factors such as skill mastery, social learning, and social persuasion with emotional, spiritual, and physical states (Archiopoli et al., 2016; Bandura, 2006; Sheeran et al., 2016). The importance of increased self-efficacy lies in its strong correlation with action. Research has found that individuals with increased self-efficacy demonstrate higher levels of goal achievement (Archiopoli et al., 2016; Bandura, 2006). Communication between the client and provider is a strong predictor of increased self-efficacy and enhances adherence to the prescribed treatment plan (Archiopoli et al., 2016).

Intra- and Interprofessional Education

Interprofessional education (IPE) occurs when students from two or more disciplines learn about the role each profession has in the delivery of client services. The goal of IPE is to improve communication, harmonization of services, and the quality and safety of patient care (Brunt, 2015). IPE is an essential step in preparing a collaborative health care provider workforce. Early exposure to the concepts of interprofessional practice enhances team functioning in the clinical setting as it empowers all team members to share information and helps mitigate perceptions of hierarchical differences between professions (Dirks, 2019). Increasingly, academic institutions are incorporating IPE into their program curricula through the use of simulation or case study approaches. IPE enhances information dissemination, which can lead to instructional and organizational improvements (Vogel et al., 2019). It also strengthens mentorship of the health care team and supports transition into practice for novice providers, including NPs (Hart & Bowen, 2016).

Nurse Practitioner Education

NP education in Canada includes both theoretical and clinical instruction. The theoretical component is delivered using online, on-campus, or a blended/hybrid approach. The clinical component is typically facilitated using a preceptorship model placing students with clinical experts, including NPs and physicians (Staples & Sangster-Gormley, 2018). This model not only allows NP students to apply theory to practice, but it socializes the NP student into the role, which supports the development of APN practice competencies (Donley et al., 2014; Staples & Sangster-Gormley, 2018). Nurse practitioner preceptors are key members in the educational preparation of new NPs and there is an urgent need to address their recruitment and retention to sustain current student placements and the expansion of NP programs across Canada (Staples & Sangster-Gormley, 2018).

Preceptors are critical members of the education team. They help ensure NP students graduate with the required knowledge, skills, and abilities to provide safe and competent patient care. They also model the role of preceptor. Staples and Sangster-Gormley (2018) reported that the benefits of preceptorship include "growth as a professional and the ability to influence NP education through linkages with faculty and students" (p. 116). They further identified several barriers that influence the retention of NP preceptors such as insufficient infrastructure, demands of clinical practice, lack of remuneration, and increased demands related to higher numbers of NP students. Some of these barriers could be mitigated when the employer creates an environment that facilitates the NP preceptor role. In order to promote this important educational service to the profession, academic institutions, employers, and other key stakeholders must address these barriers. The following case study exhibits how educational competencies are operationalized in the clinical setting.

CASE STUDY

The Story of Kay

Kay, a 68-year-old widowed female, living in a small rural community in Saskatchewan, presented with a three-week history of shortness of breath and cough. Jules, an NP-PHC student, assessed Kay and collected the following subjective and objective data.

History of Present Illness: The client stated that she developed a cold and cough approximately three weeks ago. Although the cold symptoms had resolved, the cough persisted and worsened. She felt mildly short of breath all the time and stated she could not walk more than one block without stopping to rest. Her cough was productive for moderate amounts of greenish sputum. She denied fever. She had tried over-the-counter antitussives with minimal relief. She stated she used puffers in the past, but ran out and had not used them for over a year.

Allergies: None known

Past Medical History: Chronic obstructive pulmonary disease (COPD)

Medications: Acetaminophen 500 mg 1 to 2 tablets qid; over-the-counter cough syrup at bedtime prn

Social History: Smoker x 44 years; denied alcohol use, no recreational drug use, no influenza vaccine for the past seven years, retired widow, lives on fixed income, does not drive or own a car

Family History: Non-contributory

Relevant Physical Examination Findings:
On examination, the client appeared thin and pale. She was afebrile, tachycardic at 103 beats per minute, tachypneic at 26 breaths per minute with an oxygen saturation of 90%. Her blood pressure was mildly elevated at 152/96.
Respiratory: Inspection revealed increased use of accessory muscles, no cyanosis or paradoxical chest wall movements noted; auscultation revealed a prolonged expiratory phase and wheezing (inspiratory and expiratory throughout); palpation revealed decreased tactile fremitus and percussion demonstrated hyperresonance.
Cardiovascular: Inspection revealed no jugular venous distention; regular S1 and S2, no S3 or S4 or murmurs on auscultation, and no peripheral edema noted to palpation.
Pertinent Diagnostic Tests: Spirometry results, completed three years ago, confirmed diagnosis of COPD.
Review of Systems:
No fever, chills, or night sweats.
HEENT: Denied headache, sinus pain, nasal discharge or symptoms of acute pharyngitis.
Cardiac: Denied chest pain.
Respiratory: Shortness of breath that increased with activity, productive cough for greenish sputum.
GI: Denied nausea, had stated a decreased appetite for solids, but was drinking adequate amounts of fluids.
  All other systems were within normal limits.

Discussion

Following the assessment of the client, Jules, the NP student, provided a synopsis of the findings to the preceptor, an experienced NP, and a list of potential differential diagnoses, including community-acquired pneumonia, upper respiratory viral illness, and acute exacerbation of COPD (AECOPD). Following the debriefing with the preceptor, a working diagnosis of AECOPD was proposed and a related plan of care was developed. The plan of care, as per best practice, included pharmacotherapy with bronchodilators, inhaled corticosteroid, and antibiotics. Client education related to the diagnosis was also discussed. The NP preceptor highlighted that understanding the client's goals was critical to improving outcomes and that based on these goals, resources available to COPD clients could be provided. She advised Jules that typically, management of these types of clients requires a scaffolded approach. The need to address the chief complaint first in order to alleviate symptoms is then followed by subsequent visits to address how to prevent exacerbations in the future. Kay was provided with education on how to influence disease progression. Using this approach, Jules administered a salbutamol nebulizer treatment, which Kay stated provided immediate relief for her shortness of breath.

Under the NP preceptor's direction, a return demonstration teaching method was utilized. Jules instructed Kay on the proper use of the inhalation devices she would be using at home. A follow-up visit in seven days' time was arranged with instructions to access care sooner if any symptoms worsened or she became febrile. Following the client's discharge, the NP preceptor advised Jules to add Kay's name to the interprofessional rounds agenda for discussion. These rounds, a quality improvement initiative developed by the clinic, have an overarching goal to support care of clients with chronic ambulatory care–sensitive conditions like COPD. The current interprofessional team includes an NP, a chronic disease nurse educator, a pharmacist, and a counsellor. During these rounds, Jules is informed that a COPD group education program is set to start in two weeks' time, and Jules was encouraged to discuss this with Kay at her follow-up visit.

The following week, Kay returned for reassessment and her symptoms had almost completely resolved. Her vital signs had improved, and her oxygen saturation was now 94%. Auscultation of her chest revealed scattered wheezes in the lung bases. Jules proceeded to discuss services available for the management of COPD. Kay agreed to attend the group education session, which would provide information on different topics over the course of six weeks. The NP preceptor advised Jules that as a learner she would also benefit from attending these classes. Following discussion on the benefits of this interprofessional opportunity and agreement by Jules's faculty member, the NP preceptor was able to facilitate this learning opportunity. Following the six-week course, Jules developed a greater understanding of COPD, community resources available to manage the disease, and developed relationships with other disciplines that could lead to future opportunities for collaboration. All of this had been made possible by a knowledgeable and engaged NP preceptor.

Conclusion

NPs have a broad scope of practice. The demands of their clinical practice can, at times, overshadow the development and integration of competencies related to the other domains of practice, including education. The case study demonstrated how the NP preceptor is an integral partner in NP student education. Continued and potentially increased demand for NPs to meet the health care needs of Canadians requires innovative approaches to further developing and supporting the preceptor role. Maintaining a robust NP workforce requires the willingness of clinical experts to become preceptors, which can be achieved only when identified barriers are addressed.

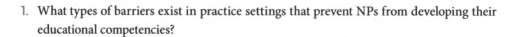

Critical Thinking Questions

1. What types of barriers exist in practice settings that prevent NPs from developing their educational competencies?

2. What opportunities exist for NP students to participate in IPE events? What could NP students do to promote IPE?
3. What behaviours should NPs role model to enhance and promote the preceptor role?

References

Archiopoli, A., Ginossar, T., Wilcox, B., Avila, M., Hill, R., & Oetzel, J. (2016). Factors of interpersonal communication and behavioral health on medication self-efficacy and medication adherence. *AIDS Care, 28*(12), 1607–1614. https://doi.org/10.1080/09540121.2016.1192577

Bandura, A. (2006). Toward a psychology of human agency. *Perspectives on Psychological Science, 1*(2), 164–180. doi: 10.1111/j.1745-6916.2006.00011.x

Brunt, B. (2015). Interprofessional education to promote collaboration. *Ohio Nurses Review, 90*(4), 20–21.

Canadian Council of Registered Nurse Regulators (CCRNR). (2015). *Practice analysis study of nurse practitioners.* Beaverton, ON: CCRNR. Retrieved from http://www.ccrnr.ca/assets/ccrnr-practice-analysis-study-of-nurse-practitioners-report---final.pdf

Canadian Nurses Association (CNA). (2019). *Advanced practice nursing: A pan-Canadian framework.* Ottawa, ON: CNA. Retrieved from https://cna-aiic.ca/-/media/cna/page-content/pdf-en/apn-a-pan-canadian-framework.pdf

College of Nurses of Ontario (CNO). (2018). *Entry-to-practice competencies for nurse practitioners.* Toronto, ON: CNO. Retrieved from https://www.cno.org/globalassets/docs/reg/47010-np-etp-competencies.pdf

Dirks, J. L. (2019). Effective strategies for teaching teamwork. *Critical Care Nurse, 39*(4), 40–47. https://doi.org/10.4037/ccn2019704

Donley, R., Flaherty, M. J., Sarsfield, E., Burkhard, A., O'Brien, S., & Anderson, K. M. (2014). Graduate clinical nurse preceptors: Implications for improved intra-professional collaboration. *Online Journal of Issues in Nursing, 19*(3), 9.

Hart, A. M., & Bowen, A. (2016). New nurse practitioners' perceptions of preparedness for and transition into practice. *The Journal for Nurse Practitioners, 12*(8), 545–552. https://doi.org/10.1016/j.nurpra.2016.04.018

Hessler, D. M., Fisher, L., Bowyer, V., Dickinson, L. M., Jortberg, B. T., Kwan, B., … Dickinson, W. P. (2019). Self-management support for chronic disease in primary care: Frequency of patient self-management problems and patient reported priorities, and alignment with ultimate behavior goal selection. *BioMed Central (BMC) Family Practice, 20*(1). https://doi.org/10.1186/s12875-019-1012-x

Melnyk, B. M., Gallagher-Ford, L., Long, L. E., & Fineout-Overholt, E. (2014). The establishment of evidence-based practice competencies for practicing registered nurses and advanced practice nurses in real-world clinical settings: Proficiencies to improve healthcare quality, reliability, patient outcomes, and costs: EBP competencies for practice. *Worldviews on Evidence-Based Nursing, 11*(1), 5–15. https://doi.org/10.1111/wvn.12021

Saskatchewan Registered Nurses Association (SRNA). (2017). *Registered nurse (nurse practitioner) entry-level competencies.* Regina, SK: SRNA. Retrieved from https://www.srna.org/wp-content/uploads/2018/01/RNNP-Entry-Level-Competencies-2017.pdf

Sheeran, P., Maki, A., Montanaro, E., Avishai-Yitshak, A., Bryan, A., Klein, W. M. P., ... Rothman, A. J. (2016). The impact of changing attitudes, norms, and self-efficacy on health-related intentions and behavior: A meta-analysis. *Health Psychology, 35*(11), 1178–1188. https://doi.org/10.1037/hea0000387

Staples, E., & Sangster-Gormley, E. (2018). Supporting NP education: Preceptorship recruitment and retention. *International Journal of Nursing Sciences, 5*(2), 115–120. https://doi.org/10.1016/j.ijnss.2018.03.005

Vogel, M. T., Abu-Rish Blakeney, E., Willgerodt, M. A., Odegard, P. S., Johnson, E. L., Shrader, S., ... Zierler, B. (2019). Interprofessional education and practice guide: Interprofessional team writing to promote dissemination of interprofessional education scholarship and products. *Journal of Interprofessional Care, 33*(5), 406–413. https://doi.org/10.1080/13561820.2018.1538111

Chapter

17A

Research Competencies

Clinical Nurse Specialist

Cheryl Forchuk

CHERYL FORCHUK is the Beryl and Richard Ivey Research Chair in Aging, Mental Health, Rehabilitation and Recovery, a Distinguished University Professor at the Arthur Labatt Family School of Nursing, Scientist and Assistant Director of the Lawson Health Research Institute, and Professor in the Department of Psychiatry, Schulich Medicine & Dentistry, Western University, London, Ontario. Cheryl also holds an appointment as Associate Clinical Professor at McMaster University, School of Nursing, Hamilton, Ontario. She has practiced as a CNS in mental-psychiatric settings, public health, and private practice. She is currently President of the Clinical Nurse Specialist Association of Canada.

KEY TERMS

continuous improvement
evidence-informed
knowledge translation (KT)
research competency

OBJECTIVES

1. Describe the differences between being a user of research findings and a generator of research findings.
2. Summarize key reasons for advanced practice nurses to engage in research.
3. Identify strategies for implementing the research competency in practice.

Introduction

Advanced practice nurses (APNs) have often described the **research competency** as one of the more challenging roles to enact (Fitzgerald et al., 2003; Gullick & West, 2016; Lewandowski & Adamle, 2009). Part of the challenge relates to differences in roles, timelines, and perceived priorities. Clinical issues are often urgent where problems are apparent and require an immediate response. Research involves a much slower, more drawn-out process with potentially fewer tangible outcomes. However, there is a risk in being so caught up with various everyday crises that questions about why these crises occur, how they can be prevented, and what interventions are best to address them do not get framed into researchable questions. Another challenge APNs face is they may not perceive having enough time to engage in research. This situation is similar to the seminal paper on upstream-downstream thinking in nursing (Butterfield, 1990). People may be so busy pulling others from the bottom of the stream that they forget to send someone upstream to find out what factors are causing people to keep falling in.

The Research Competency

As part of the clinical nurse specialist (CNS) role, the research competency can be described as having different levels of intensity. At the most basic level, an APN is expected to be able to be an educated consumer of research. However, as baccalaureate education has become the entry-level standard for all registered nurses (RNs) in Canada, it is expected that all RNs graduate as educated consumers of research. Generally, all nurses are expected to know how to critically appraise the literature in order to inform practice changes. However, the sheer volume of new research, combined with insufficient experience in using database search engines and a skills deficit in formulating researchable questions (Tracy, 2014), impedes nurses from being able to access, critique, and suggest evidence-informed practice changes in a timely fashion. These impediments make it challenging for APNs to stay apprised of new research.

Core competencies for evaluating the research roles of the CNS across Canada have recently been set out by the Canadian Nurses Association (CNA; 2014), which includes the CNS role expectation of dissemination and integration of evidence. A CNS will frequently receive consultations or requests to provide education on issues that are often well covered in the literature. During practice changes, a CNS identifies research topics for study, reviews literature evidence, and utilizes expert judgment to establish the most effective approach of a specific practice (CNA, 2016). The research dissemination role in these situations is fairly straightforward. Literature can be retrieved, summarized, and discussed with colleagues and staff. Research findings can be disseminated by leaving copies of articles for staff to read, referenced in the consultation report, or incorporated within an educative handout. With best practice guidelines, such as those available from the Registered Nurses Association of Ontario (RNAO) website, as well as other research synthesis sites, including the Cochrane Library, the hard work of collecting, critiquing, and synthesizing information is often already complete (see Table 17a.1).

As an example, during the process of developing the RNAO Best Practice Guideline, *Establishing Therapeutic Relationships* (RNAO, 2002), team members identified and reviewed over 2,000 research papers related to the topic. Now that this guideline has been developed, all of the relevant information, fully synthesized and interpreted from a nursing perspective, can be easily accessed.

Producing research knowledge involves a different level of engagement than simply retrieving and sharing knowledge, and it is this level of involvement that APNs are more likely to struggle with. Before discussing how APNs produce knowledge, it is first useful to consider

TABLE 17A.1: Websites for Gathering Best Practices

Organization	Summary of Website	Web Address
Registered Nurses Association of Ontario (RNAO)	Provides best practices in nursing that includes common nursing concerns	http://www.rnao.org/bestpractices/index.asp http://rnao.ca/bpg
The Cochrane Library	A collection of databases in medicine and other health care specialties	http://www.cochranelibrary.com
Joanna Briggs Institute	Provides examples of nursing best practices	http://joannabriggs.org/

why it is necessary to take on this challenge. Consider this: Who else would be expected to be in an ideal situation to identify and generate knowledge about the clinical aspects of nursing? Are academics in a position to do so? Nurses working in clinical practice can identify gaps between what academics describe as clinical nursing issues and what practitioners actually struggle with. Table 17a.2 provides an example of how a CNS can take an issue from practice to research and how this research can impact future practice.

TABLE 17A.2: Example of Taking an Issue from Practice to Research and Back to Practice

Phase of Process	Issues and Activities	Products
Problem identification	Some mental health patients were being discharged from psychiatric wards to homelessness or "no fixed address"	Task group with mental health, housing, shelters, and income support
Review of literature	Very little literature on subject; academic literature at times called this a myth	Decided we need to look at our own data locally
Baseline data	Looked at hospital and shelter administrative data to see how frequently in a year this actually happened (almost 200 times a year)	Forchuk et al. (2006)
Pilot project to address	Piloted an intervention partnering with income support agencies and housing supports	Forchuk et al. (2008)
Large-scale implementation of intervention	Incorporated pilot approach, including internet access to income support agency data and housing data on vacancy across city at both city hospitals	Forchuk et al. (2013b)

CASE STUDY

The Story of Saad

Saad is a CNS on a busy orthopedic unit. The unit has recently experienced significant turnover of nursing staff. There have been several incidents related to postoperative delirium that have impacted patient outcomes (prolonged hospitalization, increased health care costs) and contributed to high stress levels among nurses.

In critically appraising the literature, Saad found that some researchers indicated that education programs for nurses could improve outcomes for patients experiencing post-operative delirium. Many studies identified a lack of nursing knowledge in recognizing and managing delirium, but only one research study specifically assessed nurses' knowledge of delirium.

Saad, in consultation with the nurse manager, conducted a research study to examine delirium knowledge levels before and after delivering a tailored educational intervention using the Nurses' Knowledge of Delirium Questionnaire (Hare, Wynaden, McGowan, Landsborough, & Speed, 2008).

The pretest scores found that nurses' knowledge of delirium was poor. The nurses were unaware of the fluctuating nature of delirium and its clinical presentation. Post-test scores suggested the educational program had a positive impact on the orthopedic nurses' knowledge level of delirium, especially in the area of cognitive assessment and delirium specifically.

In response to the study, plans were incorporated in the orthopedic unit to provide ongoing in-service education to increase and reinforce team members' knowledge levels and to increase the identification of delirium, reduce the potential for negative outcomes of delirium, improve health outcomes for patients experiencing delirium, and ultimately, cost efficiencies.

Discussion

CNSs, in their clinical role, are aware of the concerns of practicing nurses from multiple information sources. They receive nursing consultations for input on issues that nurses or other members of the health care team find challenging, requests for education on areas where current practice is perceived as not working well enough, and invitations from leadership in hospital or health care agencies to help resolve systemic issues related to care. In everyday practice, a CNS may come across multiple scenarios that give insight where further knowledge was needed. As a critical appraiser of research, the CNS can determine where knowledge already exists to address issues of concern or interest by incorporating the use of evidence in practice environments. Unfortunately, there are occasions when the required information is either unavailable or is available but has not been systematically evaluated. Some CNSs may not have systematic review skills, and in situations where the literature is extensive, they may not have the time to do full reviews on their own.

Canada has been criticized as a country of perpetual pilot projects (Bégin, Eggertson, & Macdonald, 2009; Martin et al., 2018; Zelmer, 2015); however, pilot projects that are implemented, evaluated, and published are a valuable way to build upon and add to the existing pool of knowledge. Even within a single hospital or health care organization, the CNS may observe similar projects taking place without researchers being aware of each other's work, and therefore they are unable to build upon what has already been achieved.

Nurses, in general, are now being asked to make decisions that are **evidence-informed** within their own practice settings (Wu et al., 2018; Yost et al., 2014), which includes incorporating evidence from empirical research, as well as the preferences of patients; however, the extent to which research findings are integrated into practice remains questionable (Leach & Tucker, 2018; Squires et al., 2011). In this context, the APN is well positioned to act as a mentor to others by providing **knowledge translation** interventions, which aim to enhance research utilization (Abdullah et al., 2014). A knowledge translation intervention is one that promotes the consumption of research evidence into practice and/or policies and can be attributed to research utilization (Tricco et al., 2016). Table 17a.3 demonstrates examples of knowledge translation interventions that APNs, including CNSs, can lead or participate in.

What prevents CNSs from generating new knowledge? Two possible belief systems may be involved: the belief that CNSs lack the required training or expertise to undertake research, and the belief that they have neither the time nor material resources to do research.

TABLE 17A.3: Examples of Knowledge Translation Interventions

Intervention	Research Utilization	Level of Influence	Reference
Evaluating effectiveness of an advanced practice nurse-led interprofessional collaborative chronic care approach for transplant patients with CKD using interventions such as disease self-management, shared decision-making, and health care system reorganizations	• An APN-led approach, based on the chronic care model, suggested patients were able to attain targeted clinical outcomes, and have fewer ER visits and hospital readmissions, compared to physician-led approaches • The APN-led approach organized a distinct clinic for transplant patients with CKD, separate from transplant patients without CKD, to better organize management and care	Patient, System	Bissonnette (2011)

(Continued)

TABLE 17A.3: Continued

Intervention	Research Utilization	Level of Influence	Reference
Clients diagnosed with psychiatric illness who were being discharged from acute and tertiary care hospitals received two sources of support: assistance from an Ontario Works (OW) worker who had direct access to the OW database, and assistance from a housing advocate to locate available housing. Participants had to be willing and able to seek employment on OW	• The intervention was provided as a drop-in service within the hospital, where clients had direct access to assistance • Prevented discharge to homelessness for both groups; however, tertiary care clients experienced more system-level barriers • Intervention eased workload among staff • Relationships among the stakeholders within the study grew stronger • Required the intervention team to have knowledge of one another's responsibilities and role • Still requires coordination with other policy efforts at the system level	Patient, System	Forchuk et al. (2013a)
Individuals being discharged from the acute care setting were able to access a drop-in service that provided support in attaining housing prior to discharge from the hospital	• Intervention reduced the number of people discharged to no fixed address • Costs were saved with implementing and sustaining the intervention compared to discharging individuals to shelters	Patient, System	Forchuk et al. (2013b)
Intervention involves receiving support from an individual who has had a psychiatric illness and has completed a peer-support training program, as well as continued support from a hospital-based health care professional until a therapeutic relationship has been developed in the community	• Nine hospitals in Ontario implemented the transitional discharge model in 2013 • The number of hospital readmissions, lengths of stay, and hospital spending all improved • Implementation over six months' time produced an estimated cost savings of $3 million • Future research will look at testing this model in clients with other long-term health conditions	Patient, Hospitals, Health care system	Forchuk et al. (2019)

TABLE 17A.3: Continued

Intervention	Research Utilization	Level of Influence	Reference
Implementing NP role as case managers in a Healthy Bones Program at a hospital with high rates of hip fractures among older patients	• NPs identified patients at risk for hip fractures by ordering DXA scan treatments appropriately • Additional patients were prescribed anti-osteoporosis medications • New "Just in Time" Program developed to enable NPs to immediately treat patients and provide services after a DXA scan	Patient, System	Greene & Dell (2010)
Integrating explicit sexual health assessments in tertiary care hospitals for individuals with psychiatric disorders	• Assisted psychiatric patients to identify sexual health needs and concerns • Findings from staff questionnaires and client interviews suggest nurses could go on to explicitly consider sexuality needs of patients within their nursing assessments	Patient, Nurse	Park Dorsay & Forchuk (1994)
Telephone contact intervention in women undergoing treatment for breast cancer	• Integrated practice of calling patients shortly after initiation of chemotherapy • Patients found the phone calls valuable as the calls provided contact information, symptom management assistance, reassurance, and support • Future research would look at nurses' perceived value of phone calls and how they could best implement it	Patient	Smithies, Bettger-Hahn, Forchuk, & Brackstone (2009)

Addressing Expertise to Conduct Research

One factor that impacts why APNs vary in their level of expertise related to research is because coursework on research methods often differs substantially between academic programs. Programs also vary on whether or not a thesis or major research project is required. It is not uncommon for APNs to feel they are experts in clinical practice, but novices in research. The most practical solution to amend this deficit is to collaborate with others who have greater research expertise.

There are multiple potential collaborators for the CNS. These may include:

1. Partnering with other APNs who have more research experience can help APNs new to research develop confidence in building these skills. When meeting with other APNs, it is beneficial to use this opportunity to identify common areas of concern that could be mutually addressed. For example, healthy sexual function can be adversely affected by a history of sexual abuse, as well as by the use of psychiatric medications. As these issues are commonly encountered in mental health settings, assessment of sexual health is an important mutual concern. One example of a collaborative initiative on this topic involved a quality improvement project undertaken across a number of mental health clinical areas. A small research project was established, and this work succeeded in producing a publication from the process (Park Dorsay & Forchuk, 1994).

2. Partnering with academics can also be a useful strategy. In particular, beginning academics often struggle with identifying issues of importance to the profession and in gaining access to clinical populations for research purposes. An APN, who has access to the clinical area, is ideally situated to be a research partner for academics. APNs can also link with clinically based educators, health care in-service trainers, and health care librarians (Tracy, 2014) who may also be aware of other resources or partners to engage with. For example, a CNS in oncology, an oncologist, and a CNS in psychiatric and mental health nursing collaborated to evaluate a telephone support program for women undergoing chemotherapy for breast cancer. Although this specialty was not the primary area of expertise of the CNS in psychiatry and mental health nursing, the research methodology supported the nurse's contribution to the research process. As well as completing the initial evaluation of the intervention, a publication resulted (Smithies, Bettger-Hahn, Forchuk, & Brackstone, 2009).

3. Partnering with colleagues from different disciplines, especially those with more active research portfolios, should not be an overlooked strategy to gain valuable research skills. Within the clinical setting, other members of the interprofessional team who have more background in research can be approached for partnership. If the researcher has a planned project or one that is currently funded, it can be a matter of just adding an additional tool to address other issues relevant to that provider. This strategy would be much easier than doing a completely separate project and allows for the opportunity to learn research skills through active participation in research, rather than passively learning pure theory.

4. Working with staff nurses and others on a collaborative learning project by learning together to evaluate something that is already happening. For example, a new intervention, assessment form, patient educational material, or practice protocol may have been recently introduced or about to be introduced. The CNS can take advantage of this opportunity to work with staff to evaluate the change. This strategy will integrate the research, educator, and change agent role competencies. Collaborating with staff nurses is also an excellent way to boost staff morale as they consequently have increased opportunities to present research results and/or co-author papers.

Strategies to Address Lack of Time and Resources

The most fundamental and simplest way to address the perception of the lack of time is not to view research as separate from the other roles, but rather entwined within them. If research is seen as a separate activity to be completed when there is time, it simply will not happen. Examples of how the CNS can address perceived lack of time or material resources include:

1. Building in a valid evaluation component to everyday activities. Part of the Accreditation Canada certification process requires the self-evaluation of **continuous improvement** and/or quality assurance standards. Evaluation may often be done without the rigour demanded of the research process. Some considerations must be taken into account. If the initial evaluation utilizes "homemade" as opposed to valid and reliable tools or does not utilize pre- and post-test assessments or a comparison group, there is no purpose in generalizing a study without considering the sampling strategy. With just a little more effort, a more valid evaluation can be completed that might also contribute to advancing nursing knowledge. Table 17a.4 includes a list of what is needed for a quality assurance project and what extra steps are needed to convert this work into a research project.
2. Setting aside time for evaluation and research. This can be achieved by making self-appointments or appointments with others and scheduling research time in a calendar. Ideally, negotiating to have time away from the clinical area or program to work on research reduces possible distractions and the risk of being recalled to handle emerging clinical issues as they arise.
3. Consider looking at what could be delegated to others in order to reduce the workload. For example, could a student do a literature review as part of an assignment or retrieve data as part of a project? An underused resource that directly relates to time is the opportunity for employing staff who are working on modified job duties. Employers often struggle to find suitable activities for staff on modified job duties, which can often be frustrating for the staff member, and it doesn't help with the recovery process or developing positive self-image. Staff have the ability to assist with literature reviews, data collation, and chart reviews. Furthermore, this work can be an incentive for staff making positive career changes, such as those going back to graduate school after the experience of a modified job duty placement.

4. A CNS with an academic appointment may be eligible to take work-study students. These students work for faculty as part of a financial assistance program and are paid by the government, not the academic faculty. Work-study students may be from nursing programs, but they can come from any university program. For example, depending on the needs of specific research projects, this author has offered computer science students, engineering students, and law students the opportunity to be involved in the research process. It is here that the strategies to address the issue of time and material resources overlap, since the more resources that can be identified, the less personal time it will take from the CNS to participate in the research.

Other strategies for resources include:

1. Identifying financial resources of support, such as hospital or community foundations and organizations that address the specific clinical area of concern. Small seed grants for projects are often available.

TABLE 17A.4: Moving from Continuous Improvement to Research

Issue	Continuous Improvement/ Quality Assurance	Research
Purpose	To understand problem or solution in local context	To understand problem or solution
Ethics approval	Local approval or inferred if part of program evaluation	Local approval and communication with Research Ethics Board (if using data that you already have access to by virtue of role, formal ethics approval may not be necessary)
Measurement tools/ scales	Often use own instruments Questionnaires designed in-house Often interested in patient satisfaction	Use standardized tools where possible. Often interested in outcome measures
Qualitative approaches	Often open-ended responses on questionnaires that would have a basic summary or content analysis	More in-depth, open-ended items or focus groups and formal qualitative analysis method employed
Dissemination of results	Usually an in-house purpose; may be used for accreditation or as part of a quality process; shared with clinical team and management primarily	Can be used for presentation locally, regionally, nationally, or internationally; can be published in academic literature

2. If an administrative request for a project is being made, negotiate resources upfront, such as funds to support statistical analysis or the creation of a summer student position to help with writing a research report.
3. Depending on the nature of the project being proposed, potential industry partners could be considered; however, consult administrative policies first.

Conclusion

The research role is an important and necessary competency of any CNS's professional practice. Collaborating with others is one useful strategy to develop confidence and skills in this area, but specific strategies to address time and resource factors can help CNSs to fully adopt this role. Most important is the ongoing need to incorporate the research competency into all APN roles, rather than seeing research as a separate, stand-alone activity.

Critical Thinking Questions

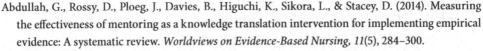

1. What are some potential strategies that might assist CNSs to disseminate research findings or to promote evidence-informed practice?
2. How might collaborating with others on clinical questions enhance the research-related skills of the CNSs and improve patient outcomes?
3. Time and resource issues are often identified as barriers to engaging in research-based activities. In what ways can this perception be altered to fully integrate the research role of CNSs into their everyday practice?

References

Abdullah, G., Rossy, D., Ploeg, J., Davies, B., Higuchi, K., Sikora, L., & Stacey, D. (2014). Measuring the effectiveness of mentoring as a knowledge translation intervention for implementing empirical evidence: A systematic review. *Worldviews on Evidence-Based Nursing, 11*(5), 284–300.

Bégin, M., Eggertson, L., & Macdonald, N. (2009). A country of perpetual pilot projects. *Canadian Medical Association Journal, 180*(12), 1185–1185.

Bissonnette, J. (2011). Evaluation of an advanced practice nurse led inter-professional collaborative chronic care approach for kidney transplant patients: The TARGET study. *The Journal of Clinical and Translational Research, 27*(2), 232–238.

Butterfield, P. G. (1990). Thinking upstream: Nurturing a conceptual understanding of the societal context of health behavior. *Advances in Nursing Science, 122*, 1–8.

Canadian Nurses Association (CNA). (2014). *Pan-Canadian core competencies for the clinical nurse specialist.* Ottawa, ON: CNA. Retrieved from http://cnaaiic.ca/~/media/cna/files/en/clinical_nurse_specialists_convention_handout_e.pdf

CNA. (2016). *Position statement: Clinical nurse specialist.* Ottawa, ON: CNA. Retrieved from https:// www.cna-aiic.ca/-/media/cna/page-content/pdf-en/clinical-nurse-specialist-position-statement_2016.pdf

Fitzgerald, M., Milberger, P., Tomlinson, P. S., Peden-McAlpine, C., Meiers, S. J., & Sherman, S. (2003). Clinical nurse specialist participation on a collaborative research project. Barriers and benefits. *Clinical Nurse Specialist, 17*(1), 44–49.

Forchuk, C., Godin, M., Hoch, J., Kingston-MacClure, S., Jeng, M., Puddy, L., ... Jenson, E. (2013a). Preventing homelessness after discharge from psychiatric wards: Perspectives of consumers and staff. *Journal of Psychosocial Nursing and Mental Health Services, 51*(3), 24–31.

Forchuk, C., Godin, M., Hoch, J., Kingston-MacClure, S., Jeng, M., Puddy, L., ... Jenson, E. (2013b). Preventing psychiatric discharge to homelessness. *Canadian Journal of Community Mental Health, 32*(3), 31–42.

Forchuk, C., MacClure, S. K., Van Beers, M., Smith, C., Csiernik, R., Hoch, J., & Jensen, E. (2008). Developing and testing an intervention to prevent homelessness among individuals discharged from psychiatric wards to shelters and "no fixed address." *Journal of Psychiatric and Mental Health Nursing, 15*(7), 569–575.

Forchuk, C., Martin, M.-L., Corring, D., Sherman, D., Srivastava, R., Harerimana, B., & Cheng, R. (2019). Cost-effectiveness of the implementation of a transitional discharge model for community integration of psychiatric clients: Practice insights and policy implications. *International Journal of Mental Health, 48*(3), 1–14. doi: 10.1080/00207411.2019.1649237

Forchuk, C., Russell, G., Kingston-MacClure, S., Turner, K., Lewis, K., & Dill, S. (2006). From psychiatric wards to the streets and shelters. *Journal of Psychiatric and Mental Health Nursing, 13*(3), 301–308.

Greene, D., & Dell, R. M. (2010). Outcomes of an osteoporosis disease-management program managed by nurse practitioners. *Journal of American Academy of Nurse Practitioners, 22*, 326–329.

Gullick, J. G., & West, S. H. (2016). Building research capacity and productivity among advanced practice nurses: An evaluation of the Community of Practice model. *Journal of Advanced Nursing, 72*(3), 605–619.

Hare, M., Wynaden, D., McGowan, S., Landsborough, I., & Speed, G. (2008). A questionnaire to determine nurses' knowledge of delirium and its risk factors. *Contemporary Nurse, 29*(1), 23–31.

Leach, M. J., & Tucker, B. (2018). Current understandings of the research-practice gap in nursing: A mixed-methods study. *Collegian, 25*(2), 171–179.

Lewandowski, W., & Adamle, K. (2009). Substantive areas of clinical nurse specialist practice: A comprehensive review of the literature. *Clinical Nurse Specialist, 23*(2), 73–90.

Martin, D., Miller, A. P., Quesnel-Vallee, A., Caron, N. R., Vissandjee, B., & Marchildon, G. P. (2018). Canada's universal health-care system: Achieving its potential. *The Lancet, 391*(10131), 1718–1735.

Park Dorsay, J., & Forchuk, C. (1994). Assessment of the sexuality needs of individuals with psychiatric disability. *Journal of Psychiatric and Mental Health Nursing, 1*(2), 93–97.

Registered Nurses Association of Ontario (RNAO). (2002). *Establishing therapeutic relationships.* Toronto, ON: RNAO.

Smithies, M., Bettger-Hahn, M., Forchuk, C., & Brackstone, M. (2009). Telephone contact intervention in women undergoing treatment for breast cancer. *Canadian Oncology Nursing Journal, 19*(3), 122–128.

Squires, J. E., Hutchinson, A. M., Boström, A. M., O'Rourke, H. M., Cobban, S. J., & Estabrooks, C. A. (2011). To what extent do nurses use research in clinical practice? A systematic review. *Implementation Science, 6*(21), 1–17.

Tracy, M. F. (2014). Competencies of advanced practice nursing: Direct clinical practice. In A. B. Hamric, C. M. Hanson, M. F. Tracy, & E. T. O'Grady (Eds.), *Advanced practice nursing: An integrative approach* (5th ed., pp. 147–182). St. Louis, MO: Elsevier Saunders.

Tricco, A. C., Ashoor, H. M., Cardoso, R., MacDonald, H., Cogo, E., Kastner, M., … Straus, S. E. (2016). Sustainability of knowledge translation interventions in healthcare decision making: A scoping review. *Implementation Science, 11*(55), 1–10. doi: 10.1186/s13012-016-0421-7

Wu, Y., Brettle, A., Zhou, C., Ou, J., Wang, Y., & Wang, S. (2018). Do educational interventions aimed at nurses to support the implementation of evidence-based practice improve patient outcomes? A systematic review. *Nurse Education Today, 70*, 109–114.

Yost, J., Thompson, D., Ganann, R., Aloweni, F., Newman, K., McKibbon, A., & Ciliska, D. (2014). Knowledge translation strategies for enhancing nurses' evidence-informed decision making: A scoping review. *Worldviews on Evidence-Based Nursing, 11*(3), 156–167.

Zelmer, J. (2015). Beyond pilots: Scaling and spreading innovation in healthcare. *Healthcare Policy/ Politiques de Santé, 11*(2), 8–9.

Chapter

17B

Research Competencies

Nurse Practitioner

Kathleen F. Hunter

KATHLEEN F. HUNTER is Professor and Coordinator for MN Entry to Practice as a nurse practitioner (NP) in the Faculty of Nursing, and Adjunct Professor, Faculty of Medicine, Division of Geriatric Medicine at the University of Alberta, Edmonton, Alberta. She has practiced in both the CNS and NP roles and is currently practicing as an NP-Adult in a continence clinic.

KEY TERMS

critical appraisal
knowledge mobilization
knowledge translation (KT)
patient outcomes
quality improvement
research
research competency

OBJECTIVES

1. Identify key quality improvement and research activities embedded in the Canadian nurse practitioner (NP) competencies.
2. Differentiate between quality improvement initiatives and research and how the NP participates in these activities.
3. Discuss the concepts of knowledge translation (KT) and knowledge mobilization, and the role of the NP in leading practice change.
4. Identify challenges and strategies to address enacting the NP research competency.

Introduction

As advanced practice nurses (APNs), it is imperative that nurse practitioners (NPs) integrate evidence-informed practice into client care. The development of NP entry to practice competencies in 2015 by the Canadian Council of Registered Nurse Regulators' (CCRNR) national practice analysis (CCRNR, 2015) expanded the focus of the original **research competency** to include **quality improvement** as well. The commitment to both quality improvement and research echoes the Canadian Nurses Association's (CNA; 2016) position statement on the NP role. Quality improvement is often directed toward specific processes/practices within an organization using systematic, data-guided activities (sometimes called a quality improvement cycle or continuous quality improvement) to identify solutions to process issues (Gregory, 2015). The knowledge generated is often specific to the organization or system and not generalizable, but is sometimes published to share information on improving outcomes. Research involves the generation of new knowledge using systematic steps of assessing relevant literature; identification of a research problem or question; development of study methods; data collection; and use of a data analysis plan (Gregory, 2015). Disseminating results with the broader research community, stakeholders, and the public through publication and other novel approaches is important. In conducting research, researchers obtain ethical approval for research and informed consent from participants. In both quality improvement and research, confidentiality of patient data is paramount.

What remains essential in the NP entry to practice competency of quality improvement and research are the activities. These include critical appraisal and application of relevant research and best practice guidelines; development and evaluation of processes that address client outcomes and contribute to the development of knowledge; identification and implementation of research-based innovations; evaluation of advanced nursing practice on client outcomes practice; engagement in research as a researcher or collaborator; and assuming the role of knowledge broker to facilitate evidence-informed practice (CCRNR, 2015; CNA, 2019). NP education programs must provide learning opportunities that foster increasing competence in systematic inquiry, knowledge development and translation at the graduate level, and prepare graduates to be lifelong learners (CASN, 2015). A competent NP is expected to act as an ongoing consumer of research, working toward improvements in client care at both the individual and systems levels through participation in quality improvement initiatives and research and acting as a change agent. The focus of the quality improvement and research competency is improvement of patient outcomes.

Development of critical appraisal and critical thinking skills to support evidence-informed practice has been one of the central factors underscoring the necessity of graduate preparation of APNs, including NPs. Central to APN in Canada is the expectation for analysis and synthesis of knowledge; an ability to understand, interpret, and apply nursing theory and research; and for the development and advancement of nursing knowledge (CNA, 2019). Although the focus of the NP is predominantly clinical, a key component of clinical client care is health care system transformation (CNA, 2016). This is disseminated through knowledge translation (KT) and knowledge mobilization. As NPs move from novice to more experienced practitioners, increasing responsibilities in quality improvement and research evolve to include leadership roles on projects and research.

Knowledge Translation: Changing Practice

KT includes synthesis of research findings, dissemination, exchange of knowledge between researchers and knowledge users, and ethically sound application of knowledge (Canadian Institutes for Health Research [CIHR], n.d.), but this process has been criticized as being too linear (Langley, Wostenholme, & Cooke, 2018). More recently, the concept of knowledge mobilization has been introduced, which goes beyond sharing information to engagement and participation of end users in both research and practice-based evidence (i.e., quality improvement) to shift cultures and improve client outcomes; a model of "collective making" within complex health systems (Langley et al., 2018). Aspects of KT and mobilization are threaded across the NP quality improvement and research competencies. Effective knowledge mobilization draws on the ability of the NP to critically appraise literature, synthesize research findings, and engage stakeholders and clients in the process of applying knowledge to the setting in which they practice. Branham, DelloSritto, and Hilliard (2014) reported that acute care/tertiary care–based NPs supported the concept of evidence-informed practice, but identified mitigating factors to implementation of recommendations, including patient needs and preferences. Broadening to a strategy of knowledge mobilization allows NPs to conceptualize the inclusion of the client in decision-making.

Maintaining currency of knowledge is an essential first step to best practice and evidence-informed care. The ability to synthesize evidence and translate knowledge to the care setting supports achievement of the best possible client outcomes and in building a positive relationship with clients. The knowledge base of NPs provides a valuable contribution to the health care teams, leading to changes in practice. In a study of long-term care settings, Sangster-Gormley et al. (2013) reported that managers valued the NP role for the expertise in care of complex residents, potential for capacity building, and staff development. All these factors require that the NP maintain a current base of knowledge related to best practices in client care.

APNs move through a process of development throughout their careers, moving from novices to more experienced and expert practitioners (Brykcaynski, 2014). Development of expertise to meet NP research competencies supports the need to develop skills as a change agent. For the novice NP focused on gaining clinical experience, assuming the role of change agent may seem daunting. It is necessary to build systematically on critical appraisal skills learned in the NP education program by reviewing current research and appraising best practice guidelines relevant to the practice area. Guidelines can be discussed with colleagues and mentors on the care team to identify potential areas of practice change. Another starting point for the novice and intermediate experienced NPs is to begin with quality improvement approaches to evaluate patient outcomes for local use, rather than a formal research project. Focusing on local practice, the developing NP may elect to present information on guideline recommendations formally or informally to unit staff, identify the practice gaps, and develop procedures or patient education materials focused on closing the gaps and improving client outcomes.

As the NP gains experience and confidence in the role, opportunities to participate in more structured and formal research appraisal within the team or other groups such as professional or special interest associations may present. This could include participation in scoping or systematic reviews of literature for the development of best practice guidelines. An experienced NP would be well situated to lead or share leadership within the interprofessional team in the practice setting with regard to practice change initiatives, quality improvement projects, and, potentially, research projects that involve evaluation of patient outcomes.

The Nurse Practitioner as Researcher

Today, more Canadian NPs are seeking doctoral education to develop their research skills and knowledge. These NPs may assume positions that involve joint academic and clinical roles, enabling more sophisticated research studies to be undertaken and having a key role to play in mentoring students or practicing NPs in research.

The involvement of the NP in research initiatives for KT and mobilization, practice transformation, and development of new knowledge must evolve over time as experience is gained in the role. At the entry to practice level, NPs should seek opportunities to identify potential research questions and join research collaborations in their area of practice in order to gain confidence and skill in research. For early career NPs, one strategy is to take advantage of opportunities to participate in research initiatives being undertaken by their team. This could include working with the team to identify research questions stemming from practice, participating in data collection, and participation in KT strategies.

CASE STUDY

The Story of Mrs. Pratt

Liz is an NP-PHC in a primary care clinic seeing 79-year-old Mrs. Pratt.

Presenting Complaint: Possible urinary tract infection (UTI)

History of Present Illness: Has had vaginal/periurethral itching and intermittent irritation, sometimes with urination, for 2–3 years, which she believes are recurrent UTIs. Urine is now smelly, and she states that "it's another UTI." Denies urinary increased frequency/urgency, fever, suprapubic or flank pain. Previous providers prescribed antibiotics (3x in past year), this helped somewhat but symptoms do not resolve.

Past Medical History: Hypertension, arthritis (knees, hips)

Drugs/Alcohol/Smoking: No illicit drug use; smoked 1/2 pack/day until age 40; alcohol 1–2 glasses of wine on weekends at dinner

Childhood: Measles, mumps

Surgical: Hysterectomy age 37 for bleeding

Psychiatric: None

Health Maintenance: Flu vaccine yearly; Pneumovax in 2011; unsure of others

Screening Tests: Vision check yearly, hearing test last year

Sexual History: Not sexually active; no vaginal exam for over 10 years

Social History: Widowed, lives in condo, no home care; daily phone contact by phone with daughter, sees weekly; independent with ADLs, IADLs

Family History: Three living children, all healthy; parents died of heart disease and "old age"

Review of Systems:
General: Feels well other than the vaginal itching, no fevers, sleeping well
HEENT: No recent changes in hearing or vision; new glasses 6 months ago
Respiratory: No cough or shortness of breath
CVS/PVS: No chest pain or palpitations; mild lower-limb edema self-managed with non-prescription support hose
GI: Occasional reflux, uses an OTC antacid; tends to constipation, managed by diet (fibre)
Urinary/genital: Ongoing mild urgency; can get to toilet on time; occasional urine loss (small volume) with coughing, wears panty liner; vaginal itchiness as above
MSK: Some long standing pain in hips/knees, relieved with acetaminophen
CNS: No headaches or seizures; no numbness or tingling of limbs
Mood: No concerns

Focused Physical Examination:
General: Healthy, appearing well groomed. Gait even, using cane in right hand.
Vital Signs: RR: 18; HR 82, regular; Temp 36.5; Serial BP #1 144/84 #2 138/77 #3 136/79
Abdomen: Obese, soft, no tenderness on palpation, no masses, bowel sounds x4
Pelvic Exam: Normal female genitalia. Small leak on cough in lying position. Vaginal tissues pale, dry, urethral caruncle present. Grade 1 anterior wall prolapse. Able to contract pelvic floor muscles, graded 4/5 on modified Oxford scale held 4 seconds.
Digital Rectal Exam: No lesions/masses/stool in rectum, sphincter tone intact
Post-void residual: 54 mL
Pertinent Diagnostic Tests: No recent lab work. Previous urine cultures 3 and 5 months ago showed no growth.
Allergies: None known
Medications: Metoprolol 25 mg daily; Acetaminophen 500 mg prn

Plan: Most likely diagnosis is urogenital atrophy. Urinalysis and urine culture ordered to rule out a urinary tract infection came back negative. In reviewing results with the patient a few days later, Liz explains symptoms of urogenital atrophy and Mrs. P. agrees to try a course of vaginal estrogen rather than another round of antibiotics.

Discussion

From the information obtained from Mrs. P.'s history of present illness, Liz identifies a larger concern. Mrs. P. has been prescribed repeated courses of antibiotics in the absence of evidence of UTI. She questions the consistency of the clinic approach and raises her concern for discussion at the next team meeting. At the meeting, Liz provided recent practice guidelines on the management of urogenital atrophy and for antibiotic stewardship in the context of UTI assessment and treatment. The clinic team agrees to develop a quality improvement project to examine practices related to UTIs in post-menopausal women, monitor practices for three months, and then utilizing the data obtained and the guidelines, develop a best practice approach for the clinic.

Challenges to Enacting the Research Competencies

Although there is considerable variation in role enactment, the NP role is often acknowledged as a clinical practice role, with the focus being direct patient/client care and less time spent on other role activities, including research (CCRNR, 2015; Kilpatrick et al., 2015). Barriers to implementation of the NP role stem from many levels, including the health system, organization, and practice setting (Sangster-Gormley, Martin-Misener, Downe-Wamboldt, & DiCenso, 2011). Such barriers can affect the ability of the NP to fully enact and engage in research competency–related activities. Specific barriers to the research competencies include lack of dedicated time/role expectations, lack of confidence in research skills, and lack of access to current literature and practice guidelines.

Lack of Dedicated Time/Role Expectations

With the emphasis on direct clinical care associated with the role, NPs have little or no dedicated time for research-related activities, even at the level of having time to access and appraise new research and guidelines. The CCRNR (2015) practice analysis reported on average 75.7% of NP work time was spent in client care, with only 4.8% in quality improvement and research. Kilpatrick et al. (2012) reported on two cases of NP practice in acute care (two Canadian hospitals), which suggested variability in the amount of time spent in the research role component, with the NPs in the first case spending 10.2% of time on research and the NPs in the second case only 0.9%. Some of these studies included NPs in teaching hospitals, which usually have an increased prevalence of research activity. Little is known about the time spent in research activities by Canadian NPs outside academic hospital settings, such as those in primary care, where time for research-related activities may be even scarcer. Economic evaluations of the NP role have focused on comparing equivalency of care in terms of patient outcomes, resource use, and costs to other health care providers such as physicians and medical residents (Kilpatrick et al., 2015). Understanding of the outcomes of the non-clinical activities, including research and quality improvement, requires further research.

NPs, managers, and physicians may have differing and conflicting views of how the NP should focus their time. The study by Kilpatrick et al. (2012) illustrates differences that can exist between practice settings with regard to the NPs' ability to enact the research competencies, and the influence of nursing and medical leadership for this activity.

Strategies

Implementation of the NP role in a way that is inclusive of all the domains of APN, such as research-related activities, must involve the stakeholders, including physicians and managers, who potentially influence role enactment. Inclusion of stakeholders in implementation of the role facilitates coming to a common understanding as well as shared vision of the NP role. As well, delineating the intention of what the role is meant to accomplish (role definition) and acceptance of the role by the team are important aspects of NP role implementation (Sangster-Gormley et al., 2011).

Lack of Confidence in Research Knowledge and Skills

It has been suggested that some NPs may not feel prepared or confident with their research skills. This could be due in part to educational preparation and limited opportunity to utilize skills in research and quality improvement. Education standards support graduate education for NPs with graduate-level coursework in research (CASN, 2012) to prepare for the breadth of the role.

Another influence on research skills is experience. Lack of confidence in research skills may be more acutely felt by the novice NP, who is often focused on consolidating new and expanded clinical skills and less focused on the other domains of practice. Even with graduate coursework in research, the research experience of novice NPs may be limited and affect confidence as many graduate-level nursing programs now offer a choice of thesis or course-based programs. Graduates of course-based programs will have preparation in research critique and evaluation, but may not have experience in conducting formal research. Whether there is a difference in NPs who have completed course-based versus thesis-based graduate programs in terms of enacting the NP research competencies has not been studied.

Strategies

As the NP develops in their role, mentoring in research skills and having the opportunity to participate in both quality improvement and research studies are essential to the growth of skills and confidence. Practice residencies for new NPs that support development of scholarly activities as well as clinical skills and knowledge have shown positive outcomes (Wirtz Rugen, Speroff, Zapatka, & Brienza, 2016). Other strategies may include continuing education related to development of skills and knowledge in research-related skills included in the competencies.

Lack of Access to Current Literature and Best Practice Guidelines

In some settings, NPs may lack access to library services, other information sources, current research, and best practice guidelines, limiting the ability to address the quality improvement and research competencies. This may be more pronounced in rural settings (Hunter,

Murphy, Babb, & Vallee, 2016); however, a rigorous comparison of urban versus rural NP access to research in Canada has not been published. Although discussed anecdotally, NP access to current literature and practice guidelines as a barrier to addressing the research competencies requires further investigation.

Strategies

Managers need to ensure—and it is incumbent that NPs request—that they have access to current evidence-informed literature. Provincial nursing professional associations and regulatory bodies may also have a role to play in facilitating access.

Conclusion

Fundamental to the quality improvement and research competency is improving practice and evaluating the outcomes of evidence-informed care. There is variation in how this competency is enacted, and the ability of the NP to meet the competency is based on experience and education, as well as system and organizational influences such as the nursing and medical leadership understanding of the NP role within the practice setting. Barriers to enacting the competency are only partially understood, and further research on how to support NPs in meeting this competency is needed. Different expectations for the novice NP compared to the more experienced NP need to be established. In the future, the increase in the number of NPs with doctoral preparation will support mentorship as well as a growth in research activity.

Critical Thinking Questions

1. What are key differences between quality improvement and research projects?
2. Novice NPs often focus on their clinical practice competencies as they gain confidence and experience. How can the novice NP be supported in developing quality improvement and research competencies? Why is this critical to patient outcomes?
3. Nursing and medical leadership often influence enactment of the NP role. What other influences (system, organizational, and practice setting) might facilitate or impede the NP from enacting the quality improvement and research competencies?

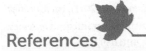

References

Branham, S., DelloSritto, R., & Hilliard, T. (2014). Lost in translation: The acute care nurse practitioners' use of evidence based practice: A qualitative study. *Journal of Nursing Education and Practice,* 4(6), 53–59. doi: 10.5430/jnep.v4n6p53

Brykcaynski, K. A. (2014). Role development of the advanced practice nurse. In A. B. Hamric, C. M. Hanson, M. R. Tracy, & E. T. O'Grady (Eds.), *Advanced practice nursing: An integrative approach* (5th ed., pp. 86–111). St. Louis, MO: Saunders Elsevier.

Canadian Association of Schools of Nursing (CASN). (2012). *Nursing masters education in Canada: Final report 2012*. Ottawa, ON: CASN. Retrieved from https://casn.ca/wp-content/uploads/2014/12/20121213ENMNescanFinalReport2.pdf

CASN. (2015). *National nursing education framework: Final report*. Ottawa, ON: CASN. Retrieved from https://www.casn.ca/wp-content/uploads/2018/11/CASN-National-Education-Framwork-FINAL-2015.pdf

Canadian Council of Registered Nurse Regulators (CCRNR). (2015). *Practice analysis study of nurse practitioners*. Beaverton, ON: CCRNR. Retrieved from http://www.ccrnr.ca/assets/ccrnr-practice-analysis-study-of-nurse-practitioners-report---final.pdf

Canadian Institutes for Health Research (CIHR). (n.d.). *Knowledge translation at CIHR*. Ottawa, ON: CIHR. Retrieved from http://www.cihr-irsc.gc.ca/e/29418.html#2

Canadian Nurses Association (CNA). (2016). *Position statement: The nurse practitioner*. Ottawa, ON: CNA. Retrieved from https://www.cna-aiic.ca/-/media/cna/page-content/pdf-en/the-nurse-practitioner-position-statement_2016.pdf

CNA. (2019). *Advanced practice nursing: A pan-Canadian Framework*. Ottawa, ON: CNA. Retrieved from www.cna-aiic.ca/-/media/cna/page-content/pdf-en/advanced-practice-nursing-framework-en.pdf

Gregory, K. E. (2015). Differentiating between research and quality improvement. *The Journal of Perinatal & Neonatal Nursing, 29*(2), 100–102. doi: 10.1097/JPN.0000000000000107

Hunter, K. F., Murphy, R. S., Babb, M., & Vallee, C. (2016). Benefits and challenges faced by a nurse practitioner working in an interprofessional setting in rural Alberta. *Canadian Journal of Nursing Leadership, 29*(3), 61–71. doi: 10.12927/cjnl.2016.24893

Kilpatrick, K., Lavoie-Tremblay, M., Ritchie, J. A., Lamothe, L., Doran, D., & Rochefort, C. (2012). How are acute care nurse practitioners enacting their roles in healthcare teams? A descriptive multiple-case study. *International Journal of Nursing Studies, 49*, 850–862. doi: 10.1016/j.ijnurstu.2012.01.011

Kilpatrick, K., Reid, K., Carter, N., Donald, F., Bryant-Lukosius, D., Martin-Misener, R., ... DiCenso, A. (2015). A systematic review of the cost-effectiveness of clinical nurse specialists and nurse practitioners in inpatient roles. *Nursing Leadership, 28*(3), 56–76. doi: 10.12927/cjnl.2016.24456

Langley, J., Wostenholme, D., & Cooke, J. (2018). "Collective making" as knowledge mobilization: The contribution of participatory design in the co-creation of knowledge in healthcare. *BioMed Central (BMC) Health Services Research, 18*, 585. doi: 10.1186/s12913-018-3397-y

Sangster-Gormley, E., Carter, N., Donald, F., Martin Misener, R., Ploeg, J., Kaasalainen, S., ... Wickson-Griffiths, A. (2013). A value-added benefit of nurse practitioners in long-term care settings: Increased nursing staff's ability to care for residents. *Nursing Leadership, 26*, 24–37.

Sangster-Gormley, E., Martin-Misener, R., Downe-Wamboldt, B., & DiCenso, A. (2011). Factors affecting nurse practitioner role implementation in Canadian practice settings: An integrative review. *Journal of Advanced Nursing, 67*, 1178–1190. doi: 10.1111/j.1365-2648.2010.05571.x

Wirtz Rugen, K., Speroff, E., Zapatka, S. A., & Brienza, R. (2016). Veterans affairs interprofessional nurse practitioner residency in primary care: A competency-based program. *Journal for Nurse Practitioners, 12*(6), e267–e273. https://doi.org/10.1016/j.nurpra.2016.02.023

Chapter 18A

Leadership Competencies

Clinical Nurse Specialist

Mary-Lou Martin

MARY-LOU MARTIN is a clinical nurse specialist-Mental Health in the Forensic Program at St. Joseph's Healthcare Hamilton in Hamilton, Ontario. She also holds an appointment as an Associate Clinical Professor in the School of Nursing at McMaster University, Hamilton, Ontario. She is currently President of the Clinical Nurse Specialist Association of Canada.

KEY TERMS

leaders
leadership
systems leadership
   competencies

OBJECTIVES

1. Describe the clinical nurse specialist (CNS) systems leadership competencies.
2. Describe the evidence related to CNS leadership in Canada.
3. Describe characteristics of an effective CNS leader.

Introduction

Clinical nurse specialists (CNSs) make a difference to the health outcomes of Canadians by demonstrating clinical leadership and evidence-informed practice with spheres of influence at the individual, aggregate, community, organizational, and health systems levels (Canadian Nurses Association [CNA], 2013). A nurse leader has attributes such as being an advocate for quality care, a collaborator, an effective communicator, a mentor, a risk taker, a role model, and a visionary (CNA, 2020). Leadership is an important component of CNSs' multi-dimensional advanced practice nursing (APN) role. CNSs have expertise in a clinical specialty and competencies that lead to the delivery of innovative and evidence-informed care (CNA, 2014).

As leaders and change agents, CNSs use systems thinking to enhance safety, cost effectiveness, and quality of care. CNSs provide leadership in managing change, influencing clinical practice, and engaging in political strategy at all systems levels to achieve accessibility to care and to advance nursing services (CNA, 2008). This leadership includes engaging in problem-solving, organizational strategic thinking, solution-focused outcomes, ethical decision-making, and advocacy. This chapter will describe and explore leadership competencies of the CNS, evidence of CNS leadership, and a case study demonstrating how a CNS can lead people, teams, and systems.

Leadership Competency

In Canada, and in response to the growing complexity of nursing practice, the need for leadership at the point of care and the need for continuity of care across the health care system were part of the creation of the CNS role (CNA, 2006, 2009, 2013). Leadership is a key aspect of CNSs' scope of practice and the strength of the CNS is the ability to combine clinical expertise with leadership and research (CNA, 2012; Schreiber et al., 2005). The leadership role of the CNS is important for patients, families, communities, populations, the nursing profession, and the health care system. CNSs who are prepared at the graduate or doctoral level are educated in leadership competencies (Heinen, van Oostveen, Peters, Vermeulen, & Huis, 2019). In 2013, CNA suggested that national CNS competencies and certification would bring clarity and consistency across all practice settings in Canada. National CNS competencies were published in 2014; however, certification and regulation remain elusive (CNA, 2014).

The CNS influences health care at three levels; client, practice setting, and organizational/systems (CNA, 2014). Four categories of core competencies were identified: clinical care, system leadership, advancement of nursing practice, and evaluation and research (CNA, 2014). Additionally, CNA identified 14 systems leadership competencies that reflect diverse specialty areas and practice environments (CNA, 2014). In 2019, CNS as well as nurse practitioner (NP) competencies were amalgamated into a pan-Canadian APN framework (2019). The Clinical Nurse Specialist Position Statement (CNA, 2016) identified system leadership as one CNS competency category and it was further identified that the CNS can decrease the length of hospital stays by promoting evidence-based interventions to prevent adverse events and lessen complications, prepare clients and their families more fully for discharge, and strengthen clients' self-care abilities (Canadian Centre for Advanced Practice Nursing Research [CCAPNR], 2012).

The CNS provides expert care and leadership in practice by working collaboratively at the point of care with nurses and other health care professionals. CNSs lead practice changes and promote the use of best practices and evidenced-informed care so that the best possible outcomes are achieved. As change agents, CNSs demonstrate their system-level competencies at the individual, unit, and organizational levels (Pauly et al., 2004; Schreiber et al., 2004). The CNS can practice across system boundaries and they work at both micro- and macro-system levels to influence stakeholders (Thompson & Lutham, 2007). The collaborations between CNSs and others in the same health care agency, across agencies, and system boundaries are important to the improvement of local, national, and global health care.

Where improvements need to be made at the point of care, CNSs identify and lead collaborative teams in quality improvement and safety outcomes and develop and test innovative nursing interventions and programs of care. They disseminate knowledge by presenting at conferences and engaging in research initiatives, and contribute to knowledge about patient care, CNS practice, and health care systems issues by publishing their research in peer-reviewed journals. As leaders, CNSs are critical thinkers and influencers who embrace involvement in health care policy decisions through educating, coaching and mentoring others about leadership, and being involved in developing policy and influencing policy decisions at different levels of health care (CNA, 2008; Canam, 2005; Fulton, 2010; Seenandan-Sookdeo, 2012). In academia, CNSs can take a lead role in developing nursing curriculum and policy in graduate nursing programs. The literature supports the CNS role as improving client and health system outcomes; decreasing hospital admissions; decreasing emergency department visits; decreasing length of stay; decreasing readmissions; and promoting practice innovations (CNA, 2012).

Evidence of Clinical Nurse Specialist Leadership

In relation to the leadership role, the CNS requires competencies that lead to improved health outcomes. In 2014, CNA stated, "the CNS improves client, population and health system outcomes by integrating knowledge, skills and expertise in clinical care, research, leadership, consultation, education and collaboration" (p. 1). Unfortunately, the literature about CNS leadership competencies and outcome in Canada is limited due to lack of regulation and certification of the role. An annotated bibliography of 70 studies was published that reported the care by CNSs was associated with improved staff nurse knowledge and improved patients' functional performance, mood state, quality of life, and satisfaction (Fulton & Baldwin, 2004). Often the CNS role is credited for reduced length of hospital stays, readmissions, emergency room visits, and costs. Regrettably, most of this research is conducted outside Canada (Bryant-Lukosius et al., 2010).

A Canadian qualitative study of 16 CNSs sought to understand CNS practice when they worked with families and children with complex health care needs. The results demonstrated that CNSs focused on the systems of health care, health needs of the population, program development, consultation, education outreach, clinical guidelines, and policies. CNSs were aware of their potential to influence the cost and quality of health care (Canam, 2005).

An historical overview of CNS and NP role development in Canada was published and found that the CNS role was often challenged by role confusion and limited administrative support (Kaasalainen et al., 2010). Bryant-Lukosius et al. (2010) utilized the results of a decision support synthesis to examine APN roles in Canada. Limited integration of CNSs in the health care system, insufficient research on CNS role implementation, lack of vision for the CNS role, limited designated CNS graduate education, and lack of CNS credentialing were all found to be challenges.

An integrative literature review of 12 studies examining CNS leadership competencies revealed that others perceived that CNSs had a positive influence at the systems level with policy and guideline development, and effective use of resources (Axen, 2011). Similarly, a qualitative study explored 11 CNSs' practice and found that CNSs were engaged in the health care system with policy development at clinical, institutional, and systems levels (Rourke, 2012).

In the Netherlands, Heinen et al. (2019) conducted an integrative review of the international literature to determine which APN leadership competencies and attributes were expected in master's-prepared CNSs, NPs, and clinical nurse leaders. Fifteen studies and seven competency frameworks were reviewed leading to the identification of 30 core competencies under the domains of clinical leadership, professional leadership, health systems leadership, and health policy leadership.

Kilpatrick et al. (2013) conducted a survey to identify the practice patterns of Canadian CNSs. The findings indicated that CNS practice patterns varied depending on the clinical specialty and graduate-level education. They also found that the lack of administrative structures/resources to support CNS role development and the lack of a protected CNS title led to confusion and was a barrier in identifying the number of CNSs in Canada.

Bryant-Lukosius et al. (2015) undertook a systematic review of 13 randomized controlled trials (n = 2,463) across four populations to evaluate the clinical effectiveness and cost effectiveness of CNSs involved in hospital-to-home transitional care. The CNSs who provided transitional care improved patient outcomes, delayed re-hospitalization, and reduced length of hospital stays and re-hospitalization rates and costs. An ICN Policy Brief by Bryant-Lukosius and Martin-Misener (2015) summarized the key outcomes of CNS care as improved access to supportive care; improved quality of life; improved health promotion practices; improved recruitment and retention; and reduced hospital admission and visits to the emergency department.

CNSs are a good health care investment for changing the Canadian health care system because the outcomes include better care for individuals, better health for the populations, and lower health care costs. CNSs are essential to leading future challenges in the system transformation of health care.

CASE STUDY

The Story of Sierra

Sierra is a CNS who has a doctoral degree in nursing and a master's degree in applied psychology and counselling. She is employed by an urban academic health care facility and has a clinical appointment with the university's faculty of nursing. Sierra has been a CNS for 15 years in the clinical specialty of mental health and addiction. She recently completed advanced courses in palliative care and pain management. Sierra's clinical practice time is allocated into four domains: clinical care (30%), advancement of nursing practice (25%), evaluation and research (20%), and leadership (25%).

Jakub, 47 years old, was born to parents who immigrated in 1976 from Poland, where his father had worked as a labourer and his mother stayed at home. Jakub and his mother were physically and emotionally abused by his father. His mother died of pneumonia when Jakub was nine. Jakub had a challenging time in elementary and high school due to bullying and difficulty in completing schoolwork. He drop-ped out of school when he was in grade 10. At 20, he was diagnosed with schizo-phrenia. He was hospitalized multiple times due to psychosis and risk for self-harm. Antipsychotic medication did not reduce or eliminate his auditory hallucinations. He experienced a voice or voices telling him, "You are stupid," "You are no good," and "You smell bad."

These auditory hallucinations caused Jakub to experience distress and negative emotions; however, he was able to complete activities of daily living. He reported that he had no close friends, and when hospitalized or living in the supervised boarding home, he stayed mainly in his room. Jakub rarely approached any of his clinicians and he interacted only if others approached him. Jakub enjoyed walking and he would routinely walk 6 km from his boarding home to the hospital for his outpatient appointments. He was knowledgeable about hockey and baseball, he was an avid fan, and he would watch the games on the TV. Most recently Jakub's father was unemployed and living in subsidized housing. His father's only contact with his son was when he was under the influence of alcohol and seeking money.

Discussion

Skyler was a new registered nurse (RN) on the in-patient mental health unit. He connected with the CNS, Sierra, to request consultation and clinical supervision to establish a thera-peutic relationship with his client, Jakub. Sierra met regularly with Skyler and introduced him to the concept of therapeutic use of self, the value of peer support, Peplau's interpersonal theory, and best practice guidelines. Sierra demonstrated therapeutic techniques to engage Jakub in a collaborative relationship. Sierra observed Skyler's interactions with Jakub and provided feedback. Sierra supported Skyler to self-reflect and develop a patient-centred plan of care. Sierra also demonstrated to Skyler and provided Jakub with trauma counselling and intervention for voice hearing. The outcomes for Sierra, Skyler, and Jakub were satisfaction, an effective therapeutic relationship, and reduced auditory hallucinations.

Jakub lived successfully in the community for many years, but this was intermittently interrupted by brief psychiatric hospitalizations. Three years ago, Jakub was diagnosed with colon cancer. While in the early palliative care phase, when he was ambulatory and able to function relatively well, Jakub remained an outpatient of the mental health program working with a different RN, Rashida. The oncologist informed Jakub that there had been a posi-tive response to the chemotherapy regime he had been taking, and that he would be moni-tored regularly in the future. A few months later, at a mental health outpatient appointment, Jakub indicated to Rashida he was experiencing constipation, loss of appetite, nausea, pain, dyspnea, anxiety, and tiredness. Following a physical examination by Jakub's oncologist, and undergoing diagnostic tests, he was told the cancer had metastasized and that chemotherapy would not be advised.

The CNS, Sierra, engaged in collaborative relationships with stakeholders across various systems so that Jakub's needs related to health, social services, spirituality, housing, and transportation could be met. She collaborated with the RN, Rashida, and Jakub to determine how quality care could be provided. Rashida was learning how to use a recovery approach; however, she had not been trained in using strength-based approaches. Sierra knew that the use of strengths in a client's care is inherent in recovery, trauma-informed, and palliative care approaches. Sierra mentored and taught Rashida how to assess and support the client to identify their strengths and past successes. Understanding Jakub's strengths informed the plan of care and supported his resiliency under his current condition of stress. When Jakub identified his strengths, he felt empowered and it enhanced his therapeutic relationships with the CNS and the outpatient nurse.

Sierra maintained her therapeutic relationship with Jakub and confirmed that his goals were being met and that he was satisfied with his care. She also provided therapeutic support to Jakub in preparing for his death. Jakub chose the care he would prefer at the end of his life. His end-of-life wishes for his care were comfort measures with no CPR and no intubation. Unfortunately, his boarding home was unable to provide end-of-life care and there was a waiting list for hospice care. Jakub identified that he did not want to die in an acute hospital bed, but instead he preferred to die in an in-patient mental health unit. Jakub said he would feel more comfortable where he was familiar with the people. When Jakub was admitted to the unit, he was still ambulatory; however, his day-to-day functioning was reduced, and he required some assistance with activities of daily living. When Jakub was in the terminal palliative phase, he spent his time in bed or in a recliner chair and required total care.

Sierra worked in partnership with the hospice's nurse practitioner (NP), Nikita. They were uniquely positioned to share leadership so that they could collaboratively coordinate with Jakub and the health care team. Nikita monitored Jakub's physical health status, pharmacological treatment, and discussed with Jakub his end-of-life wishes and also consulted with the oncologist, palliative care CNS, and a physician with palliative care expertise.

Many of the in-patient mental health nurses felt anxious and unprepared to meet the palliative care needs of Jakub. The nurses believed that palliative care is for the last days or weeks of life when instead the palliative care approach should be introduced early when a life-limiting illness is identified to be progressive and not curable. Sierra met with the nurses and debunked the myths about palliative care. Evidence-informed guidelines for palliative care, trajectories of dying, and a prognostic indicator guide were introduced to the nurses. A holistic framework for client care and evidenced-based tools for symptom management and daily functioning were taught. Sierra and the NP shared their expertise when they met with clinicians to plan the anticipated death of Jakub based on his end-of-life wishes and death management. During the downward trajectory of Jakub's health, there were regular team debriefings with support and reflection. Sierra supported the nurses when some experienced moral distress. Sierra also reinforced with staff the importance of self-care to promote health, well-being, and life balance.

Sierra and the NP were successful in advocating, collaborating, and providing leadership to ensure quality care for Jakub to the end of his life. Together, they provided evidence-informed resources; developed an educational plan; and established interprofessional partnerships across systems (i.e., health care, social services, housing). Through this clinical situation the CNS and NP demonstrated that nurses in a mental health setting require basic competence about palliative care.

The roles of the CNS and the NP often intersect, and competencies and scope of practice may overlap. Collaboration between the health care team and Jakub was critical to ethical decision-making and the delivery of high-quality palliative care in a non-traditional palliative care setting. The CNS and the NP shared responsibility and were accountable in the delivery of safe and effective care with the client.

Sierra reflected on the feedback from the client and the clinical team. This reflection identified strategies for sustaining collaborative practice between the CNS, NP, and the clinical team. Strategies included Sierra working with the nurses to assess team dynamics, develop a plan, and implement the Best Practice Guideline on Collaborative Practice. The implementation of the guideline benefited the clinicians by offering them an opportunity to learn effective ways to communicate, resolve conflict, and work collaboratively to promote teamwork and a healthy workplace. It also benefited the unit and the organization by contributing to their mission of excellence, improving team effectiveness, enhancing quality of work life, and creating opportunities for further change. Creating organizational cultures to support safer and healthier health care environments is part of the CNS leadership role.

Sierra developed a plan to determine where patient care and system improvements needed to be made. Sierra used her expert competencies to lead a quality improvement project. Change initiatives helped to implement new practices and policies and improve safety and quality of care. Nurse- and CNS-sensitive outcomes were also identified. She invited colleagues to engage in a systematic review of the literature with a plan to identify knowledge gaps so that research questions could be identified and a research proposal could be developed. The findings of the review were disseminated through presentations at conferences and publications in peer-reviewed journals. Sierra used the evidence to influence decision-making about hospital policy and how to provide the best care to mental health patients with life-limiting illnesses.

In her early years as a CNS, Sierra observed that her health care organization and the health care system were ever-changing. She joined some professional groups such as her province's professional nursing group, the Mental Health Nursing Group, the Nurse Educators Group, and the Nursing Research Group. She also joined her provincial Clinical Nurse Specialist Association, and later she was elected to the executive as a member-at-large. Sierra enjoyed the increased opportunities for professional networking. She was also involved in developing position papers about CNS issues, learning about health care policy, and being an editor for the newsletter. These networking opportunities allowed her to connect and advocate with other leaders in nursing, health care, government, and other sectors. Other involvement included planning a national CNS conference and becoming a member of the conference's scientific committee. She recognized that as part of a professional group, she could promote a national voice for CNSs, network with other CNSs, be politically engaged, and advocate for systems changes. She was also able to promote the understanding of the CNS role to others and advocate for CNSs having a protected title. She was able to make a difference by sharing her experiences, communicating evidence about the value of CNSs, and influencing change in practice and policy.

Sierra was a lifelong learner who needed to continue her development of competence in all aspects of her scope of practice. Self-reflection and self-assessment of her learning needs, strengths, leadership skills, and personal resources were important to Sierra. For Sierra, the ongoing development of competencies in leadership and health information technology was particularly important for her career development because she wanted to be involved in health care policy decisions and improving the health care system.

Conclusion

Ten years ago, it was suggested that if the CNS role was to survive, there would need to be a national voice representing CNSs as clinical leaders in the health care system. This has been only partially achieved. The Clinical Nurse Specialist Association of Canada has been a national voice for CNSs since 2016 and they are working to make CNSs, as health care leaders, more visible to the public and other stakeholders.

Having the leadership competencies to collaborate and develop partnerships with people and systems, CNSs are prepared to lead change and to challenge the status quo in improving patient and system-level outcomes. In order to demonstrate the true value of their leadership, CNSs must engage in their full scope of practice so that they can lead and contribute to effective system-level changes. Evidence supports the significance and necessity of interprofessional and multi-system collaboration as a way of providing evidence-informed, cost-effective, and sustainable health care.

There is some concern that the future of the CNS role is at risk if the job title is not protected. The CNS role would be strengthened if there was specific CNS credentialing and regulation. Additional research is needed to gain a more complete understanding of leadership outcomes of CNS practice within the Canadian health care system. With increasing globalization of health care, it will be important to explore the potential of CNS competencies being developed for a global marketplace. CNSs are essential to meeting future challenges and they offer a unique and positive leadership contribution to the health and health care system of all Canadians.

Critical Thinking Questions

1. Compare and contrast the 2014 CNS competencies and 2019 APN competencies.
2. How would you describe the CNS leadership role to others? Give examples.
3. What are the dynamic and contextual factors that influence CNS leadership?
4. What strategies can be employed that strengthen the CNS role in the Canadian health care system?

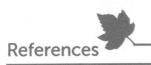

References

Axen, L. (2011). *Does graduate education grant greater visibility to the work of the nurse? A literature review of perceptions of the CNS role* (Unpublished MSN thesis, University of Victoria, Victoria, BC). Retrieved from https://dspace.library.uvic.ca:8443/bitstream/handle/1828/4014/Axen_Linda_MN_2011 .pdf?sequence=1&isAllowed=y

Bryant-Lukosius, D., Carter, N., Kilpatrick, K., Martin-Misener, R., Donald, F., Kaasalainen S., ... DiCenso, A. (2010). The clinical nurse specialist role in Canada. *Nursing Leadership, 23*(Special Issue), 140–166.

Bryant-Lukosius, D., Carter, N., Reid, K., Donald, F., Martin-Misener, R., Kilpatrick, K., ... DiCenso, A. (2015). The clinical effectiveness and cost effectiveness of clinical nurse specialist-led hospital to home transitional care: A systematic review. *Journal of Evaluation in Clinical Practice, 21*, 763–781.

Bryan-Lukosius, D., & Martin-Misener, R. (2015). *ICN policy brief: Advanced practice nursing: An essential component of country level human resources for health.* Geneva, CH: ICN. Retrieved from https://fhs.mcmaster.ca/ccapnr/documents/ICNPolicyBrief6AdvancedPracticeNursing_000.pdf

Canadian Centre for Advanced Practice Nursing Research (CCAPNR). (2012). *The clinical nurse specialist: Getting a good return on healthcare investment* [Briefing note]. Hamilton, ON: CCAPNR. Retrieved from http://international.aanp.org/Content/docs/CNS_EN.pdf

Canadian Nurses Association (CNA). (2006). *Report of 2005 dialogue on advanced nursing practice.* Ottawa, ON: CNA.

CNA. (2008). *Advanced nursing practice: A national framework.* Ottawa, ON: CNA.

CNA. (2009). *Position statement: Clinical nurse specialist.* Ottawa, ON: CNA.

CNA. (2012). *Strengthening the role of the clinical nurse specialist in Canada: Background paper.* Ottawa, ON: CNA. Retrieved from https://www.cna-aiic.ca/~/media/cna/files/en/strengthening_the_cns_role_background_paper_e.pdf

CNA. (2013). *Strengthening the role of the clinical nurse specialist in Canada: Pan-Canadian roundtable discussion summary report.* Ottawa, ON: CNA. Retrieved from https://www.cna-aiic.ca/-/media/cna/page-content/pdf-fr/clinical_nurse_specialist_role_roundtable_summary_e.pdf

CNA. (2014). *Pan-Canadian core competencies for the clinical nurse specialist.* Ottawa, ON: CNA. Retrieved from http://cna-aiic.ca/~/media/cna/files/en/clinical_nurse_specialists_convention_handout_e.pdf

CNA. (2016). *Position statement: Clinical nurse specialist.* Ottawa, ON: CNA.

CNA. (2019). *Advanced practice nursing: A pan-Canadian framework.* Ottawa, ON: CNA. Retrieved from https://www.cna-aiic.ca/-/media/cna/page-content/pdf-en/apn-a-pan-canadian-framework.pdf

CNA. (2020). *Leadership.* Ottawa, ON: CNA. Retrieved from https://www.cna-aiic.ca/en/download-buy/ leadership

Canam, C. (2005). Illuminating the clinical nurse specialist role of advanced practice nursing: A qualitative study. *Nursing Leadership, 18*(4), 70–89.

Fulton, J., & Baldwin, K. (2004). An annotated bibliography reflecting CNS practice and outcomes. *Clinical Nurse Specialist, 18*(1), 21–39.

Fulton, J. S. (2010). Evolution of clinical nurse specialist's role: Practice in the United States. In J. S. Fulton, B. L. Lyon, & K. A. Goureau (Eds.), *Foundations of clinical nurse specialist practice* (pp. 3–13). New York, NY: Springer.

Heinen, M., van Oostveen, C., Peters, J., Vermeulen, H., & Huis, A. (2019). An integrative review of leadership competencies and attributes in advanced nursing practice. *Journal of Advanced Nursing, 75*, 2378–2392. https://doi:10.1111/jan.14092

Kaasalainen, S., Martin-Misener, R., Kilpatrick, K., Harbman, P., Bryant-Lukosius, D., Donald, F., … DiCenso, A. (2010). A historical overview of the development of advanced practice nursing roles in Canada. *Nursing Leadership, 23*(Special Issue), 35–60.

Kilpatrick, K., DiCenso, A., Bryant-Lukosius, D., Richie, J. A., Martin-Misener, R., & Carter, N. (2013). Practice patterns and perceived impact of clinical nurse specialist roles in Canada: Results of a national survey. *International Journal of Nursing Studies, 50*(11), 1524–1536.

Pauly, B., Schreiber, R., MacDonald, M., Davidson, H., Crickmore, J., Moss, L., … Hammond, C. (2004). Dancing to our own tune: Understanding of advanced nursing practice in British Columbia. *Nursing Leadership, 17*(2), 47–57.

Rourke, S. N. (2012). *Canadian clinical nurse specialists: Understanding their role in policy within a British Columbian context* (Unpublished MSN thesis, University of Victoria, Victoria, BC).

Schreiber, R., MacDonald, M., Pauly, B., Davidson, H., Crickmore, J., Moss, L., … Hammond, C. (2005). Singing in different keys: Enactment of advanced nursing practice in British Columbia. *Nursing Leadership, 18*(2), 1–17.

Seenandan-Sookdeo, K. I. (2012). The influence of power in the Canadian healthcare system. *Clinical Nurse Specialist, 26*(2), 107–112.

Thompson, P., & Lutham, K. (2007). Clinical nurse leader and clinical nurse specialist role: Delineation in the acute care setting. *Journal of Nursing Administration, 37*(10), 429–431.

Chapter

18B

Leadership Competencies

Nurse Practitioner

Tammy O'Rourke

TAMMY O'ROURKE is an Assistant Professor at Athabasca University, Athabasca, Alberta. She is a nurse practitioner (NP)-PHC and led the development of one of the initial NP-Led Clinics in Belleville, Ontario, and served as the clinic's Chief NP/Clinic Director for four years. More recently she co-led the development of a new primary health care model for seniors in Edmonton, Alberta. Tammy has also held appointments at University of Alberta in Edmonton, Alberta, and Loyalist College in Belleville, Ontario.

KEY TERMS

leaders
leadership

OBJECTIVES

1. Discuss the importance of the nurse practitioner's (NP) role as a leader in today's complex health care environment.
2. Explore the Canadian Nurses Association's (CNA) NP leadership competency.
3. Discuss the outcomes associated with NP leadership.

Introduction

After decades of investments, innovation, and intent to reform Canada's health care system, the country continues to face multiple challenges in its efforts to redesign health care services. These challenges are becoming more evident with new financial constraints, and the ever-increasing incidence of chronic disease. Despite multiple attempts and pilot projects, Canada continues to lag behind other countries in progress to realizing a vision for primary health care and demonstrates a lack of a shared vision to support long-term health care reform. Strong, visible, and committed **leadership** could support the development of a shared vision; however, there are not enough **leaders** in Canada to support such a large system redesign.

Several factors can complicate the ability to increase leadership capacity and engage health care providers in leadership activities to support widespread system transformation.

In Canada, these factors include the following: the relationship between leadership activities and system outcomes are not well established; leadership programs and initiatives are not well established; and current Canadian health care system arrangements confound the situation. Progress is being made, but it is slow (Lavis, Moat, & Rizvi, 2014).

Leadership is a critical contributing factor in the success of health system redesign (Ham et al., 2011). It is also critical to the development of healthy workplaces and continued quality improvement initiatives in health services (Scammel et al., 2020). As Canada moves toward delivering new and improved primary health care services that are patient-centred and relevant to the social determinants of health, we need nurse practitioners (NPs) to demonstrate leadership in clinical practice environments. NPs are well positioned to provide leadership and there are several examples of NPs leading change to better care, better value, and better health in Canada's health care system.

When looking across Canada, Ontario and Alberta have appointed NPs as Provincial Nursing Officers. Twenty-seven Ontario NP-Led Clinics continue to provide sustainable primary health care services to over 70,000 patients and new models of NP leadership are emerging in the west. Two NP leaders in Sudbury, Ontario, developed this particular model of care in 2007 (Butcher, 2015). British Columbia announced a new compensation model for NPs who want to contract with existing health teams or develop new health teams. These NPs will be contractors and receive an annual fee for their services in addition to administration cost funding. In Alberta, Sage Seniors Association was the first academic faculty practice in the country to focus specifically on the primary health care needs for seniors embedded within a social service agency. An NP leader led the development of the successfully funded government proposal and an NP was hired to be the clinic director. In Quebec, SABSA (Services À Bas Seuil d'Accessibilité), a multi-stakeholder clinic, works with vulnerable populations who have difficulty in obtaining care in the conventional network. In this model of care, walk-in clinic users do not meet with a physician, but rather with a primary health care nurse practitioner, who can perform many of the competencies of APNs such as collaboration, consultation, and leadership (Carter, Dabney, & Hanson, 2019).

This chapter describes the role that NPs can play as leaders and innovators in Canada's health care system and provides recommendations pertaining to the activities important to enacting the CNA's core leadership competencies for all NPs.

Leadership Competency

Leadership is well defined by the CNA (2019); however, in practice, NPs can find it difficult to enact these competencies due to organizational constraints and/or limited resources to support leadership activities. Enacting the CNA leadership competencies in today's complex health care system can be a challenging yet rewarding experience for NPs. Leadership requires perseverance and NPs must engage in activities aimed at influencing important stakeholders in order to initiate and sustain change. NP leaders frequently face opposition as they challenge the status quo and seek to improve health care systems through activities aimed at shaping, sharing, and protecting visions for change in their organizations, communities, and/or provinces. Table 18b.1 depicts the leadership competencies CNA has delineated for all APNs.

TABLE 18B.1: Leadership Competencies

APNs are leaders in the organizations and communities where they work. They are agents of change, consistently seeking effective new ways to practice, improve care, and promote APN. They are able to:

- Demonstrate self-awareness, participate in professional development, and exhibit character and behaviour that is aligned with ethical values
- Evaluate programs in the organization and community and develop innovative approaches to complex issues
- Apply theories and principles of project and change management
- Develop and clearly articulate a vision for nursing practice, influence and contribute to the organization's and the health care system's vision, and implement approaches to realize that vision
- Identify problems and initiate change to address challenges at the clinical, organizational, or system level
- Advise clients, colleagues, the community, health care institutions, policy-makers and other stakeholders on issues related to nursing, health, and health care
- Advocate for enhanced access to health care by promoting APN to nurses and other health professionals, the public, legislators, and policy-makers
- Promote nursing and APN roles through involvement in academic pursuits, professional associations, and special interest groups

Source: CNA. (2019). *Advanced practice nursing: A pan-Canadian framework.* Ottawa, ON: CNA. Retrieved from https://www.cna-aiic.ca/-/media/cna/page-content/pdf-en/apn-a-pan-canadian-framework.pdf

The incorporation of leadership theory and opportunities for NPs to practice leadership activities during their education program are important. However, a well-accepted theory for nursing leadership has yet to emerge in the literature, and opportunities for NP students to practice leadership skills in current clinical contexts is inconsistent. Despite increasing knowledge in the area of outcomes associated with leadership in nursing practice, the strength of the evidence is limited to mostly correlational studies (Cummings, 2013; Wong, Cummings, & Ducharme, 2013). The story of Kateri demonstrates how NP leadership can have an impact on health care system change.

CASE STUDY

The Story of Kateri

Kateri is an NP-PHC living in a small community that is having issues attracting experienced primary health care providers. Grassroot efforts to successfully obtain government funding for team-based primary health care have been unsuccessful. As a result, Kateri found herself unemployed, while at the same time, local decision makers were supporting physician relocation at the cost of $150,000 per physician.

Kateri was travelling 45 minutes return trip to provide primary health care services in an adjacent community, while patients in her community were forced to seek access to primary health care services via the emergency room (ER) of the local hospital and urgent care clinics. These patients required care that would best be provided by an interprofessional team. Kateri desperately wanted to provide leadership in her community and to respond to their need for access to appropriately funded primary health care services. She decided to embark on her quest to make the vision for an NP-Led Clinic in her community a reality. The anticipated outcome for the introduction of this new service was improved access to team-based primary care and decreased utilization of high-cost emergency and urgent care medical services. After months of hard work, the proposal for the community's clinic received funding and today it continues to serve over 3,200 patients through the support of an interprofessional primary care team.

As you self-reflect on your knowledge of the change process and initial steps to providing leadership in the development of a new nurse practitioner role with the health care system, I challenge you to answer the following questions:

1. Are you prepared to initiate leadership and provide this type of change? If yes, how will you approach the task? And if no, what can you do to prepare yourself to provide this type of leadership?
2. What strategies can be used to engage community stakeholders to assess and plan for the introduction of an NP-led model of care?
3. How will you articulate the NP role with health care funders?

Discussion

The story of Kateri demonstrates how NP leadership competencies can have an impact on health care system change to achieve positive outcomes for her community, her profession, and the patients who were lacking access to primary health care services. Kateri was successful in introducing and implementing an innovation, an NP-Led Clinic. Her journey to innovation was like the model adapted by the Advisory Panel on Healthcare Innovation (see Figure 18b.1). Successful leaders transform systems through their innovation journey, including activities and initiatives identified in the model.

Kateri's leadership activities were aimed at generating strategic change and these activities required a certain level of sophistication. She took several steps to gain in-depth knowledge of the change process and develop skills used to engage several key stakeholders in the decision-making process relevant to the change.

The type of leadership required to make change in the preceding case study requires a strong spirit of commitment to change and the courage to face substantial opposition. Kateri demonstrated critical thinking, encouraged and supported the introduction of innovation, and positioned herself to be successful in the future and championed change. She saw a brighter, different future for her community's health care system and was optimistic that change

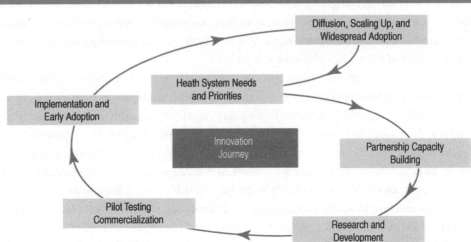

FIGURE 18B.1: Innovation Journey

Source: Advisory Panel on Healthcare Innovation. (2015). *Unleashing innovation: Excellent healthcare for Canada.* Ottawa, ON: Government of Canada. Adapted from Ivey International Centre for Health Innovation, London, ON: UWO. Used with permission.

could occur in her community. She anticipated issues and identified tools and strategies to encourage stakeholders to think positively about the change. Canada's health care system needs leaders who are enthusiastic about change and possess the drive and credibility to get things done.

Throughout the process, Kateri learned several lessons about stakeholder engagement/partnership and capacity building. One of the key lessons was that physicians need to be engaged early in the process and the need to recognize and support teamwork in health care environments. Early in the development phase of the project, Kateri spoke to multiple physicians in the community to educate them about the model and garner support for the project. Unfortunately, many local physicians were supportive of a different model of care, namely physician-led health teams. Physician-led health care teams are like NP-Led Clinics; however, these teams are led and managed by physicians. Kateri worked diligently to identify physician champions both locally and provincially who would assist in developing the clinic. She was successful in her efforts and two physicians came forward to support the work of the clinic.

Once the clinic was funded, Kateri was required to engage in activities such as human resource recruitment and management, policy development, and team building for the purpose of improving clinical services to change patient outcomes. At times, this was more challenging than the activities required to get funding for the clinic. These leadership skills were essential to ensure that patient outcomes would be improved using this type of care model. Key drivers to the development of clinical leadership in practice settings include highlighting the importance of the NP role, evidence-based practice, clinical outcome measurement, empowering clinicians, and supporting NP participation in clinical decision-making

(Davidson, Elliott, & Daly, 2006; O'Byrne, Hollett, & Campbell, 2020). In the case study, the NP-Led Clinic was in the spotlight for several reasons; it was the second clinic of its kind in the province and it had received funding despite competition from a physician-led model proposal for the same community. Kateri was now faced with the challenge of developing an interprofessional team while everyone watched.

NPs play important leadership roles in the development of interprofessional teams. Their purpose as leaders within these teams is to design strategies to support colleagues' efforts to achieve higher levels of functioning that contribute to health care system efficiency (McComiskey, Tyler, & Rowen, 2013; Rigolosi, 2005). Clinical leadership contributes to the development of effective teams and NP clinical leaders lead the way for their teams into the future, an entity that is often unknown (Davidson et al., 2006; McComiskey et al., 2013). Very little is known about clinical leadership in primary health care; it is hard to define and often difficult to measure in relation to NP practice (Nieuwboer, van der Sande, van der Marck, Rikkert, & Perry, 2019; Watson, 2008). However, most NPs are clinical leaders who are eager to enact their obligation of advocacy for patients at all system levels (Carryer, Gardner, Dunn, & Gardner, 2007).

In the case study, Kateri had to set the direction for a group of health care providers and build an integrated system of patient-centred care out of fragmented parts. She was self-motivated and goal-oriented. Kateri worked to create a collegial environment where everyone was engaged and felt supported to do their best work. It was the biggest challenge in her career to date and although she made mistakes, as many do when setting out for the first time, she continued to learn throughout the process and she used her authority to make decisions that were in the best interest of the providers and patients she served. She decided to engage the assistance of experts in human resource management. These experts supported the team's development and each member grew from increasing their knowledge of self and others. These management experts assisted Kateri in her recruitment efforts with strength-based assessments and team-building sessions.

During the same time that Kateri was developing and supporting the newly formed interprofessional team, she was focused on crossing boundaries into national and international arenas. She was able to influence others who had the decision-making capacity to enact change at the macro-system level and contribute to the development of the profession. Kateri took the time to engage with her professional organizations. She attended several teleconferences and meetings for both the RN and NP associations in her province as well as becoming a board member for her professional nursing association.

This position provided her with the opportunity to engage with multiple provincial decision makers. These decision makers included the executive director of the Association of Family Health Teams in Ontario, the provincial chief nursing officer, the provincial minister of health, and others. Professional NP leaders should hold memberships in their professional organizations and volunteer on local, provincial, and national committees because as a professional NP leader, this allows for ongoing contributions on a macro-systems level (Elliott et al., 2012). Kateri demonstrated strong professional leadership skills as she led the way to professional recognition and increased autonomy using her socio-political savvy. This type of savvy requires NPs to possess an increased level of confidence in the value of their profession and the ability to recognize opportunities for both silence and the use of voice.

Kateri's enactment of the CNA leadership competencies was crucial to the introduction and sustainability of the NP-Led Clinic in her community. She led the way to the development of an interprofessional team, which now provides primary health care services for over 3,200 patients. The clinic she developed is well known for adopting innovation and high-functioning team-based performance and has been recognized provincially and nationally for its work.

Conclusion

NPs require strong leadership skills as they lead the way to the development and introduction of NP-led service models that will provide cost-effective, high-quality alternatives to outdated models of care for Canadian citizens. As NPs advance the profession, more leaders will be required to enact the leadership competencies delineated by the CNA. Their leadership work should focus on addressing the sustainability of the NP role, the elimination of NP pilot projects, leadership of interprofessional team-based health care in various environments, and showing that NPs demonstrate better value, better care, and better health for the Canadian population.

Critical Thinking Questions

1. What characteristics and education do NP leaders require to develop and sustain shared visions for long-term health care reform?
2. What factors will contribute to NPs acquiring the leadership skills required to influence health care system changes in order to increase the number of permanent NP positions in all areas of practice?
3. Are there opportunities within your organization, community, and/or province/territory for the introduction of an NP-led innovation? How would this impact on "better value, better care, and better health" for the Canadian population?

References

Advisory Panel on Healthcare Innovation. (2015). *Unleashing innovation: Excellent healthcare for Canada*. Ottawa, ON: Government of Canada.

Butcher, M. (2015). Ontario's first nurse practitioner-led clinic. In C. Mariano (Ed.), *No one left behind: How nurse practitioners are changing the Canadian health care system* (pp. 21–34). Victoria, BC: Friesen Press.

Canadian Nurses Association (CNA). (2019). *Advanced practice nursing: A pan-Canadian framework.* Ottawa, ON: CNA. Retrieved from https://www.cna-aiic.ca/-/media/cna/page-content/pdf-en/apn-a-pan-canadian-framework.pdf

Carryer, J., Gardner, G., Dunn, S., & Gardner, A. (2007). The core role of the nurse practitioner: Practice, professionalism and clinical leadership. *Journal of Clinical Nursing, 16,* 1818–1825. doi: 10.111/j.1365-2702.2006.01823.x

Carter, M., Dabney, C., & Hanson, C. M. (2019). Collaboration. In M. F. Tracy & E. T. O'Grady (Eds.), *Hamric and Hanson's advanced nursing: An integrative approach* (6th ed., pp. 286–309). St. Louis, MO: Elsevier.

Cummings, G. (2013). Nursing leadership and patient outcomes. *Journal of Nursing Management, 21*(5), 707–708.

Davidson, P., Elliott, D., & Daly, J. (2006). Clinical leadership in contemporary clinical practice: Implications for nursing in Australia. *Journal of Nursing Management, 14,* 180–187. doi: 10.1111/j.1365-2934.2006.00555.x

Elliott, N., Higgins, A., Begley, C., Lalor, J., Sheerin, F., Coyne, I., & Murphy, K. (2012). The identification of clinical and professional leadership activities of advanced practitioners: Findings from the specialist clinical and advanced practitioner evaluation study in Ireland. *Journal of Advanced Nursing, 69*(5), 1037–1050. doi: 10.1111/j.1365-2648.2012.06090.x

Ham, C., Baker, R., Docherty, D., Hockey, P., Lobley, K., Tugendhat, L., & Walshe, K. (2011). *The future of leadership and management in the NHS. No more heroes.* Retrieved from http://www.kingsfund.org.uk/sites/files/kf/future-of-leadership-and-management-nhs-may-2011-kings-fund.pdf

Lavis, J., Moat, K., & Rizvi, Z. (2014). *Issue brief: Fostering leadership for health-system redesign in Canada, 4.* Hamilton, ON: McMaster Health Forum. Retrieved from http://www.mcmasterhealthforum.org/docs/default-source/Product-Documents/issue-briefs/fostering-leadership-health-system-redesign-canada-ib.pdf

McComiskey, C., Tyler, R., & Rowen, L. (2013). Developing a model for centralize nurse practitioner leadership. In M. Bahouth, K. Blum, & S. Simone (Eds.), *Transitioning into hospital-based practice: A guide for nurse practitioners and administrators* (pp. 69–88). New York, NY: Springer.

Nieuwboer, M., van der Sande, R., van der Marck, M., Rikkert, M., & Perry, M. (2019). Clinical leadership and integrated primary care: A systematic literature review. *European Journal of General Practice, 25*(1), 7–18. doi: 10.1090/13814788.2018.1515907

O'Byrne, P., Hollett, M., & Campbell, B. (2020). A nurse practitioner leadership model for a sexual health clinic in Canada: Staff feedback about implementation and operations. *Nurse Leader.* https://doi.org/10.1016/j.mnl.2019.11.016

Rigolosi, E. (2005). *Management and leadership in nursing and health care: An experiential approach* (2nd ed.). New York, NY: Springer.

Scammell, J., Apostolo, J., Bianchi, M., Costa, R., Jack, K., Kuiking, M., & Nilsson, S. (2020). Learning to lead: A scoping review of undergraduate nursing education. *Journal of Nursing Management, 28*(3), 756–765. https://doi.org/10.111/jonm.12951

Watson, C. (2008). Assessing leadership in nurse practitioner candidates. *Australian Journal of Advanced Nursing, 26*(1), 67–76.

Wong, C., Cummings, G., & Ducharme, L. (2013). The relationship between nursing leadership and patient outcomes: A systematic review update. *Journal of Nursing Management, 21*(5), 709–724. doi: 10.1111/jonm.12116

Chapter 19A

Consultation and Collaboration Competencies

Clinical Nurse Specialist

Marcia Carr

MARCIA CARR is a clinical nurse specialist (CNS)-geriatric medicine and geriatric psychiatry in Delta, British Columbia. She has adjunct faculty appointments at the University of British Columbia School of Nursing, Vancouver, British Columbia; Simon Fraser University Gerontology Research Centre, Vancouver, British Columbia; University of Victoria School of Nursing, Victoria, British Columbia; and is a clinical assistant at McMaster University, School of Nursing, Hamilton, Ontario. She is also a visiting professor at Fujian Medical University School of Nursing, Fuzhou, Fujian, China. Marcia is currently President-Elect for the Clinical Nurse Specialist Association of British Columbia (CNSABC) and was the first President of the Clinical Nurse Specialist Association of Canada (CNS-C), past Secretary for CNS-C, and remains the British Columbia and Yukon Territory's provincial representative on the Board for CNS-C. She was a member of advisory committees that developed the Pan-Canadian CNS Competencies (CNA, 2014) and *Advanced Practice Nursing: A Pan-Canadian Framework* (CNA, 2019).

KEY TERMS

collaboration
collaborator
consultant
consultation

OBJECTIVES

1. Explore the clinical nurse specialist (CNS) role of consultant.
2. Explore the CNS role of collaborator.
3. Apply CNS consultant and collaborator role competencies for complex patient, health care system, and specialized population issues.

Introduction

A fundamental part of clinical nurse specialist (CNS) practice, embedded within the role, is the **consultant** competency, which is enacted using a collaborative practice approach. The Pan-Canadian Core Competencies for the CNS articulates four overarching competencies that include clinical care, systems leadership, advancement of nursing practice, and evaluation and research (Canadian Nurses Association [CNA], 2014). These competencies have been expanded advanced practice nursing (APN)–wide in Canada, and further validate the importance of the consultant role to influence and impact care for individuals, direct-care health care providers, and organization system levels (CNA, 2019; Schreiber et al., 2005). Furthermore, the scope of practice for the CNS also incorporates these levels when assessing, planning, implementing, and evaluating strategies to construct micro and macro processes that are aimed at facilitating safe, quality of care, and positive health outcomes (CNA, 2014). The CNS utilizes the **collaborator** role to facilitate inclusiveness in the building of respectful and trusting partnerships that will improve care and practice changes among all care stakeholders and providers.

Consultation

Consultation as it applies to the CNS enactment of the competencies is defined as meeting with key informants and/or care providers to discuss the complex care and practice issues requiring an advanced practice nursing expertise in order to achieve measurable care improvement outcomes.

The CNS Role and Function as Consultant

The CNS applies expert advanced practice competencies, based on Benner's levels of clinical competence (Benner, 1982), when completing the advanced assessment, critical analysis and synthesis of root causes, and system care gap processes. Additionally, through a systematic process, the CNS in the consultant role provides evidence-informed, fiscally accountable strategies that have measurable outcomes to improve the system and care gaps.

Why and When Is the CNS Asked to Consult?

The CNS is asked to consult when a patient presents with complex problems requiring specialized APN expertise; when the health care system requires a clinical lens that scopes broadly at the direct care, system-wide, and external stakeholder levels for resolution of care gaps; and when specialized population needs are at risk for negative impacts and outcomes. The CNS can facilitate a systematic review that includes a root cause analysis and provides best practice strategies to improve and/or resolve the presenting problem. The CNS role additionally is positioned to influence changes and improvements at the patient/family, direct care provider, and internal/external system level.

Who Approaches the CNS to Consult?

Any member of the health care team and/or health care system may call upon the CNS to discuss a presenting patient/population/system or clinical care problem, concern, or issue. However, the CNS may independently determine the need to provide consultation beyond the original request because of discoveries made during the consultation process. Furthermore, the CNS may self-initiate a consultation through information acquired from other resources like the media, new policy statements from nursing associations, or government.

The CNS Consultation Process

One method that is often utilized in the consultation process is to initiate the Appreciative Inquiry (AI) framework in order to clarify and establish desired outcomes from the consultation (Bushe, 2011). From this process, the CNS can analyze, assist with decision-making, and create strategic change among the targeted stakeholders. This strength-based approach facilitates the building of change strategies that are received more positively by those who will be affected. Therefore, the people who are directly affected are needed (i.e., patients, families, communities) to gather their subjective perceptions along with the objective facts. A systematic gap analysis reveals actual and potential root causes that help synthesize data that can be used to evaluate outcomes (Gomez-Mejia, Balkin, & Cardy, 2008).

Collaboration

Collaboration as it applies to the CNS enactment of the competencies is a process through which the CNS methodically builds relational partnerships with key informants and stakeholders to achieve measurable outcomes. It means more than gathering participants and talking. It is building a foundation of mutual trust among the partners from which respectful realistic improvements and change can be realized. How the CNS applies the collaborative process ultimately can determine outcomes for individuals, population groups, and systems affected. Furthermore, each one of the collaborations has the potential to build a resource network that the CNS may call upon to influence and impact other desired improvements.

The following case study demonstrates how a CNS role was instrumental in targeting specific strategies by collaborating with others in the health care team to improve the health outcomes for other patients.

CASE STUDY

The Story of Esther

Esther was a vital, bright, and articulate 77-year-old retired schoolteacher living in British Columbia (BC). She was planning to go on a European trip with her husband following elective hip arthroplasty at her community hospital. During her preoperative work-up with anaesthesiology, she stated that she did not react well to general anaesthesia. From previous experiences, she stated that she became very confused post-operatively on opioids and that codeine had caused her significant constipation. She also stated that although she had some heart problems, she was normally quite well despite having part of her lung removed for cancer.

During the pre-operative work-up, the anaesthesiologist reassured her that she would receive local anaesthesia, not a general anaesthetic. Additionally, he noted that the analgesic ordered post-operatively would be hydromorphone. On the day of surgery, a different anaesthesiologist administered her anaesthesia, resulting in Esther receiving a general anaesthetic and post-operatively was written an order for meperidine rather than hydromorphone. Since she was experiencing low oxygen saturations and hypotension in the post-anaesthetic care unit, Esther was transferred to the intensive care unit (ICU) for stabilization. She experienced episodes of confusion and agitation while in the ICU. On day four, she was transferred to a medical unit for a few days and then transferred to the activation unit, where her restlessness and confusion continued. Staff put up her bedside rails while she was in bed and she had restraints on when in a chair. Her family tried to be with her as much as possible to reassure and calm her and to advocate for her care. Esther kept stating that she had terrible abdominal pain for which she received additional analgesia.

Subsequently, Esther was found on the floor beside her bed. The on-call physician gave a telephone order for lorazepam 1 mg po to sedate her. A few hours later, Esther was found on the floor again beside her bed. Initially, she was unresponsive, but later did become responsive but considerably more restless and agitated. There was bruising on the side of her face and eye. On seeing Esther like this, the family asked that a physician evaluate Esther as soon as possible. Diagnostic tests were ordered; however, Esther's condition continued to decline rapidly. The physician spoke with the family about a do-not-resuscitate order, which the family agreed to. Esther had sporadically received stool softeners and laxatives throughout her hospitalization, but there had not been a consistent tracking of whether she was having any bowel movements. Esther continued to complain about abdominal pain. An abdominal X-ray was ordered, but despite medical intervention, Esther passed away the next day.

Since her death was classified as unexpected, the case was referred to the provincial coroner. Two years later the coroner's inquest concluded that death was attributed to ischemic infarction of the bowel due to profound fecal impaction and cerebral ischemia due to prolonged post-operative oxygen desaturation and hypotension. All the findings contributed to her cognitive and functional changes and decline. The coroner directed that the College for Registered Nurses of British Columbia (CRNBC) and the College of Physicians and Surgeons of British Columbia address the clinical care issues that contributed to Esther's death.

Family, nursing, and allied health staff were all devastated by Esther's death. She had been well known in her small community and a number of staff knew her because she had taught them. The morale at the hospital was impacted as there was a feeling of shame and blame being perceived due to the directive for a coroner's inquest. The family considered litigation, but decided to be true to what they believed would be Esther's wishes, so they decided to participate in preventing the same thing from happening to anyone else.

Discussion

Esther's story is an example of a patient's hospitalization journey that should have been straightforward, but went terribly awry. This was due to several clinical care and system issues that resulted in Esther tragically dying within two weeks of her elective admission.

The BC provincial nursing regulator, CRNBC, consulted with the practicing CNS in geriatric psychiatry/geriatric medicine where Esther was hospitalized to review Esther's case and initiate the necessary steps to improve the hospital's care of acutely ill older adults. At the same time, the provincial regulatory body for physicians and surgeons was also directed to address these concerns in relation to communication and transitions of care between physicians. The CNS worked in collaboration with the nursing regulator, the nursing unit managers, and the interprofessional health care team to identify the possible root causes and care gaps contributing to this adverse patient outcome.

Prior to proceeding with any plans, the CNS formed a collaborative working group composed of unit managers, hospital directors, and direct care nursing staff to establish mutual respect and trust with those affected. The CNS purposefully built the working group's agenda and acted primarily in the consultant role to aid them in their development of the strategic plan. The CNS used the AI process (Bushe, 2011) with the working group to enable open and respectful group formation as well as enable the gathering of vital information on their wants and desired outcomes.

In order to have a concrete kick-off point from which the group was able to develop the strategic plan, the CNS developed an environmental scan tool derived from the least restraint and fall/injury prevention literature. This included identifying characteristics (i.e., no clutter, non-glare accessible lighting, low-rise beds, half-only bed railings, and fall-prevention equipment, including bed/chair alarms, and hip protectors) of what the hospital environment should look like in order to be an older adult–friendly hospital unit. The CNS additionally assessed the staff's knowledge, abilities, and attitudes about delirium, dementia, depression, fall prevention strategies, de-conditioning effects on mobility, pain, and bowel management. The CNS was highly mindful in ensuring a non-blame approach to support the already "hurting" staff, including senior administrators, who decided that the approaches and plans needed to be hospital-wide and not just the units that participated in Esther's care. The working group decided not to use surveys or questionnaires to determine staff's knowledge, abilities, and attitudes to caring for older adults as they believed it did not reflect how they currently worked together. They also decided that one of them would act as the guide/host for the CNS so that introductions and observations could be facilitated in an unobtrusive fashion. This approach meant that the CNS could not only meet but also open up informal in-the-moment conversations with the staff about their thoughts and feelings related to caring for older adults in order to set the foundation upon which relational trust could be built.

As part of the plan, the CNS completed a full chart review, including timelines of seminal events during Esther's hospitalization. Having knowledge of the findings of the coroner's inquest, the CNS paid particular attention to documentation and current nursing forms in place. From a macro-level lens, the CNS reviewed hospital policies related to post-operative care pathways, pain management, restraints, bowel management, and fall prevention.

An analysis of the data gathered from the various sources informed the identification of areas of strength and areas for improvement. The CNS presented the findings to the working group. The major strength revolved around staff expressing their desire to contribute to improving their ability to care for acutely ill older adults. They were seeking pragmatic and feasible actions that they could implement immediately as well as ones that they could work on. The overall assumption that care for any adult was the same as caring for older adults became the dominant root cause of the overall care issues that arose with Esther's hospitalization. Staff readily admitted that there were knowledge gaps in caring for acutely ill older adults. This resulted in not knowing whether a problem even existed, let alone how to articulate or address the problem. The staff agreed that if they didn't know what they should know, then how could they know that it was or could be a problem? Additionally, the need to prioritize revisions to policies and clinical practice guidelines on post-operative care, pain management, bowel management, least restraint, and fall prevention required improvements in order to facilitate clear, consistent communication and documentation. The working group decided that staff education was essential and was to be the first part of the remediation plan.

Concurrently, communication with staff required a plan that was purposefully designed by the CNS to focus on "What are they doing well? What would they suggest may need improving? What would they like to start working on first?" Building trust and credibility among the staff was mindfully evaluated throughout all interactions as it was essential that the CNS be perceived as a positive partner in helping them achieve their desired outcomes. By continually using the AI process, this assisted the facilitation process that reinforced the consultation role and how the CNS could aid with advanced clinical assessments, care planning, and evaluation of outcomes. Furthermore, this provided the CNS with opportunities to demonstrate timely support and education, which further built credibility and trust among the staff.

To address the identified targeted knowledge gaps, the CNS developed a hospital-wide, interprofessional education program. The hospital's management team committed to supporting quality and safety improvements, including staff attendance at education, equipment changes and purchasing, and environmental revisions (i.e., de-cluttering, cleaning over-the-bed lights). Working in close co-operation with a network of CNS colleagues in surgery and critical care enabled consistency of care and practices across the hospital. In addition to nursing competencies specifically focusing on the care of acutely ill older adults, interprofessional competencies were developed to ensure alignment of all providers' scopes of practice to achieve the quality improvement goals.

The CNS provided four 3.5-hour education sessions, which were repeated several times to capture most staff and management. Clinical nurse educators (CNEs) were an integral partner in the education process as they provided direct education support on the various units on an ongoing basis. This supported sustainment of practice changes on the units and provided the CNE material to use during new staff orientation. As the CNS was regionally positioned rather than single hospital or unit-based, there was a requirement to ensure the new structure could be sustained at this hospital and be replicated at other hospitals where other acutely ill older adults were cared for. The opportunity to build and pilot the strategic plan that was developed at this hospital provided the CNS with valuable information and lessons learned to apply for the whole health authority. The CNS consultant role expanded the sphere of influence and impacted the care outcomes of other complex older adult patients.

Reviewing and revising, and in some cases streamlining communication and documentation practices, can help prevent care gaps (i.e., one location to record bowel movements rather than having several different places; pre-hospital cognitive and functional status to prevent assumption of dementia rather than delirium). Clearly, CNEs and CNSs have a synergetic relationship complementing each other's practice. With the CNE's primary focus on staff education, the CNSs were able to support their abilities through ensuring currency for knowledge translation with their staff related to best practice clinical guidelines, protocols, policies, and procedures. The hospital's commitment to a never-again attitude helped to facilitate everyone's abilities and strengths to improve and sustain best practice care for acutely ill older adults.

Outcome measurement is vital to sustainability. Random audits of direct care were observed, and chart reviews were completed based upon the working group's strategic plan to review areas for improvement and to assist with future care planning and reinforcement of best practices for acutely ill older adult care.

Esther's family was an integral part of the improvement process that took place in the hospital. It was very important to engage and communicate with the family throughout all processes and activities. Their support in joining in the never-again attitude provided a stronger message because of their learning and insights of how families' voices can be better heard. The family developed and currently maintains a website telling Esther's story to support other families and, in this way, continues to honour both Esther and other older adults. Esther's daughter personally responds to any member of the public who reads and wants to know how their voice as a family member can be heard. (www.esthersvoice.com). Esther's daughter states, "Esther was always a teacher to her core, and she would want her legacy to be about learning, not blaming." The CNS continues to work with Esther's daughter to ensure that the family's voice remains heard.

Collaboration produces networks that enable CNSs to innovatively intersect with different stakeholders to create more opportunities and greater impact. The CNS continues to engage with expert partners in geriatric medicine, geriatric psychiatry, and interactive media development from two universities to collaborate and consult with Esther's daughter's computer software development company to create programs that will help patients, families, and staff. The "Mindful Garden" computer program, which is in beta-testing, is utilizing visual cues to facilitate an environment that is reassuring and calming. The structure and concept for the computer program is focused on anxious, restless, and agitated behaviours seen when an older adult is experiencing responsive behaviours related to a delirium, dementia, and/or depression. The proof of concept testing on five patients whose decision makers consented to showing their loved one "The Mindful Garden" resulted in the stimulus to now move forward with further research to validate its effectiveness. If only Esther could have seen the "The Mindful Garden" program showing her prairie wheat fields with the wind blowing through the stalks and allowing her to imagine the smell of the clean air, the research development team believes that Esther's agitation and restlessness might have been calmed and that the final outcome would have had a greater potential for recovery and going home again.

Esther is but one example of the need for health care systems to improve the quality and safety of care for acutely ill older adults. The BC Ministry of Health, and the Nursing Directorate at this pivotal time, enabled the engagement and collaboration of all the BC Health Authorities to improve care of acutely ill older adults throughout BC. Their provision of grants for five years to a group of five CNSs from three different health authorities provided funds for the collaborative development of the Acute Care Geriatric Nurse Network (ACGNN) in years one to four and the Geriatric Emergency Nurse Initiative (GENI) in the fifth year. The ACGNN and GENI work continues to support care of acutely ill older adults through the www.acgnn.ca website. During the grant-funding years, the group travelled throughout BC, especially to rural and remote areas, to educate and disseminate best practices for acutely ill older adults as CNS expertise is not available in every area. All disciplines and administration are included in learning sessions and their attendance adds greater understanding of the need to collaborate. The yearly evaluations, which include participants' wish lists, enabled the CNSs to advocate with and inform the health authorities' Chief Nursing Officers and the Ministry of Health about system changes required. The Geriatric Giants Quick Reference (ACGNN, 2020) continues to help sustain the knowledge translation fostered by the CNSs. The ACGNN CNSs have a viable and robust network sustained through volunteering of their own time to ensure availability of information and resources to influence and impact improvements in the care of acutely ill older adults provincially and nationally. The resources and information have spread to Japan, Ireland, and the United States, to name a few.

Conclusion

The CNS role and functions, which are now clearly articulated in the Pan-Canadian Core Competencies for the CNS as well as the pan-Canadian APN framework (CNA, 2014, 2019), are illustrated in Esther's story. By applying consultant and collaborator approaches, CNSs demonstrate how they can influence and impact direct patient care, the health care system, and policy decisions. CNSs strive continually to ensure and facilitate safe, best practice care for individuals, populations, and health care delivery services.

Critical Thinking Questions

1. Why would a regulatory nursing body choose to consult with a CNS in responding to a coroner's recommendation?

2. What impact can the CNS competency of consultant and collaborator have in improving best practices at the individual, population, and health care system levels?
3. What key characteristics differentiate the CNS role and function from the CNE and manager's roles and functions to enable best practices?

References

Acute Care Geriatric Nurse Network (ACGNN). (2020). *Geriatric giants quick reference* (4th ed.). Burnaby, BC: ACGNN. Retrieved from http://www.acgnn.ca/

Benner, P. (1982). From novice to expert. *American Journal of Nursing, 82*(3), 402–407.

Bushe, G. R. (2011). Appreciative inquiry: Theory and critique. In D. Bouje, B. Burnes, & J. Hassard (Eds.), *The Routledge companion to organization change* (pp. 87–103). Oxford, UK: Routledge.

Canadian Nurses Association (CNA). (2014). *Pan-Canadian core competencies for the clinical nurse specialist*. Ottawa, ON: CNA. Retrieved from https://cna-aiic.ca/~/media/cna/files/en/clinical_nurse_specialists_convention_handout_e.pdf

CNA. (2019). *Advanced nursing practice: A pan-Canadian framework*. Ottawa, ON: CNA. Retrieved from https://www.cna-aiic.ca/-/media/cna/page-content/pdf-en/apn-a-pan-canadian-framework.pdf

Gomez-Mejia, L. R., Balkin, D. B., & Cardy, R. L. (2008). *Management: People, performance, change* (3rd ed.). New York, NY: McGraw-Hill.

Schreiber, R., MacDonald, M., Pauly, B., Davidson, H., Crickmore, J., & Moss, L., … Hammond, C. (2005). Singing in different keys: Enactment of advanced nursing practice in British Columbia. *Canadian Journal of Nursing Leadership, 6*, 1–17. Retrieved from http://www.longwoods.com/content/19026

Chapter 19B

Consultation and Collaboration Competencies

Nurse Practitioner

Monica Parry

MONICA PARRY is an Associate Professor at the Lawrence S. Bloomberg Faculty of Nursing, University of Toronto, Toronto, Ontario. Her teaching focuses on interesting patient cases encountered as a practicing nurse practitioner-Adult with over 35 years of cardiovascular clinical experience. Her clinical experience has laid the foundation for a program of research to reduce the burden of cardiovascular disease and its complications.

Acknowledgement: HAFSA ANSARI is a registered nurse and recent graduate of the Lawrence S. Bloomberg Faculty of Nursing, University of Toronto, Toronto, Ontario, who assisted with updating the literature search.

KEY TERMS

collaboration
consultation
referral
transfer-of-care

OBJECTIVES

1. Explain the essential components of collaboration.
2. Discuss the difference between a consultation and a referral.
3. Recognize when a consultation results in a transfer-of-care.

Introduction

Nurse practitioners (NPs) are regulated independent health care professionals licensed by provincial regulatory authorities to optimize the health of individuals, families, communities, and populations in Canada. Provincial authorities define the scope and standards of practice for NPs, which can vary across jurisdictions. NPs practice within their scope of practice and within the limits of their experience, and are expected to collaborate, consult, and refer when a clinical issue is beyond their knowledge, skill, and competence.

This chapter section describes the core entry-to-practice collaboration, consultation, and referral competencies of NPs as defined by the Canadian Nurses Association (CNA; 2019) and the Canadian Council of Registered Nurse Regulators (CCRNR; 2015). Nurse practitioners must identify when collaboration, consultation, and referral are necessary for safe, competent, and comprehensive client care. Specific components of the *Consultation and Collaboration Competencies* (CNA, 2019), including *referral* competency, are:

- Initiate timely and appropriate consultations and referrals and provide recommendations in response to consultation and referral suggestions
- Engage with clients and collaborate with other team members at individual and organizational levels to develop quality-improvement and risk-management strategies
- Synthesize qualitative and quantitative evidence on key determinants of health; build coalitions and partnerships
- Apply group dynamic and organizational theories and utilize these theories to assist with communication, negotiation, change, and conflict prevention, management, and resolution
- Coordinate interprofessional, intraprofessional, and intersectoral teams
- Articulate the role of the advanced practice nurse to key stakeholders (CNA, 2019, pp. 33–34)

In addition, NPs must identify when collaboration, consultation, and referral are necessary for safe, competent, and comprehensive client care. Specific components of the NP collaboration, consultation, and referral competency as defined by CCRNR (2015) include the following:

1. Establish collaborative relationships with healthcare providers and community-based services (e.g., school, police, child protection services, rehabilitation, home care)
2. Provide recommendations or relevant treatment in response to consultation requests or incoming referrals
3. Identify need for consultation and/or referral (e.g., to confirm a diagnosis, to augment a plan of care, to assume care when a client's health condition is beyond the NP's individual competence or legal scope of practice)
4. Initiate a consultation and/or referral, specifying relevant information (e.g., client history, assessment findings, diagnosis) and expectations
5. Review consultation and/or referral recommendations with the client and integrate into plan of care as appropriate (CCRNR, 2015, p. 35)

The collaboration, consultation, and referral competencies apply across three streams of NP practice (Family/All-Ages, Adult, and Pediatrics) and are grounded in the philosophy of primary health care as defined by the Canadian Nurses Association (CNA, 2015, 2019). This philosophy is based on a Peoples First model of care that is grounded in the World Health Organization's (WHO) five principles of primary health care: (1) accessibility, (2) public participation, (3) health promotion and chronic disease prevention and management, (4) use of appropriate technology and innovation, and (5) intersectoral co-operation and collaboration (WHO, 2010). An integrated primary health care model seeks to improve the health of populations through illness prevention, health promotion, and chronic disease self-management across acute, community, long-term, rehabilitative, hospice, and corrections care (CNA, 2015, 2019).

Collaboration

The word *collaborate*, derived from the Latin word *collaborare*, means *to labour together* (Henneman, Lee, & Cohen, 1995). The WHO suggests that collaborative practice occurs when multiple health workers from different professional backgrounds provide comprehensive quality services across settings to patients, families, caregivers, and communities (WHO, 2010). The CNA believes that interprofessional collaborative models for health service delivery are critical for improving access to client-centred care (2011). Collaboration is composed of four essential components: (1) separate and unique roles or scope of practice, (2) common goals, (3) shared power, and (4) mutual concerns (Kuehn, 2018). Key attributes of successful collaboration include open and honest communication, mutual trust and respect, confidence in the knowledge and skills of each collaborating partner, and ability to prioritize tasks and care delivery (Fleischmann, Geister, Hoell, Hummers-Pradier, & Mueller, 2017). Barriers to effective collaboration include educational isolation, interpersonal differences, professional dissonance, renumeration structures, legislation and/or institutional policies/procedures, and role ambiguity (Kuehn, 2018; Schadewaldt, McInnes, Hiller, & Gardner, 2016). Collaboration implies a non-hierarchical relationship where power is shared; it is not synonymous with supervision or oversight of another's professional practice (i.e., physician oversight of an NP's practice). Clients are the priority focus; the services NPs provide must be responsive to their needs, and clients must be engaged in decisions about the management of their health. Effective collaboration promotes interprofessional cohesiveness, increased satisfaction, and better client outcomes. When interdisciplinary collaboration is present, clients have access to the "right service," at the "right time," in the "right place," and by the "right health professional."

In Ontario, NP-Led Clinics form part of the primary health care system. NPs manage clinics to provide primary health care services that focus on preventive, curative, rehabilitative, and supportive/palliative care to improve accessibility, public participation, health promotion, appropriate technology, and intersectoral collaboration (CNA, 2000). A recent qualitative evidence synthesis identified factors that influenced the substitution of physicians with nurses in primary care (Karimi-Shahanjarini et al., 2019). Although only 17.1% of the sample were NPs, the integration of nurses and task shifting of responsibilities required collaboration between the physicians and nurses to increase client access and improve the quality and continuity of care. Trust, mutual respect, and close working relationships were essential for collaboration.

Consultation

Consultation is an explicit request from one health care professional to another to provide guidance or advice in the care of a client. NPs consult other health care professionals when client care extends beyond their legal scope of practice, beyond their individual competence, when the diagnosis or treatment plan is unclear, or when the client would benefit from the expertise of another health care professional (College of Nurses of Ontario [CNO], 2019; College of Registered Nurses of Prince Edward Island [CRNPEI], 2019). NPs also provide consultations to other health care professionals when their expertise will improve quality or reduce risk for clients.

Consultations can be informal (i.e., patient care rounds) or formal (i.e., written request for an opinion or recommendation) and can occur during the assessment, diagnosis, or in the therapeutic management of a client. During any consultative process, the NP must describe the level of involvement and the reason for and the level of urgency of the consultation (British Columbia College of Nursing Professionals [BCCNP], 2020). Formal consultations with other health care providers require client information that describes demographics, medications, allergies, past health history, pertinent family or social history, diagnostic test results, relevant other consultations, and a summary of the current problem. It is the responsibility of the NP to follow up on the consultation findings to ensure resolution or advocate for any outstanding issues impacting the client's health. It is also expected that the NP clearly document the consultative process within the client's medical record.

When the consultation results in the need to transfer care, the decision for this transfer is jointly made between the NP, the receiving health care professional, and the client as appropriate. Transfer-of-care is a process whereby an NP transfers management for some or all of a client's care to another health care provider who explicitly agrees to accept this responsibility. With a transfer-of-care there is a clear transfer of accountability and clear communication with the client about this transfer-of-care. The NP must ensure that the accepting health care provider has the necessary clinical information to assume care, which would include a summary of the active medical issues and a treatment plan for the client. A transfer-of-care can be temporary or permanent. Usually a transfer-of-care occurs when the primary care responsibilities required for appropriate care of the client fall outside the NP's scope of practice, or in the case of medical assistance in dying, the transfer-of-care is due to conscientious objection. Changes to the Criminal Code in June 2016 enabled eligible individuals to receive medical assistance in dying and permitted NPs to administer medications to cause the death of a client. The law does not compel the NP to provide medical assistance in dying if the NP is not comfortable, or if the values and beliefs of the NP differ from those of the client. Conscientious objection by an NP typically results in a referral and a transfer-of-care to another NP or physician to address the client's needs (Centre for Effective Practice [CEP], 2017; CNO, 2018).

Referral

A referral is an explicit request from one health care professional to another to provide time-limited, client-specific health services (CNO, 2019). A referral is a form of consultation that is episodic or concurrent; it is distinctly different from a consultation because it implies time-limited treatment (Goolsby, 2002). In Canada, different professions and organizations have different referral processes. All physician/specialist referrals require a consultation letter that outlines the reason for the referral, the client's history, and pertinent physical and diagnostic findings. In Ontario, the Schedule of Benefits for Physician Services was amended in May 2015 to reduce barriers for efficient access to specialist services. At present, payments are now permitted under the Ontario Health Insurance Plan to physicians for consultation when patients are referred by an NP. The consulting physician/specialist is also required to write a report back to the NP who generated the referral. Restrictions on NP-generated referrals to private health service providers (physiotherapists, registered massage therapists, and occupational therapists) or provincial programs and services (for example, diabetes education) in Canada are dependent on provincial funding models and extended health insurance plans.

CASE STUDY

The Story of Franko

Franko is a 61-year-old male who lives with his 63-year-old wife in a low-income rental apartment in southeastern Ontario.

Chief Complaint: Presented with increasing shortness of breath on exertion, worsening over the past 3 months.

History of Present Illness: Bicuspid aortic valve, ejection fraction 53%, with moderate concentric left ventricular hypertrophy. On wait list for cardiac surgery, admitted and underwent aortic valve replacement surgery (tissue).

Past Medical History: T2DM x 14 years (HbA1c 8.1%), osteoarthritis, morbid obesity, peripheral vascular disease, TIA 2 years ago, previous stent to his left anterior descending coronary artery, permanent pacemaker for complete heart block 6 years ago, and hypertension x 14 years.

Family History: Father 78 years with chronic back pain. Mother 77 years with T2DM. Franko has no children.

Social History: His wife also underwent urgent cardiac surgery 3 months ago and is experiencing persistent postoperative sternal pain with costochondral mobility.

Neither Franko nor his wife have extended health benefits; they receive Canada Pension Plan (CPP) disability with CPP retirement benefits, and do not qualify for the Ontario Disability Support Program benefits. Franko is not active, does not walk regularly, likes to watch television most of the day.

Physical Examination: Post-operatively, vital signs stable, heart sounds normal, grade II/VI systolic ejection murmur, normal breath sounds, no nausea/vomiting, no urinary symptoms, and blood sugars 12–14 mmol/L.

Diagnostics: CXR-left lower lobe atelectasis with small pleural effusion, ECG paced rhythm at 80 beats per minute, regular.

Allergies: No known allergies.

Medications: ECASA 81 mg po daily, Clopidogrel 75 mg po daily, Enalapril 20 mg po daily, HCTZ 25 mg po daily, Rosuvastatin 40 mg po daily, Hydromorphone 2 mg po q3h prn, Metformin 1,500 mg qam and 1,000 mg qpm, and Glyburide 2.5 mg po bid.

Plan: Consult pharmacist and social work to assist with discharge planning; discharge home with wife.

Discussion

This case study illustrates how in-hospital consultation to pharmacy and social work optimizes discharge planning. The Canadian Diabetes Association's Clinical Practice Guidelines (2018) emphasize an aggressive approach to the prevention and management of diabetes. However, affordability and access to diabetes medications, devices, and supplies vary depending on where you live in Canada, which is not unlike prescription medication, device, or supply costs associated with other chronic illness conditions. Approximately 57% of Canadians with diabetes do not comply with their prescribed management plan because of affordability. Out-of-pocket expenses for Franko's medications depend on costs related to pharmacy mark-ups, dispensing fees, and public and private insurance coverage. Consultation with pharmacy and social work helped to ensure Franko's individual needs were met. Consultation with pharmacy and social work also assisted in determining the least expensive medication to prescribe, and to determine if Franko would qualify for a lower deductible from a Drug Benefit Program.

Franko's hyperglycemia post-operatively warranted the addition of a second antihyperglycemic agent. With the assistance of the pharmacist, the NP coordinating his care was able to add a relatively inexpensive second agent. The pharmacist also assisted in choosing the second agent based on the Health Canada–approved medications available across formularies. Medications "listed" were available as a full benefit to Franko. Medications that were "restricted" (i.e., available only to those who are eligible under the public drug plan and who meet specific eligibility criteria) and "not listed" (i.e., not available on the public drug plan) were not ideal medications to prescribe for him. If Franko were eligible for the Ontario Trillium Drug Program, he would have received coverage for selected blood glucose strips, and oral medications, but he would have been required to pay a deductible based on his income. If he required insulin to manage his hyperglycemia post-operatively, he would not have received assistance to cover the costs of lancets or a glucose meter in Ontario. In consultation with the pharmacist and social worker, the NP coordinating Franko's care was able to estimate the daily cost of his medication to be $16.81, or approximately $525 per month. The NP was able to make recommendations to manage costs and improve adherence to his recommended diabetes management regime.

In consultation with the collaborating cardiac surgeon, it was decided that Franko would be referred to an endocrinologist. Although the ongoing management of his care coordination would remain with his primary care provider, the endocrinologist would assist in the ongoing evaluation and management of his diabetes and diabetes-related complications. Diabetes is one of the most prevalent and costliest diseases in Canada with much of the cost and suffering attributed to diabetes complications such as retinopathy, nephropathy, neuropathy, and cardiovascular disease.

This integration and coordination of services ensured Franko received specialist services to maximize his health outcomes. This case illustrates the importance interdisciplinary collaboration with medicine, pharmacy, social work, and the client/family. It reinforces the "right care, right time, right place, and right cost" strategy embraced by many provinces in Canada.

Conclusion

Consultation, collaboration, and referral are essential components to NP practice. Clients are the priority focus; the services provided must be responsive to their needs, and clients must be engaged in decisions about the management of their health. When NPs focus on client engagement, access, trust and respect, effective communication, provision of the best possible care and services, and a population health approach, clients will have access to the "right service," at the "right time," in the "right place," and by the "right health professional." Collaboration is a complex process that requires confidence, competence, trust, and respect from all individuals. A lack of collaboration contributes to fragmentation of care, client dissatisfaction, and poor client outcomes.

Critical Thinking Questions

1. Compare and contrast the concepts of collaboration and teamwork.
2. Describe the organizational and systems-level policies that would facilitate collaborative practice environments in your province/territory.

3. Discuss possible strategies for negotiation and conflict resolution in managing restrictions to NP-generated referrals to specialist physicians, private health service providers, and provincial programs and services in Canada.
4. What elements would you incorporate into your toolkit to integrate the NP role into a collaborative practice environment?

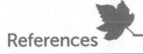

References

British Columbia College of Nursing Professionals (BCCNP). (2020). *Scope of practice for nurse practitioners: Standards, limits and conditions.* Vancouver, BC: BCCNP. Retrieved from https://www.bccnp.ca/Standards/RN_NP/NPScopePractice/scope/Pages/Default.aspx

Canadian Council of Registered Nurse Regulators (CCRNR). (2015). *Practice analysis study of nurse practitioners.* Beaverton, ON: CCRNR. Retrieved from http://www.ccrnr.ca/assets/ccrnr-practice-analysis-study-of-nurse-practitioners-report---final.pdf

The Canadian Diabetes Association. (2018). *2018 guidelines.* Toronto, ON: Canadian Diabetes Association. Retrieved from http://guidelines.diabetes.ca/cpg

Canadian Nurses Association (CNA). (2000). *The primary health care approach.* Ottawa, ON: CNA. Retrieved from https://www.cna-aiic.ca/-/media/cna/page-content/pdf-en/fs02_primary_health_care_approach_june_2000_e.pdf

CNA. (2011). *Position statement: Interprofessional collaboration.* Ottawa, ON: CNA. Retrieved from http://www.cna-aiic.ca/~/media/cna/page-content/pdf-en/interproffessional-collaboration_position-statement.pdf

CNA. (2015). *Primary health care position statement (press release).* Ottawa, ON: CNA. Retrieved from https://www.cna-aiic.ca/-/media/cna/page-content/pdf-en/primary-health-care-position-statement.pdf

CNA. (2019). *Advanced practice nursing: A pan-Canadian framework.* Ottawa, ON: CNA. Retrieved from https://www.cna-aiic.ca/-/media/cna/page-content/pdf-en/apn-a-pan-canadian-framework.pdf

Centre for Effective Practice (CEP). (2017). *Medical assistance in dying.* Toronto, ON: CEP. Retrieved from https://cep.health/clinical-products/medical-assistance-in-dying/

College of Nurses of Ontario (CNO). (2018). *Guidance on nurses' roles in medical assistance in dying.* Toronto, ON: CNO. Retrieved from https://www.cno.org/globalassets/docs/prac/41056-guidance-on-nurses-roles-in-maid.pdf

CNO. (2019). *Practice standard: Nurse practitioner.* Toronto, ON: CNO. Retrieved from https://www.cno.org/globalassets/docs/prac/41038_strdrnec.pdf

College of Registered Nurses of Prince Edward Island (CRNPEI). (2019). *Nurse practitioner standards for practice.* Charlottetown, PE: CRNPEI. Retrieved from https://immediac.blob.core.windows.net/crnpei/pdf/Standards%20for%20Practice%20NP%20-%202019-08-07.pdf

Fleischmann, N., Geister, C., Hoell, A., Hummers-Pradier, E., & Mueller, C. (2017). Interprofessional collaboration in nursing homes (interprof): A grounded theory study of nurse experiences of general practitioner visits. *Applied Nursing Research, 35,* 118–125. doi: 10.1016/j.apnr.2017.02.021

Goolsby, M. (2002). *Nurse practitioner secrets: Questions and answers to reveal the secrets to successful NP practice.* Philadelphia, PA: Hanley & Belfus.

Henneman, E., Lee, J., & Cohen, J. (1995). Collaboration: A concept analysis. *Journal of Advanced Nursing, 21*, 103–109.

Karimi-Shahanjarini, A., Shakibazadeh, E., Rashidian, A., Hajimiri, K., Glenton, C., Noyes, J., … Colvin, C. (2019). Barriers and facilitators to the implementation of doctor-nurse substitution strategies in primary care: A qualitative evidence synthesis. *Cochrane Database of Systematic Reviews,* (4). doi: 10.1002/14651858.CD010412.pub2

Kuehn, A. (2018). The kaleidoscope of collaborative practice. In L. A. Joel (Ed.), *Advanced practice nursing: Essentials for role development* (pp. 116–142). Philadelphia, PA: F. A. Davis Company.

Schadewaldt, V., McInnes, E., Hiller, J., & Gardner, A. (2016). Experiences of nurse practitioners and medical practitioners working in collaborative practice models in primary healthcare in Australia—A multiple case study using mixed methods. *BioMed Central (BMC) Family Practice, 17,* 1–16. doi: 10.1186/s12875-016-0503-2

World Health Organization (WHO). (2010). *Framework for action on interprofessional education and collaborative practice.* Geneva, CH: WHO. Retrieved from https://apps.who.int/iris/bitstream/handle/10665/70185/WHO_HRH_HPN_10.3_eng.pdf

Chapter 20

Professional Liability Protection

Elaine Borg

ELAINE BORG is Legal Counsel with the Canadian Nurses Protective Society (CNPS). She received her undergraduate degree in nursing from Queen's University in Kingston, Ontario. She worked in the infant neurosurgery unit at The Hospital for Sick Children in Toronto, Ontario, prior to focusing on her main interest, obstetrics, which she practiced at Mount Sinai Hospital, Toronto, Ontario, and the Ottawa Civic Hospital, Ottawa, Ontario. Her interest in ethical decision-making led to a position on a hospital clinical ethics committee, and from there to a career in law after graduating from law school at the University of Ottawa, Ottawa, Ontario. Elaine is a member of the College of Nurses of Ontario (CNO), the Registered Nurses Association of Ontario (RNAO), and the Law Society of Ontario. She was on the working group that drafted the National Disclosure Guidelines published by the Canadian Patient Safety Institute and the Advisory Council for Queen's University Master of Science in Healthcare Quality (MSCHQ) program.

KEY TERMS

advanced practice nursing (APN)
damages
liability
negligence
professional liability protection (PLP)

OBJECTIVES

1. Understand what is meant by professional liability protection.
2. Understand the successful defence to an allegation of negligence.
3. Understand the distinction between standards of nursing practice and the standard of care.
4. Understand the jurisdiction of your nursing regulatory body.

Introduction

The challenge in writing a chapter about **negligence** and **professional liability protection (PLP)** is not to intellectualize and decontextualize the topic. For context, consider that **advanced practice nursing (APN)** encompasses traditional work in established health care institutions but also newer and evolving ways of working (telecommunication technology, new models of care like organizations transitioning into health care teams), and types of service requests to health care professionals (medical assistance in dying, cannabis for medical purposes, cosmetic/aesthetic services). Additional complexity occurs with multi-jurisdictional practice and independent practice (or both). With these new opportunities comes the need to be vigilant in understanding the legal implications of such arrangements. This chapter will underline that legal risks can be anticipated, allowing proper practices and safety nets to be put in place so when a dispute arises, one's professional practice continues while the dispute is addressed and eventually resolved.

Professional Liability Protection

Liability means legal responsibility for one's own conduct. For the purposes of this chapter, PLP means a source of legal defence funding that will respond to civil lawsuits alleging negligent professional nursing services. The legal defence funding can be through a policy of insurance, a not-for-profit legal defence fund, or a nurse's own financial resources (if there is no other source of insurance/protection). Legal defence costs consist of legal fees and disbursements, like the cost of retaining expert witnesses, settlement monies, and **damages** awards. Damages are monetary compensation the law awards to one who has suffered damage, loss, or injury by the wrongdoing of another, such as a breach of contract or tort. A successful defence to a negligence lawsuit needs two things: evidence of having acted as a reasonable nurse in the circumstances to avoid foreseeable harm to the patient; and a source funding for legal defence costs.

The rationale for health care professionals having PLP is that it avoids an "empty judgment." An empty judgment occurs when the plaintiff (the person starting the lawsuit) has proven their case, the Court has ordered damages to be paid, but the unsuccessful defendant (the person defending against the lawsuit) does not have the money to pay the judgment. This is a hollow victory for the plaintiff and does not fulfill one of the primary purposes of tort law, compensation for harm done. For a fuller appreciation of the importance of PLP, it is helpful to understand how Courts decide medical malpractice cases, types of liability, and types of working relationships and their impact on liability risk and protection.

How Courts Decide Civil Lawsuits in Negligence

Patients are entitled to non-negligent professional health care services. If a patient believes they have received negligent care, a malpractice or negligence lawsuit may be initiated. A negligence lawsuit is a formal dispute resolution mechanism. Its processes and procedures are governed by the rules of Court. The rules of Court are provincial and territorial statutory law (i.e., written law created by the respective legislative assemblies and parliaments). The lawsuit will be resolved by the law of tort. Tort law aims to achieve compensation for the plaintiff who proves wrongful injury; justice; education; and deterrence of negligent acts. The Supreme Court of Canada made the following statement about deterrence:

> One of the primary purposes of negligence law is to enforce reasonable standards of conduct so as to prevent the creation of reasonably foreseeable risks. In this way, tort law serves as a disincentive to risk-creating behaviour. (*Stewart v. Pettie*, 1995)

Canada is a bi-juridical country, meaning it has two formal judicial systems. Quebec has retained the French Civil Code as its comprehensive, written provincial law, which governs disputes such as allegations of professional negligence. The rest of the country adheres to the common law system, which applies the province or territory's statutory law and judicial precedence to the facts in order to resolve lawsuits. Both judicial systems adhere to the same overriding principle of fairness; like cases are to be decided in a like manner. This allows people to know the law and to act within the law, thereby avoiding legal penalty.

A civil lawsuit is commenced with the issuance and service of the plaintiff's Statement of Claim. In this document, the plaintiff identifies the defendants, typically the health care institution where the care took place and the health care professionals who cared for the patient in a certain time frame, and the details of the allegations against them. The most common allegation against health care professionals is that of negligence (Picard & Robertson, 2017).

The Statement of Claim may be served on the health care institution, which would then notify its insurer. Typically, the insurer will retain a law firm to represent and defend the health care institution and its defendant employees. If you are named as a defendant, you are entitled to a copy of the Statement of Claim. If you are served with a Statement of Claim, immediately notify the source of your legal defence funding. This sounds daunting, but the key is to quickly identify what legal defence assistance you have for the claim. It may be:

- Your employer's policy of insurance by contacting your employer's risk management or legal department
- A not-for-profit legal defence fund like the Canadian Nurses Protective Society (CNPS)
- Your own insurer if you purchased professional liability insurance, i.e., if you are self-employed
- Your own lawyer if you are using your own financial resources, i.e., if you are self-employed and uninsured for the matter claimed

Negligence is the failure to take the care that a reasonable nurse in similar circumstances would have taken through actions or omissions. To be successful, the plaintiff patient must introduce evidence to prove there was a duty of care between the plaintiff and defendant;

a breach of the standard of care by the parties being sued; and foreseeable harm that was caused by a breach in the standard of care. The defendants work with their own lawyers to rally their evidence. This necessitates your co-operation with the lawyer retained to defend you so that they understand your evidence about your practice and documentation. There is a deadline by which to file the defendant's response, which is a document called a Statement of Defence.

There is a distinction between the standards of nursing practice and the standard of care referred to in the negligence analysis. Standards of nursing practice are authoritative statements written by a provincial or territorial nursing regulator that describe the required behaviour of every regulated nurse. A standard of nursing practice serves to further define responsibilities set out in legislation (written law, both Acts and regulations) and is used by the nursing regulator to evaluate individual performance. The standard of care, in the law of negligence, is a legal determination made by the Court and is that degree of care which a reasonably prudent nurse should exercise in the same or similar circumstances. The Court has found that nursing is its own distinct profession, situated within the health care team, with the same legal duties as other health care professionals:

> Nurses are professionals who also possess special skills and knowledge and the same principles apply as in the case of doctors, residents and interns. They have a duty to use those skills in making appropriate assessments of patients and to communicate accurately those assessments to physicians. (*Granger [Litigation Guardian of] v. Ottawa General Hospital*, 1996)

Advanced practice nurses may be held to a higher standard than a generalist, as observed in this Supreme Court of Canada case, which is cited as a precedent to this day in malpractice cases:

> Every medical practitioner must bring to his task a reasonable degree of skill and knowledge and must exercise a reasonable degree of care. He is bound to exercise that degree of care and skill which could reasonably be expected of a normal, prudent practitioner of the same experience and standing and, if he holds himself out as a specialist, a higher degree of skill is required of him than one who does not profess to be so qualified by special training and ability. (*Crits v. Sylvester*, 1956)

The Court will analyze the evidence submitted to it about the relevant standard of care at the time of the incident giving rise to the litigation, including evidence of APN. That evidence will be found in legislation, legal precedents about the same kind of claim, standards of professional practice, clinical practice guidelines, health care institutional policies and procedures, and expert opinions. Evidence is primarily in the form of verbal testimony of the people involved, documents, and the opinions of expert witnesses (Borg, 2004). Evidence is sought to illuminate two different issues: if there was a failure to meet the standard of care that caused the harm alleged; and the value of the harm to the plaintiff(s), called damages.

The vast majority of civil lawsuits will not be decided by a judge following a trial but will end by way of settlement or dismissal prior to a trial. One of the first steps in litigation is the exchange of relevant information between the parties, in part to encourage early resolution of the dispute. The first time the parties testify under oath is at Examinations for Discovery (CNPS, 2004) or Questioning (the title of this event is determined by the rules of civil procedure). The lawyers for the parties will be present during this, but it is the plaintiffs and defendants who respond to questions about the issues set out in the Statement of Claim and Statement of Defence.

It is typically after Examinations for Discovery or Questioning that the lawyers for the parties have their best understanding of the evidence and therefore the strengths and weaknesses of their case and will advise their clients accordingly. If the defence evidence is weak, including the inability to obtain an expert opinion that supports the defendant's care, settlement negotiations may result in the plaintiffs accepting an offer, which will bring the case to a close by way of a written agreement. The written agreement will set out the terms of the settlement, principally the amount of money to be paid to the plaintiffs, that the claim is settled once and for all, and that the parties are not to disclose the contents of the agreement, i.e., a confidentiality clause. If the defence evidence is strong, an agreement may be reached to dismiss the claim. Additionally, it is possible that the claim may be dismissed against one or several defendants as the case evolves and negligence cannot be proved against that defendant. The case would continue between the remaining parties.

If the matter does go to trial, the Court must weigh the (conflicting) evidence on what is referred to as a balance of probabilities, i.e., more likely than not, and make a determination of the facts, then apply the relevant law in order to render a judgment. If the Court determines that negligence occurred, additional evidence is needed about the value of the harm and what compensatory damages are sufficient to put the successful plaintiff in the position they would have been in if the harm had not occurred. Then the Court will identify which defendant is responsible for the payment of which damages according to the following principles:

1. *Direct Liability:* Each defendant, health care institution or health care professional, is accountable for its own actions and omissions. A defendant employer or health care facility may be found negligent and held directly liable for breaching duties it owed to the patient. These could include the duty to select professional staff using reasonable care; review staff performance on a regular basis; have and enforce appropriate policies and procedures; provide reasonable supervision of staff; and provide adequate staffing, equipment, or resources. The health care institution would rely on its insurance to pay the damages award. If a practitioner is found to have been negligent, a Court may award damages to the plaintiff that are to be paid by that individual defendant. This form of liability is called direct liability. Insurance contracts for PLP and the PLP provided by the Canadian Medical Protective

Association (CMPA) and the Canadian Nurses Protective Society (CNPS) are designed to assist with a Court finding or judgment of direct liability.

2. *Vicarious Liability:* The legal doctrine of vicarious liability holds an employer, which may be an individual or an institution, financially responsible for the negligence of its employees committed within the scope of their employment. This is a business liability. An employment relationship must have existed at the time of the incident and the defendant employee must have been sued for work done within the scope of his or her employment. It will be up to the Court to decide, based on all the facts and circumstances, whether an employer-employee relationship existed (*Bazley v. Curry*, 1999).

3. *Joint and Several Liability:* When the Court finds more than one defendant negligent, the Court will assess the amount of damages (often expressed as a percentage of the total damage award) to be paid by each defendant. Defendants can be jointly and individually liable for the damages awarded. This means the plaintiff may recover full compensation from any one of the negligent defendants, even though that defendant may then be paying for more than their share of the damages. That defendant may then seek contribution from the other negligent defendant(s).

At present, the law in Ontario (*Regulated Health Professions Act*) and in Alberta (*Health Professions Act*) requires that their member nurses self-report to the College of Nurses of Ontario (CNO) and the College and Association of Registered Nurses of Alberta respectively if a Court makes a finding against them of professional negligence. This will trigger an investigation by the nursing regulator. The nursing regulator's legal duty is to regulate nursing to protect the public so it will want to understand if the nursing practice standards and professional ethics were upheld. The civil lawsuit was about determining if the plaintiff proved they were owed compensation.

Types of Work Relationships: Employee or Self-Employed?

There are two ways to work: as an employee or as a self-employed individual, known in legal terms as an independent contractor. Historically, most nurses have been employees, and this remains the case today. But the health care environment is in a state of flux; with the rise of nurse practitioners, the creation of new health care teams, and the unsettled issue of privatization, more nurses may become independent contractors. Although there is no one test to determine if an employment relationship exists, decided tax and tort cases provide factors that Courts look at in combination to make this determination. What follows are not exhaustive lists of factors and there is no set formula for their application. The relative weight of each factor will depend on the particular facts and circumstances of each case. The Court is not bound by the characterization of parties to an agreement or contract as independent contractors if the facts reveal an employment relationship. Canada Revenue Agency has written on this subject in the following way (CRA, 2019):

1. Indicators showing that the worker is an employee
   - The relationship is one of subordination. The payer will often direct, scrutinize, and effectively control many elements of how and when the work is carried out;
   - The payer controls the worker with respect to both the results of the work and the method used to do the work;
   - The payer chooses and controls the method and amount of pay. Salary negotiations may still take place in an employer-employee relationship;
   - The payer decides what jobs the worker will do;
   - The payer chooses to listen to the worker's suggestions but has the final word;
   - The worker requires permission to work for other payers while working for this payer;
   - Where the schedule is irregular, priority on the worker's time is an indication of control over the worker;
   - The worker receives training or direction from the payer on how to do the work. The overall work environment between the worker and the payer is one of subordination.
2. Indicators showing that the worker is a self-employed individual
   - A self-employed individual usually works independently;
   - The worker does not have anyone overseeing his or her activities;
   - The worker is usually free to work when and for whom he or she chooses and may provide his or her services to different payers at the same time;
   - The worker can accept or refuse work from the payer;
   - The working relationship between the payer and the worker does not present a degree of continuity, loyalty, security, subordination, or integration, all of which are generally associated with an employer-employee relationship.

It is the right of the payer to exercise control that is relevant, not whether the payer exercises this right. It is the control of a payer over a worker that is relevant and not the control of a payer over the end result of a product or service purchased.

Perhaps the most difficult or contentious issue when considering whether or not nurses are employees is the issue of control. Because of their education, skill, and awareness of their professional accountability, nurses may require little, if any, direction and control of their daily practice. The important feature of control in an employment relationship is that the employer has the power to exercise control over the subordinate employee, not whether they do so in a particular instance.

Employers and owner/operators of health care facilities tend to prepare for the Court's application of the doctrine of vicarious liability, but nurses work at a broad spectrum of venues and under various work arrangements. Unless there is a statute or contract requiring the employer or owner/operator to have insurance coverage for its professional employees, it is their decision to make. A pragmatic effect of such insurance coverage is the strategic advantage of a united defence of the employer and its defendant employees, with the employer's defence lawyer having early and easy access to the evidence of the employees.

Another layer to this is that a plaintiff may initiate a claim involving a nurse regarding actions that were not within the scope of an employed nurse's employment. In this case, the employer's insurance can decline coverage for the claim. The nurse would then be reliant on other sources of legal defence funding, such as his or her eligibility for professional liability protection with a legal defence fund, membership in an association that has as a benefit of membership professional liability insurance, or the nurse's own financial resources. An understanding of these issues allows appropriate liability protection to be put in place by all parties to the provision of professional health care services.

Requirement to Have Professional Liability Protection

The provincial or territorial legislation governing nursing or the bylaws of a provincial or territorial nursing regulatory body may require its members to have professional liability protection in order to avoid an empty judgment. The following example is from the CNO:

> 44.4.01 Every member holding a certificate of registration in the General, Extended, Temporary, Emergency Assignment or Special Assignment class shall maintain professional liability protection to indemnify the member for all errors and omissions that may occur while practising nursing in Ontario. (CNO, *By-Laws*, 2019)

The legislation or bylaw requiring nurses to have PLP may include options of sources of funding that will fulfill the PLP requirement. There may also be set minimum amounts and deductibles. Nurses must comply if PLP is required in their home jurisdiction, but also in any other province or territory they want to work. Do not assume that the rules in your home jurisdiction are the same elsewhere. Start by reviewing what each provincial or territorial nursing regulator has written about PLP.

If PLP is required, it is sensible to first understand if you already have a source of PLP, and if so, its scope, i.e., what it will assist with and what it will not. It is important not to make assumptions about PLP, i.e., eligibility for it, the variety of legal proceedings it responds to, or its operation (traditional claims-made insurance where the threatened or actual claim is made within the policy period versus occurrence-based where eligibility at the time of the incident governs). If you are interested in a source of assistance with a legal matter that your existing or potential PLP does not include, seek out an additional service or product.

Independent Practice

Working autonomously, on your own, can be a significant change from practicing while surrounded by your colleagues and governed by your employer's management. Independent practice means not operating under the control of another health care professional, employer, or health care institution. Independent practice nurses are legally accountable for the professional services provided and for business matters, and are subject to various types of law and legal proceedings: professional discipline; civil lawsuits for professional negligence and for breach of contract, i.e., lease of premises, and privacy law to name two.

It is the independent practice nurse's responsibility to address the professional, business, liability, and risk management issues that arise. Be prepared to replicate some of the safeguards found in health care institutions, such as having policies and procedures that are reviewed periodically. Establishing a professional network of trusted peers and mentors for consultation, perhaps referral, can also help maintain your currency with best practices and ongoing learning.

Nursing regulatory bodies tend to have a written guideline on the subject of independent nursing practice. Reviewing these in advance of considering independent practice is helpful. Certain issues may not have played a role in your prior employment, such as advertising nursing services, conflict of interest, and proper use of nursing titles, but they take on new significance if you do embark on independent practice.

Prior to embarking on independent practice, consider the implications of working this way with a business advisor prior to making any final decisions, and/or taking a course on running a small business or entrepreneurship. You may consult with a business lawyer and/or an accountant to review business structure options (i.e., sole proprietorship), and their tax and legal implications, and any business regulations or bylaws, for example, business license requirements. Generally, professionals are not permitted to use incorporation to avoid professional liability to their patients. Consider consulting your financial advisor about your plans.

Working independently may also create additional legal responsibilities as a tenant, landlord, or employer, all of which justify specific business and legal advice to the business owner. When nursing services are provided through a business entity, large or small, a plaintiff alleging harm caused by the care or services provided may start legal proceedings against a nurse who provided the care or against the business entity or both.

Businesses may also face legal issues unrelated to the practice of nursing: employment disputes, contractual disputes, equipment failure, property damage, etc. Consequently, it is important for the business to be adequately insured for both aspects of the business: professional services to be rendered and the potential business liabilities. Keep in mind that no one insurance product or service will assist with every possible legal matter. Different types of insurance are available to respond to different risks. What is adequate will vary according to the circumstances, which may change over time. Insurance may be purchased through a group insurance plan or through an insurance broker in the commercial insurance market.

Independent practice nurses will most likely be considered as the health information custodians or trustees of their patient health records, unless a contract has identified another party, for example, a long-term care facility, as the health information custodian in compliance with the governing privacy legislation. Health information custodians or trustees have certain legal obligations concerning the collection, use, disclosure, retention, and disposal of a patient's personal health information. Confidential health records must be stored in a secure place and retained for any mandatory period required by law in your province or territory. It is highly recommended that independent practice nurses consult with their lawyer to determine whether they are health information custodians and to ensure that they are establishing appropriate policies and procedures consistent with the privacy legislation in their jurisdiction. The provincial or territorial Privacy Commission or Ombudsman may have useful resources designed to ensure compliance with privacy legislation.

When an independent practice nurse enters a contract to provide services, the contract will generally be prepared by the party seeking those services. Alternatively, the nurse's lawyer may draft a contract to describe the terms of the professional services that will be provided to the patient or the other contracting party. Professional contracts or service agreements vary in length and content (some taken off the internet and originally intended for work far removed from nursing), and typically include provisions that favour the interests of the party that drafted it. The contract should stipulate the professional nursing services that are to be rendered; contain provisions that support professional obligations, for example, confidentiality; and anticipate how and when the contractual relationship between the parties might end. You should have a business lawyer review the document prior to signing any agreement.

Independent contractors must decide on the type and amount of liability protection or insurance needed to protect their personal assets. While many Canadian nurses automatically become eligible for professional liability protection (but not business liability protection) from the CNPS upon registration with their nursing regulatory body, there may be options about the sources of additional legal defence funding for professional and business liabilities. If decisions about the source of legal defence funding are not addressed when health care professionals begin to work together, and on an ongoing basis, they risk discovering after a lawsuit is commenced that their assumptions about liability protection were incorrect. This could result in unnecessary professional and personal financial jeopardy.

Complaints to a Nursing Regulator

The focus of PLP is civil litigation but negligence lawsuits are not the only legal proceedings nurses may encounter. Nurses learn as undergraduates that once they are a member of a nursing regulatory body, anyone can lodge a complaint with that body regarding standards of nursing practice, professional ethics, and fitness to practice. Indeed, some such reports are required by law, an example of which can be a mandatory report by an employer who fires a nurse due to substandard nursing care. The best defence to a complaint is to ensure your nursing practice gives life to the nursing practice standards and professional ethics written and endorsed by your nursing regulator, as amended from time to time. If you are a union member, you can inquire as to what help, if any, the union provides with complaints to the nursing regulator. You may consider subscribing to a legal defence fund designed to defend against complaints to your nursing regulator.

If a complaint is made to your nursing regulator, you will be notified by them and they will also inform you of how they wish to hear from you. Remember that you have always known such a complaint was possible. Notify any source of assistance you may have for complaints (i.e., union, legal defence fund, etc.) and refresh your knowledge of the regulator's jurisdiction: practice standards, ethics, and fitness. Evidence of your compliance with the standards and ethical principles can be used in your defence.

Conclusion

It can be nerve-wracking to talk about legal disputes since no one can offer the assurance that it will never happen to you. However, you can take some steps to position yourself well in case you have to defend your nursing practice. Throughout your career, prioritize your currency with clinical (administrative, education, or research) best practices, and with nursing practice standards, as amended from time to time by your nursing regulator. Understand what sources of legal guidance and legal defence funding you already have, and if there are gaps, i.e., no assistance with complaints to your nursing regulator, research the options that are available to you. Finally, if you are notified that you are involved in legal proceedings, do not discuss your evidence with your colleagues but turn to the resources designed to assist you with legal matters.

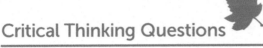

Critical Thinking Questions

1. Reflecting on your most recent challenging clinical situation, how would you explain to a lawyer retained to defend you how you upheld nursing practice standards, practiced ethically, and acted reasonably in the circumstances?
2. Does you nursing regulator require its members to have PLP and if so, how do you obtain it?
3. What are the two aspects of independent practice that self-employed nurses must plan for?

References

Bazley v. Curry. (1999). 2 S.C.R. 534.

Borg, E. (2004). The nurse as an expert witness. *Canadian Nurse, 6*, 38–39.

Canada Revenue Agency (CRA). (2019). *Small businesses and self-employed income.* Ottawa, ON: CRA. Retrieved from https://www.canada.ca/en/revenue-agency/services/tax/businesses/small-businesses-self-employed-income.html

Canadian Nurses Protective Society (CNPS). (2004). *infoLAW examinations for discovery.* Ottawa, ON: CNPS.

College of Nurses of Ontario (CNO). (2019). *Revised by-law no. 1, general (December 2019), s.44.4.* Toronto, ON: CNO.

Crits v. Sylvester. (1956). S.C.R. 991.

Granger (Litigation guardian of) v. Ottawa General Hospital, [1996] O.J. No. 2129 (Ont. Gen. Div.).

Health Professions Act, R.S.A. 2000, c H-7, s.127.1(1)(3), *Reporting by regulated members.* Edmonton, AB: Government of Alberta. Retrieved from http://www.qp.alberta.ca/documents/Acts/H07.pdf

Picard, E. T., & Robertson, G. B. (2017). *Legal liability of doctors and hospitals in Canada* (5th ed.). Toronto, ON: Carswell.

Regulated Health Professions Act, 1991, S.O. 1991, c. 18, s. 85.6.2. *Reporting by members re: professional negligence and malpractice.* Toronto, ON: Government of Ontario. Retrieved from https://www.ontario.ca/laws/statute/91r18/v6

Stewart v. Pettie. (1995). 1 S.C.R. 131.

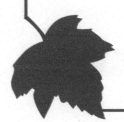

SECTION IV

Advanced Practice Nursing Specialty Roles in Canada

This section provides a picture of some of the advanced practice nursing (APN) roles found across Canada. The clinical nurse specialist (CNS) specialty roles that contribute to the Canadian health care system that are discussed in this section include the fields of geropsychiatry, mental health, and ambulatory care. These are by no means representative of all the CNS roles that exist. The focus for discussion of the nurse practitioner roles is organized around primary health care/family/all ages, and tertiary care roles. At the core, all APN roles build and expand upon the foundation of the registered nurse role with an overall goal of facilitating timely and accessible care within fiscally challenging and changing environments to provide optimal health services for Canadians.

Chapter

21

Clinical Nurse Specialist: Geropsychiatry

Gloria McInnis-Perry

GLORIA MCINNIS-PERRY is an Associate Professor in the Faculty of Nursing at the University of Prince Edward Island, Charlottetown, Prince Edward Island. She is a specialist in seniors' mental health in acute and long-term care, in community and hospital-based settings in Canada and the United States.

KEY TERMS

clinical nurse specialist (CNS)
geropsychiatric clinical nurse specialist (GPCNS)
mental illnesses
older adults

OBJECTIVES

1. Describe the role of the geropsychiatric clinical nurse specialist (GPCNS).
2. Explore the role functions of the GPCNS.
3. Identify the unique challenges in providing mental health care to the older adult.

Introduction

In Canada, persons aged 65 years and older account for approximately 17.2% of the population; 25% of these older adults are immigrants; less than 1% are in same-sex partnerships; and 10.6% are visible minorities. The proportion of older adults is estimated to continue to rise and one in five Canadians should be aged 65 and older in 2024 (Statistics Canada, 2019a). Concurrently, Canadian men and women are living longer with a life expectancy of 80 and 84.1 years respectively (Statistics Canada, 2019b). Despite improvements in technology and public health measures, which support an increase in life expectancy, many older adults live with chronic health conditions, with four out of five older adults living at home with a chronic health problem. Approximately, 75% of Canadians aged 65 and over report having at least one of the seven most common health problems (arthritis, cancer, chronic obstructive lung disease, diabetes, heart disease, high blood pressure, and mood disorders), with many reporting the coexistence of multiple chronic conditions (MCC), which are two or more of these conditions (Health Council of Canada, 2010). Physical disability and associated pain and functional impairment are also more prevalent in later life (Meisner, Linton, Seguin, & Spassiani, 2017). Unfortunately, older adults with high comorbidity who have MCC report poorer health, take more prescriptions, have an increased risk of functional dependency, a higher number of health care visits (Canadian Institute for Health Information [CIHI], 2011; Ploeg et al., 2017) and more negative psychological health outcomes (Steptoe, Deaton, & Stone, 2015).

Living a long and healthy life is a desire for most older adults. For others, coping with changes—such as retirement, relocation, social losses, and normal decline in physical health—poses risks to mental health at a time when strengths and resources can be reduced. Over 20% of adults aged 60 and over suffer from a mental or neurological disorder (World Health Organization [WHO], 2017). Moreover, the prevalence of mental illness increases after the age of 69 up to 42% by the age of 90 (Mental Health Commission of Canada [MHCC], 2016). Elder abuse (physical, verbal, psychological, financial, and sexual) and neglect are estimated to occur in one in six older adults, which can lead to physical injuries and sometimes long-lasting psychological consequences such as depression and anxiety (WHO, 2017). Being an older adult who identifies as lesbian, gay, bisexual, transgender, or queer (LGBTQ) increases the likelihood of mental and health disparities (Driscoll & Gray, 2017).

The most common **mental illnesses** after age 65 are mood and anxiety disorders, cognitive and mental disorders due to a medical condition (including dementia and delirium), substance misuse (including prescription drugs and alcohol), and psychotic disorders (MacCourt, Wilson, & Tourigny-Rivard. 2011). Older adults commit suicide less; however, this group has the highest rate of successful attempts (Lindner, Foerster, & von Renteln-Kruse, 2014). Depressive episodes, agoraphobia, and panic disorder can present as first-episode disorders for the 60 years and over age group (Kessler, Amminger, Aguilar-Gaxiola, Lee, & Üstün, 2007). Older adults with depressive symptoms have poorer functioning compared to those with chronic medical conditions and have an increased perception of poor health resulting in increased utilization of health care services. Of increasing concern is that the baby boomer cohort, those born between 1946 and 1966, will have their own specific challenges (Bristow, 2016) such as family care conflict, intimate and social networking needs, and embodiment issues (O'Connor & Kelson, 2018).

Mental health problems are under-identified by older adults and health care professionals worldwide (WHO, 2017). In Canada, seniors' mental health specialized treatment programs, support services, research, and knowledge are lacking (MacCourt et al., 2011). Furthermore, non-physician mental health care professionals who care for seniors with MCC are challenged in providing care within a fragmented health care system, overcoming stigma, and dealing with seniors' mental health care knowledge gaps (Perrella, McAiney, & Ploeg, 2018). Nonetheless, most older adults' mental health problems can be managed with adequate preventive strategies, timely recognition and diagnosis, and delivery of person-centred or recovery-focused philosophy of care with corresponding interventions.

This chapter examines the role of the geropsychiatric clinical nurse specialist that includes a discussion of the educational preparation for the role, consideration of aging issues, and advanced mental health nursing care of mentally ill older adults and their families. A case study will demonstrate how the advanced practice nursing (APN) role competencies are integrated into the daily practice of the geropsychiatric clinical nurse specialist.

Geropsychiatric Clinical Nurse Specialist

The **geropsychiatric clinical nurse specialist (GPCNS)** is a **clinical nurse specialist (CNS)** with a specialty in the mental health of older adults and has expert knowledge in normal age-related changes, common psychiatric, cognitive, and co-morbid medical disorders occurring in later life. The GPCNS has a high level of expertise in assessing, making nursing diagnoses, and treating complex health responses of individuals, groups, and communities. Role functions of the GPCNS include educating and coaching patients, families, and nurses; performing in-depth physical, social, and psychological assessments; providing direct physical and psychological interventions; consulting and collaborating with family caregivers, nursing staff, physicians, and other disciplines to plan and evaluate individualized care based on assessments; managing interprofessional care over a defined period of time; serving as leaders by changing practices or directing interprofessional teams; and conducting or participating in research activities (Bourbonniere & Evans, 2002).

Issues Related to Aging in Canada

GPCNSs are aware of the current issues facing the older adult. Understanding the biological changes related to normal aging and aging well, as well as the social, cultural, spiritual, and religious context of mentally ill older adults and their families are central to person-centred and recovery-focused care. The aging process is universal, highly complex, diverse, and influenced by changes in the biological, psychological, social, ethno-cultural, and spiritual aspects of the individual. Grouping older adults based on chronological age remains the most common means of assessing the elderly and determining their suitability for a wide variety of programs and age categories. However, the GPCNS must consider cohort effects that take into account the influence of historical time and the attributes of a particular generation and how events may be experienced differently between and within different cohorts.

Ageism, Stigma, and Discrimination

Older adults face issues of ageism, stigma, and discrimination. Ageism is the existence of negative attitudes toward persons based on their chronological age. Older adults with mental health problems face overlapping stigma: the stigma of mental illness, as well as the stigma of being older (MHCC, 2012; Perrella et al., 2018; WHO, 2017). Self-imposed stigma, and not wanting to admit one has a psychological weakness and/or admitting one has a problem, can become a self-imposed barrier to accessing mental health care and increase the risk for mental health complications such as suicide (Diggle-Fox, 2016). Older adults who live with serious and persistent mental illness most likely experience extrapyramidal symptoms due to the use of conventional antipsychotics whose side effects can be quite disabling for the older adult and lead to further social stigmatization (Robison, McInnis-Perry, Weeks, & Foley, 2017). Many older adults with serious and persistent mental illness have greater difficulty accessing age-related services such as a nursing home. Conversely, older adults' age may limit access to certain health care services. Addressing these issues of ageism, stigma, and/or discrimination is part of the recovery philosophy and a part of the GPCNS's ethical practice.

Aging Well

Aging well is "a lifelong process optimizing opportunities for improving and preserving health and physical, social, and mental wellness; independence; quality of life; and enhancing successful life-course transitions" (Peel, Bartlett, & McClure, 2005, p. 115). Emphasizing a wellness perspective of aging encourages one to consider the person's strengths, resilience, resources, and capabilities (Touhy, Jett, Boscart, & McCleary, 2018). The social determinants of health such as income and social status, social support networks, physical health and social environments, personal health practices, coping skills, and health services are all factors that impact older adults' well-being.

Social, Cultural, and Spiritual/Religious Context

Consideration of the social, cultural, spiritual, and religious contexts in which older adults live and how those shape their world view is essential to ensure a holistic approach when providing psychiatric mental health care. These fundamental areas along with the physical aspects determine how mental health and mental illness are understood. Moreover, evidence suggests that there are differences in aging expectations across racial/ethnic groups of older adults, which supports the need for more culturally competent care (Menkin et al., 2017). Most older adults prefer to age in place in their own home, supported by family and friends with the necessary professional health care.

Social support is important to human health (Gottlieb & Bergen, 2010), and has been defined as the resources that persons perceive to be available or that are actually provided to them by non-professionals in the context of both formal support groups and informal helping relationships (Cohen, Gottlieb, & Underwood, 2000). Social support can be emotional, such as intimacy and attachment; instrumental, such as direct financial aid or services; informational, such as assistance with problem-solving or the provision of feedback; companionship; and esteem support (Barrera, 1986). Age and gender differences in social support needs must be considered, especially in factors such as social assessments, strengthening relationships, addressing social isolation, and providing opportunities for older adults to participate in meaningful activities (McInnis-Perry, Weeks, & Stryhn, 2013).

Nonetheless, many older adults who live alone are women (Newall et al., 2009), and are lonely (Victor, Scambler, Bowling, & Bond, 2005). Most are without the social support of their immediate family, friends, and community (Aday, Kehoe, & Farney, 2006). Social isolation among older adults has been termed a significant public health concern (Glass, 2016) and can lead to adverse physical and mental health issues such as loneliness (Finlay & Kobayashi, 2018), depressive symptoms (Taylor, Wang, & Morrow-Howell, 2018), poor self-rated health, cognitive decline (Shankar, Hamer, McMunn, & Steptoe, 2013), and decreased quality of life

(Bedney, Goldberg, & Josephson, 2010). On the contrary, older adults who perceive themselves as having higher levels of support have a higher life satisfaction, which can buffer the impact of depressive symptoms, reduce stress, and is inversely related to social isolation (Adams et al., 2015).

Among older Canadians, there is great cultural and ethnic diversity (i.e., First Nations, LGBTQ, immigrants, refugees, and other ethno-culture groups) that present challenges in the provision of a comprehensive recovery-focused mental health care system. Culture and ethnicity are often linked; however, culture is a way of life (behaviours, values, attitudes, and geographic and political factors) that is attributed to a group of people, while ethnicity refers to race, origin or ancestry, identity, language, and religion (Phinney, 1996). The expression, interpretations, and care of mental illness vary within and among culture groups.

Spirituality is expressed and understood in a cultural context. The GPCNS's understanding of the older adult's beliefs, values, and spirituality is an essential aspect in providing holistic nursing care. The term *religion* is often used interchangeably with spirituality; however, the two are distinct. Religion is "the organized set of beliefs, traditions, and behaviors that relate to some greater entity outside the self," and spirituality is "the inner life of personal development, the search for meaning that may or may not be a part of any religion or a relationship to a higher power" (Chandler, 2012, pp. 578–579). The importance of religion and spirituality as a source of protection is well documented as it affects older adults' mental health and positive health outcomes, such as higher quality of life, lower rates of depression, substance use/abuse, cognitive decline (Lucchetti, Barcelos-Ferreira, Blazer, & Moreira-Almeida, 2018), anxiety, suicide (Baetz & Bowen, 2011), mental health status, and treatment effects (Weber & Pargament, 2014). The importance of taking a brief spiritual history is an essential aspect of mental health care (Harrington, 2016; Lucchetti et al., 2018). However, the expression of one's religion/spirituality may pose challenges in mental health care as these experiences may be seen as a "normal cultural experience," "sacred," or a "blessing" versus a delusional symptom. Often negative psychological outcomes are related to negative religious coping, spiritual struggle, misunderstanding, miscommunication, or negative beliefs (Weber & Pargament, 2014).

The GPCNS needs to understand how older adults define and describe their religious/spiritual beliefs and experiences, and how these may differ from the GPCNS's personal beliefs. Several spiritual history/assessment/screening approaches are found in the literature (Harrington, 2016); all attempt to recognize the person's spiritual needs and the role that religion and spirituality play in the older adult's life and how they influence their day-to-day functioning. If the older adult's preoccupation with religion and religious rituals becomes so destructive that the person cannot function with daily life, then the consideration of an underlying psychopathology must be assessed.

Recovery-Focused Care

A mental health system that addresses the complex interaction between the individual and social dimensions that influence mental health outcomes must be both person-centred and comprehensive in its approach to recovery and well-being. Much effort is needed to promote

TABLE 21.1: Applying Recovery Principles to the Assessment of the Older Adult

Considerations When Assessing Older Adults

1. Always assess and consider the older adult's strength and ability to function.
2. Distinguish between normal and abnormal aging. Older adults are more likely to have somatic complaints and attribute these to physical problems rather than mental health problems. To the older adult, these symptoms are real and the GPCNS needs to acknowledge these feelings. Exploring the temporal context of the symptoms will provide the GPCNS with a better understanding of the history, possible triggers, and whether or not the symptoms are part of normal worry versus a mental health disorder.
3. Consider the effect that medical illnesses and medication have on the presentation of mental illness.
4. Some older adults exhibit subsyndromal symptoms of an illness, in which severity and symptoms are not high enough to be diagnosed with a formal psychiatric diagnosis, however, therapeutic interventions may relieve symptoms, improve functional status, prevent a more serious illness and improve overall quality of life.
5. The loss of a loved one, status, pet, or object may be quite a significant loss to the older adult as the ability to replace these losses may be more difficult than for a younger person.
6. Always assess for suicidal ideation, complete a risk assessment and consider the personal context of the older adult. Implement safety measures and inform appropriate persons.

Source: McInnis-Perry, 2019.

the mental health of older adults and to prevent mental illness. Good physical health, meaningful activities, and secure and supportive relationships all contribute to good mental health and quality of life for older adults. In a recovery-oriented system, persons who experience mental health problems and illnesses are treated with dignity and respect, where personal recovery is accepted and transformation of the person is supported (Rankin & Petty, 2016). The concept of recovery is built on the principles of choice, respect, hope, empowerment, self-determination, person-centred, and responsibility (MHCC, 2009). Older adults living with mental illness who participate as fully as possible in their own care and well-being make informed choices with the support of health care professionals, family, and friends. Essential to recovery is the removal of all barriers in order for the person to have access to the right mix of evidence-informed service at the right time (MHCC, 2009). Early intervention at the first indication of mental illness and/or addiction symptoms is important as it can shorten the recovery journey.

Geropsychiatric Clinical Nurse Specialist Competencies

Clinical

Caring for the older adult who exhibits signs and symptoms of a mental health disorder can present some unique challenges. The GPCNS must consider the bio-psycho-social-cultural-spiritual influences on the older adult and integrate this knowledge with individualized treatment of the various mental disorders. The GPCNS must also consider the most common mental illnesses in the older adult, the clinical considerations of providing evidence-informed holistic care, and keep abreast of relevant and ongoing research in this area. Growing older for some means living longer with a recurrent serious and persistent mental illness; experiencing late-onset mental illnesses; living with behavioural and psychological symptoms associated with dementia; and living with chronic medical problems with known correlations with mental illness, such as Parkinson's disease, cerebral vascular disease, and chronic obstructive lung disease (Horgan et al., 2009).

Assessment

The GPCNS assesses clients, develops and contributes to the plan of care, and intervenes in complex health care situations within the specialty of geropsychiatry. The process begins with a comprehensive mental health assessment based on the GPCNS's underlying philosophy, theoretical framework, experience, access to electronic charting, assessment databases, and workplace policy. The GPCNS collects, documents, and analyzes client information and draws conclusions supported by this information. Since most older adults being cared for by the GPCNS present with complex mental health issues, a high level of clinical reasoning skills supported by evidence must guide the care.

The GPCNS considers both the process and the content of the assessment. This includes engaging the client into a therapeutic relationship, maintaining appropriate boundaries, and utilizing recovery principles and techniques (see Table 21.1). The GPCNS must be alert to inconsistencies in the interview and consider the ongoing nature of the assessment process. It is important for the older adult to feel valued, listened to, and safe. The assessment should consider the interview environment, whether the interview is formal or informal, structured, semi-structured, or unstructured, and whether the older adult has communication deficits or barriers requiring modifications.

The GPCNS completes an assessment, which targets various aspects of functioning such as physical performance, cognitive functioning, psychological functioning, affective, social, and psychosocial abilities. The GPCNS reviews already existing medical (diagnostic and laboratory tests, medications) and general nursing data (activities of daily living, nutrition, sleep hygiene, etc.) in addition to collecting new information from the older adult, family, significant others, and formal caregivers over the course of caring for the older adult. In assessing the older adult, social support systems, both quality and quantity, should be considered, with more emphasis on the latter. Quality of support should include whether the persons in the older adult's life are getting along, are geographically close, and are supportive. The older adult's religious/spiritual beliefs and cultural traditions should be included. More focused screening such as assessing suicidal ideation may be warranted for those older adults deemed high risk. Screening tools may be used to assist in the assessment and monitoring of mental illness; however, one must consider the selection and use of tools on factors such as the characteristic of the situation, the presenting problem, and the older adult's abilities to self-report. Many diagnostic criteria and instruments used for defining and identifying mental illnesses have been developed and validated in younger adults, which in turn may not adequately capture the older adults' experience, subclinical symptoms, and influence of race, cultural, and educational level. It is recommended that where possible, the GPCNS purposely select screening and assessment tools that have been validated for older adults.

Nursing Diagnoses

Assessment skills are used to identify nursing diagnoses and to develop nursing interventions that reduce symptoms, risks, or functional decline. The use of nursing diagnoses with consideration of medical diagnoses, including those related to the *Diagnostic Statistical Manual of Mental Disorders*-5 (DSM-5; American Psychological Association [APA], 2013) will assist in the identification of specific interventions.

Interventions and Outcomes

Nursing interventions should be based on a comprehensive assessment and be evidence-informed, while patient/client outcomes should be nurse-sensitive, desirable, achievable, and measurable. There are many interventions available to the GPCNS in the care of the older adult living with a mental illness. The use of evidence-informed nursing protocols and guidelines should be considered. Often the GPCNS provides formal and informal education to the client, family, and nursing staff or provides advocacy. There are many educational opportunities for the GPCNS while fulfilling the competencies inherent in the role. As a clinician, the GPCNS educates the client and family about mental illness, mental health issues, and care practices. As part of an interprofessional team, the GPCNS can develop continuing education programs, orientation, and mentor programs to support the team process. As a mentor/coach/trainer the GPCNS supervises and educates other nurses to strengthen psychiatric mental health nursing, gerontological competencies, and promotes the standards of practice.

A step-by-step approach to care is individualized to the older adult's present needs, mental health disorder, symptoms of the illness, functional level, existence of comorbidities, present and past medication usage, and access to available resources and a collaborative team. Depending on these factors, the GPCNS will begin with the least intrusive approach to care. Non-pharmacological interventions are suggested as the first step, such as individual and group activity (stress management, music, art, exercise, use of humour, relaxation, mindfulness, reminiscence, dietary factors, sleep hygiene, reality orientation), environmental factors (therapeutic and safe, sensory-sensitive, and orienting), addressing caregiver issues (communication, care practices, stress, and grieving) through education and supportive therapy (self-help groups or formal therapy).

After prompt identification and assessment provision of education about the mental health issue or illness is provided, advice on self-medication use and risk of over-the-counter medications is given. Active monitoring of symptoms and functioning is of prime importance to the GPCNS. If no improvement is evident, then individual, group, and/or self-help groups are suggested before moving on to more formalized psychotherapeutic interventions. The use of medications may come into play if the prior interventions do not work or if the older adult's functioning level declines and/or the risk of self-harm increases. More intense and multiagency services such as community mental health or in-patient care may be necessary.

Psychopharmacotherapy used in conjunction with psychotherapy is a common practice in treating the older adult.

Researcher

As a researcher, the GPCNS disseminates research findings and educates patients/clients, families, students, health care providers, and policy-makers. The GPCNS generates and synthesizes and is an expert in leading evidence-based practice, evidence-informed practice, and professional practice at all levels based on multiple sources of knowledge (Canadian Nurses Association [CNA], 2019). The research competencies are integral components of the role of the GPCNS, as every aspect of the advance practitioners' role is influenced by research.

Leadership

Leadership is a hallmark of the GPCNS's practice (Lyon, 2014). The GPCNS is a transformational leader, one who appeals to others' sense of values, helps them see a higher vision, and encourages them to exert themselves in helping to achieve the vision. The GPCNSs possess leadership skills necessary to transform the mental health system, and specifically older adults' mental health care. They participate in professional organizations, present and act as role models, which impact on geropsychiatric mental health care (Tringali, Murphy, & Osevala, 2008). The GPCNSs lead, coach, and mentor direct-care nurses in providing evidence-informed care to older adults living with mental health issues. As well, they design and provide mental health promotion and risk-reduction programs and initiatives. The GPCNSs work collaboratively within the interprofessional team to provide older adults' mental health care. Many GPCNSs lead or become part of initiatives such as strategic planning, the development and/or revision of policies and procedures, and the education of patients, staff, and families.

Consultation and Collaboration

Consultation and collaboration are integral parts of the GPCNS's role (CNA, 2009). Consultation is the indirect provision of care through helping others implement change (Pearson, 2014). The GPCNS has expertise and may be consulted on a complex patient case, group specific to staff or patients or organizational specific issues with the purpose of improving health care. The GPCNS "collaborates with other health-care providers and other interested parties to maximize health benefits being provided, while recognizing and respecting the knowledge, skills and perspectives of all" (CNA, 2017, p. 10). Collaborative practice is envisioned as an interprofessional process of communication and decision-making that enables the separate and shared knowledge and skills of health care providers to synergistically influence the client/patient care provided (Way, Jones, & Busing, 2006).

Depending on where the GPCNS practices and whether the CNS has a practice base versus an independent external consultant role (Doody, 2014), consultation and collaboration may be a more common role or a more selective role; for example, being the CNS of an older adult's mental health community team versus the director of the team. Whether based in the community, long-term care centre (LTC), or hospital setting, the role of the consultant will depend on the reason for the consult, the patient, available resources, and level of expertise of the CNS. The GPCNS completes a thorough assessment, identifies problems, suggests interventions, and evaluates outcomes. Interventions usually involve the client, family, and health care providers. Important in a recovery-focused philosophy is the client-provider collaborative care plan, in which clients are engaged and participate in treatment decisions. Collaborative care can take many forms and can include setting goals for treatment, preparing a treatment or action plan, and having patients participate in treatment decisions.

Often the GPCNS is a facilitator of interprofessional teams, which requires strong team building and communication skills. Communicating the plan of care to all involved is essential. If further medical or diagnostic testing is required, referral or consultation to medicine may be required. The GPCNS may make specific recommendations to nursing staff, such as medication monitoring, completion of behavioural checklists, and implementation of behavioural management strategies. Other interventions may require referral to other health care professionals such as social workers, occupational therapists, and nutritionists.

CASE STUDY

The Story of Bea

Bea, an 85-year-old widow who moved to a nursing home three months ago, was recently referred by her general practitioner (GP) for assessment of changes in her behaviour (restlessness, agitation, argumentative, yelling, verbal abuse toward nursing staff, social withdrawal, crying, insomnia, and refusal to attend group activities). Bea has a diagnosis of dementia (vascular and probable Alzheimer's disease), herpes zoster, hypertension, hyperlipidemia, previous hip fracture, and osteoarthritis in both hips. She is on Aricept, Zocor, Lopressor, Neurontin, and Aspirin.

The GPCNS visits the nursing home and begins a comprehensive nursing assessment, which includes a review of Bea's health status as documented in her health file. The GPCNS notes that Bea's pre-admission cognitive screening on the Mini Mental State Exam (MMSE) was 20/30, and the Geriatric Depression Scale (GDS) was 3/10. The GPCNS completes the geropsychiatric mental health assessment tools (repeated MMSE and GDS) and a social/environment assessment. She coordinates a meeting with Bea, Bea's GP and family, nursing, and other care providers. The GPCNS findings are: MMSE 19 (moderate CI); GDS 9/15 (moderate depression). No SI nor HI. Laboratory tests were normal. Bea has an unsteady gait and walks with a walker. She has a hearing deficit, has pain in her hips and upper torso. She has had a reported weight loss of 2.2 kg over the last two weeks and has a positive Behavioural Monitoring Checklist.

Bea's room is located at the end of a long dimly lit and poorly oriented corridor. She has infrequent visits from her family and friends. Bea expresses anger toward her family for sending her to LTC and for not visiting. She misses working in the garden and attending daily mass. Bea seems frustrated with the inconsistency in staff care, and not receiving adequate pain relief during the night makes it difficult to sleep comfortably.

Bea's nursing diagnoses include chronic confusion, alteration in mood, grief, pain, disturbed sensory perception (auditory), self-care deficit, imbalanced nutrition (less), impaired physical mobility, disturbed sleep pattern, ineffective individual coping, insomnia, risk for loneliness and family alteration.

Subsequent to these findings, the GPCNS requests a Behavioural Monitoring Checklist and more laboratory tests. Working collaboratively with the interprofessional team, it is determined that the geropsychiatrist is to see Bea to rule out major depression/dysfunctional grieving. The GP is to assess pain management and make referrals for a hearing test, nutritionist, and physiotherapy to assess gait. The GPCNS will provide education to the staff on person-centred care, depression, relocation issues, pain management and comfort measures, effective communication issues, self-care, and diversional activities. As well, the GPCNS will provide individual supportive therapy to help Bea with the transitional stress to LTC and help her cope with the responses to her depression, monitor her response to the antidepressant and pain medication, and repeat the GDS. The GPCNS will involve Bea's family and caregivers and attend Bea's case conferences for six months.

Conclusion

The GPCNS provides expert advanced nursing care for older adults living with complex mental health issues across the health care continuum. Education and support of older persons, their family, nurses, interprofessional staff, and the facilitation of change are all components of a GPCNS's practice. The GPCNS is an evolving specialty in an ever-evolving health care system, which requires the development and use of evidence-informed knowledge and skills in order to keep abreast of changing holistic care practices when caring for mentally ill older adults and their families.

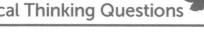

Critical Thinking Questions

1. What are the roles of GPCNS?
2. What unique factors must the GPCNS consider when working with older adults?
3. What modifications of the comprehensive mental health assessment are necessary when caring for the mentally ill older adult?

References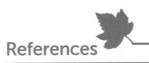

Adams, T. R., Rabin, L. A., Da Silva, V. G., Katz, M. J., Fogel, J., & Lipton, R. B. (2015). Social support buffers the impact of depressive symptoms on life satisfaction in old age. *Clinical Gerontologist, 39*(2), 139–157.

Aday, R. H., Kehoe, G. C., & Farney, L. (2006). Impact of senior center friendships on aging women who live alone. *Journal of Women & Aging, 18*(1), 57–73.

American Psychological Association (APA). (2013). *Diagnostic and statistical manual of mental disorders* (5th ed.). Arlington, VA: APA.

Baetz, M., & Bowen, R. (2011). Suicidal ideation, affective lability, and religion in depressed adults. *Mental Health, Religion and Culture, 14*(7), 633–641.

Barrera, M. (1986). Distinction between social support concepts, measures and models. *American Journal of Community Psychology, 14*, 413–445.

Bedney, B., Goldberg, R. B., & Josephson, K. (2010). Aging in place in naturally occurring retirement communities: Transforming aging through supportive service programs. *Journal of Housing for the Elderly, 24*, 304–321.

Bourbonniere, M., & Evans, L. (2002). Advanced practice nursing in the care of frail older adults. *Journal of American Geriatrics, 50*(12), 2062–2076.

Bristow, J. (2016). The making of Boomergeddon: The construction of the baby boomer generation as a social problem in Britain. *The British Journal of Sociology, 67*(4), 575–591.

Canadian Institute for Health Information (CIHI). (2011). *Health care cost drivers: The facts.* Ottawa, ON: CIHI. Retrieved from https://secure.cihi.ca/free_products/health_care_cost_drivers_the_facts_en.pdf

Canadian Nurses Association (CNA). (2009). *Position statement: Clinical nurse specialist.* Ottawa, ON: CNA. Retrieved from https://www.cna-aiic.ca/~/media/cna/page-content/pdf-en/clinical-nurse-specialist_position-statement.pdf

CNA. (2017). *Code of ethics for registered nurses.* Ottawa, ON: CNA. Retrieved from http://www.cna-aiic.ca/~/media/cna/files/en/codeofethics.pdf

CNA. (2019). *Advanced practice nursing: A pan-Canadian framework.* Ottawa, ON: CNA. Retrieved from https://www.cna-aiic.ca/-/media/cna/page-content/pdf-en/apn-a-pan-canadian-framework.pdf

Chandler, E. (2012). Religious and spiritual issues in DSM-5: Matters of mind and searching of the soul. *Issues in Mental Health Nursing, 33*, 577–588.

Cohen, S., Gottlieb, B. H., & Underwood, L. G. (2000). Social relationships and health. In S. Cohen, L. G. Underwood, & B. H. Gottlieb (Eds.), *Social support measurement and intervention: A guide for health and social scientists* (pp. 3–25). New York, NY: Oxford University Press.

Diggle-Fox, B. (2016). Assessing suicide risk in older adults. *The Nurse Practitioner, 41*(10), 28–35.

Doody, O. (2014). The role and development of consultancy in nursing practice. *British Journal of Nursing, 23*(1), 32–39.

Driscoll, M., & Gray, K. (2017). Special consideration in mental health evaluation of LGBT elders. *The American Journal of Psychiatry: Residents' Journal, 12*(5), 4–6.

Finlay, J., & Kobayashi, L. (2018). Social isolation and loneliness in later life: A parallel convergent mixed-methods case study of older adults and their residential contexts in the Minneapolis metropolitan area, USA. *Social Science Medicine, 20*, 25–33.

Glass, A. P. (2016). Resident managed elder intentional neighborhoods: Do they promote social resources for older adults? *Journal of Gerontological Social Work, 59*(7–8), 554–571.

Gottlieb, B., & Bergen, A. (2010). Social support concepts and measures. *Psychosomatic Research, 695,* 511–520.

Harrington, A. (2016). The importance of spiritual assessment when caring for older adults. *Aging and Society, 36,* 1–16. https://doi.org/10.1017/S0144686X14001007

Health Council of Canada. (2010). Helping patients help themselves: Are Canadians with chronic conditions getting the support they need to manage their health. *Canadian Healthcare Matters,* January, Bulletin 2, Toronto, ON. Retrieved from http://publications.gc.ca/collections/collection_2011/ccs-hcc/H173-1-2-2010-eng.pdf

Horgan, S., LeClair, K., Donnelly, M., Hinton, G., MacCourt, P., & Kreiger-Frost, S. (2009). Developing a national consensus on the accessibility needs of older adults with concurrent and chronic mental and physical health issues: A preliminary framework informing collaborative mental health care planning. *Canadian Journal on Aging, 28*(2), 97–105.

Kessler, R. C., Amminger, G. P., Aguilar-Gaxiola, S., Lee, S., & Üstün, T. B. (2007). Age of onset: A review of recent literature. *Current Opinion in Psychiatry, 20*(4), 359–364.

Lindner, R., Foerster, R., & von Renteln-Kruse, W. Z. (2014). Physical distress and relationship problems. *Gerontological Geriatrics, 47*(6), 502–507.

Lucchetti, A., Barcelos-Ferreira, R., Blazer, D. G., & Moreira-Almeida, A. (2018). Spirituality in geriatric psychiatry. *Current Opinion Psychiatry, 31,* 373–377.

Lyon, B. L. (2014). Transformational leadership as the clinical nurse specialist's capacity to influence. In J. S. Fulton, B. L. Lyon, & K. A. Goudreau (Eds.), *Foundations of clinical nurse specialist practice.* New York, NY: Springer.

MacCourt, P., Wilson, K., & Tourigny-Rivard, M. F. (2011). *Guidelines for comprehensive mental health services for older adults in Canada.* Calgary, AB: MHCC. Retrieved from https://www.mentalhealthcommission.ca/sites/default/files/2017-09/mhcc_seniors_guidelines_0.pdf

McInnis-Perry, G., Weeks, L., & Stryhn, H. (2013). Age and gender differences in emotional and informational social support insufficiency in older adults in Atlantic Canada. *Canadian Journal of Nursing Research, 45*(4), 50–68.

Meisner, B., Linton, V., Seguin, A., & Spassiani, N. A. (2017). Examining chronic disease, pain related impairment, and physical activity among middle-aged and older adults in Canada. *Topics in Geriatric Rehabilitation, 33*(3), 182–192.

Menkin, J. A., Guan, S., Araiza, D., Reyes, C., Trejo, L., Choic, S. E., ... Sarkisian, C. (2017). Racial/ethnic differences in expectations regarding aging among adults. *The Gerontological Society of America, 57*(S2), S138–S148.

Mental Health Commission of Canada (MHCC). (2009). *Towards recovery and well-being: A framework for a mental health strategy for Canada.* Calgary, AB: MHCC. Retrieved from https://www.mentalhealthcommission.ca/sites/default/files/FNIM_Toward_Recovery_and_Well_Being_ENG_0_1.pdf

MHCC. (2012). *Changing directions changing lives: The mental health strategy for Canada.* Calgary, AB: MHCC. Retrieved from http://strategy.mentalhealthcommission.ca/pdf/strategy-images-en.pdf

MHCC. (2016). *Making the case for investing in mental health in Canada.* Calgary, AB: MHCC. Retrieved from https://www.mentalhealthcommission.ca/sites/default/files/2016-06/Investing_in_Mental_Health_FINAL_Version_ENG.pdf

Newall, N. E., Chipperfield, J. G., Clifton., R. A., Perry, R. P., Swift, A. U., & Ruthig, J. C. (2009). Causal beliefs, social participation, and loneliness among older adults: A longitudinal study. *Journal of Social and Personal Relationships, 26*(2–3), 273–290.

O'Connor, D., & Kelson, E. (2018). Boomer matters: Responding to emotional health needs in an aging society. *Journal of Gerontological Social Work, 61*(1), 61–77.

Pearson, G. S. (2014). Consultation in the clinical nurse specialist role. In J. S. Fulton, B. L. Lyon, & K. A. Goudreau (Eds.), *Foundations of clinical nurse specialist practice* (pp. 269–276). New York, NY: Springer.

Peel, N., Bartlett, H., & McClure, R. (2005). Healthy ageing: How is it defined and measured? *Australian Journal on Ageing, 23*(3), 115–119.

Perrella, A., McAiney, C., & Ploeg, J. (2018). Rewards and challenges in caring for older adults with multiple chronic health conditions: Perspectives of seniors' mental health case managers. *Canadian Journal of Community Mental Health, 37*(1), 65–79.

Phinney, J. (1996). When we talk about American ethnic groups, what do we mean? *American Psychologist, 51*(9), 918–927.

Ploeg, J., Matthew-Maich, N., Fraser, K., Dufour, S., McAiney, C., Kaasalainen, S., ... Emili, A. (2017). Managing multiple chronic conditions in the community: A Canadian qualitative study of the experiences of older adults, family caregivers and healthcare providers. *BioMed Central (BMC) Geriatrics, 17*(1), 40. doi: 10.1186/s12877-017-0431-6

Rankin, S., & Petty, S. (2016). Older adult recovery: What are we working towards? *Mental Health Journal, 21*(1), 1–10.

Robison, D., McInnis-Perry, G., Weeks, L., & Foley, V. (2017). Dignity in older adults living with schizophrenia. A phenomenological study. *Journal of Psychosocial Nursing, 56*(2), 20–28.

Shankar, A., Hamer, M., McMunn, A., & Steptoe, A. (2013). Social isolation and loneliness: Relationships with cognitive function during 4 years of follow-up in the English longitudinal study of ageing. *Psychosomatic Medicine, 75*(2), 161–170.

Statistics Canada. (2019a). *Project population by age group according to three projection scenarios for 2006, 2011, 2016, 2021, 2031 and 2036.* Ottawa, ON: Statistics Canada. Retrieved from https://www150.statcan.gc.ca/t1/tbl1/en/tv.action?pid=1710005701

Statistics Canada. (2019b). *Table 13-10-0389-01: Life expectancy, at birth and at age 65, by sex, three-year average, Canada, provinces, territories, health regions and peer groups.* Ottawa, ON: Statistics Canada.

Steptoe, A., Deaton, A., & Stone, A. A. (2015). Subjective wellbeing, health, and ageing. *Lancet, 385*(9968), 640–648. doi: 10.1016/S0140-6736(13)61489-0

Taylor, H. O., Wang, Y., & Morrow-Howell, N. (2018). Loneliness in senior housing communities. *Journal of Gerontological Social Work, 61*(6), 623–639.

Touhy, T., Jett, K., Boscart, V., & McCleary, L. (2018). *Ebersole and Hess' gerontological nursing and healthy aging* (2nd Cdn. ed.). Toronto, ON: Elsevier.

Tringali, C. A., Murphy, T. H., & Osevala, M. L. (2008). Clinical nurse specialist practice in a care coordination model. *Clinical Nurse Specialist, 22*, 231–239.

Victor, C., Scambler, S., Bowling, A., & Bond, J. (2005). The prevalence of, and risk factors for, loneliness in late life: A survey of older people in Great Britain. *Aging and Society, 25*, 357–375.

Way, D., Jones, L., & Busing, N. (2001). *Implementation strategies: Collaboration in primary care— family doctors and nurse practitioners delivering shared care,* 1–11. Toronto, ON: Ontario College of Family Physicians. Retrieved from http://citeseerx.ist.psu.edu/viewdoc/download?doi=10.1.1.458.383&rep=rep1&type=pdf

Weber, S., & Pargament, K. (2014). The role of religion and spirituality in mental health. *Current Opinion in Psychiatry, 27*(5), 358–363.

World Health Organization (WHO). (2017). *Mental health of older adults.* Retrieved from https://www.who.int/news-room/fact-sheets/detail/mental-health-of-older-adults

Chapter

22

Clinical Nurse Specialist: Mental Health

Josephine Muxlow and Bernadine Wallis

JOSEPHINE MUXLOW is a clinical nurse specialist (CNS)-Mental Health with Indigenous Services Canada, First Nations and Inuit Health Branch, Atlantic Region, Halifax, Nova Scotia. She was a pioneer of the CNS role at First Nations and Inuit Health Branch and holds an appointment as Adjunct Professor at Dalhousie University, School of Nursing, Halifax, Nova Scotia.

BERNADINE WALLIS is an Instructor at the University of Manitoba, College of Nursing, Faculty of Health Sciences, Winnipeg, Manitoba, and previously was a clinical nurse specialist (CNS)-Mental Health with the First Nations and Inuit Health Branch, Health Canada, Winnipeg, Manitoba.

KEY TERMS

advanced practice nursing
(APN) role
clinical nurse specialist
(CNS)-mental health
direct care
indirect care
system leadership

OBJECTIVES

1. Understand the role of the CNS-mental health in the Canadian health care system.
2. Analyze and evaluate how the CNS-mental health functions independently and collaboratively within a health care setting.
3. Understand how the Canadian Nurses Association Pan-Canadian Clinical Nurse Specialist Core Competencies (2014) become the pillars of CNS-mental health practice.
4. Identify strategies the CNS-mental health utilizes for advancing nursing, system leadership, and quality management in a mental health care setting.

Introduction: Mental Health in Canada

Mental health and substance use remain key public health care issues for Canadians nationwide from a health and wellness perspective. Although the demographics and the population have shifted slightly since the first edition of this chapter, one in five Canadians continues to experience mental illness with an increase to one in two by the age of 40 (Mental Health Commission of Canada [MHCC], 2017). In 2017, suicide rates among males in Canada tripled the rate from among females (Public Health Agency of Canada [PHAC], 2019a, 2019b). The current mental health care situation in Canada is compounded by the recent opioid crisis that resulted in 2,142 opioid-related deaths between January and June 2019. The PHAC (2019a, 2019b) data on opioid-related harms in Canada stated that 13,900 Canadians died of an apparent opioid overdose between January 2016 and June 2019, and 17,050 were hospitalized between January 2016 and March 2019 for opioid-related poisoning.

Mental health is an integral component of health and well-being. Canada, like other global countries, has yet to equate mental health on the same level as physical health. The MHCC's (2017) latest figures show that 7.2% of Canada's health care budget is designated to mental health care in comparison to 13% in England. A Statistics Canada (2018) survey on disability reported anxiety, depression, bipolar disorder, and severe stress disorder as the most frequent reported mental health conditions related to disabilities. Lang et al. (2018) also found that mental and substance use disorders were the leading cause among all ages' disability-adjusted life years. In addition, over 2 million Canadians over the age of 15 have a mental health–related disability; it is most common among youth. They project that by 2020, depression, which is currently ranked fourth, will become the second cause of disability for males and females of all age groups. In the work environment, 30% of disability claims and 70% of disability costs can be attributed to mental health care issues. The Canadian Alliance on Mental Illness and Mental Health (CAMIMH; 2016) found that 500,000 Canadians in any given week are absent from work due to mental health, mental illness, or psychological health care issues. The reported lost productivity in the workplace pertaining to absenteeism or pre-senteeism is over $6 billion annually. In Canada, the yearly economic cost of mental illness and psychological health care issues is over $50 billion with $20 billion of this attributed to workplace health.

Statistics Canada (2018) reported that over one million Canadians with a mental health disability require psychological counselling and only half were able to receive the health care services required. Over the last decade, mental health, mental illnesses, and subs-tance use harm have been brought to the forefront in Canada by several reports and ini-tiatives (CAMIMH, 2016; Canadian Mental Health Association [CMHA], 2014, 2018, 2020; Employment and Social Development Canada, 2016; MHCC, 2009, 2012; PHAC, 2019a, 2019b). The following outlines the evidence of the impact of mental health and substance use in our society:

- Suicide is the second leading cause of death within the age group of 15 to 43 and the ninth leading cause of death in Canada in 2017.

- The majority of the 4,000 Canadians who die by suicide each year experienced a mental health problem or issue.
- Depression is the fourth cause of disability and by 2020 will rank second.
- Over 2 million Canadians over the age of 15 have a disability related to mental health issues.
- As high as 70% of young adults with mental health problems experienced issues from childhood.
- Illegal drugs and other toxic substances are contributing factors to many of the deaths related to opioid overdose.
- 500,000 Canadians are absent from work on a weekly basis due to a psychological health issue.

The **clinical nurse specialist (CNS)-mental health** in an **advanced practice nursing (APN) role** has the opportunity to contribute to clients' health care outcomes from a holistic approach through utilizing evidence and research findings to inform clinical practice, a trauma-informed lens in day-to-day practice, and in system transformational leadership to contribute to an efficient, effective patient-centred mental health care system. An equitable and efficient mental health care system not only aligns health care and services with clients' holistic needs but enhances the quality of health care outcomes related to wellness and recovery. Given the complexity of access to timely integrated mental health care services, the CNS-mental health can also contribute to health care outcomes through mental health promotion activities and interventions.

This chapter focuses on the role of the CNS-mental health. It is important to acknowledge that there are other health care professionals with various titles and classifications who practice in various psychiatric and mental health care settings across Canada.

The Role of the Clinical Nurse Specialist-Mental Health

The CNS-mental health is a registered nurse (RN) who holds a graduate degree in nursing and has a high level of expertise in the clinical speciality of psychiatric mental health nursing and demonstrates characteristics including essential leadership, facilitation and change management skills to achieve patient outcomes, organization strategic goals, and system outcomes (Canadian Nurses Association [CNA], 2019).

The CNS-mental health analyzes, synthesizes, and applies nursing knowledge, theory, and research evidence to foster system-wide changes and advance psychiatric mental health nursing care (CNA, 2014). Within this context, the CNS-mental health plays a pivotal role in the transformation of the mental health care system by enhancing care and services, promoting better health, reducing cost, and promoting equity and social justice in mental health care.

The CNS-mental health practice within the provincial or territorial scope of practice for RNs has no formal legislation or regulation required for the CNS role. There is also no national credentialing for the CNS role, although the CNA has a National Certification Examination available to all practicing psychiatric and mental health nurses and other nursing specialty groups. The two national professional associations that support the CNS-mental health and promote quality improvement are the Clinical Nurse Specialist Association of Canada/ Association des infirmières et infirmiers cliniciens specialisés du Canada (CNS-C/ICS-C) and the Canadian Federation for Mental Health Nurses.

Fulton, Lyon, and Goudreau (2014) described developmental differences between an experienced RN and a CNS pertaining to the "breadth and depth of the specialty area, clinical practice, **system leadership**, the understanding of inner self, emotions and inner leadership, ethical practice, and professional practice and affiliation" (p. 19). One key difference is the CNS consultation role and system leadership skills related to coaching, mentoring, and analysis of ethical issues.

The CNS specific core competencies include clinical care, system leadership, and advancement of nursing practice, evaluation, and research (CNA, 2014; see Figure 22.1). Canada's APN framework was recently published with six categories of competencies: (1) direct comprehensive care, (2) healthy system optimization, (3) education, (4) research, (5) leadership, and (6) consultation and collaboration (CNA, 2019). The CNS competencies, as part of APN, are also embedded in the framework regardless of the area of specialty and practice setting. In addition, the CNS-mental health provides both **direct** and **indirect care** and uses a variety of approaches and strategies in providing client-centred care, APN, system leadership, and evaluating and critically appraising nurse-sensitive outcomes (see Figure 22.1). The new competencies complement and enhance the CNS-specific competencies and provide a pathway to elaborate, reconstruct, and build stronger pillars on them.

Clinical Care

In order to provide client-centred care, the CNS-mental health integrates trauma-informed practice in conjunction with holistic and public health nursing approaches, as well as psychotherapeutic care, the nursing process, and broad theoretical mental approaches. The integration of trauma-informed practice enables the CNS-mental health to apply the advanced knowledge of pathophysiology within the context of the ripple effect of a traumatic event on the physical, emotional, mental, spiritual, and relationship aspects of the client's life. The knowledge of the impact of a traumatic event on regulating emotions, manifestation of trauma through feelings of shame, guilt, powerlessness, helplessness, self-esteem, and loss of identity become an integral part of the therapeutic intervention. An essential component of developing a care plan with the client is the identification of the client's strengths, resilience, meaning, and goals.

The CNS-mental health promotes mental health/mental wellness by integrating public health care approaches and the social determinants of mental health in clinical practice. The evidence demonstrates that key determinants of mental health are employment, education, housing and income, supportive relationships (peer), involvement in social activities, community engagement, and freedom from discrimination and stigma (CMHA, 2014; World Health Organization [WHO], 2004, 2015). Many Canadians living with mental health problems and mental illness fail to experience these key determinants of health and therefore have difficulties achieving goals to increase resilience and decrease risk factors.

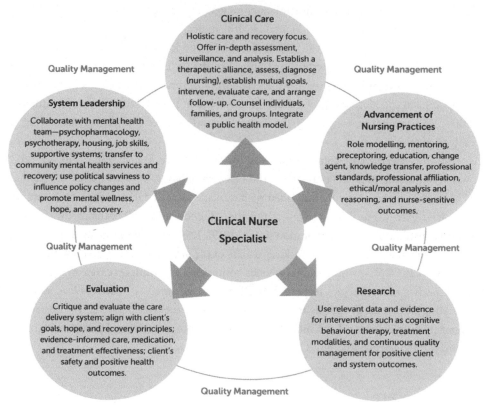

FIGURE 22.1: Clinical Nurse Specialist: Domains, Role, and Functions

This figure describes the domains of clinical care, advancement of nursing practice, research, evaluation, and system leadership as they pertain to the roles and functions of the clinical nurse specialist with the focus of a quality management perspective.

Source: Muxlow, J. (2014).

The direct and indirect care provided by the CNS-mental health is grounded in cultural competence, which integrates the client's ways of knowing and doing, and the meaning of care, the reality of the client's life, as well as the ability to engage and interact effectively with the client regardless of the client's mental health status. The CNS incorporates best practices and critical analysis during the holistic assessment, monitoring, and intervention phases of care to achieve positive health care outcomes. Likewise, the CNS applies system-level and leadership skills when consulting and collaborating with other health professionals to improve the health of the population.

Direct Care

The CNS-mental health utilizes a holistic model (see Figure 22.2) demonstrating expert knowledge, skills and competencies, integrating values and beliefs, building interpersonal relationships and therapeutic alliance (trust, respect, dignity, engagement, and communication skills), and analyzing the social and cultural determinants of health so that they are

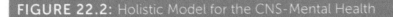

FIGURE 22.2: Holistic Model for the CNS-Mental Health

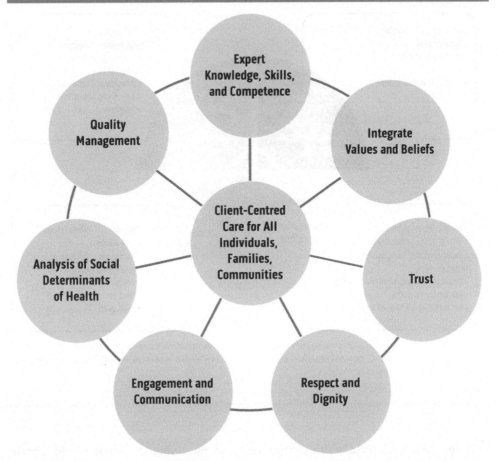

This figure illustrates the components of holistic care used by the CNS-mental health to provide client-centred care to individuals, families, and communities.

Source: Muxlow, J. (2014).

meaningful to the client. Knowledge of political competence is also required to navigate both the internal and external mental health care system for client safety and positive health care outcomes. Likewise, the CNS-mental health applies system-level and leadership skills when consulting and collaborating with other health professionals to improve the health of the population.

The percentage of the CNS-mental health's practice activities related to direct care varies with the organization and practice setting. Components of direct care provided include comprehensive holistic assessment (i.e., validation, implementation, and evaluation) with a systematic approach using problem-solving skills and techniques to manage a wide range of clients with compounding mental, physical, social, and economic issues. Direct care also includes monitoring the effect of medication(s); counselling (individual, families, and group); co-therapy with other health professionals; crisis intervention and stabilization; and psycho-educational activities related to promoting mental health, wellness, and recovery. Knowledge

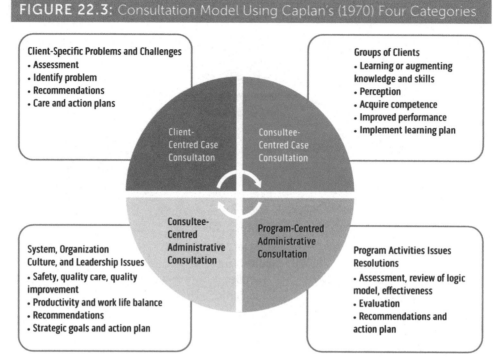

FIGURE 22.3: Consultation Model Using Caplan's (1970) Four Categories

This figure uses Caplan's (1970) four categories of consultation with additional clarifications of CNS activities related to client-specific problems, system, organization culture, and leadership issues, as well as groups of clients and programs activity issues and resolutions.

Source: Adapted by Muxlow, J. (2014).

and application of public health nursing enhances the ability to address complex health care–related issues, health care inequities, and social justice issues while providing direct care. In addition, the CNS-mental health incorporates clinical inquiry, system theory, and research to evaluate and critically appraise nurse-sensitive outcomes and continuous quality-improvement initiatives under the umbrella of quality management. Other relevant aspects of practice include working with clients to attain goals and to promote positive mental health care activities to achieve mental wellness, hope, and recovery. This is accomplished by integrating knowledge and information gained through engagement and communication into policy and clinical guidelines whenever there are identifiable risks for client safety, quality care, continuous quality improvement, and positive health care outcomes.

The evidence of the increasing need for mental health care services discussed earlier in the chapter demonstrates the need for the CNS-mental health to continue to advocate for a full scope of practice in hospital and community mental health care settings. At the forefront of the mental health care system, the CNS's practice is improving the health care status of clients whose health and well-being are compromised as a result of physical, emotional, and psychosocial problems with or without complex and persistent mental health care issues and concurrent disorders.

Indirect Care

Consultation and Collaboration

Consultation and collaboration are two key components of any CNS's indirect practice. It is important to differentiate between providing direct care to clients with complex health care issues and providing consultation on complex and persistent mental health care issues to health care providers and decision makers. Depending on the practice setting, both direct and indirect health care fall under the CNS role. It is also important to acknowledge that the CNS-mental health becomes a consultee with the psychiatrist, pharmacist, and other health care team members when addressing risk management and psychopharmacology issues. At this time, prescribing rights are not available to CNSs working in the Canadian health care system, although they are generally available to the larger community of CNSs practicing in the United States and mental health nurses in the United Kingdom (Hemingway & Ely, 2009; MacLure et al., 2014).

Consultation is interwoven in all aspects of the CNS role. Keltner, Schwecke, and Bostrom (1999) defined consultation as an interactive process between two professionals to discuss a work-related problem at the individual, family, group, program, or system level. This core competency is widely acknowledged in the CNS community (CNA, 2008; National Association of Clinical Nurse Specialist [NACNS], 2010).

The CNS-mental health functions as an expert consultant in psychiatric/mental health care nursing and is instrumental in assisting nurses and mental health care practitioners in addressing complex and persistent mental health issues within or outside their own full scope of practice. Inherent is having a clear understanding of the issues, knowledge, skills, and competence in teaching and learning techniques, issues management and resolution, and individual, group, and system dynamics. The CNS-mental health provides advanced knowledge when consultation is requested by a health care provider for an issue or a problem that is outside the health care provider's scope of practice or level of competence. Erchul and ABPP (2009) described Caplan's four types of mental health consultation (see Figure 22.3).

Keltner, Schwecke, and Bostrom (1991) found that the psychiatric consultant nurse used their expertise to provide three types of consultation: patient-focused, consultee-focused, and system- or organization-focused and listed the following as key factors in the consultation process:

- Consultant should be in a staff position rather than a supervisor/management position to promote open communication.
- Consultees accept the consultant's recommendations with free will.
- Issues addressed are work-related and remain professional, not personal.
- Consultee remains responsible for the client.
- Consultant and consultee develop a professional peer relationship for problem-solving rather than one of the staff supervisor/managers. (p. 152)

In the Canadian health care system, the CNS-mental health provides consultation mainly on an informal basis without the formal contractual agreement advocated by Caplan (1963). In a publicly funded in-patient mental health care setting, the CNS-mental health provides consultation services as a member of the mental health care team in the organization. There may be variation from province to province based on provincial mandates, outreach services affiliated with the organization, service delivery contracts, and memorandum of understanding for clinical mental health care services between the health authority and specific community health care agencies. The CNS affiliated with a community-based mental health care setting may extend consultation services to include interprovincial organizations such as correctional services and community health care centres within the catchment or zone area.

Regardless of the type of consultation and principles adhered to during the consultation process, Keltner et al. (1991) describe six phases of the consultation process, which are like the nursing process, as:

1. Opening and contracting: clarification of roles, expectations, anticipated outcomes and contractual agreement;
2. Assessment and diagnosis: perceptions of the issue, previous interventions and current expectations;
3. Setting of specific, realistic and time sensitive mutually agreed goals with recommended actions and anticipated outcomes;
4. Implementation of the recommended actions performed by the consultee;
5. Evaluation of outcomes: assess for goal attainment and anticipated outcomes; and
6. Closing, disconnecting and documentation. (p. 158)

The CNS-mental health has the unique opportunity to facilitate formal and informal consultations of all types for both health care and non-health care staff, policy-makers, and administrators whose portfolios have an indirect effect on clients with mental health care problems and illness. The CNS-mental health uses evidence to augment knowledge to influence policy development and changes at the local and political level, and contributes to mental wellness initiatives to improve client health care outcomes. The areas of consultation include but are not limited to suicide prevention, crisis intervention and crisis stabilization, safety and use of restraints, capacity building in communities, staff professional development, and promoting community wellness across the lifespan.

Collaboration is also a function of the CNS's indirect care practice. The CNS-mental health works collaboratively with members of the interprofessional team to meet the client's desired goals and is a part of the mental health care team. Case management is utilized that facilitates collaboration among health care sectors and community agencies in advocating for health care, services, and support to meet the client's identified biopsychosocial, and cultural needs. It also focuses on the client's strengths and holistic approaches in the collaborative relationship with the client, families, and mental health care team. An integral component to collaboration is the coordination of care and services on a continuum for client safety (personal and environmental), and the promotion of mental wellness and recovery.

Open communication with colleagues, other health care sectors, and community agencies and the ability to appreciate each team member's contribution is essential in a collaborative relationship.

CASE STUDY

The Story of Jay

Jay, a 38-year-old male who lives in a small halfway house, was admitted to the in-patient unit two weeks ago with a psychotic episode. The information documented on his intake assessment included a CT scan to rule out a brain tumour. He has had a supra pubic catheter in situ for the last three months. In the past, he has been treated for substance misuse; his drug of choice was opioid, and he had been on an antidepressant for the past year. A home and community care nurse visits him at the group home once per week.

Mary, the CNS-mental health, assesses and evaluates Jay's current mental health status, milieu, and psychopharmacology interventions effects. Mary feels that a holistic model of care that is respectful is foundational to working with Jay. She works collaboratively with the halfway house staff, home and community care, addiction services, and other members of the in-patient mental health care team to address Jay's primary and mental health care needs

Mary used knowledge, skills, and knowledge transfer for a comprehensive assessment, interpersonal skills for interactions and relationships with Jay and the interprofessional team, and political competence for consulting with the addiction health care sector.

Jay's neurological scan was normal. Mary considered that the management of a psychotic episode should include insight-oriented therapy, diagnostic and laboratory results. Jay will be returned to the halfway house in two weeks. Case management and discharge planning processes commenced for follow-up and positive outcomes. A plan for his return home was developed and implemented in collaboration with Jay, home and community care, members of the in-patient health care team, and addiction services.

System Leadership

The CNS-mental health requires knowledge on addiction and the interrelationship between mental health, addiction, and chronic physical diseases. The evidence on mental health, mental illness, and addiction published by the MHCC (2012) strengthens the call for changes and transformation of the current mental health care system. The mental health care system is a complex open system with competing inputs and outputs that feed back into the environment. The system provides services and/or programs for clients across the lifespan, although the level of service or program varies from province to province. Programs and/or services are provided in an acute care unit, general psychiatric unit, assessment and short-stay unit, specialized units for clients with serious and persistent mental illness, forensic units, and community-based clinics/health care centres with or without assertive and intensive community and mobile crisis teams.

The current emphasis and initiatives on mental health, mental illness, and mental health care strategies provincially, nationally, and globally target mental health care promotion and prevention, and the reduction of health care inequities. The CNS-mental health, as a transformational leader and change agent, leads and influences changes within the system for continuous quality improvement, promoting mental wellness and fostering recovery.

The CNS-mental health influences and leads change at a clinical level, program level, and a system level. Interpersonal and communication skills are central to motivate, inspire, and influence system changes. At the clinical level, the CNS-mental health facilitates collaboration with the interprofessional team across health care services and sectors in promoting teaching and learning for safe quality care and positive health care outcomes. In addition, the CNS-mental health creates an environment for the professional growth of the health care team through role modelling, mentoring, and team building.

At the program level, the CNS-mental health analyzes and synthesizes evidence and leads the development and implementation of clinical guidelines and policies for continuous quality improvement. Similar processes are used with the addition of program management skills to develop and implement programs and activities such as mental wellness, managing symptoms, suicide prevention, managing behaviour, and stress management.

At the system level, the CNS-mental health conducts environmental scans and uses other evaluation tools to evaluate gaps in the system that affect client and staff safety, presents findings to senior management, and develops strategies to reduce risk and enhance quality management. System leadership, within a mental health care setting, includes the promotion of a safe environment and maintaining a supportive and healthy work environment. The CNS-mental health intervenes by creating a safe space (physical and emotional) through open communication, shared power, activities that foster hope, peer support, and provision of required tools and resources, therapeutic milieu, psychoeducation, negotiation, and policy.

Advancing Practice Nursing

The CNS-mental health, as a member of the interprofessional mental health care team, advances nursing practice through role modelling, mentoring, and coaching. The CNS-mental health demonstrates the importance of professional development through continuous learning, professionalism, ethical and moral conduct in keeping with nursing standards of practice and code of ethics, reflective practice, professional affiliation, and academic affiliation. The CNS-mental health utilizes knowledge and evidence to facilitate learning with clients and families, mentoring members of the interprofessional team, and as a preceptor for undergraduate and graduate students.

It is important to recognize different learning styles and tailor teaching principles and techniques to accommodate learners' needs. The CNS-mental health, as an educator, assesses the learner's readiness, motivating factors, and is flexible in approaches to engaging the client or staff member. Two key success factors include understanding the learner's readiness for change and applying adult learning principles when working with adults.

The CNS-mental health mentors staff members using formal or informal processes on an ongoing basis to acquire knowledge, skills, and competencies. Mentoring occurs in assessment and evaluation of anticipated outcomes, and the provision of treatment modalities and liaising with other health care disciplines internally or externally across the continuum of care.

Evaluation and Research

The CNS-mental health researches, retrieves, critically appraises, and synthesizes systematic reviews and other research literature relevant to mental health care and addiction as part of their competencies. Evidence is integrated into clinical practice for assessments, interventions, developing strategies, quality management, and evaluation of positive health care outcomes. Interventions include strategies used in case management and building therapeutic relationships.

In addition, the CNS-mental health utilizes evidence from a variety of key data sources such as Statistics Canada's Community Health Survey, the Canadian Institute of Health Information (CIHI), RNAO's Best Practice Guidelines related to mental health, the Centre for Addiction and Mental Health, and the Mental Health Commission of Canada to shape interventions, outcome evaluation, policy revisions, and program redesign. It is essential that the CNS-mental health demonstrates competence to measure and evaluate health care outcomes.

The CNS-mental health, as a system leader, utilizes research and evaluations to demonstrate cost analysis and cost containment related to safe quality care and positive health outcomes. Leading and/or participating in research at the organization level and/or the university level is important as well as engaging and disseminating evidence as a knowledge translator to members of the interprofessional team through face-to-face presentations, journal clubs, video conferences, and publications in organizational newsletters and nursing journals.

Conclusion

The CNS-mental health is involved in creating a safe environment for the client and staff through the creation of therapeutic relationships and the promotion of positive mental health and recovery. Promoting positive mental health requires that the CNS-mental health appraise, synthesize, and apply evidence that informs practice utilizing a client-centred, holistic-based model of health care, and develops and implements initiatives and strategies that would increase protective factors, reduce risk factors, and foster resilience.

The CNS-mental health demonstrates specialized knowledge, skills, and competence at the expert level as a role model, mentor, and a consultant to members of the interprofessional team for complex mental, physical, and addiction issues. The CNS-mental health also utilizes advanced and specialized knowledge and skills for problem-solving, ethical dilemmas, and issues resolution.

The pillars of the CNS-mental health practice are the CNS core competencies whereby quality management is interwoven through every aspect of care and service delivery. The CNS-mental health is required to demonstrate in-depth knowledge, skills, and competencies in pathophysiology, psychotherapeutic approaches, and psychopharmacology in addressing the stigma, system inefficiencies, and complex and persistent issues within a health care setting.

Finally, the CNS-mental health leads and influences change in the health care system that supports the client in achieving their goals and health care outcomes through transformational leadership. The CNS-mental health promotes best practices, evidence-informed care, and client safety to advance the nursing profession by developing clinical guidelines, policies and protocols, and measurement tools for continuous quality improvement. As a transformational leader, the CNS develops and implements initiatives that align with the organization's strategic goals for positive health care outcomes.

Critical Thinking Questions

1. Analyze and evaluate the impact of the CNS-mental health role in a health care setting. What are the linkages to a holistic model of care, client safety, advancing nursing care, and quality improvement?
2. A client living with a mental illness and co-occurring addiction issues is admitted to a mental health unit. What theoretical framework would determine the practice of a CNS-mental health with this client? Why?
3. A mental health nurse is working with Jay, the client identified in the case study. Describe how you would implement the consultant role of the CNS.

References

Canadian Alliance on Mental Illness and Mental Health (CAMIMH). (2016). *Mental health now! Advancing the mental health of Canadians: The federal role.* Ottawa, ON: CAMIMH. Retrieved from https://www.camimh.ca/wp-content/uploads/2016/09/CAMIMH_MHN_EN_Final_small.pdf

Canadian Mental Health Association (CMHA). (2014). *Social determinants of health: Enabling minds.* Toronto, ON: CMHA. Retrieved from http://www.enablingminds.ca/resource-library/managers-guide/social-determinants-mental-health/#.XiUtw8hKjcc

CMHA. (2018). Concurrent mental illness and substance use problems. Toronto, ON: CMHA. Retrieved from https://cmha.ca/documents/concurrent-mental-illness-and-substance-use-problems

CMHA. (2020). *Mental illness and addiction: Facts and statistics.* Toronto, ON: CMHA. Retrieved from
    https://www.camh.ca/en/driving-change/the-crisis-is-real/mental-health-statistics

Canadian Nurses Association (CNA). (2008). *Advanced nursing practice: A national framework.* Ot-
    tawa, ON: CNA. Retrieved from https://www.cna-aiic.ca/en/~/media/nurseone/page-content/
    pdf-en/anp_national_framework_e

CNA. (2014). *Pan-Canadian core competencies for the clinical nurse specialist.* Ottawa, ON: CNA. Retrieved
    from http://cna-aiic.ca/~/media/cna/files/en/clinical_nurse_specialists_convention_handout_e.pdf

CNA. (2019). *Advanced practice nursing: A pan-Canadian framework.* Ottawa, ON: CNA. Retrieved from
    https://www.cna-aiic.ca/-/media/cna/page-content/pdf-en/advanced-practice-nursing-framework-en.pdf

Caplan, G. (1963). Types of mental health consultation. *American Journal of Orthopsychiatry, 33*(3),
    470–481.

Employment and Social Development Canada. (2016). *Psychological health in the workplace.* Ottawa,
    ON: Government of Canada. Retrieved from https://www.canada.ca/en/employment-social-deve-
    lopment/services/health-safety/reports/psychological-health.html

Erchul, W. P., & ABPP. (2009). Gerald Caplan: A tribute to the originator of mental health consultation.
    Journal of Educational and Psychological Consultation, 19, 95–105. doi: 10, 1080/10474410902888418

Fulton, J. S., Lyon, B. L., & Goudreau, K. (Eds.). (2014). *Foundations of clinical nurse specialist nurse
    practice* (2nd ed.). New York, NY: Springer.

Hemingway, S. J., & Ely, V. (2009). Prescribing by mental health nurses: The UK perspective. *Perspec-
    tives in Psychiatric Care, 45*(1), 24–35.

Keltner, N. L., Schwecke, L. H., & Bostrom, C. E. (1991). *Psychiatric nursing: A psychotherapeutic ma-
    nagement approach.* St. Louis, MO: Mosby.

Keltner, N. L., Schwecke, L. H., & Bostrom, C. E. (1999). *Psychiatric nursing* (3rd ed.). St. Louis,
    MO: Mosby. Retrieved from https://www.archive.org/stream/psychiatricnursi00kelt#page/340/
    mode/2up

Lang, J. J., Alam, S., Cahill, L. E., Drucker, A. M., Gotay, C., Kayibanda, J. F., ... Orpana, H. M. (2018).
    Global burden of disease study trends for Canada from 1990 to 2016. *Canadian Medical Association
    Journal, 190*(44), E1296–E1304. doi: 10.1503/cmaj.180698

MacLure, K., Johnson, G., Diack, L., Bond, C., Cunningham, S., & Stewart, D. (2014). Views of the Scot-
    tish general public on non-medical prescribing. *International Journal of Clinical Pharmacy, 35*(5),
    704–710. doi: 10.1007/s11096-013-9792-x

Mental Health Commission of Canada (MHCC). (2009). *Toward recovery & well-being: A framework
    for a mental health strategy for Canada.* Ottawa, ON: MHCC. Retrieved from https://www.mental-
    healthcommission.ca/sites/default/files/FNIM_Toward_Recovery_and_Well_Being_ENG_0_1.pdf

MHCC. (2012). *Changing directions changing lives: The mental health strategy for Canada.* Ottawa, ON:
    MHCC. Retrieved from https://www.mentalhealthcommission.ca/sites/default/files/MHStrategy_
    Strategy_ENG.pdf

MHCC. (2017). *Strengthening the case for investing in Canada's mental health system, economic consi-
    derations.* Ottawa, ON: MHCC. Retrieved from https://www.mentalhealthcommission.ca/sites/de-
    fault/files/2017-03/case_for_investment_eng.pdf

National Association of Clinical Nurse Specialist (NACNS). (2010). *Clinical nurse specialist core com-
    petencies: Executive summary 2006–2008. The National CNS Competency Task Force.* Wakefield,
    MA: NACNS. Retrieved from https://www.nacns.org/wp-content/uploads/2017/01/CNSCoreCom-
    petenciesBroch.pdf

Public Health Agency of Canada (PHAC). (2019a). *Joint statement from the co-chairs of the special advisory committee on the epidemic of opioid overdoses on new data related to the opioid crisis.* Ottawa, ON: PHAC. Retrieved from https://www.canada.ca/en/public-health/news/2019/12/joint-statement-from-the-co-chairs-of-the-special-advisory-committee-on-the-epidemic-of-opioid-overdoses-on-new-data-related-to-the-opioid-crisis.html

PHAC. (2019b). *Suicide in Canada: Key statistics.* Ottawa, ON: PHAC. Retrieved from https://www.canada.ca/content/dam/phac-aspc/documents/services/publications/healthy-living/suicide-canada-key-statistics-infographic/pub-eng.pdf

Statistics Canada. (2018). *A demographic, employment and income profile of Canadians with disabilities aged 15 years and over, 2017.* Ottawa, ON: Statistics Canada. Retrieved from https://www150.statcan.gc.ca/n1/pub/89-654-x/89-654-x2018002-eng.htm

World Health Organization (WHO). (2004). *Promoting mental health: Concepts, emerging evidence, practice: Summary report.* Geneva, CH: WHO. Retrieved from http://www.who.int/mental_health/evidence/en/promoting_mhh.pdf

WHO. (2015). *Mental health: Strengthening our response. Media Fact Sheet, No 220.* Geneva, CH: WHO. Retrieved from http://www.who.int/mediacentre/factsheets/fs220/en/

Chapter 23

Clinical Nurse Specialist: Ambulatory Care

Jennifer Price

JENNIFER PRICE is Chief Nursing and Professional Practice Executive at Women's College Hospital, Toronto, Ontario. She has held roles as both a clinical nurse specialist (CNS) and an acute care nurse practitioner (ACNP) at Women's College Hospital's Women's Cardiovascular Health Initiative. Jennifer has focused on evaluating the clinical efficacy of the cardiac rehabilitation and primary prevention program designed specifically for women, including behavioural therapy for depression.

KEY TERMS

ambulatory care
ambulatory care nursing
  (ACN)
chronic disease management
self-management
self-management support

OBJECTIVES

1. Define ambulatory care nursing.
2. Explore the rationale for ambulatory care.
3. Explore the role of the clinical nurse specialist (CNS) in ambulatory care.

Introduction

To understand the role of advanced practice nurses (APNs) in **ambulatory care**, we need to consider the roots of ambulatory care. This chapter will explore the shift from in-patient to ambulatory care and highlight the importance of the clinical nurse specialist (CNS) as a key provider in the ambulatory setting.

The Shift to Ambulatory Care

Shifting health care services to the community has been a long-standing political priority in Canada (Royal College of Nursing [RCN], 2014; van Soeren, Hurlock-Chorostecki, Pogue, & Sanders, 2008). With our population living longer, more people are living with comorbidities and require ongoing complex interventions, which they prefer to receive within their own community (Rich, Lipson, Libersky, & Parchman, 2012; Vlasses & Smeltzer, 2007). Rapid changes in the provision of care such as evidence-based pre- and post-operative care have decreased hospital length of stay and moved care out of the hospital and into the ambulatory setting. Transitioning health care out of acute care facilities into the ambulatory setting not only delivers positive health outcomes but also frees up hospital beds and resources to provide the most acute and specialized care to individuals with high acuity levels (Negley, Cordes, Evenson, & Schad, 2016).

The shift to increasing ambulatory volumes occurred over time, but the early 1990s saw a definite movement of care from the hospital setting into the community. Several factors have contributed to the expansion of ambulatory care services. Financial policies during the late 1980s and early 1990s dictated the closing of acute care hospital beds, causing patients to be discharged earlier into the community (Canadian Institute for Health Information [CIHI], 2005; Hastings, 1986; Katz, Martens, Chateau, Bogdanovic, & Koseva, 2014). These patients were often acute and required more intensive care in the community. Fortunately, as fiscal caps for hospital care moved patients into the ambulatory care setting, advances in technology enabled more care and diagnostics to be delivered through minimally invasive or non-invasive procedures (Vlasses & Smeltzer, 2007). Pharmacotherapy has also evolved as a treatment that can more easily be managed in the ambulatory setting allowing, for example, the management of post-operative pain at home or the infusion of intravenous antibiotics (Nevius & D'Arcy, 2008). In addition, improved technology has facilitated the management of care by becoming seamless and portable through the use of electronic patient records (Vlasses & Smeltzer, 2007).

Today, most health care in Canada occurs outside hospital walls. This applies to both physician services and services provided by other health care practitioners, including nurses. While this seems obvious as the Canadian health care system is widely acknowledged for having a strong primary care focus, what is not as well understood is the increasing volume of specialty care, including surgery, interventional procedures, and diagnostics delivered in the community (Katz et al., 2014).

The CIHI reports on hospital stays and ambulatory care visits within the hospital sector using the National Ambulatory Care Reporting System (see Figure 23.1). This contains data for day surgery, outpatient and community-based clinics, and emergency departments. Ambulatory, as well as emergency care, is one of the largest volume patient activities in the country, which makes it a significant health care service in Canada (CIHI, 2019). In 2019, the CIHI found that hospitals continued their shift to outpatient care with growth in ambulatory care (74%) and community health care services (140%) outpacing nursing in-patient services (60%) since 2005–2006 (CIHI, 2019).

In relation to complex care, as technology and treatments have improved, people with cancer are relying more on ambulatory cancer services for diagnosis and treatment, and even incorporating supportive services. In Canada, the shift to community-based cancer care and ambulatory services has significantly expanded. As an example, more than half of all

FIGURE 23.1: The Continuing Shift from In-patient to Outpatient Care

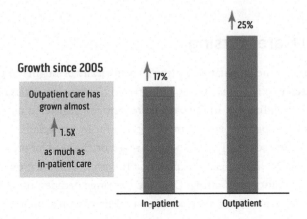

Growth since 2005

Outpatient care has grown almost

↑ 1.5X

as much as in-patient care

↑ 17% In-patient

↑ 25% Outpatient

Cases are becoming more complex

2013–2014 to 2017–2018

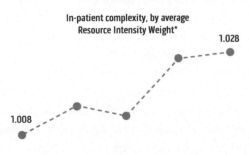

In-patient complexity, by average Resource Intensity Weight*

1.008 ... 1.028

2013–2014   2014–2015   2015–2016   2016–2017   2017–2018

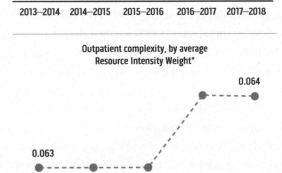

Outpatient complexity, by average Resource Intensity Weight*

0.063 ... 0.064

2013–2014   2014–2015   2015–2016   2016–2017   2017–2018

Note: *Resource Intensity Weight is based on the 2018 Case Mix Group+ (CMG+) and the 2018 Comprehensive Ambulatory Classification System (CACS) methodologies.

Source: CIHI. (2019). *Hospital spending: The continuing shift from inpatient to outpatient care.* Ottawa, ON: CIHI. Retrieved from https://www.cihi.ca/en/the-continuing-shift-from-inpatient-to-outpatient-care

chemotherapy is delivered outside of hospitals in Ontario, British Columbia, and Alberta, which provides better access to cancer care services that are close to home (Garland, 2015).

Ambulatory Care Nursing

Mastal (2010) describes the ambulatory setting as historically belonging to physicians. Most outpatients were seen in physicians' offices and referred to other specialties or different levels of service such as hospitalization. In the past, there were few registered nurses (RNs) in ambulatory care settings as patients were primarily cared for by physicians. As health care has shifted to the ambulatory setting from the acute care sector, the need for professional **ambulatory care nursing (ACN)** has increased exponentially with a resultant growth in the number of nurses in the ambulatory care setting. Over the last three decades, these nurses have also grown in their ability to distinguish themselves as a specialty with a unique set of skills (Mastal, 2010) as evidenced by the two associations founded by professional ambulatory nurses.

ACN has been recognized as a specialty nursing role in the United States for several decades with their professional group, the American Academy of Ambulatory Care Nursing (AAACN), founded in 1978 as an educational forum for administrators. Today, membership is open to all nurses, as well as other health professionals who are interested in ambulatory care and telehealth nursing (AAACN, 2014).

In 2012, the Canadian Association of Ambulatory Care (CAAC) was founded to highlight the groundbreaking work in ambulatory care in Canada. The CAAC provides a forum for all professionals working in any area of ambulatory care to share their knowledge and skills through networking and education (CAAC, 2012). Both organizations define ACN in similar ways, stating that these professionals care for individuals, families, groups, communities, and populations. The setting for ambulatory nursing is distinctively different from other nurses as they practice in the home, primary and specialty outpatient venues, and non-acute surgical and diagnostic outpatient settings, all in the community.

The patient flow in ambulatory care is vastly different from the hospital setting. ACN is characterized by RNs caring for high volumes of patients in a relatively short time period (always less than 24 hours), dealing with issues that can be both unknown and unpredictable. While assessments can be rapid and focused, the nurse/patient/family relationships are typically developed over the long term. Unlike in the hospital, the ambulatory care nurse frequently works in isolation. While they may provide direct patient care, the ambulatory care nurse is more likely to be an organizer or manager of care, directing patients in self-care or helping them make behavioural changes. The ambulatory care nurse addresses patients' wellness, acute illness, chronic issues, and end-of-life requirements. These nurses are patient advocates, navigators, and coordinators of all health care (AAACN, 2014, 2017; CAAC, 2012). This type of working environment requires a strong clinical background, leadership skills, and an autonomous critical thinking ability.

Nurses in the community often work with fewer resources, making it more difficult to receive feedback from a nursing colleague. In addition, ambulatory care nurses interact with patients face to face and via telephone or internet. This lack of direct contact with patients often demands different assessment and communication skills, as such, the direct, non-verbal sensory input of facial expressions and body language is lost.

With the increasing complexity of the care required, the AAACN recognizes the requirement for all levels of nursing in the ambulatory setting, including the APN roles of the nurse practitioner (NP), CNS, and nurse researcher (AAACN, 2014).

The Role of the APN in Ambulatory Care

Throughout history, nurses have developed, refocused, and expanded their roles to meet patient and population requirements. The emergence of APNs, which include both the CNS and the NP, is an excellent example of this. A more recent example is the emergence of APNs in the ambulatory setting. Specifically, there has been widespread adoption of the CNS in chronic disease management. With their advanced preparation and clinical expertise, they are well positioned to provide education, clinical care, guidance, and support care given by families and other providers as well (Abraham & Norful, 2019).

At the heart of chronic disease management is self-management, a term used widely in the health care literature with no gold standard definition (Barlow, Wright, Sheasby, Turner, & Hainsworth, 2002). Self-management includes the work individuals assume to live well with their ongoing medical conditions. This includes physical tasks as well as role management and the confidence to carry out this work (Adams, Greiner, Corrigan, & Institute of Medicine, 2004).

Self-management support is critical to the development of self-management and emphasizes the patient's central role in managing and being responsible for their health because the locus of responsibility rests with them. In addition, self-management support involves collaborative relationships with patients and their families and goes beyond the provision of education and support. Patients and providers work together to define problems/barriers, develop priorities, and set goals while the provider offers problem-solving support and strategies to build confidence. While self-management support can be provided by a variety of health care professionals, APNs in ambulatory care are ideally positioned to provide self-management support to their patients and families.

Self-management approaches have been shown to have positive impacts on the well-being of individuals with chronic illness (Barlow et al., 2000, 2002; Warsi, Wang, LaValley, Avorn, & Solomon, 2004). In addition, Lorig's work suggests improved health behaviour, health status, and decreased health care use in patients participating in a chronic disease self-management program (CDSMP; Lorig & Holman, 2003; Lorig, Ritter, Laurent, & Fries, 2004; Lorig, Ritter, Laurent, & Plant, 2008; Lorig & Visser, 1994).

Several studies have specifically examined the role of APNs in ambulatory care as they provide self-management support or assist patients' transition to the home setting. A randomized controlled trial in patients with rheumatoid arthritis compared a CNS ambulatory intervention with in-patient care and a multidisciplinary daycare team. No significant differences were identified between the groups during the two-year follow-up with the exception that visits to the CNS occurred more often and home help was less frequent in this group.

The authors concluded that the CNS intervention was effective in this patient population and a useful alternative to other multidisciplinary strategies in the setting of the complex care requirements of individuals with rheumatoid arthritis (Tijhuis, Zwinderman, Hazes, Breedveld, & Vlieland, 2003).

Brooten et al. (2001) examined prenatal, infant, and maternal outcomes over a one-year period post-delivery where half the prenatal care was delivered in the home by CNSs. Results showed that the group cared for in the home by the CNS had fewer fetal/infant deaths, fewer preterm infants, and fewer re-hospitalizations. The researchers also identified that the CNS prenatal home care saved hospital days, which translated to a cost savings of $2.5 million during that year.

Brooten, Youngblut, Deatrick, Naylor, and York (2003) examined five clinical trials of APN interventions with the intent to describe the APN interventions, patient problems, and time and type of intervention. All the trials were examining APN transitional care, that is, comprehensive discharge planning and home follow-up. Groups with greater mean APN time and contacts per patient had better health outcomes and greater health care cost savings. Of all the APN interventions, surveillance was the most predominant in all patient populations, accounting for over 50% of the 150,131 interventions. Health teaching, guidance, and counselling were the second most frequent category of APN intervention in four of the five trials. Treatments and procedures accounted for less than 1% of all the interventions across all groups. Case management, the final category of interventions, accounted for 12–25% of the interventions, depending on the trial. The authors concluded that to provide this type of transitional care, APNs had to have advanced skills and competencies in assessment, collaboration, teaching, counselling, communications, and managing health behaviours. These trials support the value of the APN role in ambulatory care, demonstrating improved health care outcomes in the setting of improved cost savings.

CASE STUDY

The Story of Kety

Kety is a 40-year-old woman with a primary diagnosis of coronary artery disease who was referred to cardiac rehabilitation (CR) following her ST-elevation myocardial infarction (STEMI) and percutaneous coronary intervention (PCI). She was seen initially by the CNS for assessment and for decisions concerning which team members needed to be included in her care plan.

A review of Kety's history revealed that she had been recently well, but that in her late 20s and early 30s she had been followed for hypertension and hyperlipidemia. She increased her activity and with the assistance of a dietitian, lost 45 kg. This brought her blood pressure and cholesterol values within normal range.

She is a smoker and admits to occasional marijuana use. Kety has a significant family history of cardiac disease with both parents having been diagnosed with premature coronary artery disease as well as aunts, uncles, and cousins all with premature disease.

Two months before the consultation, Kety experienced 4 days of shortness of breath accompanied by heartburn. She then spent an entire day snowshoeing, followed by a large dinner, and subsequently awoke at 5 a.m. with crushing retrosternal chest pain. She presented to the emergency department and was taken for angiography where she was found to have 95% blockage of her right coronary artery.

Attempts to open the artery were unsuccessful and a decision was made to treat her medically. She continued to experience chest pain and 4 days later, a second angioplasty attempt was successful, at which time a drug-eluting stent was placed in the distal right coronary artery. She was discharged home and does not describe any chest pain or discomfort since the procedure, but reports an overwhelming feeling of fatigue and noted her heart "pounding" in her chest.

Today, Kety is alert and oriented, but appears anxious. She complains that she is unsure of what she should be doing for activity and feels that her clinicians judge her for her smoking and marijuana use. Initial vital signs are BP right arm sitting 120/80, apical HR 60, RR12; weight 84 kg, height 1.36 m, BMI 45.2, and waist circumference 94 cm. On physical examination, her air entry is equal to the bases and clear. She has normal heart sounds with no murmurs. She appears sad. Utilizing the Beck Depression Inventory screening tool reveals a score of 20 and it is noted she self-scores as pessimistic. A review of Kety's medications reveals she is taking acetylsalicylic acid, clopidogrel, metoprolol, rosuvastatin, pantoprazole, and nitroglycerin prn. She is not taking any over-the-counter medications and states that she is taking all her prescribed medications routinely.

An initial problem list for Kety included hypertension, hyperlipidemia, obesity, activity intolerance, anxiousness/frightfulness, and depression. While this seems like a routine problem list for a cardiac patient, we must consider Kety's age, which brings complexity to her care and supportive needs. From the literature, we understand that young women with coronary artery disease have different needs than their male counterparts, and research has shown that they may indeed have worse outcomes. Patients with complex medical and psychosocial issues are routinely assessed and treated in ambulatory care. Referrals to social work, pharmacy, and the dietitian are made.

The CNS focuses on assisting Kety in understanding and coming to terms with her diagnosis of coronary artery disease. This includes open discussions concerning medications to control her hypertension and hyperlipidemia. The importance of preventing blockage of her stent and the prevention of a secondary cardiac event were also addressed. Kety will benefit from ongoing follow-up to assist with self-management support. Learning how to recognize symptoms is an important surveillance skill that patients with chronic diseases require to help them manage their chronic condition. Developing healthy behaviours around exercise and nutrition will also be part of the long-term plan for Kety. Due to Kety's age, she was also referred to gynecology for expert advice concerning appropriate birth control and the management of her menses while on blood thinners.

Discussion

In the case study, the CNS utilizes many of the advanced skills described by Brooten et al. (2003). Assessment must be timely and focused as the individual is usually scheduled for a short appointment. Collaborating with the interprofessional health care team was critical to managing Kety's anxiety and fear in the outpatient setting as well as the diagnosis and treatment of medical issues. In Kety's case, health education and counselling were key to helping her understand her condition and work toward caring for herself to ensure the best quality of life.

While the CNS in ambulatory care can provide excellent self-management support, another important component of the role is teaching and coaching of nursing colleagues. This part of the practice is an excellent way to disseminate evidence-based practice to our health care colleagues. CNSs often act as role models for other nursing staff as well as conducting formal and informal education sessions. In Kety's case, her primary care nurses and physician were unaware of the unfavourable health care outcomes women with coronary disease face and the issue with excessive bleeding during menses due to her blood thinners. This was an important teaching moment for the CNS with the primary care colleagues.

Conclusion

In Canada, health care is shifting from in-patient acute care to a variety of outpatient ambulatory and community health care settings. This movement and shifting of resources have been a political priority in Canada since the 1980s. This shift has been facilitated by advancements in minimally invasive surgery, improved diagnostics, pharmaceutical therapies, and technology enhancing the transfer of patient information. These advancements in medical and health technology have also enabled the population to live longer. As a result, many more individuals are living longer with multiple complex comorbidities requiring ongoing complex care interventions.

The increasing complexity of patients being cared for in the ambulatory setting has resulted in the increased need for professional nursing care. These nurses have been able to articulate a unique realm of practice founded on two national ambulatory care organizations.

The role of APNs, including the CNS, in ambulatory care has grown as well, with research evidence to support improved health outcomes and health care cost savings in the setting of APN interventions. As health care continues to move out of the hospital, opportunities for APNs in ambulatory care will grow as they provide their expert skills in assessment, education, counselling, and research within this diverse and multi-faceted setting.

Critical Thinking Questions

1. What is the impact of the shift to ambulatory care on the health care system and/or patients/families?
2. What is the impact of the APN role in ambulatory care now, and what might you anticipate in the future?

References

Abraham, C. M., & Norful, A. A. (2019). Cost-effectiveness of advanced practice nurses compared to physician-led care for chronic diseases: A systematic review. *Nursing Economics, 37*(6), 293–305.

Adams, K. M., Greiner, A., Corrigan, J., & Institute of Medicine. (2004). *The 1st annual crossing the quality chasm summit: A focus on communities.* Washington, DC: National Academies Press.

American Academy of Ambulatory Care Nursing (AAACN). (2014). *About American Academy of Ambulatory Care Nursing.* Pitman, NJ: AAACN. Retrieved from https://aaacn.org

AAACN. (2017). American Academy of Ambulatory Care Nursing position statement: The role of the registered nurse in ambulatory care. *Nursing Economics, 29*(2), 1–9. Retrieved from https://www.aaacn.org/sites/default/files/documents/RNRolePositionPaper.pdf

Barlow, J. H., Turner, A. P., & Wright, C. C. (2000). A randomized controlled study of the Arthritis Self-Management Programme in the UK. *Health Education Research, 15*(6), 665–680.

Barlow, J., Wright, C., Sheasby, J., Turner, A., & Hainsworth, J. (2002). Self management approaches for people with chronic conditions: A review. *Patient Education and Counseling, 48*(2), 177–187.

Brooten, D., Youngblut, J. M., Brown, L., Finkler, S. A., Neff, D. F., & Madigan, E. (2001). A randomized trial of nurse specialist home care for women with high-risk pregnancies: Outcomes and costs. *American Journal of Managed Care, 7*(8), 793–803.

Brooten, D., Youngblut, J. M., Deatrick, J., Naylor, M., & York, R. (2003). Patient problems, advanced practice nurse (APN) interventions, time and contacts among five patient groups. *Journal of Nursing Scholarship, 35*(1), 73–79.

Canadian Association of Ambulatory Care (CAAC). (2012). *About CAAC.* Toronto, ON: CAAC. Retrieved from http://www.canadianambulatorycare.com/about-us.html

Canadian Institute for Health Information (CIHI). (2005). *Hospital trends in Canada: Results of a project to create a historical series of statistical and financial data for Canadian hospitals over twenty-seven years.* Ottawa, ON: CIHI.

CIHI. (2019). *Hospital spending: The continuing shift from inpatient to outpatient care.* Ottawa, ON: CIHI. Retrieved from https://www.cihi.ca/en/the-continuing-shift-from-inpatient-to-outpatient-care

Garland, S. (2015). *Health interventions in ambulatory cancer care centres.* Ottawa, ON: CADTH. Retrieved from https://www.cadth.ca/health-interventions-ambulatory-cancer-care-centres

Hastings, J. E. (1986). Organized ambulatory care in Canada: Health service organizations and community health centers. *Journal of Public Health Policy, 7*(2), 239–247.

Katz, A., Martens, P., Chateau, D., Bogdanovic, B., & Koseva, I. (2014). Do primary care physicians coordinate ambulatory care for chronic disease patients in Canada? *BoMed Central (BMC) Family Practice, 15*, 148. doi: 10.1186/1471-2296-15-148

Lorig, K. R., & Holman, H. (2003). Self-management education: History, definition, outcomes, and mechanisms. *Annals of Behavioral Medicine, 26*(1), 1–7.

Lorig, K. R., Ritter, P. L., Laurent, D. D., & Fries, J. F. (2004). Long-term randomized controlled trials of tailored-print and small-group arthritis self-management interventions. *Medical Care, 42*(4), 346–354.

Lorig, K. R., Ritter, P. L., Laurent, D. D., & Plant, K. (2008). The internet-based arthritis self-management program: A one-year randomized trial for patients with arthritis or fibromyalgia. *Arthritis and Rheumatism, 59*(7), 1009–1017. doi: 10.1002/art.23817

Lorig, K. R., & Visser, A. (1994). Arthritis patient education standards: A model for the future. *Patient Education and Counseling, 24*(1), 3–7.

Mastal, M. F. (2010). Ambulatory care nursing: Growth as a professional specialty. *Nursing Economics, 28*(4), 267–269.

Negley, K. D., Cordes, M. E., Evenson, L. K., & Schad, S. P. (2016). From hospital to ambulatory care: Realigning the practice of clinical nurse specialists. *Clinical Nurse Specialist, 30*(5), 271–276.

Nevius, K. S., & D'Arcy, Y. (2008). Decrease recovery time with proper pain management. *Nursing Management, 39*(11), 26–32. doi: 10.1097/01.NUMA.0000340815.21271.a2

Rich, E., Lipson, D., Libersky, J., & Parchman, M. (2012). *Coordinating care for adults with complex care needs in the patient-centered medical home: Challenges and solutions. White paper.* Rockville, MD: Agency for Healthcare Research and Quality.

Royal College of Nursing (RCN). (2014). *Moving care to the community: An international perspective.* London, UK: RCN. Retrieved from http://www.rcn.org.uk/__data/assets/pdf_file/0006/523068/12.13_Moving_care_to_the_community_an_international_perspective.pdf

Tijhuis, G. J., Zwinderman, A. H., Hazes, J. M., Breedveld, F. C., & Vlieland, P. M. (2003). Two-year follow-up of a randomized controlled trial of a clinical nurse specialist intervention, inpatient, and day patient team care in rheumatoid arthritis. *Journal of Advanced Nursing, 41*(1), 34–43.

van Soeren, M., Hurlock-Chorostecki, C., Pogue, P., & Sanders, J. (2008). Primary healthcare renewal in Canada: A glass half empty? *Healthcare Papers, 8*(2), 39–44.

Vlasses, F. R., & Smeltzer, C. H. (2007). Toward a new future for healthcare and nursing practice. *Journal of Nursing Administration, 37*(9), 375–380. doi: 10.1097/01.NNA.0000285140.19000.f5

Warsi, A., Wang, P. S., LaValley, M. P., Avorn, J., & Solomon, D. H. (2004). Self-management education programs in chronic disease: A systematic review and methodological critique of the literature. *Archives of Internal Medicine, 164*(15), 1641–1649.

Chapter 24

Nurse Practitioner: Family/All Ages

Laura Johnson and Jane MacDonald

LAURA JOHNSON has worked as a nurse practitioner since 2005. At present, she is working as an independent contractor with Bayshore Home Health in Winnipeg, Manitoba. Laura has taught extensively in undergraduate and graduate nursing education.

JANE MACDONALD has worked as a nurse practitioner since 2001. She recently transitioned from primary health care in Winnipeg, Manitoba, to long-term care in Vernon, British Columbia. Her urban-based primary care practice included patients across the lifespan with an emphasis on the elderly and chronic disease management. While most of her work involves clinical care of patients, she is also engaged in clinic-based quality improvement projects and precepting nurse practitioner students.

KEY TERMS

advanced practice nursing (APN)
core competencies
direct clinical care
primary health care nurse practitioner (PHCNP)

OBJECTIVES

1. Describe the role of the primary health care nurse practitioner (PHCNP).
2. Describe the key competencies fundamental to the nurse practitioner (NP) role.
3. Evaluate critical trends in the health care system and their implications for the PHCNP.
4. Explore the barriers and facilitators of PHCNP practice.
5. Engage in dialogue regarding the role of the PHCNP in the primary health care (PHC) setting.

Introduction

The **primary health care nurse practitioner (PHCNP)** has been one of the fastest-growing **advanced practice nursing (APN)** roles in Canada (Donald et al., 2010) and continued optimization is helping to further integrate it across all Canadian jurisdictions (Canadian Nurses Association [CNA], 2019). The role is also known as family/all ages, reflecting the population-based focus of the Canadian Nurse Practitioner Examination (CNPE). To be consistent with current nomenclature from the Canadian APN literature, the chapter will refer to the role as PHCNP.

PHCNPs apply advanced nursing and medical theory acquired for the provision of clinical care for all age groups and a wide variety of health conditions. While the foundation of the PHCNP role is **direct clinical care**, the non-clinical domains of consultation, collaboration, reflective practice, research, and leadership also define the role. Nurse practitioner (NP) **core competencies** developed by the CNA (2010a) provide guidance and structure for PHCNPs in the operationalization of the role. Federal and provincial governments, regulatory bodies, and grassroots initiatives also contribute to role actualization. The CNA's 2019 pan-Canadian framework supports a coordinated approach for APN implementation and integration while permitting flexibility among jurisdictions for role development.

Primary Health Care Nurse Practitioner Education

The educational entry to practice preparation of the PHCNP in Canada has fluctuated from post-baccalaureate diploma to a graduate degree (CNA, 2019; Kaasalainen et al., 2010). At present, NP education remains available at graduate and postgraduate levels with the minimum educational preparation being a graduate degree in nursing (CNA, 2019). The majority of NP educational programs in Canada focus on PHC. Core courses in NP educational programs' curricula include topics of roles and responsibilities, advanced health assessment, health promotion, diagnostic reasoning, pathophysiology, advanced pharmacology, and management of acute episodic and chronic health conditions across the lifespan (Canadian Council of Registered Nurse Regulators [CCRNR], 2015). The development of role competence and autonomy is a hallmark of NP curricula related to diagnostic reasoning and decision-making (Duff, 2019; Mick & Ackerman, 2000), where the legal authority to order diagnostic tests, treatments, and prescribe medication is within the NP scope of practice (CNA, 2019; Duff, 2019). Once advanced education has been completed, graduate NPs must pass a credentialing examination demonstrating NP competencies in order to obtain licensure for the jurisdiction in which they are pursuing employment. All jurisdictions in Canada have NP legislation and regulations in place (CNA, 2019). In most jurisdictions, graduates write the CNPE, which is administered by the provincial or territorial regulatory body. Reciprocity between jurisdictions for licensure exists except for British Columbia and Quebec, where the inclusion of an objective structured clinical exam is required (British Columbia College of Nursing Professionals [BCCNP], 2019; Ordre des infirmières et infirmiers du Québec [OIIQ], 2018).

The education of NPs consists of academic as well as extensive clinical experiences. Although NP education readies students for the clinical practice role, there is a lack of standardization in the number of clinical placement hours required, and in the qualifications clinical preceptors should possess (Canadian Association of Schools of Nursing [CASN], 2012; Contandriopoulos et al., 2015; DiCenso et al., 2007). Clinical hours provide the opportunity to put into practice the knowledge acquired in the classroom setting. Preceptors are central to clinical education by assisting the student to bridge the gap between clinical practice and theory. Mentoring through preceptorship prepares the NP graduate student to autonomously and independently provide care for conditions within the scope of practice of the NP, as a novice NP. PHCNP clinical practice synthesizes a number of competencies and standards of practice that are acquired through the NP education program and reinforced through clinical practice. The novice PHCNP practice may look vastly different from the practice of a more experienced NP, yet the core standards and competencies are the same (CASN, 2011). The combination of graduate education and direct comprehensive care provides the depth and breadth for NP students to develop competencies of APN for health promotion, treatment, and management of medical conditions.

Primary Health Care Nurse Practitioner Role Description

The APN role, such as the NP, is delineated from basic nursing roles and is defined by educational preparation, direct clinical practice, and in-depth nursing knowledge and expertise, allowing one to meet the needs of individuals, families, groups, and/or populations (CNA, 2019). NPs are advanced practice nurses (DiCenso et al., 2007, 2010), and NP competencies are outlined as specific knowledge, skills, and personal attributes required for safe and ethical practice (CNA, 2019). Nursing practice competencies are essential for NP education and the development of work roles. Role competencies are a means to define work (CNA, 2019), and generally confidence is the most frequently mentioned characteristic with respect to facilitating effective work (Jones, 2005). The CNA competencies have applicability across practice settings and are integral to NPs' safe and ethical practice (CNA, 2019; Duff, 2019). Not only do they provide the basis for educational programs and guide the regulation and registration of NPs, they help guide novice and experienced NPs alike in actualizing direct clinical practice and other aspects of the NP role. The Canadian Nurse Practitioner Core Competency Framework outlines the following initial NP core competencies, which provide the basis for educational programs, NP regulation, and guide the NP in the work setting:

- professional role, responsibility and accountability
- health assessment and diagnosis
- therapeutic management
- health promotion and prevention of illness, and injury (CNA, 2010a)

The 2019 APN Framework (CNA, 2019) has revised and expanded core competencies for both CNSs and NPs:

- direct comprehensive care
- optimizing health system
- education
- research
- leadership
- consultation and collaboration
- continuing competence
- professional liability protection
- unique NP competencies are based on client population needs and context of practice, including age, developmental stage, health condition and complexity of clients (CNA, 2019)

PHCNPs focus on health promotion, preventative care, diagnosis, treatment, and management of common acute and stable chronic conditions through the utilization of evidence-based nursing and medicine.

A national consensus-based definition of the NP role was developed in 2006, which stated that NPs were "registered nurses with additional educational preparation and experience who possess and demonstrate the competencies to autonomously diagnose, order and interpret diagnostic tests, prescribe pharmaceuticals, and perform specific procedures within their legislated scope of practice" (CNA, 2016b). Formally in 2006, CNA's Canadian Nurse Practitioner Initiative (CNPI) report advocated for title protection for NPs, and since then across the country, in conjunction with scope of practice regulations, provinces and territories have legislated this title protection (CNPI, 2006a, 2006b; CNA, 2016a).

The introduction of the PHCNP role is linked to nationwide health reform efforts to improve the accessibility and quality of PHC (CNA, 2019; Donald et al., 2010). Major health care reform initiatives in the 1990s identified the potential impact nursing and other health care professionals could have on patient care, which led to the reframing of PHC in Canada (CNA, 2019; Donald et al., 2010). Federal and provincial initiatives aimed to enhance health promotion, support equitable access to service, and increase quality of care. This allowed for the re-introduction of the PHCNP role that was lost in the 1980s (Donald et al., 2010). Legislation, regulations, remuneration, and education strategies were developed to aid in role implementation (Donald et al., 2010). The number of NPs in Canada has more than tripled in the past decade to over 5,000 across a variety of settings (CIHI, 2018).

Clinical Practice: The Foundation of Primary Health Care Nurse Practitioner Practice

As direct care providers, NPs synthesize research, education, clinical expertise, leadership, and consultation to provide comprehensive health care. A unique aspect of the work of NPs is the provision of direct patient care in a primary care setting within an advanced scope of practice (title and scope of practice are protected by legislation). The comprehensive activities provided by the NP improve quality of care and facilitate the patients' optimal progression through the health care system.

The PHCNP role allows for the provision of care to individuals across the lifespan in the management of acute episodic illnesses and chronic conditions. The foundation of NP practice is "direct clinical practice ... which unfolds around the premise that individuals seek care for a broad range of health care concerns over time and across the life span" (Pohl & Kao, 2014, p. 403). Direct clinical care by a PHCNP requires the critical application of health assessment followed by diagnosis and therapeutic management skills for patients pursuing care. As an autonomous health professional with a graduate education, the PHCNP builds on the registe-red nurse (RN) foundation of health promotion, illness prevention, and health management by integrating advanced nursing and medical theory in providing comprehensive health ser-vices (CNA, 2010a). PHCNPs work collaboratively with patients and other health care profes-sionals to provide care to diverse populations in a variety of settings (CNA, 2010a).

Although there is variation between provincial/territorial jurisdictions, the legislated authority allows for NPs to autonomously order and interpret diagnostic tests, perform minor surgical procedures, and prescribe medications (CNA, 2010a). PHCNPs are accountable to patients regarding their care in terms of clinical findings, diagnoses, and management plans including testing, referrals, pharmaceutical management, and rehabilitation (CNA, 2010a).

PHCNPs work in a variety of settings from government-funded community clinics, private clinics, family health networks, emergency rooms, and outpatient clinics attached to hospitals (CNA, 2016b). The NP role has also been utilized for innovative approaches to health care provision such as in Ontario, where the creation of NP-Led Clinics operates on the strengths of the NP role: autonomous provision of care for those with acute episodic and chronic health needs (Heale & Butcher, 2010). Other innovative methods, including virtual health care visits and mobile bus services, are becoming more common. Mobile buses travel to communities on a set rotation (Dinh, 2012a), breaking down a barrier to health care access and offering a unique and profound opportunity to improve health and expand health care.

The majority of PHCNPs work in community clinics funded through a variety of fun-ding models. The structure, function, governance, and funding vary regionally across Canada, but can be broadly categorized into four models: physician-led practices, NP-led practices, community-led practices, and integrated primary care networks. Community-led clinics (known as community health centres in British Columbia, Manitoba, and Nova Scotia, or family care clinics in Alberta) are the most common settings in which PHCNPs are employed and have a mandate to serve the needs of the community. They feature interprofessional health care teams, in which PHCNPs have patients registered to them either directly or through a col-laborating physician. Physician-led clinics may incorporate a variety of health care disciplines within their structure, of which the PHCNP role may be one. NP-Led Clinics are relatively new on the PHC landscape, with models operating in Ontario, Manitoba, and Saskatchewan (Dinh, 2012a). Ontario continues to lead this innovative model of NP-Led Clinics (Heale & Butcher, 2010; Stewart, 2018). An example of an NP-Led Clinic is featured in Box 24.1.

BOX 24.1

Example of an NP-Led Clinic: The Lakehead NP-Led Clinic

The Lakehead NP-Led Clinic opened in November 2010 and serves the city of Thunder Bay and area, Ontario. It provides PHC to 4,800 patients, with a NP-to-patient ratio of 1:800. The interprofessional (IP) team includes six NPs, one RN, two registered practical nurses (RPNs), two social workers (1.2 full-time equivalent), one registered dietitian (1.0 full-time equivalent), and one pharmacist (0.2 full-time equivalent).

The NPs provide health promotion, disease and injury prevention, treatment, re-habilitation, and other support services. The NP-Led Clinic's collaborating physician has medical directives in place for the NPs for some controlled acts and is a source for consultation on complex cases. He comes to the clinic on a monthly basis to see pa-tients at the clinic. As well, a collaborating psychiatrist comes once per month.

The roles of the dietitian, social worker, and pharmacist in the NP-Led Clinic are similar to other IP collaboration team models. The dietitian provides nutrition edu-cation to individuals and groups for health promotion and management of chronic diseases. The social worker not only provides counselling support to clinic patients, addressing issues such as depression, anxiety, grief, and chronic pain, but also makes referrals to appropriate community services; helps patients navigate systems; and completes paperwork required to access social supports. The pharmacist conducts individual patient assessments to identify, prevent, and resolve medication-related problems; and reviews health histories, identifies problems, and develops and moni-tors care plans, which are then communicated to the patient and the interprofessional team (Dinh, 2012a; Nurse Practitioners' Association of Ontario [NPAO], 2019).

Depending on the type of clinic, new patients may be registered to a PHCNP through a screening process tailored to each clinic's needs. The first point of contact for a patient must be a person who is knowledgeable of both the NP and physician role in order to appropriately match that individual to a provider, depending on a patient's health needs and the strengths, experience, and scope of practice of the NP and physician. An individual not familiar with the NP role may require education about the PHCNP.

Within the community clinic setting, patients seeking care of a PHCNP are usually looking for a regular health care provider whom they can access as necessary for identified health concerns across the lifespan. This could be a parent seeking a provider for a new infant, a teenager transitioning from care provided by a pediatrician, a patient's previous provider has retired or moved, a woman requiring prenatal care, or someone who is unhappy with their current provider. There is an identified shortage of providers across Canada resulting in Canadians being unattached to a provider. The integration of the PHCNP into the health care system by a variety of funding mechanisms allows for these types of individuals to become patients of a PHCNP (CNA, 2010b). Further work is needed on how to best remunerate interdisciplinary teams as the delivery of primary health care evolves in Canada (Canadian Federation of Nurses Unions [CFNU], 2018; Wranik et al., 2015).

As is the case for most health care professionals, variety and complexity is routine for PHCNPs in community settings. While the basic structure of a typical day may be standardized, the patients booked on that day provide NPs with challenges, excitement, and rewards. A mix of acute episodic, health maintenance, and chronic presentations comprise most days. The ratio varies depending on the day, the community, urban versus rural setting, and community demographics. The ages of the patients booked on a day-to-day basis may range from predominantly elderly/very elderly to an equal mix of young and old to predominantly young. Typically, in NP-Led Clinics, an NP will have their own patient caseload, but most clinics work in a team environment, therefore the team supports each other. A large percentage of the PHCNP's days are spent in clinical practice with a patient panel ranging between 500 and 1,000 individuals (Dinh, 2012a). There is a paucity of literature regarding NP caseload size, but what does exist indicates rosters ranging from 400 up to 1,000 patients per NP (Martin-Misener et al., 2015). Standardized assessment to measure and monitor NP workload is needed in order to understand factors that influence workload independent of regulatory and employer influence (O'Rourke, 2019).

Characteristics of a PHCNP interaction include awareness of scope of practice and operating appropriately within legislation, regulations, and standards. It also requires the integration of applicable cultural elements, awareness of determinants of health while carrying out either a focused history/physical examination or a comprehensive well-person examination. The well-person history and examination for a teenager will look very different than that for an elderly person and the NP must integrate the developmental and life stages into overall management (CNA, 2010a). PHCNPs must also be able to adapt quickly to change and apply critical thinking to verbal and non-verbal cues of a presentation.

Patient Relationship

The privilege of the PHCNP role is the development of a relationship with a patient as it allows for a deeper, richer understanding of the patient and fosters mutual trust and respect. PHCNP patient visits may be longer than those of their physician counterparts (Dierick-van Daele, Metsemakers, Derckx, Spreeuwenberg, & Vrijhoef, 2009), thereby potentially addressing more than one health concern in a visit. Patient satisfaction with NPs is often related to the time element (Heale & Pilon, 2012; Williams & Jones, 2006), which allows for relationship building to occur. The evolution between a patient and PHCNP is an inherent part of the role with mutual trust and respect enhancing relationship development (Pohl & Kao, 2014). A longitudinal study examining NP and patient interactions validated the importance of patient-centred care in the APN of PHCNPs. Patient-centred care and the element of time allowed for more concerns identified by either the patient or the PHCNP to be negotiated and managed by the PHCNP. The art of embracing and managing issues ultimately resulted in achievement of goals for the patient. There is value to PHCNPs holding on to their nursing roots as a foundation for their approach to patient care while at the same time blending the medical model into practice style (de Leon-Demare, MacDonald, Gregory, Katz, & Halas, 2015).

An understanding of the complexities of a person's personal life, appreciating the social, lifestyle, and functional challenges, can allow for a more comprehensive and personalized health care management plan (Pohl & Kao, 2014). It is often the long-standing nature of the NP-patient relationship that creates that understanding (Pohl & Kao, 2014).

Commonly Seen Conditions

A typical clinic day will involve a variety of presentations ranging from acute episodic presentations such as respiratory or genitourinary infections to the management of chronic stable health conditions such as diabetes or hypertension. Chronic disease management is a priority and management of this requires an approach that is multi-faceted and interdisciplinary. All presentations require the PHCNP to perform a focused health assessment using assessment tools and techniques based on the individual's needs and relevance to stage of life (CNA, 2010a). Competent NPs will identify limits of their scope of practice. Maturation in the role leads to role evolution and increasing comfort with complexity of care management.

Patient Populations Served

Patient populations vary depending on the community and demographics. Age, gender, and ethnicity are all relevant factors in providing care and shape the vision of a primary care clinic. Pediatrics may comprise a large percentage of some PHCNPs' practices whereas in other communities the practice may be largely built around a geriatric population. Cultural awareness and sensitivity are also integrated within the PHCNP role and may be more present in some clinic populations than others. In this increasingly global world, the ease of travel requires the NP to be informed of global health and political concerns as well.

Primary and Secondary Prevention

Health promotion and illness/injury prevention is a hallmark of the NP role (CNA, 2015) as it incorporates foundational pieces of undergraduate nursing education with the medical aspect acquired in graduate education (CNA, 2019). The PHCNP often will incorporate features of both primary and secondary prevention into clinic visits as applicable, but more so with a patient's annual physical examination, if required, which allows the opportunity to review well-person topics not normally covered during episodic visits or routine chronic condition visits. The integration of medical knowledge allows for primary and secondary prevention to be tailored by the PHCNP for each individual.

Depending on the type of clinic, PHCNPs may collaborate with the primary care nurses (PCNs) in the clinic for health promotion and injury/illness prevention strategies. The strength of primary care clinics is their interdisciplinary nature, which allows other health care professionals such as PCNs to utilize their scope of practice to its fullest by undertaking the primary and secondary prevention aspects of clinical care (DiCenso & Bryant-Lukosius, 2010).

The PHCNP educates patients about primary prevention by counselling about preventing the onset of specific diseases via risk reduction. The PHCNP may help a patient alter behaviours that potentially lead to disease such as smoking cessation or by reducing exposure to a disease through vaccination (Donovan, n.d.). Secondary prevention such as mammography, cervical cytology, and fecal occult blood testing are procedures that detect and treat pre-clinical pathological changes thereby controlling disease progression and are essential to a PHCNP's practice. Awareness of changes to primary and secondary prevention recommendations requires the PHCNP to keep current of evidence-based literature and recommendations.

Chronic Disease Management

Chronic disease management is another central element of the PHCNP role. Once a patient has developed a chronic disease such as diabetes or hypertension, the PHCNP can lessen the impact of the disease on the patient's function and quality of life through a multi-dimensional approach to care incorporating all the elements of APN. The overall coordination of care is paramount and can be complex for some chronic disease presentations; PCNs, social workers, dietitians, and specialists may all be involved to some degree with chronic disease management, and the PHCNP is often the principal coordinator.

Collaboration

Collaboration between the NP, the patient and their family, and the community is essential to PHCNP practice. Nurse practitioners must also establish collaborative relationships with all members of the health care team. As the member of the team who provides continuity and stability in the care and management of patients over the long term, PHCNPs often emerge as leaders in primary care teams in health care settings.

Within primary care clinics, foundational staff usually includes support staff, nurses, NPs, physicians, and a clinic manager. Support staff is the first point of contact for the public and require a detailed understanding of roles and responsibilities of all providers, as well as an understanding of clinic process. Other health care professionals associated with a primary clinic will vary depending on community needs and system availability. Mental health specialists (counsellors and/or psychiatrists) are often a part of the primary care team, as is dietician support. Occupational therapy, physiotherapy, pharmacy, midwifery, social work, and perhaps specialty medicine may be accessible in some form as well. PHCNPs collaborate with a variety of health care professionals within and outside clinics, depending on the community setting and its needs; for example, with local church groups or homeless shelters.

Within clinical practice, collaboration may occur multiple times throughout the day. The PHCNP must recognize and balance the needs and expectations of the patient with the boundaries of the system both within the clinic and the larger health care system as a whole. Collaboration between other health care professionals occurs, depending on the presentation. Effective collaboration is dependent on team composition, personalities, and requires effort (Pohl & Kao, 2014). Physician collaboration may be formal or informal and some days is more present than others for a PHCNP. The autonomous nature of the PHCNP's scope of practice does not require physician collaboration to occur at regular intervals, but more so when the PHCNP recognizes a condition or presentation is beyond their scope of practice. However, the requirement that NPs have a formal collaborative practice agreement with a physician remains in Quebec, New Brunswick, Nova Scotia, Prince Edward Island, and Newfoundland and Labrador (Spence, Agnew, & Fahey-Walsh, 2015).

A good portion of the PHCNP's clinical encounters may involve collaboration with the PCNs in the clinic. The PCN role is relatively new as well within the health care team for the same reasons as the NP role, as cited earlier, and is continually being broadened and reinvented as experience and opportunity allows. Maximizing the PCN's scope of practice creates opportunities for the PCN and PHCNP to work in tandem in the provision of patient care, which is specifically beneficial for primary prevention and with chronic disease presentations.

Formal interprofessional collaboration may occur in the form of daily "team huddles" or weekly team meetings, or with ad hoc meetings involving outside agencies to discuss complex case management. This may involve the team directly caring for the patient or may be an opportunity for other health professionals to hear the challenges with a patient's condition and provide input based on their professional background and expertise.

Informal collaboration is more often the reality of primary care and patient management for the PHCNP: PHCNP to PCN; PHCNP to physician or support staff, or vice versa. Informal collaboration is necessary to expedite patient management inherent in the day-to-day interaction. It may occur as a hallway huddle between an NP, PCN, and physician, and some mix thereof. These consults usually involve a patient currently in the clinic who requires change management.

A cornerstone feature of NP practice is collaboration and it is embedded into the core competencies (CNA, 2010a, 2019). Given the nature of funding of NP roles, collaboration with other health care professionals is essential. It allows for more comprehensive health care for the patient and results in high-quality, cost-effective outcomes (Cowan et al., 2006; Pohl & Kao, 2014).

Consultation

Consultation or referral to other health care professionals in the primary care clinic such as a referral to the PCN, counsellor, or dietician may be indicated in circumstances where more comprehensive, interdisciplinary care is required. Consultation with the larger system outside the clinic may also occur. A PHCNP requests consultation via the referral mechanism for those situations they identify as outside their scope of practice; the patient likely has a diagnosis that needs to be supported or clarified by a specialist; has a diagnosed complex condition for which input into ongoing care from a specialist is warranted; or fails to respond to standard, evidence-based care. The PHCNP's comfort with consultation enhances patient care and provides for more comprehensive care (CNA, 2010a) and has been identified as a core competency for APNs (CNA, 2019). A referral for surgical consult for cholelithiasis, or to gynecology for uterine fibroid complications, or to psychiatry for mental health assessment, diagnosis, and management suggestions are examples of how consultation is actualized by the PHCNP.

There are circumstances when another of the health care providers may consult the PHCNP within the clinic. The physician may seek the PHCNP's opinion, for example, regarding reproductive health or contraceptive management. There may be some role evolution occurring whereby as the NP role becomes further integrated and embedded within the health care system, physician support and acceptance continues to grow, and respect for the role enhances the collaborative relationship.

CASE STUDY

The Story of Ayana

Ayana is a 52-year-old Somalian woman who has been in Canada for two years. She is relatively new to the clinic and to the PHCNP Lori. She is accompanied by her daughter Fatmata, who translates for Ayana, even though Fatmata's command of English is poor.

Through Fatmata's translation, Lori is able to gather the following history. As a recent immigrant to Canada, Ayana lives with her two daughters and infant granddaughter in an apartment complex in the downtown area. She has been widowed for 10 years; her husband was killed due to political unrest in Somalia. She and her children spent the previous eight years in a refugee camp prior to coming to Canada. She does not work as she does not feel confident with her language and feels she will be discriminated against for both gender and race; the thought of having to enter the workforce makes her very anxious.

In Somalia, Ayana had been a self-employed businesswoman operating her own vegetable stand. Her source of income is through Employment and Income Assistance, and she is attending daily language classes to improve her English. Health care prior to coming to Canada was limited to seeking care as needed for episodic situations such as childbirth or breathing problems. Ayana is unfamiliar with and suspicious of primary and secondary prevention strategies that are commonplace in Canada. She has never had a complete physical examination.

Her current health concern is "trouble breathing." Today she has had trouble catching her breath since being outside in the cold. She experiences similar episodes a few times a week, but they usually pass within an hour or two. She was told in Somalia that she has asthma and should carry a puffer to help her, but she couldn't afford it and felt she didn't need it as the episodes usually passed on their own. She feels a bit better in the office now that she is warm. On examination, Ayana's BP is 154/92, R = 24, P = 80, T = 37.1(oral), O_2 saturation 91% room air, S1/S2RRR, no S3/S4/M. Air entry decreased to bases, expiratory wheezes throughout. No increased work of breathing observed. Lori's working diagnosis is asthma exacerbation.

Lori's management plan is comprehensive, reflecting not only the acute presentation of Ayana, but other multi-dimensional needs that have been identified:

long-term asthma management; primary and secondary prevention including immunizations, mammography, colorectal cancer screening, cervical cytology, diabetes, and cholesterol screening; exploration of anxiety; and further assessment of psychosocial needs.

In order to implement the management plan, Lori addresses Ayana's asthma exacerbation by ordering a chest X-ray, WBC & differential, and prescribing a short-acting bronchodilator and an inhaled corticosteroid. She requests that the primary care nurse see Ayana and Fatmata before leaving the clinic to review correct inhaler technique and to discuss immunizations. She requests follow-up in 48 hours with both herself and the PCN. At that time, the asthma management plan can be adjusted accordingly, but will also afford Lori and the PCN an opportunity to discuss with Ayana the importance of regular health surveillance strategies.

After Ayana leaves the clinic, Lori speaks with the clinic social worker regarding community resources for immigrant women for both job entry and counselling, with the intention of exploring Ayana's receptiveness to support at the next visit. Lori is also able to make arrangements for a health authority translator to be present for the next visit as Fatmata is unable to attend.

At her next visit, Ayana is feeling much better. She is resistant to having any further physical exam take place or any further blood work as she doesn't see the need. She is receptive to speaking with the social worker regarding counselling and community supports.

Non-Clinical Primary Health Care Nurse Practitioner Domains of Practice

Reflective Practice

Reflective practice is considered an essential attribute of health care practitioners. The goal of reflective practice is self-discovery and growth, as well as the expansion of one's knowledge (Pretorius & Ford, 2016). Reflection encourages practitioners to review an experience of practice in order to describe, analyze, evaluate, and so inform learning about practice (Jacobs, 2016). Continuing competency is a requirement of many regulatory bodies for NP registration and incorporates elements of self-reflection. It enables the NP opportunity to assess areas of strength and weakness, and the professional obligation to self-identify areas of weakness and create a self-learning plan for change (CNA, 2010a).

Reflective practice is inherent to growth as a PHCNP regardless of whether one is a novice or an expert (Tracy, 2014). Direct clinical practice requires the integration of standards of care, awareness of scope of practice, and evidence-based management (Pohl & Kao, 2014) through a level of expertise acquired through educational preparation, a supportive work environment, and self-reflection (Pohl & Kao, 2014). A novice NP may initially be more task oriented with patient presentations, but as they gain confidence and expertise with the role, they will integrate "critical thinking and skillful interviewing" (Pohl & Kao, 2014, p. 407).

Reflective practice allows the NP to explore experiences to critically analyze and improve practice (Tracy, 2014).

Research

Research is one domain considered foundational throughout most APN models (CNA, 2019; Spross, 2014) and is often an expectation cited in job descriptions (CNA, 2011). "Research-sensitive practice" (Tracy, 2014, p. 164) is an approach that incorporates research in an unstructured manner for the APN. The PHCNP is well positioned to evaluate practice and clinical outcomes, to benchmark and identify best practices, and to lead efforts designed to improve quality and patient safety. Research may be actualized at the clinic level through quality improvement projects, or at a more systemic level with research contributions to the science of nursing as a whole. It is within the professional obligation of the PHCNP to stay current with evidence-based information and building opportunities into the role for either engaging in research or reviewing research are instrumental to fulfilling this responsibility.

Leadership

Leadership is generally explained as the art and science of influencing a group toward the achievement of a goal. The NP role is derived from a strong base of clinical experience and education, which develops both extensive and extended skills and a critical awareness of the place of nursing in health service delivery. Consequently, the NP role is a leadership role in clinical practice (Carryer, Gardner, Dunn, & Gardner, 2007). Key elements of clinical leadership include the need to guide and influence care delivery systems and to act as a change agent and effectively deal with conflict by the use of skills in communication, negotiation, collaboration, and evaluation. Thus, the PHCNP lead both in the immediate clinical environment and in the wider context of health service delivery.

The leadership domain is essential to the emerging role in Canada where acting as a resource, consultant, or collaborating to shape policy or educate organizations is necessary to advance the NP role (CNA, 2019). The PHCNP may actualize this by providing leadership in the clinical area through initiation of research, or assuming the lead as a role model for the PCNs by challenging them to maximize their scope of practice. Leadership is also demonstrated by being an educator or a preceptor to other health care professionals and the public. Primary health care nurse practitioners should also advocate for quality, accessible, and cost-effective health care (Pohl & Kao, 2014) and ensure that clinical practice, as a whole, reflects evidence-based standards (CNA, 2019). The PHCNP's role as a leader in the community through memberships on boards of health and education and as an influential policy-maker is based primarily on the competency of collaboration.

Barriers to Practice

The integration of PHCNPs into the Canadian health care system has not been without its challenges and there continue to be barriers to practice. Barriers prevent full role integration and sustainability that can affect continuity of care and jeopardizes safe, effective care.

Inconsistencies in legislation and education standards have led to lack of role clarity and challenges with credibility and portability (Donald et al., 2010), although this may be less of an issue as regulatory bodies co-operate to ensure consistency across the country (CNA, 2019). Amendments of provincial and territorial legislation to optimize the NP role are necessary. This includes removing federal barriers to NP practice such as prohibiting the distribution of drug samples and requiring a formal collaborative agreement with a physician in some provinces. Restrictions to scope of practice such as prescriptive authority and medication management interfere with seamless patient care. Medication lists appropriate for the PHCNP may not be suitable for the NP working in a personal care home or in the emergency department setting. Health and social policy review are necessary to remove barriers such as the signing of death certificates, or completion of insurance forms (Donald et al., 2010).

Perceived hierarchical roles present ongoing interprofessional challenges between PHCNPs and other health care professionals (Dinh, 2012b). Settings that lack a strong governance and understanding of the NP role can lead to failure of role implementation or suboptimal utilization of the PHCNP (Dinh, 2012b). Insufficient structure for collaboration has also been cited as a barrier, as has lack of evaluation of NP role implementation (Dinh, 2012b). A national tracking system has been suggested to monitor the trend of PHCNP activity (Donald et al., 2010). National-level guidance would further integrate and promote the role and allow for a more cohesive voice in addressing the barriers that continue to exist.

Conclusion

The PHCNP role is the fastest-growing APN role in the country as the benefits of the role to accessibility and quality care are increasingly recognized by the public and various levels of governments. PHCNPs provide comprehensive health care to individuals and families across the life continuum in a multi-dimensional approach consistent with the domains of APN. Operationalization of the role is supported by the CNA's NP core competencies, which provide guidance and structure for the role. It is expected that the PHCNP role will continue to experience integration and acceptance into the health care system.

Critical Thinking Questions

1. In what manner is collaboration demonstrated in the role of the PHCNP?
2. Discuss incentives for developing and supporting interprofessional practice teams either in an NP-Led Clinic or in a general PHC practice group.
3. If you were advocating for the PHCNP role, what would you consider the strengths and contributions of the role in improving health care for Canadians?

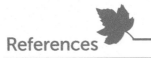

References

British Columbia College of Nursing Professionals (BCCNP). (2019). *Nurse practitioner registration*. Vancouver, BC: BCCNP. Retrieved from https://www.bccnp.ca/Registration/RN_NP/NPapplication/1EN/Pages/Step1.aspx

Canadian Association of Schools of Nursing (CASN). (2011). *Nurse practitioner education in Canada: Final report.* Ottawa, ON: CASN.

CASN. (2012). *Nurse practitioner education in Canada: National framework of guiding principles & essential components.* Ottawa, ON: CASN.

Canadian Council of Registered Nurse Regulators (CCRNR). (2015). *Practice analysis study of nurse practitioners.* Beaverton, ON: CCRNR. Retrieved from http://www.ccrnr.ca/assets/ccrnr-practice-analysis-study-of-nurse-practitioners-report---final.pdf

Canadian Federation of Nurses Unions (CFNU). (2018). *The CFNU pan-Canadian nurse practitioner retention & recruitment study.* Retrieved from https://nursesunions.ca/wp-content/uploads/2018/06/CFNU_UntappedPotential-Final-EN.pdf

Canadian Institute for Health Information (CIHI). (2018). *Regulated nurses 2017: RN and NP data tables.* Ottawa, ON: CIHI.

Canadian Nurse Practitioner Initiative (CNPI). (2006a). *Nurse practitioners: The time is now. An integrated report.* Ottawa, ON: CNA.

CNPI. (2006b). *Nurse practitioners: The time is now. A solution to improving access and reducing wait times in Canada.* Ottawa, ON: CNA.

Canadian Nurses Association (CNA). (2010a). *Canadian nurse practitioner core competency framework.* Ottawa, ON: CNA.

CNA. (2010b). *Meeting the challenges: CNA's response to promoting innovative solutions to health human resources challenges, a report of the standing committee on health.* Ottawa, ON: CNA.

CNA. (2011). *Collaborative integration plan for the role of nurse practitioners in Canada 2011–2015.* Ottawa, ON: CNA.

CNA. (2015). *Position statement: Primary health care.* Ottawa, ON: CNA. Retrieved from https://www.cna-aiic.ca/~/media/cna/page-content/pdf-en/primary-health-care-position-statement.pdf

CNA. (2016a). *The Canadian nurse practitioner initiative: A 10-year retrospective.* Ottawa, ON: CNA. Retrieved from https://cna-aiic/ca/~/media/cna/page-content/pdf-en/canadian-nurse-practitioner-initiative-a-10-year-retrospective.pdf

CNA. (2016b). *Position statement: The nurse practitioner.* Ottawa, ON: CNA. Retrieved from https://cna-aiic.ca/~/media/cna/page-content/pdf-en/ps_nurse_practitioner_e.pdf

CNA. (2019). *Advanced practice nursing: A pan-Canadian framework.* Ottawa, ON: CNA. Retrieved from https://www.cna-aiic.ca/-/media/cna/page-content/pdf-en/apn-a-pan-canadian-framework.pdf

Carryer, J., Gardner, G., Dunn, S., & Gardner, A. (2007). The core role of the nurse practitioner: Practice, professionalism and clinical leadership. *Journal of Clinical Nursing, 16,* 1818–1825.

Contandriopoulos, D., Brousselle, A., Dubois, C.-A., Perroux, M., Beaulieu, M.-D., Brault, I., ... Sangster-Gormley, E. (2015). A process-based framework to guide nurse practitioners integration into primary healthcare teams: Results from a logic analysis; Organization, structure and delivery healthcare. *BioMed Central (BMC) Health Services Research, 15*(78), 1–11. doi: 10.1186/s12913-015-0731-5

Cowan, M., Shapiro, M., Hays, R., Afifi, A., Vazirani, S., Ettner, S., & Ward, C. (2006). The effect of a multidisciplinary hospitalist/physician and advanced practice nurse collaboration on hospital costs. *Journal of Nursing Administration, 36*, 79–85.

de Leon-Demare, K., MacDonald, J., Gregory, D., Katz, A., & Halas, G. (2015). Articulating nurse practitioner practice using King's theory of goal attainment. *Journal of the American Academy of Nurse Practitioners, 27*(11), 631–636. doi: 10.1002/2327-6924.12218

DiCenso, A., Auffrey, L., Bryant-Lukosius, D., Donald, F., Martin-Misener, R., Mathews, S., & Opsteen, J. (2007). Primary health care nurse practitioners in Canada. *Contemporary Nurse, 26*(1), 104–115.

DiCenso, A., & Bryant-Lukosius, D. (2010). *Clinical nurse specialist and nurse practitioner in Canada: A decision support synthesis.* Ottawa, ON: CHSRF. Retrieved from http://www.chsrf.ca

DiCenso, A., Bryant-Lukosius, D., Martin-Misener, R., Donald, F., Abelson, J., Bourgeault, I., ... Harbman, P. (2010). Factors enabling advanced practice nursing role integration in Canada. *Nursing Leadership, 23*(Special Issue), 211–238.

Dierick-van Daele, A., Metsemakers, J., Derckx, E., Spreeuwenberg, C., & Vrijhoef, H. (2009). Nurse practitioners substituting for general practitioners: Randomized control trial. *Journal of Advanced Nursing, 65*(2), 391–401.

Dinh, T. (2012a). *Improving primary health care through collaboration: Briefing 1—current knowledge about interprofessional teams in Canada.* Ottawa, ON: Conference Board of Canada. Retrieved from http://www.integrationresources.ca/wordpress/wp-content/uploads/2013/09/D36_PrimaryHealthCare-Briefing1.pdf

Dinh, T. (2012b). *Improving primary health care through collaboration: Briefing 2—barriers to successful interprofessional teams.* Ottawa, ON: Conference Board of Canada. Retrieved from https://professionals.wrha.mb.ca/old/professionals/collaborativecare/files/IPHCTC-Briefing2.pdf

Donald, F., Martin-Misener, R., Bryant-Lukosius, D., Kilpatrick, K., Kaasalainen, S., Carter, N., ... DiCenso, A. (2010). The primary healthcare nurse practitioner role in Canada. *Nursing Leadership, 23*(Special Issue), 88–113.

Donovan, D. (n.d.). *AFMC primer on population health: A virtual textbook on public health concepts for clinicians.* Ottawa, ON: The Association of Faculties of Medicine of Canada. Retrieved from http://phprimer.afmc.ca/inner/about_the_primer

Duff, E. (2019). A structural equation model of empowerment factors affecting nurse practitioner's competence. *Nurse Education in Practice, 38*, 145–152.

Heale, R., & Butcher, M. (2010). Canada's first nurse practitioner-led clinic: A case study in health care innovation. *Nursing Leadership, 23*(3), 21–29. doi: 10.12927/cjnl.2010.21939

Heale, R., & Pilon, R. (2012). Nurse practitioner clinics: Exploration of client satisfaction. *Canadian Journal of Nursing Leadership, 25*(3), 43–55. doi: 10.12927/cjnl.2012.23056

Jacobs, S. (2016). Reflective learning, reflective practice. *Nursing, 46*(5), 62–64.

Jones, M. L. (2005). Role development and effective practice in specialist and advanced practice roles in acute hospital settings: Systematic review and meta-synthesis. *Journal of Advanced Nursing, 49*(2), 191–209.

Kaasalainen, S., Martin-Misener, R., Kilpatrick, K., Harbman, P., Bryant-Lukosius, D., Donald, F., ... DiCenso, A. (2010). A historical overview of the development of advanced practice nursing roles in Canada. *Nursing Leadership, 23*(Special Issue), 35–60.

Martin-Misener, R., Donald, F., Kilpatrick, K., Bryant-Lukosius, D., Rayner, J., Landry, V., ... McKinlay, R. J. (2015). *Benchmarking for nurse practitioner patient panel size and comparative analysis of nurse practitioner pay scales: Update of a scoping review.* Toronto, ON: MOHLTC. Retrieved from https://fhs.mcmaster.ca/ccapnr/documents/np_panel_size_study_updated_scoping_review_report.pdf

Mick, D. J., & Ackerman, M. H. (2000). Advanced practice nursing role delineation in acute and critical care: Application of the Strong Model of Advanced Practice. *Heart & Lung, 29*, 210–221.

Nurse Practitioners' Association of Ontario (NPAO). (2019). *Nurse practitioner-led clinics.* Toronto, ON: NPAO. Retrieved from https://npao.org/about-npao/clinics/

Ordre des infirmières et infirmiers du Québec (OIIQ). (2018). *Primary health care preparation guide for the primary health care nurse practitioner certification exam.* Montreal, QC: OIIQ. Retrieved from https://www.oiiq.org/documents/20147/2875928/guide-preparation-premiere-ligne-eng.pdf/50fb27e7-6b99-aa89-aea0-e6ac6e151777?version=1.0

O'Rourke, T. (2019, August 23). Telephone interview.

Pohl, J., & Kao, T. (2014). The primary care nurse practitioner. In A. Hamric, C. Hanson, M. Tracy, & E. O'Grady (Eds.), *Advanced practice nursing: An integrative approach* (pp. 396–428). St. Louis, MO: Elsevier.

Pretorius, L., & Ford, A. (2016). Reflection for learning: Teaching reflective practice at the beginning of university study. *International Journal of Teaching and Learning in Higher Education, 28*(2), 241–253.

Spence, L., Agnew, T., & Fahey-Walsh, J. (2015). *A pan-Canadian environmental scan of the scope of practice of nurse practitioners.* Toronto, ON: Ontario Nurse Practitioners' Association.

Spross, J. (2014). Conceptualizations of advanced practice nursing. In A. Hamric, C. Hanson, M. Tracy, & E. O'Grady (Eds.), *Advanced practice nursing: An integrative approach* (pp. 27–61). St. Louis, MO: Elsevier.

Stewart, N. (2018). Nurse practitioner-led clinics in British Columbia. *UBC Graduate Research Open Collections.* Retrieved from https://open.library.ubc.ca/cIRcle/collections/graduateresearch/42591/items/1.0365319

Tracy, M. (2014). Direct clinical practice. In A. Hamric, C. Hanson, M. Tracy, & E. O'Grady (Eds.), *Advanced practice nursing: An integrative approach* (pp. 147–182). St. Louis, MO: Elsevier.

Williams, A., & Jones, M. (2006). Patients' assessments of consulting a nurse practitioner: The time factor. *Journal of Advanced Nursing, 53*(2), 188–195.

Wranik, D., Korchagina, M., Edwards, J., Bower, I., Levy, A., & Katz, A. (2015). *How best to pay interdisciplinary primary care teams.* Ottawa, ON: Canadian Institutes of Health Research.

Chapter

25 — Nurse Practitioner: Adult

Rosemary Wilson and Monakshi (Mona) Sawhney

ROSEMARY WILSON is Associate Professor at Queen's University, School of Nursing, Kingston, Ontario. She is also a nurse practitioner (NP)-Adult in chronic pain management at Kingston Health Sciences Centre, Kingston, Ontario.

MONAKSHI (MONA) SAWHNEY is a nurse practitioner (NP)-Adult with a specialty practice in acute pain management at North York General Hospital, Toronto, Ontario, and chronic pain management at Kingston Health Sciences Centre, Kingston, Ontario. She is also Assistant Professor at Queen's University, School of Nursing, and Department of Anesthesia and Perioperative Medicine, Kingston, Ontario.

KEY TERMS

acute care nurse practitioner (ACNP)
clinical nurse specialist/nurse practitioner (CNS/NP)
nurse practitioner (NP)
nurse practitioner (NP)-Adult
specialty nurse practitioner (SNP)
tertiary care nurse practitioner (TCNP)

OBJECTIVES

1. Describe the NP-Adult role in acute and specialty care practice.
2. Explore the NP practice competencies for the NP-Adult role in Canada.
3. Discuss the barriers and facilitators of NP-Adult practice.
4. Explore evidence of the effectiveness of the NP-Adult role in the Canadian context.

Introduction

This chapter discusses the role of the **nurse practitioner (NP)** in the adult patient care stream. The **NP-Adult** is an advanced practice nurse who provides specialized health care, most often within a hospital setting, to adolescents, adults, older adults, and their families with particular health care conditions. Direct clinical care occupies the largest domain of NP-Adult practice while the domains of research, leadership, consultation, and collaboration also contribute to the foundation of this largely hospital-based NP role (DiCenso et al., 2010). As is the case with other NP roles, the Canadian Nurse Practitioner Core Competency Framework developed by the Canadian Nurses Association (CNA; 2010) guides the operationalization of NP-Adult across the continuum of care. Core competencies for the NP-Adult role are professional role responsibility and accountability (clinical practice, collaboration, consultation and referral, research, leadership); health assessment and diagnosis; therapeutic management; and health promotion and prevention of illness and injury.

The NP-Adult role began its evolution in the 1980s and 1990s as a blended clinical nurse specialist/nurse practitioner (CNS/NP) role (DiCenso et al., 2010) in response to increases in patient complexity and a shortage of physician coverage (Kilpatrick, 2008; Kilpatrick et al., 2010). In the years since, role titles across Canada have included acute care nurse practitioner (ACNP), tertiary care nurse practitioner (TCNP), specialty nurse practitioner (SNP), and CNS/NP. The role titles ACNP and NP-Adult will be used interchangeably to be consistent with the literature presented.

NP-Adult Education

NP-Adult education has been consistently at the graduate level since its early inception and through the CNS/NP titled role (DiCenso et al., 2010; Martin-Misener, 2010). Educational programs are offered either as a combined graduate/NP or postgraduate NP certificate or diploma. In a national survey of schools of nursing offering NP education (response rate 70%, N = 27), 15% included NP-Adult programs (Staples & Sangster-Gormley, 2018). Educational programs for the NP-Adult role provide a combination of theoretical and clinical learning consistent with the preparation for APN, providing essential content for practice in all domains. Graduate-level core courses in nursing theory, research methods, statistics, and health policy are taken with NP courses in combined programs and include pathophysiology, pharmacotherapeutics, advanced health assessment and clinical reasoning, therapeutic management, and NP roles and responsibilities. Clinical practicum hours are required in each of the programs.

The Canadian Association of Schools of Nursing (CASN) recommends the entry requirement be graduate-level education and a minimum of 700 hours of direct clinical practice, excluding laboratory time for all NP programs, regardless of the stream (CASN, 2012). All NP-Adult education programs are generalist in nature except for those offered in Quebec, where the specialties of cardiology, nephrology, and neonatology are supported by Ordre des infirmières et infirmiers du Québec (OIIQ). Table 25.1 presents the various NP-Adult programs in Canada. At successful completion of an NP-Adult program, students are eligible to write either the Adult-Gerontology Primary Care Nurse Practitioner Certification Examination offered by the American Academy of Nurse Practitioners Certification Program or the Adult Nurse Practitioner Examination offered by the American Nurses Credentialing Center for provincial or territorial registration. The CASN Task Force on NP Education

(2012) recognized that there is a paucity of doctorally prepared NPs in faculty roles and that recruitment of NPs into doctoral studies is an issue in Canada.

Overall, NP-Adult education programs are designed to meet entry to practice competencies set out by individual provincial regulatory bodies (CASN, 2012). It is important to note that similar to the primary health care nurse practitioner (PHCNP), the NP-Adult's knowledge, skills, and ability expand with practice experience and as such, there is variability in scope of practice enactment. In addition, although clinical practicums within educational programs may be specialty based, the context and detail required for autonomous specialty practice beyond entry to practice competencies often requires additional work by the NP-Adult in the early part of their practice. For example, the recommendation has been made

TABLE 25.1: NP-Adult Registration by Province/Territory

Province/Territory and Website	NP-Adult Registration/Licence
British Columbia https://www.bccnp.ca/Pages/redirect.aspx?requestedURL=www.crnbc.ca/	No
Alberta https://www.nurses.ab.ca/	Yes
Saskatchewan https://www.srna.org/	No
Manitoba https://www.crnm.mb.ca/	No
Ontario https://www.cno.org/	Yes
Quebec https://www.oiiq.org/	No
New Brunswick http://www.nanb.nb.ca/	No
Nova Scotia https://www.nscn.ca/	No
Prince Edward Island https://www.crnpei.ca/	No
Newfoundland and Labrador https://www.arnnl.ca/	Yes
Northwest Territories, Nunavut https://www.rnantnu.ca/	No
Yukon https://yukonnurses.ca/	No

that mental health education be a distinct component of all NP educational programs and/or be delivered as part of a national certification for post-registration (Creamer & Austin, 2017).

The Canadian Council of Registered Nurse Regulators (CCRNR) released a practice analysis of Canadian NPs in all categories (N = 909) in 2015. NP-Adult respondents comprised 21% of the sample and had an average of 14.3 years of nursing experience prior to completing an NP educational program; 61% of these had more than five years of experience in their role.

There can be incongruity between the NP educational stream chosen, the NP stream of registration, and with the ultimate practice/employment setting (CASN, 2012; DiCenso et al., 2010). For example, PHCNPs may be employed in acute care settings and ACNPs may be employed in primary health care settings as a result of position and resource availability in the area. Almost and Laschinger (2002) found that 90.5% of ACNPs in Canada were working in acute care settings and 82.5% were employed full time while the more recent practice analysis commissioned by CCRNR (2015) reflected that 80% of NP-Adult respondents worked in a hospital (in-patient and/or outpatient) setting and 10% in primary care.

NP-Adult Role and Scope of Practice in Canada

The NP-Adult/ACNP contributes to patient care by utilizing an expanded scope of clinical practice with activities that fall within both traditional medical and nursing disciplines (Sidani & Doran, 2010). Consistent with the early blended roles of the CNS/NP, the NP-Adult in Canada practices in the broad domains of clinical, research, education, and administration (Kilpatrick, 2008, 2013a, 2013b), and within the established competencies of APN. The NP-Adult role can be found in a multitude of specialty settings ranging from in-patient, service-based patients groups (i.e., neurosurgery, orthopedics, cardiac surgery, cardiology) and outpatient service-based groups (i.e., oncology, asthma) to consultative/concurrent care management teams in both in-patient and outpatient settings (i.e., palliative care, acute and chronic pain management, anticoagulation, diabetes; Spross, 2009). Overall, the NP-Adult provides specialty care to meet the needs of specialty populations (DiCenso et al., 2010). NPs in all Canadian provinces and territories are authorized to diagnose diseases or conditions, order and interpret diagnostic testing, and prescribe medications and treatments (DiCenso et al., 2010). The level of legislated autonomy to perform these functions varies across Canada and depends on provincial and territorial regulations.

The NP-Adult role has been found to be associated with greater clinical responsibilities than the CNS role with as much as 80% of work time spent providing clinical care (Sidani et al., 2000). Individuals in these roles have described their practice as including consultation, support, and education for both physicians and nurses in specialty areas (DiCenso et al., 2010). The hallmark of this role is its interprofessional and collaborative practice with diverse groups of health professionals in a team-based approach (Bryant-Lukosius & DiCenso 2004; Hansen et al., 2017; Hurlock-Chorostecki, Forchuk, Orchard, van Soeren, & Reeves, 2014). A study that evaluated NP role implementation in an in-patient neurosurgery service in an acute care hospital described NP enactment of the domains of advanced practice as 80%

clinical and consulting, with 20% split among education, research, and leadership (Keenan, Mutterback, Velthuizen, Pantalone, & Gossack-Keenan, 2018).

In a study of a combined group of ACNPs, physicians, administrators, and staff nurses, van Soeren and Micevski (2001) found that most staff nurses agreed that the role was an important clinical resource in their practice. Hurlock-Chorostecki et al. (2015) conducted a survey of NPs in acute care and long-term care settings to assess the processes of implementing interprofessional care, including interdependence, partnership or collaboration, collective problem-solving, professional relationships, communication, and shared decision-making. In this study, greater than 50% of the NPs in acute care engaged in all the elements of interprofessional care. Partnership or collaboration and collective problem-solving had the broadest range of activity engagement, while more than 75% of NPs reported engaging in shared decision-making, communication, and interdependence. In non-clinical activity, ACNPs report engaging in more research and academic activities than PHCNPs (DiCenso et al., 2010).

However, individual NP-Adult practice is variable in role enactment as patient care demands and existing support usually dictate workflow in the role. Kilpatrick et al. (2012a, 2012b), using a case study, mixed-methods time and motion study, found that ACNPs in an in-patient cardiology specialty experienced a faster pace of work in the morning that was reflective of patient care demands. The interaction with physician colleagues and the clarity of administrative structures in place in this group were related to participants' engagement in both clinical and non-clinical activities. For example, ACNPs with more institutional support from administration and medicine spent more time in the research domain of practice. Interestingly, those with greater practice autonomy spent less time on indirect clinical care activities such as leading rounds, discussing cases with physicians and staff nurses, but were identified as the first responder and as having an important role as the professional presence with patients. Overall, in the two cases, ACNPs spent 73% and 61.5% of time in clinical practice, 4.4% and 12.3% in educational activity, 4.2% and 16% in administrative activity, and 10.2% and 0.9% in research activity respectively. Both groups spent between 8% and 9% on activities associated with personal time (Kilpatrick, 2013a, 2013b).

In a related examination of the same group, Kilpatrick (2013a, 2013b) observed the processes surrounding patient care decision-making and communication behaviours within direct and indirect clinical care. ACNPs were observed to have initiated 40% of communications with team members and with patients: roughly double the amount of time spent by the physician on service. The average of communication behaviours/minutes recorded in the two cases were 9.5 and 13.8, a finding that illustrates the importance of this role as central to team functioning for coordination of care. Significant improvement of communication patterns post–NP-Adult role implementation on a neurosurgery in-patient unit was established by Kennan et al. (2018) with qualitative comments reflecting a dramatic change in the comprehensiveness of communication and the quality of the work environment. Additionally, medical residents surveyed in this study reported the improvement in communication was associated with a 20% reduction in patient-related calls from nursing staff.

The reliance of the clinical specialties on the presence of the NP-Adult has, however, been found to come at a price for nurses in some of these roles. Rashotte and Jensen (2010) conducted a qualitative study of ACNPs in specialty practice (N = 26). Informants described the feeling of being adrift in the early part of their practice, particularly when in mentorship with physicians rather than other ACNPs. For participants in the latter part of their practice, the theme of being pushed to do more was an aspect of addressing the needs of the clinical environment. An overall finding was the notion that ACNP informants felt they were pioneers within the context of their institutional environment. A similar result was found in the context of palliative care, where NPs highlighted the need for alignment with another specialty NP in palliative care for mentorship and guidance (Collins & Small, 2019).

Barriers and Facilitators to NP-Adult Practice

Barriers and facilitators to NP practice exist regardless of stream of registration. The effect these factors have is variable and dependent on the structure and functional aspects of the practice environment. DiCenso et al. (2010) found that initial role development, clarity, awareness and implementation, and intraprofessional and interprofessional relationships were some of the features of these roles that could be either barriers or facilitators. A discrepancy between administration and physician specialists about the amount of time ACNPs spent in directing patient care can contribute to both inter- and intraprofessional conflict.

In some cases, physicians want ACNPs to have more time in clinical practice while administrators want time protected for non-clinical activities of leadership, education, and research to ensure these roles are more aligned with nursing. The risk of alignment to other disciplines continues with the predisposition for some roles to be implemented with reporting structures to non-nursing program–level administrators or physicians. The additional impact of inconsistent titling in organizations (NP versus advanced practice nurse) complicates awareness and understanding of the role and the achievement of role clarity. Physicians, administrators, staff nurses, and ACNPs all cited role clarity as essential to the successful implementation of the ACNP role (van Soeren & Micevski, 2001).

Physician receptivity to the role has been found to be related to physician remuneration systems in place. Dimeo and Postic (2012) identified a fee-for-service billing structure to be one of the greatest barriers to role implementation in emergency room settings while alternative or salary-based funding systems facilitated success. In addition, physicians had a preference for a complementary rather than a replacement role with activities of coordination of care, patient self-management facilitation, and discharge planning being key and a value-added role in clinical practice (DiCenso et al., 2010). The understanding of the line between independent NP-Adult practice and autonomous practice can affect the impact "overlapping scopes of practice of NPs and physicians" have on improving patient access to care (p. 25). Relationships with collaborating physicians and administration have been associated with the achievement of autonomous practice and successful role implementation (Almost & Laschinger, 2002; Dimeo & Postic, 2012; Kilpatrick et al., 2012a, 2012b). Kilpatrick et al. (2012a, 2012b) identified the need for an administrative and medical champion, and Almost and Laschinger (2002) reported a statistically positive association between ACNP empowerment and collaboration with physicians that was similar to collaboration with managers.

The role of management as a conduit for organizational communication is an important link for ACNPs to function within the broader context of the organization in addition to providing the resources required for patient care.

Job strain associated with empowerment in ACNP practice is a related barrier to successful role implementation and enactment. Almost and Laschinger (2002) reported that empowerment in the ACNP role was a predictor of job strain with almost half of the variance in job strain being accounted for by the combined effect of collaboration with physicians and managers and workplace empowerment. A qualitative study by Stahlke Wall and Rawson (2016) adds that oncology NP informants struggled to have the aspects of their job that they considered nursing to be valued by colleagues and administrators in the same way as the overlapping aspects of practice with physicians.

Trust between team members, essential for collaboration, was a factor in successful role implementation and enactment in the emergency room and cardiology settings (Dimeo & Postic, 2012; Kilpatrick et al., 2012a, 2012b). For example, Dimeo and Postic (2012) assert that the traditional hierarchical relationship between physicians and the NP dissipated with the development of a collaborative and trusting professional relationship. The researchers make recommendations for ensuring NPs hired are the right fit for the clinical team and the population served, and that a 12-week orientation is necessary for implementation success. Time is required to complete the boundary work required for collaboration and role fluidity toward the improvement of patient care and the achievement of team objectives (Kilpatrick et al., 2012a, 2012b). Boundary work should also include creating space as an adjustment to making the leap to interpreting the role in day-to-day activities, loss of the valued function of interactions of experienced nurses with physicians, trust between team members and interpersonal dynamics, such as taking time to listen to others, making themselves available to staff, setting appropriate limits, and promoting work of other team members (Kilpatrick et al., 2012a, 2012b).

Evidence of NP-Adult Role Effectiveness

The impact of NP-Adult practice on continuity of care has been noted by physicians, administrators, staff nurses, and ACNPs (van Soeren & Micevski, 2001) and may be related to its clinical focus. The role of the NP-Adult has been examined for effectiveness in improving functional outcomes (Sidani et al., 2005), length of hospital stay, testing and associated cost (Sarkissian & Wennberg, 1999), team effectiveness (Kilpatrick, 2013a), and processes of care and associated patient satisfaction (Sidani & Doran, 2010). Sidani et al. (2005) investigated the outcomes of patients (N = 123) who did and did not receive care by an ACNP in a cross-sectional design in two cities in southern Ontario admitted for orthopedic, cardiac, and spinal surgery. Patients who received ACNP care reported higher levels of physical and social functioning and fewer role limitations in their physical and mental health. In reporting interim results of comparisons between physician and NP practice in an adult atrial fibrillation management service, Smigorowsky (2019) reported patients cared for by NPs were more commonly asymptomatic compared to those cared for by physicians (48% versus 25%) and trending toward improvement in quality of life and satisfaction with care.

Sarkissian and Wennberg (1999) found a reduction in hospital length of stay, decreased use of laboratory testing, and lower associated costs after the implementation of an ACNP in an epilepsy care service. The monitoring activities of this ACNP role included diagnostic functions; care planning and delivery; patient assessment and assessment of home and community resources; patient and family education; and the indirect activities of coordination of care, staff education, quality improvement, research consultation with attending and specialist staff, referrals, and discharge planning. Kilpatrick (2013a) found an improvement in team effectiveness, reporting an increase in the team's ability to meet patient needs, provide more complete follow-up, and facilitate communication made an important contribution to care coordination and patient/family-focused care. Additional, ACNPs in this study were found to have a more global view of patient care resulting in medical issues being addressed sooner. Similarly, Sidani and Doran (2010) found that patients who reported higher levels of care coordination also reported improvement in mental health. Additionally, patients in this study who reported higher levels of counselling and education reported improvements in physical function and social functioning respectively. Overall, most patients reported a reduction in the number and severity of symptoms during the study period and satisfaction with care.

CASE STUDY

The Story of Marcia

Marcia is a 42-year-old woman with long-standing chronic widespread pain. She is newly referred to the Chronic Pain Clinic, having been referred by the NP-PHC from her Family Health Team (FHT), which is near her home in the extreme northern boundary of the Local Health Integration Network 120 km away. Leanne, the NP-Adult seeing Marcia on her first visit, has many years of experience caring for patients with chronic non-cancer pain.

Leanne has planned to spend extra time assessing Marcia as the very comprehensive referral letter she has received documents the many challenges Marcia has experienced prior to coming to the clinic. Marcia had a musculoskeletal injury 10 years ago while working as a registered practical nurse (RPN) in a long-term care facility. At the time of her injury, Marcia was assessed for a vertebral fracture and intervertebral disc prolapse with imaging, and a lumbar spine MRI. The imaging results were negative and Marcia expressed being particularly frustrated with these findings, stating, "I still have pain."

Since the injury, Marcia has been unable to continue working as sitting, standing, and lifting cause increased pain. She had been receiving Workplace Safety and Insurance Board assistance, which began several months after her workplace disability coverage ceased. Marcia's treatment has included physiotherapy and massage therapy, neurofeedback, and medications such as muscle relaxants, pain and adjunctive pain medications, including opioids, and non-steroidal medications. Marcia reported that the only treatments she received that were of benefit were the massage therapy, neurofeedback, and baclofen. Marcia's health history included hypothyroidism, depression (for which she has received treatment), and she is a 30-pack/year smoker. She denies alcohol or other substance use. She is reasonably financially stable, although she finds covering the costs of transportation for clinic visits difficult. Marcia lives with her husband and two teenaged sons in a rural community. Her husband works as a farmhand in the local area. Her home relationships are solid and supportive and she has some household assistance from her mother-in-law two days a week. Marcia's current medications are as follows: acetaminophen 325 mg po prn; oxycodone 5 mg two tablets po qid prn (average 8/day); L-thyroxine 0.025 mg po daily; duloxetine hydrochloride 40 mg po daily, and PEG 3350 17 mg po daily prn.

Using her knowledge of the evidence-informed recommendations and the guidelines for the assessment and management of chronic non-cancer pain, Leanne asked Marcia to complete a number of questionnaires to provide a baseline picture of her pain. The results revealed that Marcia has moderate to severe pain-related interference with activity, the absence of depression, and a low rating for pain catastrophizing. Marcia also scores low risk on the Opioid Risk Tool (Michael G. DeGroote National Pain Centre, 2020). Descriptions of her pain were aching, tiring, gnawing, and throbbing all in her lower-back area with no radiation, and she rated her overall pain intensity as 7/10. Her focused physical examination revealed an antalgic gate with no evidence of laterality and was negative for any neurologic findings or red flags. Leanne noted that Marcia had some trigger-point tenderness in her erector spinae muscles and quadratus lumborum muscles bilaterally.

Leanne's initial plan of care included ordering baseline blood work (CBC, electrolytes, magnesium), and initiated a referral to social work, with Marcia's consent, for support and assistance with covering travel costs. She also secured Marcia's written consent to contact her primary care provider, called the referring NP-PHC from Marcia's FHT to have the imaging reports sent to assess the requirement for updated imaging. Recognizing that a review of imaging would be required prior to referral for additional physiotherapy, or to one of her physician colleagues for consideration of interventional pain management techniques, Leanne used the visit to establish a trusting relationship with Marcia, and to develop a comprehensive understanding of her current situation. Leanne collaborated with Marcia to choose a date for her next clinic appointment at a time when her husband could drive her, and that would include the social worker, Leanne, and her physician colleague. Leanne promised to ensure that any additional imaging that may be required could be performed at the same time.

Marcia left the clinic expressing a sense of relief that she had been "listened to and valued" and stated she was hopeful that working with the chronic pain team could help with her pain and improve her quality of life.

Conclusion

The NP-Adult, also referred to as CNS/NP, ACNP, TCNP, and SNP, provides care to patients with complex health care challenges in the context of collaborative teams, usually in acute care institutional settings. Practice characteristics of the role are variable and dependent on the needs of the specialty population and the organizational supports available, but include activities in both clinical and non-clinical domains. The number of these APN roles is growing in the face of increased needs for chronic disease management within an already fiscally constrained health care system. Essential to the successful scope of practice enactment of the NP-Adult role is the individual practitioner's ability to realize their own potential.

Critical Thinking Questions

1. What factors influence NP-Adult scope of practice in Canada?
2. What steps should be taken to increase role success when implementing an NP-Adult role in a specialty practice area?
3. What are the main practice differences between the PHCNP and NP-Adult roles?

References

Almost, J., & Laschinger, H. K. S. (2002). Workplace empowerment, collaborative work relationships, and job strain in nurse practitioners. *Journal of the American Academy of Nurse Practitioners, 14*(9), 408–420.

Bryant-Lukosius, D., & DiCenso, A. (2004). A framework for the introduction and evaluation of advanced practice nursing roles. *Journal of Advanced Nursing, 48*(5), 530–540. Retrieved from http://aipsq.com/_pdf/Bryant-Lukosius%20DiCenso%20A%20framework%20for%20the%20introduction%20and%20evaluation%20of%20advanced%20practice%20nursing%20roles.pdf

Canadian Association of Schools of Nursing (CASN). (2012). *Nurse practitioner education in Canada: National framework of guiding principles and essential components.* Ottawa, ON: CASN.

Canadian Council of Registered Nurse Regulators (CCRNR). (2015). *Practice analysis study of nurse practitioners.* Beaverton, ON: CCRNR.

Canadian Nurses Association (CNA). (2010). *Canadian nurse practitioner core competency framework.* Ottawa, ON: CNA. Retrieved from http://www.cno.org/globalassets/for/rnec/pdf/competencyframework_en.pdf

Collins, C., & Small, S. (2019). The nurse practitioner role is ideally suited for palliative care practice: A qualitative descriptive study. *Canadian Oncology Nursing Journal, 29*(1), 4–9.

Creamer, A., & Austin, W. (2017). Canadian nurse practitioner core competencies identified: An opportunity to build mental health and illness skills and knowledge. *The Journal for Nurse Practitioners, 13*(5), e231–e236.

DiCenso, A., Bryant-Lukosius, D., Borgeault, I., Martin-Misener, R., Donald, F., Abelson, J., … Harbman, P. (2010). *Clinical nurse specialists and nurse practitioners in Canada: A decision support synthesis.* Ottawa, ON: CHSRF/FCRSS. Retrieved from http://www.cfhi-fcass.ca/Libraries/Commissioned_Research_Reports/Dicenso_EN_Final.sflb.ashx

Dimeo, M., & Postic, M. (2012). Lessons learned in developing and implementing the nurse practitioner role in an urban Canadian emergency department. *Journal of Emergency Nursing, 38*(5), 484–487.

Hansen, K., McDonald, C., O'Hara, S., Post, L., Silcox, S., & Gutmanis, I. (2017). A formative evaluation of a nurse practitioner-led interprofessional geriatric outpatient clinic. *Journal of Interprofessional Care, 31*(4), 546–549.

Hurlock-Chorostecki, C., Forchuk, C., Orchard, C., van Soeren, M., & Reeves, S. (2014). Hospital-based nurse practitioner roles and interprofessional practice: A scoping review. *Nursing & Health Sciences, 16*(3), 403–410.

Hurlock-Chorostecki, C., van Soeren, M., MacMillan, K., Sidani, S., Collins, L., Harbman, P., … Reeves, S. (2015). A survey of interprofessional activity of acute and long-term care employed nurse practitioners. *Journal of the American Association of Nurse Practitioners, 27*(9), 507–513. doi: 10.1002/2327-6924.12213

Keenan, A. M., Mutterback, E. E., Velthuizen, K. M., Pantalone, M. E., & Gossack-Keenan, K. L. (2018). Perceptions of the effectiveness of advanced practice nurses on a neurosurgery unit in a Canadian tertiary care centre: A pre-and-post implementation design. *International Journal of Nursing Sciences, 5*(2), 138–143.

Kilpatrick, K. (2008). Praxis and the role development of the acute care nurse practitioner. *Nursing Inquiry, 15*(2), 116–126.

Kilpatrick, K. (2013a). How do nurse practitioners in acute care affect perceptions of team effectiveness? *Journal of Clinical Nursing, 22*, 2636–2647.

Kilpatrick, K. (2013b). Understanding acute care nurse practitioner communication and decision-making in healthcare teams. *Journal of Clinical Nursing, 22*, 168–179.

Kilpatrick, K., Harbman, P., Carter, N., Martin-Misener, R., Bryant-Lukosius, D., Donald, F., … DiCenso, A. (2010). The acute care nurse practitioner role in Canada. *Nursing Leadership, 23*(Special Issue), 114–139.

Kilpatrick, K., Lavoie-Tremblay, M., Ritchie, J. A., Lamothe, L., Doran, D., & Rochefort, C. (2012a). How are acute care nurse practitioners enacting their roles in healthcare teams? A descriptive multiple-case study. *International Journal of Nursing Studies, 49*, 850–862.

Kilpatrick, K., Lavoie-Tremblay, M., Ritchie, J., Lamothe, L., & Doran, D. (2012b). Boundary work and the introduction of acute care nurse practitioners in healthcare teams. *Journal of Advanced Nursing, 68*(7), 1504–1515.

Martin-Misener, R. (2010). Will nurse practitioners achieve full integration into the Canadian healthcare system? *Canadian Journal of Nursing Research, 42*(2), 9–16.

Michael G. DeGroote National Pain Centre. (2020). *Canadian guideline for safe and effective use of opioids for chronic non-cancer pain: Appendix B-2: Opioid risk tool.* Hamilton, ON: McMaster University. Retrieved from http://nationalpaincentre.mcmaster.ca/opioid/cgop_b_app_b02.html

Rashotte, J., & Jensen, L. (2010). The transformational journey of nurse practitioners in acute care settings. *Canadian Journal of Nursing Research, 42*(2), 70–91.

Sarkissian, S., & Wennberg, R. (1999). Effects of the acute care nurse practitioner role on epilepsy monitoring outcomes. *Outcomes Management for Nursing Practice, 3*(4), 161–166.

Sidani, S., & Doran, D. (2010). Relationships between process and outcomes of nurse practitioners in acute care: An exploration. *Journal of Nursing Care Quality, 25*(1), 31–38.

Sidani, S., Doran, D., Porter, H., LeFort, S., O'Brien-Pallas, L., Zahn, C., & Sarkissian, S. (2005). Outcomes of nurse practitioners in acute care: An exploration. *The Internet Journal of Advanced Nursing Practice, 8*(1). Retrieved from https://ispub.com/IJANP/8/1/12232

Sidani, S., Irvine, D., Porter, H., O'Brien-Pallas, L., Simpson, B., McGillis Hall, L., ... Redelmeir, D. (2000). Practice patterns of acute care nurse practitioners. *Canadian Journal of Nursing Leadership, 13*(3), 6–12.

Smigorowsky, M. (2019). *Outcomes of nurse practitioner-led care in adult patients with atrial fibrillation* (Unpublished doctoral thesis, University of Alberta, Edmonton, AB).

Spross, J. (2009). Conceptualizations of advanced practice nursing. In A. Hamric, J. Spross, & C. Hanson (Eds.), *Advanced practice nursing: An integrative approach* (4th ed., pp. 27–66). St. Louis, MO: Saunders Elsevier.

Stahlke Wall, S., & Rawson, K. (2016). The nurse practitioner role in oncology: Advancing patient care. *Oncology Nursing Forum, 43*(4), 489–496.

Staples, E., & Sangster-Gormley, E. (2018). Supporting nurse practitioner education: Preceptorship, recruitment and retention. *International Journal of Nursing Sciences, 5*(2), 115–120.

van Soeren, M., & Micevski, V. (2001). Success indicators and barriers to acute nurse practitioner role implementation in four Ontario hospitals. *AACN Clinical Issues, 12*(3), 424–437.

Chapter

26

Nurse Practitioner: Pediatrics

Jamie Churchill and Kevin Zizzo

JAMIE CHURCHILL is a nurse practitioner (NP)–Pediatrics in Neurology at Hamilton Health Sciences McMaster Children's Hospital, Hamilton, Ontario.

KEVIN ZIZZO is a nurse practitioner (NP)–Pediatrics and is the owner/practitioner for MyPediatricNP, an NP consulting company. He sits on the Board of Directors of the Nurse Practitioners' Association of Ontario.

KEY TERMS

family-centred care
pediatric nurse practitioner
(PNP)
transition

OBJECTIVES

1. Appraise the history of the pediatric nurse practitioner (PNP) role in Canada.
2. Discuss the current PNP role in Canada.
3. Examine barriers to PNP practice.

Introduction

The term *acute care nurse practitioner* (ACNP) was adopted widely in Canada in the 1990s to encompass those NPs working with specialized populations in an acute care setting, such as pediatrics (Kaasalainen et al., 2010). Due to this classification, the **pediatric nurse practitioner (PNP)** usually falls under the umbrella term *ACNP*, which includes the NP-Adult and the neonatal NP. A PNP works with infants, children, adolescents, and their caregivers to provide advanced health care services. They assess, diagnose, and treat patients with acute, episodic, or chronic health care conditions, and consult and collaborate with other health care team members to provide **family-centred care**. PNPs who work in areas providing ongoing care may also have the responsibility of preparing and overseeing the transition of their patients from pediatric to adult services. This chapter will discuss the history and current state of the PNP role and barriers to practice for the PNP. The chapter will present a case study that demonstrates the role in practice.

History of the Pediatric Nurse Practitioner Role in Canada

The first PNP role began in the United States at the University of Colorado, where a program was developed in 1965 (Wilson, 2005). NPs graduating from this program were educated to provide well child care and to manage common health problems seen in childhood. Later, programs for PNPs working in acute care were developed.

The ACNP role was developed in Canada in the late 1980s to offset rapidly increasing physician workloads in acute care settings and to address the lack of continuity of care for seriously ill patients and increased complexity of care delivery (Kilpatrick et al., 2010). The first Canadian educational program to address the pediatric specialty was offered at McMaster University School of Nursing in neonatology in 1986 (Kilpatrick et al., 2010).

In Ontario during the 1990s, there was a decrease in the number of medical residents from medical schools, but there was also an increase in the number and acuity of acute care admissions to hospitals (Irvine et al., 2000). The ACNP role was identified as part of the solution to address the health care needs of hospitalized patients. Subsequently, NPs were introduced to improve continuity of care for medically complex patients who required prolonged hospitalizations (Pringle, 2007). During this time, health care reform was occurring that set out to ensure more efficient use of health care resources (Kaasalainen et al., 2010). Later, in 1993, the first PNP program was developed at the University of Toronto Faculty of Nursing (Hurlock-Chorostecki, van Soeren, & Goodwin, 2008). Two streams—adult and pediatrics— were offered at the postgraduate level and graduates practiced in acute care settings with specialized populations (Kaasalainen et al., 2010).

The PNP role was to provide comprehensive advanced practive nursing (APN) care to patients and their families in general pediatrics or in subspecialty settings. The PNP role is legislated and regulated throughout Canada under the abbreviation NP-Pediatrics. Most tertiary pediatric centres in Canada today utilize PNPs in both the in-patient and the ambulatory settings.

More recently, McGill University has also launched a PNP program (McGill University Ingram School of Nursing, 2017).

The Role of Pediatric Nurse Practitioners in Canada

In Canada, PNPs work primarily in pediatric acute care facilities, in both in-patient roles and ambulatory clinics. They may work in any number of subspecialties such as cardiology, endocrinology, oncology, etc. Patient care is provided along the continuum from diagnosis, acute care management, chronic illness management, to palliative care or transition to primary or adult care.

The ACNP roles, including the PNP, have not been researched or published as widely as the NP role in primary health care, also known as NP-Family/All Ages. This is most likely due to the relatively smaller number of PNPs in practice compared to other counterparts. As of 2018, 51% of nurse practitioners in Ontario report practicing in primary care, while only 7% of nurse practitioners in Ontario held their specialty certificate in pediatrics (Mattison &

Wilson, 2018). The PNP roles in Canada are often incorporated within interprofessional teams and, theoretically, they share core competencies with other APN roles (Schober & Affara, 2009). Overarching competency domains included clinical practice, research, education, consultation and collaboration, and leadership, but have been articulated more widely in the 2019 pan-Canadian APN Framework (Canadian Nurses Association [CNA], 2010, 2019).

Even with these competencies, role confusion is prevalent in the pediatric community and the optimal use of the PNP's knowledge and skills is sometimes overlooked. A survey of ACNPs in Ontario found that 20% identified themselves as working in pediatric hospitals (Hurlock-Chorostecki et al., 2008). Direct patient care and clinical practice is variable across the spectrum of the PNP role and is dependent on the expectations of the PNP's interprofessional team members. Clinical practice in the current PNP role includes patient and family assessment, diagnosis, ordering various laboratory and diagnostic tests, developing treatment plans, patient and family education, and ongoing medical and medication management. On average, PNPs spend 80% of their daily practice time in the domain of direct patient care (Maloney & Volpe, 2005).

An Ontario survey examining NP roles in hospital settings included NPs from two pediatric hospitals (van Soeren, Hurlock-Chorostecki, & Reeves, 2011). The PNPs reported that they spent 38% of their time in the clinical domain with most of their time being spent in the consultation domain. They reported working closely with the interprofessional team, physician collaborators and specialists, to provide care to vulnerable patient populations. Health care colleagues reported that PNPs were approachable, provided continuity of care, and had a good knowledge of the patient with a deep understanding of their issues, which they were able to share with colleagues, patients, and their families. It was concluded that patient safety was improved because PNPs were able to ensure that details of care were not missed. Many consultations by the PNP were with physicians or nurses. Allied health care professionals, residents, specialty clinics, and others accounted for the remainder of the PNP consultations. The PNP role supports communication among team members across health disciplines, which was appreciated by the other professionals. The PNPs spent the remaining 20% of their time equally divided between the leadership, research, and other work categories (i.e., meetings, email, travel).

The CNA (2016) held a roundtable discussion and found that all NPs had very little opportunity to engage in research activities. As an example, a typical job description for a PNP at a tertiary care hospital states that the primary focus of the role is clinical, spending up to 80% of time in this domain (Lee & Clause, 2014). This leaves only 20% of one's time to devote to research, education, consultation, and leadership. Of course, PNPs are engaged in knowledge translation in practice, but may find it difficult to engage in actual research studies. There have been many important research studies published by PNPs related to the pediatric population. Given that most PNPs practice in tertiary care and affiliated academic centres, research opportunities may be more readily available to them as compared to, for example, NPs in primary health care.

PNPs provide education to patients, families, students, and staff as part of their role (Maloney & Volpe, 2005; McCarty & Rogers, 2012). They educate patients and families, nurses, residents, and fellows. They precept graduate NP students and may provide guest lectures at conferences and seminars. Providing education can address both health care management as well as educating others about the roles and responsibilities of the PNP. In one hospital, PNPs direct an in-patient asthma education program, promoting self-management by the patient and their parents (McCarty & Rogers, 2012). At another hospital, PNPs were asked to be part of and present at residency orientation in order to provide the medical residents with a comprehensive discussion about the role of the PNP. This type of education can mitigate future role discrepancies and increase overall job satisfaction.

In an article written about Quebec's first PNP, the PNP discussed two key aspects of her role; the latitude to order a consultation as the situation necessitated, and the confidence and self-awareness to collaborate with physician colleagues if she had reached the limits of her scope of practice. She acknowledges that her experience and knowledge had taken time to be recognized, but her role is now valued and has an important place in health care (Montreal Children's Hospital, 2019).

In 2018, APNs described their leadership in themes of patient-focused, organizational, and system-focused (Lamb, Martin-Misener, Bryant-Lukosius, & Latimer, 2018). Patient-focused leadership included managing patient-centred care, coaching and education, advocating, and initiating meaningful communication. Organization and system-focused leadership was described as improving the quality of care provided, enhancing professional nursing practice, being an expert clinician, communicating effectively, mentoring and coaching, providing leadership on internal and external committees, and facilitating collaboration. A PNP will have the responsibility to assess and utilize these themes by tailoring them to their specific specialty. For example, a PNP may have a more prominent leadership role in advocating for their clients' care if their patient population is not be able to fully advocate for themselves.

Family-Centred Care

Family-centred care incorporates the needs and wishes of both the patient and their family members. Pediatric health care centres work with both the patients and their families to address the health care needs of the patient. Decisions about the patient's diagnosis, work-up, treatment, and overall plan impact not only the patient, but their family unit as well. The PNP works in a position where they can engage with the patient and the family to identify a plan of care that works best for the entire family. The PNP forms a partnership with the patient and their caregivers to guide the patient's care. Health care planning, delivery, and evaluation are performed in collaboration with patients, families, NPs, nursing, physicians, and other care providers (American Academy of Pediatrics, 2012). The care team takes into consideration the families' cultural, ethnic, and socio-economic background when developing care plans for patients and their families.

Policies, procedures, and organizational practices need to factor in patient and family needs, beliefs, and cultural values. Patients and families should have all the information needed to effectively participate in care and decision-making and they should be able to choose their level of involvement. For hospitalized patients, the PNP and team need to regularly communicate with the family so they can make informed decisions. Supports should be in place to help a child at all stages of development. This includes both formal and informal supports. Collaboration with patients and families should be at all levels. Patient and family representatives should be involved in policy-making, committee work, education, and on advisory councils. Patients and families need to be empowered in order to participate in the care of the patient and in decision-making. The PNP must incorporate family-centred care into their practice by communicating regularly with the family, understanding their needs and concerns, and being able to provide this information to other health care team members and act as an advocate for the family.

Barriers to PNP Practice

Many barriers to the success of PNP practice are also found among other ACNP specialties. They include the inability to work to one's full scope of practice, lack of funding models, and legislation and policies that exclude NPs. Barriers unique to the PNP role are not well documented or researched, but may include limited workplace options, lack of ongoing educational opportunities, and precarious entry examinations for practice that are not standardized across Canada. Such barriers prevent PNPs from fully realizing their full capacity as NPs and can lead to frustration and decreased job satisfaction in the workplace.

A survey conducted by the Canadian Federation of Nurses Unions (CFNU; 2018) found that 26% of NPs report not being able to work to their full scope of practice. This number rose to 33% for NPs working in a hospital setting, which is where PNPs tend to practice most. When asked why they are unable to work to their full scope, the top three barriers that were reported were the way one's role was defined by their institution, employer barriers, as well as personality and philosophy of physician colleagues.

Poor professional awareness of the ACNP role has been associated with fluctuating expectations and concerns about whether the ACNP is practicing outside their scope of practice (DiCenso & Bryant-Lukosius, 2010). This suspected role ambiguity can also result in role overlap with other nursing and medical team members, thereby creating potential resentment and hostility.

One practice barrier encountered often throughout the NP community is that of legislation or policies that contain outdated language that excludes NPs from providing services and care within their ability and scope. An example is reimbursement for clients through private insurers. NPs have the competency and legal scope to write prescriptions for medications and medical devices. Even so, many private medical insurers require physician-issued prescriptions for devices and medications, which contribute to an inefficient system that does not take advantage of its workforce. In the pediatric setting, a PNP may come across this issue when attempting to obtain a specific medication. Children with cerebral palsy may benefit from the administration of botulinum toxin (Botox) injections to spastic muscles. This medication is not covered through a provincial plan in Ontario if the family has private insurance. The procedure for obtaining Botox for these children includes a letter to the insurance company outlining the rationale, dosage, and goals of the medication, and the completion of specific pre-authorization forms supplied by each insurance company. Currently, the language in some forms allows for only physicians to have the ability to complete and submit them, even though the PNP may have the ability and legal scope to order this medication.

Entry into practice as an NP in Canada requires passing an approved examination. An NP-Family/All Ages examination has been developed and utilized effectively in all 10 provinces to ensure a standard entry to practice among this large group. Unfortunately, there is no such standard entry examination in Canada for pediatrics, and all jurisdictions that license NPs in a pediatric category utilize the American Pediatric Nursing Certification Board's (PNCB's) Primary Care Pediatric Nurse Practitioner Certification Examination (CNA, 2016). As previously discussed, most PNPs tend to work in acute care settings and/ or pediatric hospitals, thereby producing an incongruity based on the examination title and purpose alone.

Though it is impractical for Canada to develop an examination for the pediatrics stream due to the limited number in the specialty, the PNCB's examination for pediatrics is based in primary care, where very few, if any, Canadian PNPs find themselves employed as primary health care centres are looking for NPs who can provide care across the life spectrum. This limitation in relation to workplace opportunities is also a barrier to PNP practice. The lack of a funding model for PNPs to work in primary health care has prevented PNPs from entering this sector to provide primary health care support to a vulnerable population. Also contributing to the decreasing quantity of PNPs is the limited choice for education. As of the 2013/2014 academic year, there were 28 NP programs across Canada, yet only two pediatric specialty certification streams (CNA, 2016).

CASE STUDY

The Story of Aubrey

Aubrey has been referred to the outpatient ambulatory neurology clinic at a local children's hospital by her family physician for evaluation of ongoing headaches. She is coming to her first appointment and will be seen by Kyan, the PNP in the clinic. She arrives at the clinic with her mother and younger sibling.

Past Medical History: Aubrey is a 14-year-old girl with no significant comorbidities. Her birth history is non-contributory. She has no chronic conditions and has had one previous surgery, a tonsillectomy, at the age of 6. She denies any allergies and has no other hospitalizations. Her immunizations are up to date.

History of Present Illness: Aubrey has been experiencing headaches for the past year. She describes approximately 2–3 headache episodes per week and in between these headaches she remains healthy and symptom-free. She does report "all-day headaches" sometimes, but more often her headaches last 30–60 minutes and tend to occur in the evening or at night. She states that she often wakes with a headache during the night. She describes the headaches as a "pressing feeling" that occurs in the front of her head. On a scale of 1 to 10 she rates the pain as an 8 or 9. She often feels nauseous before her headaches and sometimes vomits. Her mom thinks Aubrey looks pale before a headache and acknowledges that Aubrey will often retreat to her room during the headache where it is dark and quiet. She has tried ibuprofen and acetaminophen for her headaches, but denies they provide any relief.

Family History: Aubrey's immediate family consists of her mother, father, and two younger siblings. Her father suffers from high blood pressure and depression. Her two younger siblings are healthy with no noted medical conditions. Her mother states she had headaches as a young girl, but did not require any medication for them. They disappeared spontaneously as she aged.

Social History: Aubrey started high school this past year and is in an enriched stream with a heavy course load. She is an "A" student and admits feeling stressed about her academic performance. She denies drug use, but does drink alcohol with her friends on occasion. She states she will drink up to four beers/night "once in a while." She does not have a significant other and states she is not sexually active.

Physical Examination: Aubrey is 168 cm in height and 76 kg. She is pleasant and articulate during the examination and answers questions appropriately. Her vital signs are all within normal limits for her age, except for a blood pressure of 135/86. There is no fever. Examination of the skin reveals no neurocutaneous stigmata and there is no papilledema. Cranial nerves II–XII are intact. Muscle tone in all four limbs is equal and appropriate with no spasticity or laxity. She demonstrates intact sensation and coordination. She has a negative Romberg test and appropriate reflexes.

Investigations: No previous neuroimaging has been completed. She has not had any laboratory testing done.

Assessment: At this point, Kyan considers the current information he's obtained and diagnoses that Aubrey is suffering from pediatric migraine without aura. Differential diagnoses and other considerations for ongoing headaches discussed and evaluated by Kyan included headache due to infection, trauma, tension headache, space-occupying lesion, and vascular issues.

Discussion

At this point, Kyan discussed management options with Aubrey. He provided patient education on potential lifestyle factors that may influence headache severity and frequency. They discussed, in private, stresses in Aubrey's life that may be contributory, such as her schoolwork. Kyan also spent time educating Aubrey about the effects of alcohol on the developing brain. Clinically, Kyan did not find any concerning neurological findings and feels comfortable starting Aubrey with non-pharmacological interventions, such as a headache diary, increased physical activities, changes in diet (limiting caffeine intake), and relaxation techniques. Kyan consulted with a collaborating physician regarding Aubrey's case due to the night waking with headaches and elevated blood pressure. Together they agreed that up to 25% of pediatric migraines have been documented to have night waking and with no other neurological findings, and they can retake her blood pressure in three weeks to reassess. In the meantime, Kyan referred Aubrey to a dietician as her BMI is 27 and healthy lifestyle and food choices may improve her headaches. He made a follow-up appointment with Aubrey for three weeks to reassess her blood pressure and review her headache diary. He also advised Aubrey that should any neurological signs or symptoms appear, Kyan will consult and collaborate with a physician colleague for ongoing investigations. Should Aubrey remain stable, Kyan will choose to follow her at regular intervals, adjusting the treatment plan as needed, in order to ensure overall health.

Transition from Pediatric to Adult Primary Health Care

Pediatric patients many experience several transitions in their health care experience. Transition, defined as the move from one level of health care to another, may occur at one or several time points. Successful transition may require advanced preparation and engagement of the patient, their family, and involved health care providers. Time points for transition include transition at diagnosis; from childhood to adolescence to young adulthood; from pediatric tertiary care to adult tertiary care; and from tertiary care to primary health care.

PNPs work with their patients to prepare them for these transition points. In order to ensure the successful transition of patients, the health care team requires a structured approach to the transition process (O'Sullivan-Oliveira, Fernandes, Borges, & Fishman, 2014). The developmental stage of the patient must be considered when implementing transition planning. Children, adolescents, and young adults with chronic illness, or who have had childhood illnesses with potential for future illness as a result of the diagnosis or treatment, require preparation as they transition to adult care. Transition is the process of preparing adolescents and young adults for the move from one point in the health care system to another.

Clear policies on transition are needed to ensure the best outcomes for the patient (Wilkins, D'Agostino, Penney, Barr, & Nathan, 2014). This includes policies on the timing of transfer from the pediatric service, the preparation and education of the patient, and the integration of primary care providers in the transfer process. PNPs may participate in developing transition policies and programs and engaging stakeholders in the process. As well, they can work with patients to ensure they have self-advocacy skills. They can provide the patient with education related to their treatment plan, its potential short- and long-term side effects, and the need for lifelong monitoring that facilitates the development of self-advocacy skills. When preparing a patient for transition from pediatrics, the PNP participates in preparing a summary of recommendations for the team taking on the care of the patient by engaging the patient, family, and primary care or adult care providers in order to ensure a successful transition.

Several factors need to be taken into consideration that include timing the patient's needs while at the same time being flexible. The patient needs to understand their treatment plan, be aware of the risks for short- and long-term effects as a result of their disease and/or treatment, have the skills to manage their own health care, and understand the importance of lifelong risk-based monitoring (Wilkins et al., 2014). The PNP, in preparing the patient for transition, should assess the patient's capacity to engage in the process, including the patient's knowledge, skills/self-efficacy, beliefs and expectations, goals, and relationships and psychosocial functioning. The PNP, in their encounters with the patient, should evaluate the patient's physical health and function, sexual/reproductive health, mental health, social competence, health behaviours, and health education (Nathan, Hayes-Lattin, Sisler, & Hudson, 2011).

Transition assessment tools should be implemented early in the patient's continuum of care and be reassessed at defined developmental time points (O'Sullivan-Oliveira et al., 2014). Psychosocial and transitional needs must be factored in when deciding to transition a patient. The PNP can play a role in alleviating parental and patient concerns around transition, developing institutional recommendations for transition, and providing the health care providers to whom the patient is being transitioned with relevant information on the patient, their management and their treatment, and follow-up recommendations. As well, they can work with their care team to develop transition guidelines and identify research priorities for the population. The PNP can act as the liaison with the patient and the pediatric and the adult services by identifying patient, family, and health care provider barriers and facilitators to transition and creating potential solutions (Jalkut & Allen, 2009). Anticipatory guidance should be used to engage the patient and to prepare them for the adult health care experience. The conversation should include a review of the patient's disease and treatment, a discussion about career planning, a lifestyle review, and care recommendations.

Conclusion

PNPs in Canada practice primarily in pediatric tertiary care centres. They practice as part of an interprofessional team in providing family-centred care to pediatric patients and their families. PNP roles require team engagement, role integration, and intention to be successfully implemented. The PNP may be involved in the patient's care from diagnosis, throughout treatment, and to transition to adult care or primary care. They provide education on illness, management, and best practices to patients, families, colleagues, and health care learners. They practice collaboratively with health care team members and consult with other health care professionals to ensure that optimal pediatric patient care is provided. In order to ensure the future of PNPs, we must advocate for more ongoing educational opportunities, a standardized examination that reflects PNP practice in Canada, and funding models that encourage a variety of practice settings for the role. Continued education disseminated to other health care providers about the PNP role and practice competencies can assist with a united and successfully functioning team.

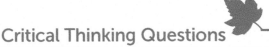

Critical Thinking Questions

1. A new PNP has just started employment with the respiratory team at a children's hospital. How can the PNP articulate their role to their colleagues?

2. As a PNP in a busy neurology clinic, you see a 16-year-old boy with epilepsy who consistently forgets to take his anti-epileptic medication. Using patient education and current research, how can you best address this situation with the client and his family?

3. In what ways can an individual PNP engage with potential NPs to consider this stream? In what ways can institutions and professional nursing organizations promote the role of the PNP?

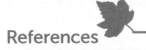

References

American Academy of Pediatrics Committee on Hospital Care and Institute for Patient and Family-Centered Care. (2012). Policy statement. Patient- and family-centered care and the pediatrician's role. *Pediatrics, 129*(2), 393–404. doi: 10.1542/peds.2011-3084

Canadian Federation of Nurses Unions (CFNU). 2018. *Fulfilling nurse practitioners' untapped potential in Canada's health care system: Results from the CFNU pan-Canadian nurse practitioner retention & recruitment study.* Ottawa, ON: CFNU. Retrieved from https://nursesunions.ca/research/untapped-potential/

Canadian Nurses Association (CNA). (2010). *Canadian nurse practitioner core competency framework.* Ottawa, ON: CNA.

CNA. (2016). *The Canadian nurse practitioner initiative: A 10-year retrospective.* Ottawa, ON: CNA. Retrieved from https://cna-aiic.ca/-/media/cna/page-content/pdf-en/canadian-nurse-practitioner-initiative-a-10-year-retrospective.pdf

CNA. (2019). *Advanced practice nursing: A pan-Canadian framework.* Ottawa, ON: CNA. Retrieved from https://www.cna-aiic.ca/-/media/cna/page-content/pdf-en/apn-a-pan-canadian-framework.pdf

DiCenso, A., & Bryant-Lukosius, D. (2010). *Clinical nurse specialists and nurse practitioners in Canada: A decision support synthesis.* Ottawa, ON: CFHI. Retrieved from https://www.cfhi-fcass.ca/Search-ResultsNews/10-06-01/b9cb9576-6140-4954-aa57-2b81c1350936.aspx

Hurlock-Chorostecki, C., van Soeren, M., & Goodwin, S. (2008). The acute care nurse practitioner in Ontario: A workforce study. *Nursing Leadership, 21*(4), 100–116.

Irvine, S., Sidani, S., Porter, H., O'Brien-Pallas, L., Simpson, B., McGillis Hall, L., … Nagel, L. (2000). Organizational factors influencing nurse practitioners' role: Implementation in acute care settings. *Canadian Journal of Nursing Leadership, 13*(3), 28–35.

Jalkut, M. K., & Allen, P. J. (2009). Transition from pediatric to adult health care for adolescents with congenital heart disease: A review of the literature and clinical implications. *Primary Care Approaches, 35*(6), 381–387.

Kaasalainen, S., Martin-Misener, R., Kilpatrick, K., Harbman, P., Bryant-Lukosius, D., Donald, F., … DiCenso, A. (2010). A historical overview of the development of advanced practice nursing roles in Canada. *Nursing Leadership, 23*(Special Issue), 35–60.

Kilpatrick, K., Harbman, P., Carter, N., Martin-Misener, R., Bryant-Lukosius, D., Donald, F., ... DiCenso, A. (2010). The acute care nurse practitioner role in Canada. *Nursing Leadership, 23*(Special Issue December), 114–139.

Lamb, A., Martin-Misener, R., Bryant-Lukosius, D., & Latimer, M. (2018). Describing the leadership capabilities of advanced practice nurses using a qualitative descriptive study. *Nursing Open, 5*(3), 400–413.

Lee, R., & Clause, R. F. (2014). *Advanced practice nursing roles at Hamilton Health Sciences (HHS).* Hamilton, ON: HHS.

Maloney, A. M., & Volpe, J. (2005). The inpatient advanced practice nursing roles in a Canadian pediatric oncology unit. *Journal of Pediatric Oncology Nursing, 22*(5), 254–257. doi: 10.1177/1043454205279290

Mattison, C. A., & Wilson, M. G. (2018). Rapid synthesis: Enhancing health system integration of nurse practitioners in Ontario. *McMaster Health Forum, 17.* Retrieved from http://hdl.handle. net/11375/23852

McCarty, K., & Rogers, J. (2012). Inpatient asthma education program. *Pediatric Nursing, 38*(5), 257–263.

McGill University Ingram School of Nursing. (2017). *Pediatric nurse practitioner.* Montreal, QC: McGill. Retrieved from https://www.mcgill.ca/peds/education-training/interprofessional-education/pediatric-nurse-practitioner-program

Montreal Children's Hospital. (2019). *A day in the life of ... a pediatric nurse practitioner.* Montreal, QC: Montreal Children's Hospital. Retrieved from https://www.thechildren.com/news-and-events/latest-news/day-life-ofa-pediatric-nurse-practitioner

Nathan, P. C., Hayes-Lattin, B., Sisler, J. J., & Hudson, M. M. (2011). Critical issues in the transition and survivorship of adolescents and young adults with cancer. *Cancer, 117*(10 Supplement), 2335–2341.

O'Sullivan-Oliveira, J., Fernandes, S. M., Borges, L. F., & Fishman, L. N. (2014). Transition of pediatric patients to adult care: An analysis of provider perceptions across discipline and role. *Pediatric Nursing, 40*(3), 114–121.

Pringle, D. (2007). Nurse practitioner role: Nursing needs it. *Nursing Leadership, 20*(2), 1–5.

Schober, M., & Affara, F. (2009). *International council of nurses: Advanced nursing practice.* Oxford, UK: Wiley.

van Soeren, M., Hurlock-Chorostecki, C., & Reeves, S. (2011). The role of nurse practitioners in hospital settings: Implications for interprofessional practice. *Journal of Interprofessional Care, 25*, 245–251.

Wilkins, K. L., D'Agostino, N., Penney, A. M., Barr, R. D., & Nathan, P. C. (2014). Supporting adolescents and young adults with cancer through transitions: Position statement from the Canadian Task Force on adolescents and young adults with cancer. *Journal of Pediatric Hematology/Oncology, 36*(7), 545–551. doi: 10.1097/MPH.0000000000000103

Wilson, K. (2005). The evolution of the role of nurses: The history of nurse practitioners in pediatric oncology. *Journal of Pediatric Oncology Nursing, 22*(5), 250–253.

Chapter

27

Nurse Practitioner: Neonatal

Mary McAllister, Marilyn Ballantyne, Amy Wright, and Amanda Symington

MARY McALLISTER is the Associate Chief, Nursing Practice, at The Hospital for Sick Children (SickKids), Toronto, Ontario, where she began her career as a neonatal nurse practitioner (NNP), and later was a clinical nurse specialist (CNS). She has held academic positions at Ryerson University, the Lawrence S. Bloomberg Faculty of Nursing, University of Toronto, both in Toronto, Ontario, and the Edith Cowan University School of Nursing, Perth, Australia. Mary is the editor for the *Practice for the Nursing Leadership Journal*. She continues to be involved in nursing professional organizations, contributing to advances in nursing practice, and being a champion for evidence-informed practice provincially, nationally, and internationally.

MARILYN BALLANTYNE is a nurse practitioner (NP)-Pediatrics and Chief Nurse Executive & Clinician Investigator at the Holland Bloorview Kids Rehabilitation Hospital, Toronto, Ontario. She has extensive clinical experience as an NP-Pediatrics in acute and outpatient settings. She has held academic positions at McMaster University, Hamilton, Ontario, the Lawrence S. Bloomberg Faculty of Nursing, University of Toronto, Toronto, Ontario, and clinical/research positions at SickKids Hospital, Toronto, Ontario.

AMY WRIGHT is a nurse practitioner (NP)-Pediatrics in the Neonatal Intensive Care Unit at McMaster Children's Hospital and an Assistant Professor in the Lawrence S. Bloomberg Faculty of Nursing at the University of Toronto, Toronto, Ontario. Dr. Wright's program of research focuses on community-engaged, participatory approaches to health equity for Indigenous families in Canada.

AMANDA SYMINGTON is a nurse practitioner (NP) in the Neonatal Intensive Care Unit at Niagara Health, St. Catharines General Hospital, St. Catharines, Ontario. She has over 30 years' experience in the field and has been involved in the education of NNPs throughout her career.

KEY TERMS

advanced neonatal nursing
(ANN)
advanced nursing practice
(ANP)
advanced practice nursing
(APN)
clinical nurse specialist/nurse
practitioner (CNS/NP)
expanded role nurse (ERN)
neonatal nurse practitioner
(NNP)

OBJECTIVES

1. Summarize the historical development of
   the neonatal nurse practitioner (NNP) role in
   Canada.
2. Understand the evolution of NNP education.
3. Understand the evolution of NNP workforce
   and human resource planning.
4. Characterize the role, credentialing, and
   scope of practice of NNPs.
5. Examine the available evidence evaluating
   NNP impact.
6. Construct a vision for the future of NNPs in
   Canada.

Introduction

Neonatal nurse practitioners (NNPs) were first introduced into Canadian neonatal intensive care units (NICUs) in 1988, almost two decades after the role was introduced in NICUs
in the United States (US; DiCenso, 1998; Faculty of Health Sciences, 1991). The history of
the NNP role offers a glimpse into the realities of an evolving health care system at a time
when medical education and the health care system were undergoing significant change. This
chapter explores the origins of the NNP role in Canada and its evolution with emphasis on
education, workforce, scope of practice, and evaluation.

Historical Development of the Neonatal Nurse
Practitioner Role in Canada

While introduced in Canada later than in the US, the impetus for introducing the NNP
role into tertiary-level NICUs was similar on both sides of the border. Proposed changes in
medical education would result in reductions in the number of funded pediatric trainees
who traditionally rotated through NICUs and provided care to critically ill and premature
newborns (Faculty of Health Sciences, 1991; Honeyfield, 2009). Given this emerging reality,
the Ontario Minister of Health and Long-Term Care (MOHLTC) asked the Ontario Council
of Administrators of Teaching Hospitals and the Council of Ontario Faculties of Medicine to
explore resident alternatives for teaching hospitals. A neonatal subcommittee was established
to consider two alternatives: an expanded nursing role and a physician assistant role. The
subcommittee agreed that nurses, with appropriate preparation, would be well positioned
to assume responsibilities traditionally designated to pediatric residents, a decision that was
consistent with the College of Nurses of Ontario's (CNO) position. Introduction of physician
assistants at that time was viewed as costly duplication of education and services, with the
potential for fragmentation in care and potential role confusion and overlap among care

providers (Faculty of Health Sciences, 1991; McMaster University School of Nursing, 1987). The MOHLTC subsequently funded a pilot project to study the need for nurses in an expanded role to fill service gaps in the tertiary level.

The feasibility of the development and implementation of an expanded role nurse (ERN) in Ontario NICUs, funded by the MOHLTC, was explored by a team of researchers from McMaster University in Hamilton, Ontario (McMaster University School of Nursing, 1987; Mitchell, Pinelli, Patterson, & Southwell, 1993). Broad consultation with key stakeholders (N = 655) was completed, including surveying postgraduate residency program directors in Ontario as well as all Ontario tertiary-level NICU medical directors and nursing leaders. Surveys were also sent to Alberta, as they were exploring NNP roles as alternatives to resident care in NICUs and to established US centres. The results of these surveys informed the decision to develop the NNP role, indicating that workload in NICUs exceeded medical staff availability and there was an openness to pursue an expanded nursing role as a suitable alternative to resident care (Paes et al., 1989). Key stakeholders envisioned a professional role that included high levels of technical expertise, autonomous decision-making, and leadership skills. In the US, NNPs were already assuming responsibility for the care of a caseload of infants, as well as having educational, research, and leadership responsibilities. This stakeholder consultation led to the definition of a new nursing role to be deployed in Ontario NICUs (Faculty of Health Sciences, 1991; Hunsberger et al., 1992; McMaster University School of Nursing, 1987).

The nature of the ERN role was explored and defined in an early unpublished background paper (McMaster University School of Nursing, 1987) and careful attention was paid to the characteristics of basic, extended, and expanded nursing practice. At the time, basic nursing practice was characterized as diploma or bachelor's educational preparation, possession of generalist skills. Extended nursing practice included the same basic educational preparation with the addition of specialty preparation (formal or informal) in a specific practice area. Extended nursing practice was described as incorporating specific skills, some of which might be traditionally performed by other disciplines. Expanded nursing practice was differentiated from basic and extended as requiring a graduate degree in nursing; expertise in a clinical nursing specialty; and knowledge and skills grounded in theory and research. The attributes of the expanded role nurse were consistent with those of advanced practice nursing (APN) roles. Given the experiences in the US, and to be consistent with the findings of the stakeholder analysis and this review of the levels of nursing practice, it was agreed that the proposed ERNs be prepared at the graduate level, in alignment with the role definition of an APN (Faculty of Health Sciences, 1991; McAllister et al., 1993; McMaster University School of Nursing, 1987).

To prepare for the first graduates of McMaster University's ERN program, regulatory organizations were required to review specific "delegated medical acts" that this new type of clinician would require authorization to perform (i.e., endotracheal intubation, umbilical arterial and venous line insertion, lumbar puncture). The Advisory Committee on Special Procedures of the College of Physicians and Surgeons, with membership from the CNO, as well as the Registered Nurses Association of Ontario, Ontario Medical Association, and Ontario Hospital Association, reviewed and approved the delegation of these specific acts to neonatal ERNs. Later, as roles proliferated in other acute care environments and with the proclamation of the Regulated Health Professions Act (1991) in Ontario as a new regulatory framework, medical directives were used as the mechanism to authorize qualified clinicians to perform controlled acts considered outside their discipline-specific scope of practice.

Once the NICU ERN role was implemented, clinicians, regulators, and professional association representatives began work to regulate this new APN role. As other acute care nurse practitioner roles were introduced, more attention was paid to the development of regulation to authorize the full scope of NP practice across all specialties, beginning with the practice of primary health care NPs and then those practicing with specific populations.

By the time the first three graduates completed their graduate program (1988) at McMaster University, the role had been renamed **clinical nurse specialist/nurse practitioner (CNS/NP)**. These graduate-prepared clinicians pioneered this new expanded neonatal nursing role in three Ontario tertiary NICUs with a vision of developing a clinical leadership role. As the program continued, the number of graduates increased and by 1992, there were 15 CNS/NPs practicing in 5 Ontario NICUs and related practice environments (i.e., neonatal follow-up programs; Hunsberger et al., 1992). By 1989, interest in this APN role was emerging in other parts of the country, with Alberta and Manitoba establishing their first positions at that time (Evanochko, 2011; D. Fraser, personal communication, March 14, 2015). Other parts of the country, including Nova Scotia and Quebec, followed suit, piloting the development and integration of this expanded nursing role in NICUs.

However, a discussion of the history of the NNP role in Canada would not be complete without acknowledging a controversy that emerged along the way. In its early iterations, the ERN role was described by some as an assistant to physicians. Expanding the scope of nursing practice was conceptualized by some authors as taking on medically delegated tasks and they questioned the need for nurses to assume such tasks when there seemed to be no shortage of physicians in Canada (Mitchell & Santapinto, 1988). These authors concluded that the ERN concept did not represent the advancement of nursing but rather the extension into medicine, thus diluting nursing impact with medical model–dependent practice. Those opposed to the ERN suggested that it was not necessary for nursing to own the problems arising from medical residency shortages (Mitchell & Santapinto, 1988). Those practicing in expanded roles offered a different perspective, presenting the development of the "expanded role nurse" as an opportunity to enhance the nursing role in order to improve the quality of patient care. The role was presented as holistic, complementary, and capable of advancing the profession of nursing, encompassing clinical care, education, and research responsibilities (Rubin, 1988).

A final historical focus is that of funding for this new role. In Ontario, funding for the establishment of the first neonatal ERN positions was provided by the MOHLTC. This allowed employing organizations to embed the role in their structures and provided a unique opportunity to evaluate the impact of the role in practice settings (Mitchell et al., 1993). However, over time and as NNP teams were established, the responsibility for securing funding to employ additional NPs has been borne by NICUs. Presently, hospitals employing NNPs are required to source funding from within their allocated budgets. This can be challenging given the large number of competing financial and clinical priorities that hospitals face.

Evolution of Neonatal Nurse Practitioner Education in Canada

In the 1970s, hospital-based "in-house training" programs were developed in the US in response to the urgent need in neonatology for expanded nursing roles. Over time, the need for a more standardized approach to nursing education became apparent. Hospital-specific neonatal education lacked connection with university programs in nursing, which created barriers for nursing mobility and career advancement. Preparation at the graduate level was increasingly viewed as essential to achieve the level of standardization and in-depth knowledge and skills required for expanded nursing practice in an academic interprofessional NICU context. Highly influential was the concurrent success of graduate-level NNP education in the US, programs that started in the early 1970s. The appropriateness of the NNP role for academically prepared nurses was controversial. NNP education was viewed as moving away from nursing core curricula to embrace the medical model. Graduate nursing education— traditionally grounded in administration, education, and research—was evolving to include advanced practice nursing curricula to the exclusion of NP-specific content.

In Canada, a multidisciplinary group at McMaster University conducted an initial feasibility study that verified the need for expanded role neonatal nurses in Ontario (Hunsberger et al., 1992; Paes et al., 1989). The program admission criteria, program objectives, course descriptions and content, educational resources, length of program, supervision, and staffing were developed based on the findings of the interprofessional role definition study (Hunsberger et al., 1992) and through faculty consultation, surveys, and site visits to existing graduate-level NNP programs in the US. Graduate-level education prepared NNPs for clinical practice with knowledge based on theories, concepts, and research, and facilitated the development of leadership, education, and research skills.

In 1986, McMaster University launched the first graduate-level program to prepare advanced neonatal nurses in Canada. The neonatal stream was incorporated into the existing 16-month Master of Health Sciences (MHSc) degree program. The neonatal component included 600 hours of theory-specific, problem-based tutorials and 720 hours of supervised clinical practice. The course content included advanced physical assessment, diagnostic reasoning, therapeutic management, pharmacology, and pathophysiology. In 1994, the program was integrated into the new thesis-based Master of Science in Nursing (MScN) program. In 1997, McMaster University recognized the neonatal courses as highly specialized and approved the creation of a separate Graduate Diploma in Advanced Neonatal Nursing (ANN). The program length was 10 months and included 3 theory-specific courses and 720 hours of clinical practice. To enrol in the Graduate Diploma program, students required or were near completion of a graduate degree in nursing. In 2011, McMaster University began to offer the program via distance education to increase access to students from across Ontario and other provinces. Education was offered using a hybrid format of synchronous on-campus and off-campus problem-based learning via web conferencing, three innovative one-week residency periods, and clinical practicums completed at home NICU sites with local qualified NNP preceptors.

The education program for ANN founded at McMaster University was evaluated extensively. Two evaluations of the educational program were conducted. Mitchell et al. demonstrated in a before-and-after study that graduating NNPs from the first three programs (1987 to 1989) acquired the expected competencies and scored higher than first-year students (Mitchell et al., 1995) and scored similarly in a cohort study with pediatric residents on knowledge, problem-solving, examination, communications, and clinical skills in the NICU (Mitchell et al., 1991). The positive findings validated the educational preparation of NNPs, which ultimately led to the expansion of programs across Canada (Mitchell et al., 1995) and set the foundation for the subsequent successful establishment of acute care advanced practice NP education in pediatrics and adults. Table 27.1 provides an overview of Canadian NNP programs, program status, and number of graduates since inception.

In Alberta, the first NNP education program was established in 1992 as a certificate of ANN Practice at the University of Alberta. The certificate program courses were offered in addition to the required Master of Nursing (MN) degree courses and thesis. The NNP courses included pathophysiology and clinical management curricula and 600 hours of supervised clinical practice. The overall program length was two full years, plus thesis. The program changed in 1996 to a course- or thesis-based MN in **Advanced Nursing Practice (ANP)** degree, including three NNP-specific pathophysiology, advanced physical assessment, and clinical management courses and 800 hours of clinical practice. The overall program length is two years, including the MN courses. In addition, a post-MN option was offered that included the same courses completed over a one-year period. In 2012, the University of Alberta program closed due to low student enrolment (C. Evanochko, personal communication, March 12, 2015). The program began admitting students again in 2018 and is currently open for MN students only. There is no postgraduate option currently offered.

In Nova Scotia, the first NNP program was established in 1998 through the Dalhousie University School of Nursing, MN program. The program length is two years with 760 clinical practice hours. The MN with integrated NNP courses was offered three times in response to the health human resources needs in the NICU at the affiliated IWK Health Centre. The program is currently inactive (M. Campbell-Yeo, personal communication, March 12, 2015).

In Quebec, the first NNP education program started in September 2003 at McGill University Ingram School of Nursing. Students complete the non-thesis Master of Science in Nursing (applied; MSc[A]) degree over a two-year period followed by a Graduate Diploma in Neonatology. The MSc(A) program consists of 45 credits (21 of 45 credits are neonatal-specific courses). The diploma is entirely clinical, including rotations to intermediate care (Level II), intensive care (Level III+), as well as antenatal consults and neonatal follow-up for 30 credits. Overall, the combined Master and Diploma program is completed over a two-and-a-half-year period with 75 credits and 980 clinical practice hours. McGill University offers the option of a post-Master certificate in the theory of neonatology (pathophysiology) for 15 credits (will be available via videoconferencing as of fall 2020). Once completed, students transition to complete the Diploma (clinical). The government of Quebec continues to offer a $60,000 bursary to students in exchange for a guarantee of three years of NNP practice in Quebec (L. Morneault, personal communication, September 9, 2019).

Workforce and Human Resource Planning

Since 2010, there has been a steady decline in the number of available and active Canadian NNP education program impacting the supply of the NNP workforce. Some programs run every other year during periods of low enrolment and/or fiscal restraint. The NNP programs at the University of Alberta and Dalhousie University were inactive for several years and recently reopened to address local education needs. Over the 2018–2019 academic year, McGill University and the University of Alberta had active NNP programs. There is a similar trend reported in the US—that of a declining number of NNP education programs and concurrent decline in the number of new NNPs entering practice, based on the survey results of NNP program directors (Bellini, 2013; Freed, Moran, Dunham, & Nantais-Smith, 2015). Since 2005, a total of 19 NNP programs have closed in the US, and since 2012, the number of online programs has decreased by 10% (Bellini, 2013). In 2014, 50% of NNPs responding to the workforce survey reported being short-staffed (Kaminski, Meier, & Staebler, 2015). In the 2016 survey, 75% of clinical NNPs and 73% of administrators reported a shortage of NNPs to cover practice needs, and shortages were projected to persist (Welch-Carre, 2018). While the number of NNPs graduating from US programs decreased by 23% over a five-year period (2009 to 2013), the most recent NNP workforce study reports a 15% increase in NP enrolment in accredited programs (Welch-Carre, 2018). Of interest is the growth of Physician Assistant (PA) programs that offer a neonatal focus. The first PA program focused on neonatology started in 2005 (Abu Jawdeh, Hardin-Fanning, Kinnard, & Cunningham, 2019) and the number of programs has since grown to five in the US (T. Mattis, Ensearch, personal communication, September 4, 2019). In fact, NNP administrators recently reported that some NNP vacancies were being filled by PAs (20%), hospitalists (13%), other APNs (23%), and neonatologists (28%; Welch-Carre, 2018). Of note, in Canada and the US, the demand for NNPs continues to grow due to increasing NICU admissions per year, expanded bed capacity, and the aging of the current NNP workforce.

To address the emerging gap in the supply and demand of NNPs, McMaster University conducted an education needs survey of Canadian tertiary care NICUs (94% response rate) in June 2014 to inform education and workforce planning (Ballantyne, 2014). Respondents indicated that 40 full-time NNPs will be needed to maintain current workforce needs and quality safe care. The survey findings may underestimate the actual need, taking into consideration the current clinical activities, total volume of patients, staffing patterns, workload, extended work hours, erosion of off-service academic time, fatigue and burnout, and impending retirements. At the time of the survey, 79% of the NICUs indicated that the current numbers of NNPs were not sufficient to provide service needs, and 57% reported vacant NNP positions. Furthermore, one-third of the existing national NNP workforce reported they intend to retire over the next 10-year period (11 within 0 to 3 years; 10 within 3 to 6 years;

and 9 within 7 to 10 years). As the number of education programs continues to decline, the supply of new NNP graduates will not adequately meet the emerging need for new NNPs.

As of March 2015, there were 109 NNPs working in Neonatology (Level 3 NICU, Level 2 and Neonatal Follow-up) in seven provinces across Canada. There are 21 in Alberta, 6 in Saskatchewan, 3 in Manitoba, 54 in Ontario, 16 in Quebec, 8 in Nova Scotia, and 1 in Newfoundland and Labrador. NPs in the neonatal specialty represent approximately 3% of the estimated 3,655 NPs in Canada in 2013 (Canadian Institute for Health Information [CIHI], 2013). Since 2015, NNP roles have continued to expand beyond the Level 3 and Level 2 NICU to Level 1 settings (Follett et al., 2017). The NNP role is well positioned in the Level 1 and 2 settings to provide appropriate care in local communities and facilitating transitions to home. As of November 11, 2019, a national NNP Health Human Resources survey quantified the current state and future needs for NPs working in neonatal services across Canada. Early results indicated that current NNP staffing was insufficient, with neonatal leaders reporting unfilled vacancies across Canada. Of the respondents thus far, 53% suggest that substitutes for NNPs are being considered (PAs, fellows, and hospitalists). There is also an anticipated wave of NNP retirements over the next three years and again in five to seven years, indicating an urgency to address the shortage of NNPs, ensuring the availability of appropriate educational programs and credentialing mechanisms (McAllister, Ballantyne, & Lamb, 2019).

TABLE 27.1: Canadian NNP Programs

University Name and Location	Year of Program Start	Program Status	Type	Length	Number of Graduates N =
McMaster University Hamilton, Ontario	1986	Closed—not active since 2014	Post-Master's Diploma	Full-time 10 months	75
University of Alberta Edmonton, Alberta	1992	Closed 2012; reopened 2019–2021	MN Post-MN	Full-time 2 years 1 year	27
Dalhousie University Halifax, Nova Scotia	1998	Not active; reopened for three cohorts, last in 2017 (local students only)	MN	Full-time 2 years	23
McGill University Montreal, Quebec	2003	Active	MScN (A) + Diploma Post-Master's Certificate	Full-time 2+ years 11 months	19 + 4 (December 2019)

Titling, Scope of Practice, and Credentialing

Titling and Scope of Practice

Even though they completed an ERN program, the first graduates from McMaster University were not called ERNs but CNS/NPs. Graduate preparation, while still controversial, was deemed necessary in order to develop advanced practitioners able to make autonomous decisions in the care of critically ill newborns and their families (Mitchell et al., 1993).

At that time, graduate-prepared nurses who focused on advancing clinical practice, predominantly in acute care, were employed as CNSs. While there were similarities between the CNS and the new CNS/NP roles, there were also differences. Both CNSs and CNS/NPs were expected to generate and use research and incorporate clinical practice, consultation, education, and leadership activities. However, while the CNS scope of practice focused on improving patient care in an issue-driven way (i.e., focusing on improvement of pain management for a patient population), CNS/NPs were expected to provide and manage patient care and had a population-driven clinical practice (i.e., providing comprehensive care for specific patients). Both roles incorporated expanded nursing knowledge and skills and leadership responsibilities, but this new neonatal role also included extended knowledge and skills (i.e., medical diagnosis, prescriptive authority; Pinelli, 1997; Wright, 1997). The CNS has always been identified as an APN role and as the CNS/NP in neonatology incorporated the three essential elements that characterized APN, including graduate education, client focus, and specialized knowledge and skills within a clinical specialty, it was also deemed an APN role (Giovannetti, Tenove, Stuart, & van den Berg, 1996).

The merged role of CNS/NP has been controversial, and the analysis has featured prominently in the literature (Kaasalainen et al., 2010). Fenton and Brykczynski (1993) reported three distinct perspectives regarding the education of CNSs and NPs. The first advocated merging the roles, a second suggested that they be kept separate, and a third proposed that core educational content become the basis for both roles with distinct content focusing on role-specific knowledge and skill development. While the analysis of the merged CNS/NP role was presented long after the title was used for the new neonatal role, the third perspective reflects the intention at the time the McMaster curriculum was developed. The CNS/NP title acknowledges shared and unique competencies as well as the core characteristics of the APN role (Pinelli, 1997).

Given the deliberate adoption of the CNS/NP title, early position descriptions reflected the role domains characteristic of current APNs: clinical practice, education, research, consultation, and leadership. These new neonatal clinicians used "advanced knowledge and skills to ensure optimal care to high risk neonates and their families in collaboration with the health care team" (The Hospital for Sick Children, 1987, 1990).

In their clinical role, they assumed responsibility for managing the care of neonates and their families from admission to discharge, including neonatal and delivery room issues, infant resuscitation and assessment, and initiation of diagnostic investigations and therapies in collaboration with a neonatologist. Initially, controlled acts traditionally authorized to physicians were delegated to CNS/NPs, but supervision was required before these acts could be performed by CNS/NPs independently. These controlled acts included making a medical diagnosis; ordering medications; and performing procedures such as intubations, lumbar punctures, and insertion of chest drains (Mitchell et al., 1991; Mitchell-DiCenso et al., 1996b). In addition, all diagnostic and treatment orders required co-signature by a physician. Despite these restrictions, these early clinicians evolved a role that offered care that complemented that provided by traditional clinicians such as clinical nurses and physicians (Canada West Foundation [CWF], 1998). They spent 80% of their time in clinical care and established themselves as leaders in advancing clinical care and quality improvement and research (Mitchell, 1998). They practice in a variety of practice sites, focusing on neonatal care, including NICUs, Level II neonatal units, neonatal follow-up clinics, and even breastfeeding support services. Currently, credentialed NNPs no longer require authorization mechanisms for many aspects of care management, including communicating a diagnosis, ordering diagnostic investigations, and prescribing medications and other treatment options.

As APNs, neonatal CNS/NPs were viewed as mentors and role models by front-line nursing colleagues, and they collaborated with other nursing leaders to provide leadership, support, and encouragement for nurses' development. Their consultation role often involved responding to requests from within their organizations, or to those from external organizations or the community, seeking information about the specialized needs of neonates. Their research role included critical appraisal of evidence as it related to clinical decision-making, identifying researchable questions, as well as participating or leading research teams. Leadership responsibilities included the development of policies and procedures to guide practice and participating in or leading quality improvement initiatives (Mitchell, 1996).

As the CNS/NP role was established as an advanced role in nursing, their position within hiring organizations reflected their nursing roots. From the first introduction of the role, neonatal CNS/NPs were hired as APNs, reporting directly to a senior nursing leader (Director, Chief Nurse, etc.) for professional practice with a matrix reporting line to neonatal medicine for the medical dimensions of their role. This reporting structure has been implemented consistently across Canada, a role feature that differentiates it from similar roles in the US, where approximately half of the NNP respondents to a survey stated they reported directly to medicine (Ruth-Sanchez, Lee, & Bosque, 1996; Samson, 2006). Medical recognition of the importance and complementary nature of APN roles in neonatal care was galvanized in 2000 with the publication of a position statement by the Canadian Paediatric Society (Fetus and Newborn Committee, 2000). Reaffirmed by the Society in 2001, this statement offers strong support for the continued development and implementation of APN roles at the graduate level to support the provision of care for critically ill newborns and their families.

As NPs became increasingly well recognized in the health care system and regulated as legitimate health care providers across Canada, the merged role title of CNS/NP faded and NPs practicing in the neonatal field transitioned to the title of NNP, the same title used for many years in the US. The roles and responsibilities of these advanced clinicians continue to evolve in alignment with the establishment of national APN frameworks and standards (Canadian Nurses Association [CNA], 2008, 2010, 2019).

CASE STUDY

The Story of Jonathan

Jonathan, a twin, was born at 27 weeks gestation to Mrs. G., a 32-year-old G4P0 mother. Jonathan received surfactant at birth and then required positive pressure ventilation to support his respiratory status. His sister, Emily, also received surfactant and required a short period of positive pressure ventilation, but quickly weaned to non-invasive ventilation. Upon admission, both Jonathan and Emily were admitted to the neonatal nurse practitioner (NNP) team in the Neonatal Intensive Care Unit (NICU).

Shortly after their admission, the admitting NNP met with the twins' parents. He confirmed the antenatal and perinatal history with them, explained what they might expect during the twins' first few days of life, and answered their parents' questions. He also asked them how they had planned to feed the twins, discussing the advantages of providing breast milk for them. Mr. and Mrs. G. told the NNP that they planned to breastfeed. As the twins were not able to breastfeed immediately, Mrs. G. was anxious to get started with milk expression. The NNP introduced Mr. and Mrs. G. to one of the NICU's breastfeeding nurse champions, who accompanied them to a private room, and oriented them to the breast pump so they could get started with milk expression.

Over the next few weeks of life, Emily continued to do well with non-invasive ventilation, but Jonathan continued to require significant oxygen and ventilator support. He experienced many desaturation and bradycardic episodes, requiring frequent adjustments in his oxygen. Jonathan's mother was very worried about him and talked to the NNP about her concerns. She didn't understand why Emily was doing so well while Jonathan was having such trouble. The NNP listened to Mrs. G.'s concerns, completed a thorough physical assessment, reviewed all of Jonathan's recent investigations and clinical data, and then sat down to discuss Jonathan's care with her.

Given Jonathan's evolving chronic lung disease and his labile respiratory status, the NNP decided to discuss a trial of diuretics to target his chronic lung disease. With the intent to partner with Mrs. G. in treatment planning, the NNP outlined how a three-day course of furosemide might help to clear excess fluid in Jonathan's lungs, and possibly reduce his need for oxygen and ventilator support. She asked Mrs. G. what she thought about this option. Mrs. G. seemed surprised by this question, and then asked the NNP what he thought. The NNP described the benefits and risks associated with the treatment option. The NNP discussed how they would know if the strategy was effective for Jonathan, specifically by seeing that his oxygen requirements would stabilize and/or decrease, resulting in a decrease in ventilator support, and fewer desaturation and bradycardic episodes. After thoughtful consideration, Mrs. G. agreed that they should try the course of furosemide, and the NNP wrote the orders for the three-day course at 2 mg/kg/day.

The next day, while the NNP was making rounds on the patients in her care, he met a very excited Mrs. G. in the hall, who stated that she thought the furosemide was working, that Jonathan had experienced far fewer desaturation and bradycardic episodes overnight, his oxygen had come down by 10%, and his ventilator rate had also been reduced. The NNP was enthusiastic when he told Mrs. G. that this sounded very positive and that he would come and see Jonathan shortly. He reflected on the partnership that had been cultivated between the NNP and Mrs. G. and was pleased that Jonathan had a solid team of nurses, respiratory therapists, physicians, NPs, and his parents on his side in monitoring his response to the treatment plan, so that the best decisions could be made to support him in his recovery.

Credentialing

In Ontario, the CNS/NP title was used for approximately 10 years when, as a result of changes to provincial legislation, the scope of practice of NPs was defined (Nurse Practitioners' Association of Ontario [NPAO], n.d.). In keeping with the early evolution of NP roles, primary care NPs were the first to be regulated, but that left practicing NNPs in regulatory limbo, requiring the use of physician-approved medical directives to authorize their practice. In Alberta, legislative changes to authorize NP practice were proclaimed in 2000, including NP title protection, but regulations for the Child (Neonatal Specialty) stream were introduced in 2004 and updated in 2017 (College and Association of Registered Nurses of Alberta [CARNA], 2017). It was not until 2008 when NP title protection was enacted in Ontario and three streams of NPs (Primary Health Care, Adult, Child) qualified for registration in the Extended Class. While a positive step forward, title protection left practicing NNPs unable to use the NP title, while pursuing new and unclear regulatory requirements to be credentialed and recognized as NPs in a subspecialty of pediatrics (NPAO, n.d.). Initially, NPs practicing in neonatology had several examination options to be credentialed provincially, but in 2010, when the US-based National Certification Corporation no longer allowed Canadian-educated neonatal NPs access to their NNP examination, a made-in-Canada alternative was sought. As of 2015, the only examination available to credential NNP program graduates was offered in Quebec, by the Ordre des infirmières et infirmiers du Québec (OIIQ) on a limited basis and it has not been deemed a national examination. As of 2019, it was reported that the OIIQ would no longer require successful completion of an NP examination to be regulated as an NP in Quebec, meaning that the NNP examination may no longer be available (L. Morneault, personal communication, September 9, 2019). However, this change in the requirement for an examination is under review again (N. Ponzoni, personal communication, November 18, 2019). The instability in access to a credentialing examination has the potential to significantly limit the availability of credentialed NNPs in Canada in the future.

Evaluation of the Neonatal Nurse Practitioner Role in Canada

The introduction of the NNP role was comprehensively evaluated in Canada. A prospective randomized controlled trial was conducted by Mitchell-DiCenso et al. to determine the safety and effectiveness, the quality of care, satisfaction with care, and associated costs of the role (Mitchell-DiCenso et al., 1996a, 1996b). All infants admitted to the tertiary-level NICU at McMaster Children's Hospital (N = 821 infants) over a one-year period were randomized to care by an NNP (n = 414) or a pediatric resident (n = 407) team. The study findings indicated that NNP care met practice standards and was equivalent to pediatric resident care on all measures of performance, including neonatal mortality, morbidity, length of stay, quality of care, parent satisfaction, long-term developmental outcomes, and costs (Mitchell-DiCenso et al., 1996a). NNPs scored significantly better in two of seven quality-of-care indicators for documentation and the care of neonates with jaundice. Neonatologists reported statistically lower time spent with NNPs than residents. Staff nurses reported overall increased job satisfaction and an increased sense of autonomy and increased participation in decision-making with NP care (Mitchell-DiCenso et al., 1996b). US-based studies using less rigorous research designs (i.e., retrospective chart review) similarly found that NNPs provided safe, cost-effective, and equivalent to or superior quality of care as compared to pediatric residents (Aubrey & Yoxall, 2001; Bissinger, Allred, Arford, & Bellig, 1997; Carzoli, Martinez-Cruz, Cuevas, Murphy, & Chiu, 1994; Karlowicz & McMurray, 2000; Lee, Skelton, & Skene, 2001; Schultz, Liptak, & Fioravanti, 1994; Woods, 2006). To date, the study conducted by Mitchell-DiCenso et al. (1996b) is the only clinical trial to validate the NNP role in tertiary-level NICUs (Donald et al., 2014). The findings from the NNP comparison studies are remarkably consistent with the broader NP literature, which has demonstrated no difference in health outcomes of patients across the lifespan with NP care as compared to physician care (Donald et al., 2014).

Future research is needed to ascertain the current state of NNPs' impact, quality of care, cost-effectiveness, retention, health, and well-being of the workforce. The initial trial was conducted when the NNPs were still in the novice phase of their roles and development (i.e., one to three years post-graduation). A similar study done today, when many of the NNPs have more than 30 years of practice experience, would capture the richness of their expertise, which would be unique in comparison to any other health care providers in the NICU.

Future Implications

The NNP role has been effectively integrated into the Canadian health care system for three decades, despite its controversial start. However, if this important and effective clinical role is to be sustained in current and future health care systems, there are several issues that must be considered, including supply and demand, credentialing, access to education programs, role satisfaction, role effectiveness, and, ultimately, role sustainability.

NNP supply and demand has been identified as an issue throughout the role's history and is multi-faceted in nature (Honeyfield, 2009). Quantifying the number of practicing NNPs, unfilled NNP positions, and NNPs joining and leaving the workforce in any given year is challenging. In Canada, we have not explored these issues consistently and with regulation being a provincial jurisdiction, the task is even more complicated. However, anecdotally we know that many NNPs who pioneered this role beginning in the late 1980s and early 1990s are beginning to retire, and the average age of NNPs is starting to decline, a reality similar to that of the US, where the average age of NPs was 49 in 2013 (Hooker, Brock, & Cook, 2016). Coupled with a shortage of pediatricians due to insufficient enrolment and graduates pursuing subspecialty certification, the retirement of experienced NNPs is contributing to the national shortage of pediatric subspecialty care (Abu Jawdeh et al., 2019; Tithecott, Levin, & Filler, 2018; Gigli, Beauchesne, Dirks, & Peck, 2019).

Given this context, the demand for NNPs is urgent as NICUs continue to provide care to smaller and more critically ill infants and their families. Recruitment, education, and credentialing of NNPs are influenced by provincial funding; provincial and organizational priorities; availability of seats in education programs; accessibility of credentialing processes that accurately evaluate the knowledge, skills, and abilities of entry-level NNPs; and acceptance of the role in the clinical environment. As most nurses now enter the profession with an undergraduate nursing degree, the pool of nurses qualified to enter graduate NNP programs is larger. However, nurses who choose to pursue this career path must see that there are employment opportunities for them. Many have been positively influenced by their experiences working with NNPs and see the role as an opportunity to remain directly involved in clinical care while also developing their leadership abilities as APNs.

Credentialing issues require attention and NNPs must be considered as part of the national NP workforce. While NPs are regulated provincially, a national body, the Canadian Council of Registered Nurse Regulators (CCRNR), announced and completed an analysis of NP entry to practice knowledge, skills, and abilities for all three NP categories: Family/All Ages, Adult, and Pediatric (CCRNR, 2013, 2015). While NNPs are registered or licensed in a pediatric or child category, there is a risk that, given NNPs' subspecialized clinical practice, they may not have been included as CCRNR developed a national examination and credentialing strategy. As of 2015, the examination offered by OIIQ in Quebec was the only examination available to credential graduates from Canadian NNP education programs. As NPs in Quebec will now receive their credential to practice as a result of completing their graduate-level NP program, the OIIQ NNP examination is no longer available to credential NNPs in Canada (L. Morneault, personal communication, 2019). As a result, a process to legitimately credential NNPs across Canada must be considered. Failure to do so will reduce credentialing options and further reduce the supply of NNPs to meet a sustained and ever-increasing need for these specialized APNs.

Access to education programs is also important to consider. As described earlier, there are currently only two active programs preparing NNPs in Canada: University of Alberta and McGill University. Programs are available in person only. Graduates of US programs can apply to have their credentials reviewed at the provincial level, but completion of a US program doesn't expose graduates to issues relevant to the Canadian context. As a result of the perceived shortage of NNP education programs, a national working group was struck in June 2017, including provincial representatives from regulatory, educational, and clinical organizations, to explore the current state and work with key stakeholders to address the educational and credentialing deficits. Given the ongoing supply-and-demand issues, the availability of NNP education programs must be closely monitored and assessed on a regular basis to ensure there are enough seats to meet the current and future demands for this role.

A reduced supply of NNPs may also be a stimulus for organizations to look at other roles to address their NICU human resource needs. Physician assistants (PAs) have been introduced in several provinces and their numbers are growing, although they are not currently practicing in NICUs in Canada. NICUs in the US have introduced PAs into NICUs as a human resource strategy largely as a result of reduced enrolment of nurses in NNP programs (Abu Jawdeh et al., 2019). This has spurred the development of neonatal PA training/residency programs across the US to adequately prepare PAs to provide care in NICU settings (Abu Jawdeh et al., 2019). While NICU leaders recognize that PAs and NPs bring unique and different approaches to neonatal care (Abu Jawdeh et al., 2019), given that the PA alternative was considered when the NNP role was first established in Canada, it now seems likely that the option of PAs in the NICU might be considered to meet neonatal care needs in Canada.

The NNP role has evolved as a fully advanced practice role with the majority of NNP time focused on direct clinical practice. However, there is a clear expectation from NNPs and employers alike that NNPs should be supported to engage in activities that reflect all elements of APN. Most NNPs have approximately 10–20% of their time allocated to these other dimensions of the role. However, when there are staff shortages or surges in patient census, this time can shrink, compromising NNP impact as nursing leaders who are charged with advancing quality improvement initiatives, leading research, teaching, and mentoring. This can lead to frustration on the part of NNPs because they are unable to achieve broader professional goals. As well, the talents and expertise of these advanced practice clinicians may not be leveraged, and their impact will not be maximized. In some cases, in Canada, the NNP role has expanded to include a hospitalist role where NNPs act as the most responsible practitioner (MRP) for well-baby nurseries. There are opportunities to evolve this NNP-hospitalist model further, as well as expand the role of the NNP into community practice. With advances in technology and treatment, medical complexity is common among infants in the NICU (Kieran et al., 2019). Upon discharge from hospital, these NICU graduates may require technological support, such as oxygen therapy, feeding pumps, ventilators, and more (Goldstein & Malcolm, 2019). Significant opportunity exists for NNPs to provide comprehensive care for technology-dependent infants and their families during the transition home from the NICU and within the home as a liaison between specialist and community care services. NNPs are well positioned to provide this type of care in community settings as they are familiar with the conditions, treatments, and technologies that NICU graduates often require following discharge and have a vast understanding of healthy growth and development (Goldstein & Malcolm, 2019).

With respect to NNP effectiveness, well-designed Canadian studies have confirmed that NNPs are safe and effective care providers in NICUs. However, there are opportunities to continue to evaluate the current impact of this role. Given recent attention to lengths of stay, patient safety, quality, and hospital-acquired conditions (such as central line–associated bloodstream infections), NNPs can play a significant clinical leadership role in reducing health care acquired conditions and consider how they might evaluate their impact on these important patient outcomes. Nurse-sensitive outcomes, such as readiness for discharge, might be explored to further substantiate the value NNPs bring to the efficient care of critically ill newborns and their families. There may also be opportunities to align NNP research and evaluation efforts with the priorities of clinical programs and organizations, strengthening interprofessional collaborative efforts.

Conclusion

The NNP role has been well established and sustained for more than 30 years in many Canadian provinces, but it cannot be assumed that its sustainability is guaranteed. While the role continues to exist across the country and these neonatal nursing leaders are well respected and valued in their regions, there may be value in developing a national community of practice for NNPs so that they can share innovative practices, research, patient safety initiatives, recruitment/retention efforts, and their collective wisdom in order to strengthen the NNP presence nationally. The Canadian Association of Neonatal Nurses (CANN) has recently created an online forum to bring NNPs from across the country together through its social media presence (A. Wright, CANN President, personal communication, September 15, 2019). This forum has the potential to promote a united national NNP voice and leverage the power of the NNP collective to further advance quality neonatal care and the NNP role, cementing it within the health care system in Canada.

In summary, the NNP role has been a positive addition to the Canadian health care system, emerging at a time when changes were being made within the medical education system. The development of the role was done in a thoughtful and planned way, ensuring that key stakeholders were engaged. The number of NNPs deployed in NICUs and related clinical environments has grown steadily, their effectiveness has been confirmed, and professional organizations have published position statements that advocate for the role in practice settings. Access to education programs and appropriate national credentialing standards are recent challenges to succession planning that must be addressed. However, the NNP role was the right role at the right time, providing care to the right population in the right way, and today it continues to be an essential APN role across the country. These nursing leaders will no doubt continue to be intellectually curious, creative, and courageous as they solidify this role within the national health care landscape.

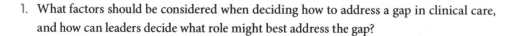

Critical Thinking Questions

1. What factors should be considered when deciding how to address a gap in clinical care, and how can leaders decide what role might best address the gap?

2. When considering CNS and NP roles, what are the advantages and disadvantages of a merged CNS/NP role?
3. What are the barriers and facilitators that influence the successful integration of a new advanced nursing role in health care?
4. Is graduate preparation necessary to provide care to critically ill newborns? Why or why not?
5. What issues should be considered when addressing sustainability of the NNP role in the Canadian health care system?

References

Abu Jawdeh, E. G., Hardin-Fanning, F., Kinnard, T. B., & Cunningham, M. D. (2019). Neonatal post-graduate training program for physician assistants: Meeting a need in neonatal care. *Journal of Perinatology, 39*(5), 746–753. doi: 10.1038/s41372-019-0350-9

Aubrey, W. R., & Yoxall, C. W. (2001). Evaluation of the role of the neonatal nurse practitioner in resuscitation of preterm infants at birth. *Archives of Diseases Child Fetal and Neonatal Edition, 85*(2), F96–F99.

Ballantyne, M. (2014). *Education needs survey of Canadian tertiary care NICUs.* Unpublished raw data.

Bellini, S. (2013). State of the state: NNP program update 2013. *Advances in Neonatal Care, 13*(5), 346–348.

Bissinger, R. L., Allred, C. A., Arford, P. H., & Bellig, L. L. (1997). A cost-effectiveness analysis of neonatal nurse practitioners. *Nursing Economics, 15*(2), 92–99.

Canada West Foundation (CWF). (1998). *Nurse practitioners and Canadian health care: Toward quality and cost effectiveness.* Calgary, AB: CWF. Retrieved from https://cwf.ca/research/publications/nurse-practioners-and-canadian-health-care/

Canadian Council of Registered Nurse Regulators (CCRNR). (2013). *CCRNR announces national nurse practitioner practice analysis.* Beaverton, ON: CCRNR. Retrieved from http://www.cno.org/globalassets/new/ccrnr/np-practice-analysis-ccrnr.pdf

CCRNR. (2015). *Practice analysis study of nurse practitioners.* Beaverton, ON: CCRNR. Retrieved from http://www.ccrnr.ca/assets/ccrnr-practice-analysis-study-of-nurse-practitioners-report---final.pdf

Canadian Institute for Health Information (CIHI). (2013). *Regulated nurses, 2013 summary report.* Ottawa, ON: CIHI. Retrieved from https://secure.cihi.ca/estore/productFamily.htm?locale=en&pf=PFC2646&lang=en

Canadian Nurses Association (CNA). (2008). *Advanced nursing practice: A national framework.* Ottawa, ON: CNA. Retrieved from https://www.cna-aiic.ca/en/~/media/nurseone/page-content/pdf-en/anp_national_framework_e

CNA. (2010). *Canadian nurse practitioner core competency framework.* Ottawa, ON: CNA. Retrieved from http://www.cno.org/globalassets/for/rnec/pdf/competencyframework_en.pdf

CNA. (2019). *Advanced practice nursing: A pan-Canadian framework.* Ottawa, ON: CNA. Retrieved from https://www.cna-aiic.ca/-/media/cna/page-content/pdf-en/apn-a-pan-canadian-framework.pdf

Carzoli, R. P., Martinez-Cruz, M., Cuevas, L. L., Murphy, S., & Chiu, T. (1994). Comparison of neonatal nurse practitioners, physician assistants, and residents in the neonatal intensive care unit. *Archives in Pediatric and Adolescent Medicine, 148*(12), 1271–1276.

College and Association of Registered Nurses of Alberta (CARNA). (2017). *Scope of practice for nurse practitioners (NPs)*. Calgary, AB: CARNA. Retrieved from https://www.nurses.ab.ca/docs/default-source/document-library/standards/scope-of-practice-for-nurse-practitioners.pdf

DiCenso, A. (1998). The neonatal nurse practitioner. *Current Opinions in Pediatrics, 10*, 151–155.

Donald, F., Kilpatrick, K., Reid, K., Carter, N., Martin-Misener, R., Bryant-Lukosius, D., ... DiCenso, A. (2014). A systematic review of the cost-effectiveness of nurse practitioners and clinical nurse specialists: What is the quality of the evidence? *Nursing Research and Practice* (Epub). doi: 10.1155/2014/896587

Evanochko, C. (2011). "Growing your own" ... Creating a neonatal nurse practitioner team. *Neonatal Network, 30*(5), 289.

Faculty of Health Sciences, McMaster University. (1991). *Expanded role nurses in neonatology*. Unpublished, Faculty of Health Sciences, McMaster University, Hamilton, ON.

Fenton, M. V., & Brykczynski, K. A. (1993). Qualitative distinctions and similarities in the practice of clinical nurse specialists and nurse practitioners. *Journal of Professional Nursing, 9*(6), 313–326.

Fetus and Newborn Committee, Canadian Paediatric Society. (2000). Advanced practice nursing roles in neonatal care. *Paediatrics and Child Health, 5*(3), 178–182.

Follett, T., Calderon-Crossman, S., Clarke, D., Ergezinger, M., Evanochko, C., Johnson, K., Mercy, N., & Taylor, B. (2017). Implementation of the neonatal nurse practitioner role in a community hospital's labor, delivery, and Level 1 postpartum unit. *Advances in Neonatal Care, 17*(2), 106–113. doi: 10.1097/ANC.0000000000000343

Freed, G. L., Moran, L. M., Dunham, K. M., & Nantais-Smith, L. (2015). Capacity of, and demand for neonatal nurse practitioner educational programs: A missing piece of the workforce puzzle. *Journal of Professional Nursing, 31*(4), 318–322.

Gigli, K. H., Beauchesne, M. A., Dirks, M. S., & Peck, J. L. (2019). White paper: Critical shortage of pediatric nurse practitioners predicted. *Journal of Pediatric Health Care, 33*(3), 347–355. doi: 10.1016/j.pedhc.2019.02.008

Giovannetti, P., Tenove, S., Stuart, M., & van den Berg, R. (1996). *Report of the CAUSN working group on advanced nursing practice*. Ottawa, ON: CAUSN.

Goldstein, R. F., & Malcolm, W. F. (2019). Care of the neonatal intensive care unit graduate after discharge. *Pediatric Clinics of North America, 66*(2), 489–508.

Honeyfield, M. E. (2009). Neonatal nurse practitioners: Past, present, and future. *Advances in Neonatal Care, 9*(3), 125–128.

Hooker, R. S., Brock, D. M., & Cook, M. L. (2016). Characteristics of nurse practitioners and physician assistants in the United States. *Journal of the American Association of Nurse Practitioners, 28*(1), 39–46.

The Hospital for Sick Children. (1987). *Job description—clinical nurse specialist—nurse practitioner (neonatal)*. Toronto, ON: The Hospital for Sick Children.

The Hospital for Sick Children. (1990). *The clinical nurse specialist—neonatal practitioner team*. Toronto, ON: The Hospital for Sick Children.

Hunsberger, M., Mitchell, A., Blatz, S., Paes, B., Pinelli, J., Southwell, D., ... Soluk, R. (1992). Definition of an advanced nursing practice role in the NICU: The clinical nurse specialist/neonatal nurse practitioner. *Clinical Nurse Specialist, 6*(2), 91–96.

Kaasalainen, S., Martin-Misener, R., Kilpatrick, K., Harbman, P., Bryant-Lukosius, D., Donald, F., & DiCenso, A. (2010). A historical overview of the development of advanced practice nursing in Canada. *Canadian Journal of Nursing Leadership, 23*(Special Issue), 35–60.

Kaminski, M., Meier, S., & Staebler, S. (2015). National Association of Neonatal Nurse Practitioners (NANNP) workforce survey. *Advances in Neonatal Care, 15*(3), 182–190.

Karlowicz, M. G., & McMurray, J. L. (2000). Comparison of neonatal nurse practitioners' and pediatric residents' care of extremely low-birth-weight infants. *Archives in Pediatric and Adolescent Medicine, 154*(11), 1123–1126.

Kieran, E., Sara, R., Claydon, J., Hait, V., de Salaberry, J., Osiovich, H., & Shivananda, S. (2019). Outcomes of neonates with complex medical needs. *Advances in Neonatal Care, 19*(4), 275–284.

Lee, T. W., Skelton, R. E., & Skene, C. (2001). Routine neonatal examination: Effectiveness of trainee paediatrician compared with advanced neonatal nurse practitioner. *Archives of Disease in Children. Fetal & Neonatal Edition, 85*, F100–F104.

McAllister, M., Ballantyne, M., & Lamb, A. (2019). Canadian neonatal nurse practitioner health human resource survey. Unpublished raw data.

McAllister, M., Fryers, M., Campbell, H., Avery, S., Haddad, M., Booth, M., Sabo, K., … Doyle, S. (1993). *The Hospital for Sick Children position paper: Enhancing, extending and expanding the role of the nurse.* Toronto, ON: The Hospital for Sick Children.

McMaster University School of Nursing. (1987). *Background paper for position-statement on the "expanded role" in nursing.* Hamilton, ON: McMaster University School of Nursing.

Mitchell, A., Pinelli, J., Patterson, C., & Southwell, D. (1993). *Utilization of nurse practitioners in Ontario (Paper 93-4).* Unpublished manuscript.

Mitchell, A., Watts, J., Whyte, R., Blatz, S., Norman, G., Guyatt, G., … Paes, B. (1991). Evaluation of graduating neonatal nurse practitioners. *Pediatrics, 88*(4), 789–794.

Mitchell, A., Watts, J., Whyte, R., Blatz, S., Norman, G. R., Southwell, D., … Pinelli, J. (1995). Evaluation of an educational program to prepare neonatal nurse practitioners. *Journal of Nursing Education, 34*(6), 286–289.

Mitchell, G., & Santapinto, M. (1988). The expanded role nurse: A dissenting viewpoint. *Canadian Journal of Nursing Administration, 1*(4), 8–10, 14.

Mitchell-DiCenso, A., Guyatt, G., Marrin, M., Goeree, R., Willan, A., Southwell, D., … Baumann, A. (1996a). A controlled trial of nurse practitioners in neonatal intensive care. *Pediatrics, 98*(6 Pt. 1), 1143–1148.

Mitchell-DiCenso, A., Pinelli, J., & Southwell, D. (1996b). Introduction and evaluation of an advanced nursing practice role in neonatal intensive care. In K. Kelly (Ed.), *Outcomes of effective management practice* (pp. 171–186). Thousand Oaks, CA: SAGE Publications.

Nurse Practitioners' Association of Ontario (NPAO). (n.d.). *Nurse practitioner history in Ontario.* Toronto, ON: NPAO. Retrieved from http://npao.org/nurse-practitioners/history/#.VQ8CdfnF8rU

Paes, B., Mitchell, A., Hunsberger, M., Blatz, S., Watts, J., Dent, P., … Southwell, D. (1989). Medical staffing in Ontario neonatal intensive care units. *Canadian Medical Association Journal, 140*(11), 1321–1326.

Pinelli, J. M. (1997). The clinical nurse specialist/nurse practitioner: Oxymoron or match made in heaven? *Canadian Journal of Nursing Administration, 10*(1), 85–110.

Rubin, S. (1988). ERN contributing to the development of the nursing profession. *Canadian Journal of Nursing Administration, 1*(2), 23–27.

Ruth-Sanchez, V., Lee, K. A., & Bosque, E. M. (1996). A descriptive study of current neonatal nurse practitioner practice. *Neonatal Network, 15*, 23–29.

Samson, L. F. (2006). Perspectives on neonatal nursing: 1985–2005. *Journal of Perinatal and Neonatal Nursing, 20*(1), 19–26.

Schultz, J. M., Liptak, G. S., & Fioravanti, J. (1994). Nurse practitioners' effectiveness in NICU. *Nursing Management, 25*(10), 50–53.

Tithecott, G., Levin, S., & Filler, G. (2018). Innovating to educate paediatric consultant generalists for the new Canadian health care. *Paediatrics & Child Health, 23*(2), 122–124.

Welch-Carre, E. (2018). *National Association of Neonatal Nurses: NNP Workforce White Paper.* Chicago, IL: National Association of Neonatal Nurses. Retrieved from http://nann.org/uploads/NNPWorkforceWhitePaper.pdf

Woods, L. (2006). Evaluating the clinical effectiveness of neonatal nurse practitioners: An exploratory study. *Journal of Clinical Nursing, 5,* 35–44. doi: 10.1111/j.1365-2702.2005.01246.x

Wright, J. (1997). *Commonalities and diversity between acute care CNSs and ACNPs.* Unpublished manuscript.

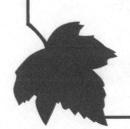

SECTION V

Critical Issues in Advanced Practice Nursing in Canada

This section provides the reader with critical issues affecting advanced practice nursing currently and in the future in Canada and globally, including sustainability of the roles. The issues relating to advanced practice nurses that are discussed include education, interprofessional practice, role management, performance evaluation and outcomes of practice, and the influence of health policy within a changing health care environment and fiscal restraint.

Chapter 28

The Advanced Practice Nurse and Interprofessional Collaborative Practice Competence

Carole Orchard

CAROLE ORCHARD is a Professor Emerita at the Arthur Labatt Family School of Nursing and for-mer Coordinator for the Interprofessional Health Education and Research Office at Western University, London, Ontario. Her work has been focused on understanding how health care providers can shift from the current multidisciplinary practice model into client-centred col-laborative practice to support the growing client populations with complex health and social issues who today often fall through the cracks in our current models of care. Carole was the co-lead in development of the Canadian Interprofessional Health Collaborative national framework for interprofessional competence. From this work, her program of research has led to publications on both instrument development and theorized models that are inter-nationally recognized. Carole has also focused on the role of nurse leaders to support the enactment by advanced practice nurses for the significant contributions they can make to the many health challenges faced by our patients and their families in today's health care.

KEY TERMS

client-centred collaborative
    practice
collaborative leadership
competence
competencies
interprofessional (IP)
    collaboration
role clarification
teamwork

OBJECTIVES

1. Explore the meaning of competence and competency.
2. Explore the application of interprofessio-nal (IP) collaboration competency domains within health care teams.
3. Gain an understanding of how IP client-centred practice can be integrated into ad-vanced nursing practice within health care teams.
4. Explore the effective roles of advanced practice nurses as members of IP client-centred collaborative teams.

Introduction

In most countries, advanced practice nurses (APNs), particularly nurse practitioners (NPs), are required to achieve a level of competence through licensing examinations and competence in enacting their roles while others, such as clinical nurse specialists (CNSs), more frequently complete advanced practice through higher education programs, and may also hold a certification in a nursing specialty before assuming their roles. Thus, they may have advanced practice knowledge but were unable to translate it into specification of actual competency in their practice, which would allow for more in-depth assessment of their impact on health care outcomes.

In interprofessional (IP) client-centred practice, health care professionals from several disciplines are brought together with their clients who are experiencing complex health and social challenges to address the needs that are beyond any one professional working in isolation. While each professional in an IP team contributes their professional knowledge, skills, and expertise in shaping a coordinated plan of care, nursing input may or may not be the first intervention that the client chooses to work on.

While the APN role is integral to client care, the degree of involvement in that care may vary across a trajectory of time in the client's needs. In today's APN practice, assessment of competence needs to focus on three levels: the professional level (the one focused on primarily today); the advanced practice nurse as an individual contributor to collaborative client-centred practice; and finally, the advanced practice nurse's contribution to the functioning of the team. The roles of individual contributor and functioning of the team will be the focus in this chapter.

This chapter will introduce the reader to a new orientation of client and practitioner roles within the envisioned IP collaborative practice where the client becomes the driver of their own care and the advanced practice nurse and other health care professionals become facilitators to assist the client in achieving agreed-upon health outcomes focusing on the steps of the Framework for Client-Centred Collaborative Practice (Orchard, Anderson, & Ford, 2018; Orchard, Anderson, Ford, & Moran, 2015). Discussion will include the meaning of competence and competency and how they are applied to the Canadian Interprofessional Health Collaborative's (CIHC) National Interprofessional Competency Framework (2010). This discussion will explore how all the CIHC competency domains can assist in an evolving role of APNs in client-centred care and for APNs to assess their own demonstration of competence in collaborative teamwork practice.

Literature Review

A literature review of recent papers (2011–2019) was carried out to update this chapter from the first edition (2016). It appears that lack of clarity around competencies associated with the APN role, outside of the NP role, is limiting studies predominantly on the role of NPs within IP teams (Hurlock-Chorostecki et al., 2013, 2014a, 2014b; Kowitlawakul et al., 2014; Lowe, Plummer, O'Brien, & Boyd, 2011). There is further ambiguity related to the education of APNs, which generally addresses the need to focus on the APN role within IP teams (Chen, Rivera, Rotter, Green, & Kools, 2016; Farrell, Payne, & Heye, 2015; Gerard, Kazer, Babington, & Quell, 2014; Giddens et al., 2014; LeFlore & Thomas, 2016; Rugen, Speroff, Zapatka, & Brienza, 2016), as collaborator and leader of IP teams (Andregard, 2015; Kilpatrick, Lavoie-Tremblay, Ritchie, Lamothe, & Doran, 2011; Lacasse, 2013; LeFlore & Thomas, 2016; McInnes, Peters, Bonney, & Halcomb, 2015; Price, Doucet, & McGillis Hall, 2014), and integrating IP competencies without any specificity of what these comprise (Farrell et al., 2015). Rugen et al. (2016) specify team-based competencies for NPs as bridging medicine and nursing in primary health care. In these teams the NP was reported to provide patient-centred care, leadership, and population health improvements (Rugen et al., 2016) and generally preparing new NPs to work within IP teams (Giddens et al., 2014). Even in articles related to APN competencies, the focus is more on the nursing role with clients than on the role within teams.

Competence and Competency

What constitutes competence in practice? Competence is often associated with the demonstration of competencies. Competencies are characterized in a variety of ways and linked to professional roles, professional domains of task, work processes, and work outcomes. They can also be associated with minimal performance and linked to entry-to-practice competence (Govaerts, 2008). Competency can be used by employers to address performance expectations in job roles; by professional regulators to specify required performance by professionals in their practice (Axley, 2008); and to determine what or how to assess the impact of care on patient outcomes, or even when to provide care to patients. Competencies often contain five dimensions, including, "cognitive knowledge (know-that), functional skills (know-how), personal behaviours (know how to behave), ethical values, and meta-competencies (ability to cope with uncertainty)" (Le Deist & Winterton, 2005, p. 35). Roegiers (2016) has reconceptualized these dimensions into "know how to think … know how to respond … [and] know how to act" (p. 12).

Competency is therefore viewed in a variety of ways, such as an outcome demonstrated by a set of behaviours, as a process leading to outcomes, as a shared approach in arriving at care decisions, and as a means to determine when performance is at an acceptable level in a job role. Rarely is it viewed consistently by those who use the term. Competence is focused on the individual's performance and not at the team level and may also be considered as minimal and not exceptional performance (Cowan, Norman, & Coopamah, 2005). The complexity of care for many patients today necessitates practitioners' interdependence of knowledge (knowing that), skills (knowing how to), and expertise of all members in a team of health care professionals (coping with uncertainty) along with the client as a contributing member of the team (Adams, Orchard, Houghton, & Ogrin, 2014). Focusing on competence within a set of outcomes and behaviours provides insight into specific application of competencies but excludes an understanding of processes adopted in arriving at care decisions. Team competence necessitates attention to assessing the integrated knowledge and tasks of each member working together (Garavan & McGuire, 2001). Roegiers (2016) concluded that "all types of content—knowledge, know-how, life skills, cross-cutting competences—are necessary to enable [teams of health care professionals] to resolve complex [patient] situations [health and social challenges]" (p. 16).

Teamwork is dependent on building relationships among its members. Team relationships act as a "glue" connecting members into a unified whole. Team competence then is a measure of team relationship effectiveness and requires a multi-dimensional approach that addresses both the processes used and the outcomes achieved from the team's relational work to determine their practice competency (Garavan & McGuire, 2001; Orchard & Rykhoff, 2015). The current popularity within health professional education and practice focuses almost exclusively on outcomes that are desirable to be demonstrated to ensure such practice is enacted. What is often missing is considering the processes taken to achieve such outcomes. Interestingly, in a review of unintended consequences or near misses in care, the process is the focus, but it is carried out backwards from the outcome to determine what might have gone wrong (Canadian Patient Safety Institute [CPSI], 2014).

In IP collaborative practice, a similar focus is used. The judgments made by the team working together are the outcome, but the focus is on the processes used to arrive at a judgment, which are the important learning steps within teamwork. The frequent competency perspective on outcomes then limits the evidence of contributions made by an individual health professional or APNs into the overall shared approaches to care. Ideally, health care today is enacted with the input of health care professionals, clients, and often their informal caregivers. This shifts the importance of how individuals provide care to how members of teams, including clients and their informal caregivers, work together to reach a shared plan of care and how it will be implemented to achieve goals set together. While in nursing such an approach to giving patients their voice in their care is often written about and taught, in reality it seems not to be a norm commonly enacted within hospital practice environments based on research studies (Henderson, 2003; Sahlsten, Larsson, Plos, & Lindencrona, 2005; Tutton, 2005; Wellard, Lillibridge, Beanland, & Lewis, 2003). Wellard et al. (2003) suggested that health care professionals, including nurses, may feel the need to exert their professional prowess rather than "allowing" the above role for their patients. A further potential for professionals feeling the need to exert their power may be associated with the ideology of evidence-based practice, which draws health care professionals' focus away from working with their clients to evidence and its integration into standardized approaches to care (Holmes, Murray, Perron, & Rail, 2006). If as nurses we wish to reassert our disciplinary ontology through its epistemology associated with our patterns of knowing (Chinn & Kramer, 2018), then IP client-centred collaborative practice can be viewed as an asset to our practicing as partners with our clients.

When APNs work together with the total IP team, including the client, then the need for team members to know how all members think, how to respond to each other's input, and how to act on what the client is willing to do are critical toward achieving effective health outcomes. Therefore, a focus on competence cannot be based only on individual health care professionals or APNs and how they enact their personal and professional knowledge, skills, and expertise. Collaborative practice necessitates a sharing of all members' perspectives on what profession-based knowledge, skills, and expertise can be combined with all their contributed ideas to become a set of potential approaches that may help clients address their chosen need(s), and not be fixed on institutional outcomes and those associated with standardized algorithms or protocols arising from evidence-based medicine (EBM) studies in isolation. Rather, knowledge, skills, and expertise should be adapted to be relevant and meaningful to clients.

Roegiers (2007) suggests making team judgments requires use of all team members' "resources" comprised of their knowledge, know-how (skill enactment), and life skills (experiential learning) to address complex situations. Therefore, in a competent IP team, perspectives of all members are shared in response to a client's shared situation. The choices are dependent on the client's agreed-upon chosen thinking processes arising from application of all members' collective resources (including the client's) associated with each member's professional standards of practice, evidence-based knowledge, experiential practice, and procedures for assessing, defining, and interpreting clients' care needs. What then comprises IP team collaboration competence?

Interprofessional Collaboration Competency Framework

The CIHC's National Interprofessional Competency Framework (2010) is one of the only frameworks that focuses on the process that teams utilize to achieve collaborative practice. It reflects an integrative pedagogy approach discussed earlier as attributed to Roegiers (2007) and Tardif (1999). In this form of competence, the focus is on the goal trying to be achieved. In this case **IP collaboration** provides the goal for competence. To achieve this goal, foundational components are identified that together can enable the goal to be achieved. The overall direction is on patient/client/family-centred care/services, which require demonstration of IP communications between and across health care professionals, necessitating an understanding of each other's roles inclusive of each person's knowledge, skills, and expertise that can be brought into their teamwork (**role clarification**), and how their team functions together (team functioning) through adoption of **collaborative leadership**, and their ability to address and resolve any IP conflicts (IP conflict resolution; see Figure 28.1).

These foundational components integrate with each other to reach the goal. Therefore, each of the competencies is referred to as a domain. Tardif provides some insight into variants that can affect health care professionals' capacity to work collaboratively in teams. He notes this capacity is dependent on the complexity of the situation: the team's ability to share and use additive application of their shared resources; integration of resources into care planning; and members' developmental capacity to work within the team (Tardif, 1999). Thus, an individual team member's capacity to work collaboratively within a team is evolutionary and depends upon their familiarity with the practice context and their teamwork experience. Each team member's competence in IP collaborative client-centred practice is always changing. Team members are in a constant self-directed learning cycle enacting their collaborative team practice competence. Table 28.1 provides the CIHC competency domains with their descriptors that integrate Tardif's variants.

FIGURE 28.1: The National Interprofessional Competency Framework

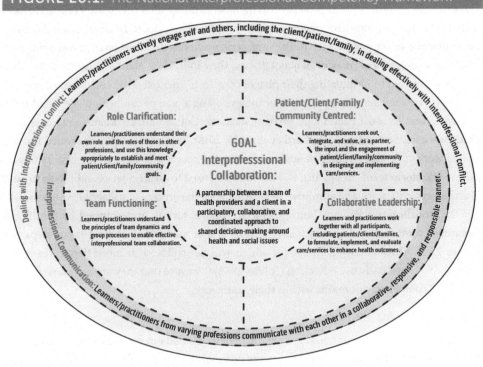

Source: CIHC. (2010). *A national interprofessional competency framework.* Vancouver, BC: CIHC. Retrieved from http://www.cihc.ca/files/CIHC_IPCompetencies_Feb1210.pdf. Reprinted with permission.

TABLE 28.1: CIHC Competency Domains and Descriptors

Competency Domain	Descriptors Learners/practitioners ...
Patient/Client/Family/Community-Centred Care	"... seek out, integrate and value, as a partner, the input and the engagement of the patient/client/family/community in designing and implementing care/services."
Interprofessional Communication	"... from different professions communicate with each other in a collaborative, responsive and responsible manner."
Role Clarification	"... understand their own role and the roles of those in other professions, and use this knowledge appropriately to establish and meet patient/client/family and community goals."
Team Functioning	"... understand the principles of team dynamics and group processes to enable effective interprofessional team collaboration."
Collaborative Leadership	"... work together with all participants, including patients/clients/families, to formulate, implement and evaluate care/services to enhance health outcomes."
Interprofessional Conflict Resolution	"... actively engage self and others, including the patients/client/family, in dealing effectively with interprofessional conflict."

Source: CIHC. (2010). *A national interprofessional competency framework.* Vancouver, BC: CIHC. Retrieved from http://www.cihc.ca/files/CIHC_IPCompetencies_Feb1210.pdf.

Since the publication of the National IP Competency Framework, further work has been carried out to assist health care professionals in understanding what changes are needed to move from the current predominant multidisciplinary model of practice to IP client-centred collaborative practice. In the former, each health professional assesses the client on their own and all the health care professionals may or may not discuss their individual plans for the client. Rarely is the client involved in formulating their plan of care. In IP client-centred collaborative practice, all health care professionals work together in developing a plan of care with a client and informal caregiver. To assist health care professionals, the Collaborative Patient-Centred Practice Framework has been created (Orchard et al., 2015, 2018). This framework was created through shared work of several IP competencies international experts who have a long history of working to transform teams in practice and is now being used to create a set of audit tools to assist practitioners, educators, and administrators in auditing the process of collaborative teamwork.

The Collaborative Patient-Centred Practice Framework is underpinned by the IP collaborative competency domains (CIHC, 2010) and is comprised of four main steps (see Figure 28.2). Throughout all the steps, which will be explored in more depth, teams are expected to continually use reflection (Schön, 1983) to ensure that they are demonstrating all the CIHC competency domains within their teamwork.

Step 1: Getting Ready

This step reflects the research and systematic reviews carried out by Salas, Cooke, and Rosen (2008) to identify the need to build teams outside their health care practice. Within this step

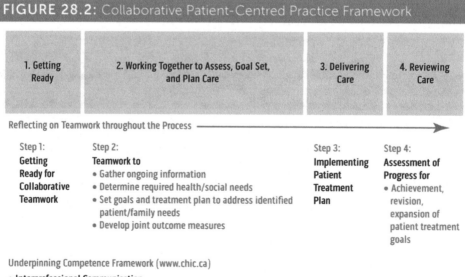

FIGURE 28.2: Collaborative Patient-Centred Practice Framework

Source: Orchard, C. A., Anderson, E., & Ford, J. (2018). *Collaborative patient-centred practice framework.* Presentation at All Together Better Health VI, September 3, 2018, Auckland, New Zealand.

the team needs to explore and develop their knowledge, skills, and expertise in enacting all the CIHC competency domains. The discussion related to the patient/client/family-centred care/service domain will be discussed in depth under step 2.

Members working within IP collaborative teams must understand and employ team dynamics to develop competence in team functioning. Often there is confusion as to what a team is and who comprises a team. A team is a group of individuals who are interdependent in their tasks, who share responsibility for outcomes, who see themselves and who are seen by others as an intact social entity embedded in one or more larger social systems, and who manage their relationships across clinic boundaries (Cohen & Bailey, 1997). In collaborative teams, all team members are responsible for its functioning. The components associated with team functioning include team context/structure, team processes, and team outcomes (Deneckere et al., 2011).

Team Context/Structure

The structure or context of a team is comprised of its culture and climate for organizing a team, team interdependence, resources, and coordinating mechanisms (Deneckere et al., 2011). IP collaborative teams can be found in any health care setting and are comprised of several members from small to large. Length of time working in a team does not necessarily lead to high levels of collaborative team functioning; the environment or climate created by its members to support their teamwork are essential elements in effective team functioning. West and Poulton (1997) identify team participation, team objectives, task orientation, clarity of tasks, support for innovation, and commitment to teamwork as effective elements in teams. Team task orientation focuses on creating an atmosphere in which all members can seek each other's input for advice, and together critically explore generated knowledge and skills that can be applied to address complex client care situations. While it has been reported that positive team environments support monitoring and reflection on team performance achievement, restructuring of an organization is required in order to develop clear shared objectives to facilitate a coordinated approach in health care delivery (West & Poulton, 1997).

Team Processes

Processes used by teams to achieve their work are necessary to support positive working environments. Teamwork processes needed to lay the foundation for effective collaborative work include learning to achieve meaningful task interdependencies; holding shared goals across the team; and using the multiple information sources available both within the team and from other sources. However, creating a team-shared process to work together can be achieved only through intensive communication processes (Salas, DiazGranados, Weaver, & King, 2008). Two competency domains are therefore key in moving toward effective team functioning, IP communication, and role clarification.

Interprofessional Communication

Collaborative interactive communication is "a continuous transactional process involving participants' exchange of messages, many of which are effected by external physiological and psychological noise" (Adler & Proctor II, 2010, p. 11). In any transaction, people have a strong likelihood of occupying different environments and using varying communication channels in which a degree of "noise" is always present. Transactions are comprised of two components: content and relational. The content of communications is what is to be discussed, while the relational aspect reflects how parties feel about each other. The relational aspect of interactions in IP teams can be further affected by four factors: affinity (connection to one another), immediacy (the interest or attention to what is being said), respect (the amount of respect shared among the team members), and control (the degree of control one team member exerts over the others during any interaction; Adler & Proctor II, 2010).

The ability to effectively use all team members' combined knowledge, skills, and expertise is associated with the team's collaborative communication skills. The patterns that health professionals use in their professional communications are unique within each profession as an outcome of their uni-professional identity formation. Health care professionals within their own professional preparation accumulate unique language and patterns of communications, as well as profession-specific approaches to clients' care. This education model limits learning beyond one's own profession; adds barriers to the effectiveness of IP interactions; and leads to missed communication due to the relational aspects of communication, long associated with patient untoward events (Institute of Medicine, 2001) and errors in care decision-making (Robinson, Gorman, Summer, & Yudkowsky, 2010).

IP communications are only as effective as the quality of the information being shared between the sender and the receiver. IP communication is about communicating between parties and is associated with each member's personality, professional, and personal interactive approaches. Effective IP communication is about ensuring shared understandings exist between the team members involved in a transaction. Effective communication is reported to occur when a message has clarity and precision and relies on verification; collaborative problem-solving; is delivered through a calm, supportive demeanour when under stress; and when the parties maintain mutual respect toward each other that arises from an authentic understanding of each other's unique role (Robinson et al., 2010). Hence, chances of missed communications are high if team members do not create a team-shared set of communication guidelines (Defenbaugh & Chikotas, 2016; Kilpatrick, 2012; Matziou et al., 2014; Wittenberg, Goldsmith, & Neiman, 2015). These guidelines must identify the types and importance of communications (i.e., degree of urgency), and then what means are to be used to convey each type (i.e., email, pager), what the content of each type needs to be, and to whom each type of message is to be conveyed. Traditionally most health care professionals depend on established systems that organizations use; however, this negates attention to the relational and most important aspect of IP communications. The importance of establishing such guidelines was stressed in a paper by Kilpatrick (2012) as a need for effective patient care.

Lack of communication training and preparation for IP teamwork among nurses working in palliative care has been reported by Wittenberg et al. (2015), and Matziou et al. (2014) reported difficulties in communication among physicians and nurses due to lack of approaches and frameworks that were common to both. In an integrative review of IP communication, Foronda, MacWilliams, and McArthur (2016) concluded that the situation-background-assessment-recommendation (SBAR) technique provided a promising approach to improvement in IP reporting. Therefore, SBAR does provide one means for the use of a consistent framework to improve IP communications in health care.

In summary, APN competence in IP communication is essential for effective interactions with health care professionals and ensuring patient safety. Effective IP communication is underpinned by the level of clarity in understanding each team member's role within the team.

Role Clarification

Attention to the importance of understanding each other's roles from their professional perspective is growing in practice. The importance of knowing about the roles of other team members is a key component in effective team functioning. Role clarification occurs at three levels: generic, focal, and functional. The generic role is the scope of practice we are licensed to enact and have been prepared in through our educational programs; the focal role relates to the selected knowledge, skills, and expertise we use when focusing care on a specific client; finally, each team member must also be prepared to assist in ensuring the team works effectively, which is the functional role.

While health care professionals learn about their own professional role, it is not the norm to seek out the knowledge, skills, and expertise of other health care professionals they work with. Yet, this is a key to working collaboratively in teams. If there is no attention given to having a fulsome discussion with other health care team members about their knowledge, skills, and expertise, misperceptions of each other's roles and inaccuracies can lead to frustrations among members and undermine trust within their team.

Learning within one's own profession creates strong in-group affiliation with their own profession and perceptions of others as out-group members who are perceived to perform at a lesser level of competence. Social psychologists associate this in-group bias with social contact theory. To overcome this in-group bias necessitates IP team members to learn about the knowledge, skills, and expertise of all members. Strategies are needed that focus on addressing three mediators identified by Pettigrew and Tropp (2008): decreasing anxiety in joining the team; receiving respect from the other team members for their knowledge, skills, and expertise; and clarifying each other's roles. Together, attention to these mediators for intergroup contact can enhance a higher quality of care than would be realized if approached by each team member independently.

Studies have been reported around the role of APNs with specific attention to that of NPs in teams (Andregard, 2015; Hurlock-Chorostecki et al., 2013, 2014b; Kilpatrick et al., 2011; Kowitlawakul et al., 2014; Morilla-Herrera et al., 2016). A recent study by Allen, Orchard, Kerr, and Adams (2019) focused on finding the means to measure role clarification using first a concept analysis followed by development and testing of the Interprofessional Role Clarification Scale (IPRCS). The IPRCS is comprised of three dimensions—knowing roles, articulating roles, and sharing roles (Allen et al., 2019)—and shows some promise for gaining a further understanding of what comprises clarification of roles in practice settings. When role clarification and IP communication are focused on within IP collaborative practice, there is a greater chance of achieving enhanced team outcomes.

Team outcomes are achieved through coordination of care processes, team effectiveness, perceived communication with client/family, satisfaction, perceived follow-up of care, and professional agreements on best practices (Deneckere et al., 2011). The focus of collaborative teamwork is always on achieving shared goals, which is associated with how the team functions or on how the team works with clients and their families to reach the healthiest state possible for clients. To achieve this level of functioning, a team requires a level of maturity in relationship building between what Howarth, Warner, and Haigh (2012) called reciprocal respect and trust of members. Shared confidence among members is dependent on an evolved perceived team credibility as members gain skill in using their collective efficacy in working toward a shared goal of client-centred care. Team credibility occurs only through members' negotiated time (the length of time they work together) and space (setting and work environment), allowing for formation of conditional partnerships with each other. The outcome is achievement of their shared goals and effective team functioning. Effective team functioning to achieve the above outcome is dependent on both collaborative leadership and IP conflict resolution processes.

Collaborative/Shared Leadership

The complexity of client care needs necessitates decentralization of leadership into the hands of those who are at the clients' care interface. No longer can health care professionals wait until administrative decision-making processes are provided to affirm care decisions. Today decision-making must occur within IP teams through collaborative leadership that occurs "when all members of a team are fully engaged in the leadership of the team and are not hesitant to influence and guide their fellow team members in an effort to maximize the potential of the team as a whole" (Pearce, 2004, p. 48).

Achievement of shared leadership can be realized only when each team member feels respected and valued as a team member; can trust others and be trusted in turn; have a say in planning, implementation, and evaluation of teamwork and care; and participate as valued members in shared work outcomes. The capacity of a collaborative team to share in collaborative team leading is an essential component to effective teamwork. Carson, Tesluk, and Marrone (2007) suggest that collaborative leadership is enacted within two forms: focused and distributed. "Focused leadership occurs when leadership resides within a single individual, whereas distributed leadership occurs when two or more individuals share the roles, responsibilities, and functions of leadership" (Carson et al., 2007, p. 1218). No matter which form of collaborative leadership is chosen within a team, effectiveness of its teamwork necessitates "development and shaping of team processes generating shared goal commitment, and shaping a constructive climate" (Balthazard, Waldman, Howell, & Atwater, 2004, p. 7).

Collaborative or shared leadership is usually supported through a formal organizational leader referred to by Pearce and Sims Jr. (2002) as the vertical leader. The collaborative team then interacts with the vertical leader to ensure their teamwork fits within the overall organization. Orchard and Rykhoff (2015) proposed a Complementary Leadership Framework (see Figure 28.3), which incorporates Pearce and Sims Jr.'s (2002) concepts of vertical and shared leadership integrated through a reciprocal building of relationships between the vertical

FIGURE 28.3: The Complementary Leadership Framework

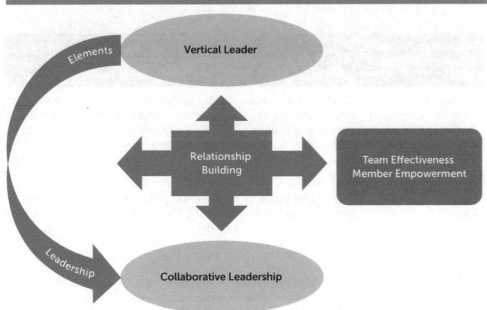

Source: Orchard, C. A., & Rykhoff, M. (2015). Collaborative leadership in the context of interprofessional patient-centred collaborative practice. In D. Forman, M. Jones, & J. Thistlethwaite (Eds.), *Leadership and collaboration* (pp. 71–94). Basingstoke, UK: Palgrave Macmillan. Reprinted with permission.

leader's transformative, transactional, and empowering leadership (Pearce, 2004) and the team members' shared leadership connected by shared relational coordination as proposed by Gittell, Godfrey, and Thistlethwaite (2013). The vertical leader's transformational leadership is comprised of "modeling the way" (clarifying their own values and validating and connecting actions to the team's shared values); "inspiring a shared vision" (helping the team to see a desired future); "enabling others to act" (seeking opportunities for them to innovate and take risks); "challenging the process" (seeking innovative ways to change, grow, and inspire); and "encouraging the heart" (recognizing others' contributions; Kouzes & Posner, 2006). See Table 28.2.

The team then complements these leadership elements as a coherent whole in its practice. Team members model leadership when they demonstrate their knowledge of their personal values and how these enhance or interfere in working with others, and when they help the team stay focused on patients' care and their own well-being. The team creates a shared vision by focusing on their patient-specified goals, brought about by collaboratively bringing all their shared ideas together to reach the goal. Team members enable others to act by being respectful of each other and ensuring goals reached are shared with their patients. Enabling others to act is shown when team members encourage other colleagues to take on assumption of and support for the team coordination role. Team members challenge the process by reflecting on their teamwork effectiveness and inclusion of patients and family members in planning for, implementing, and evaluating their care. Finally, the team recognizes each

TABLE 28.2: Comparison Enacting Kouzes and Posner's Leadership Practices

Leadership Practice (Kouzes & Posner, 2006)	Vertical Leader	Interprofessional Team Leadership
"Model the way"	Clarifying own values and validating and connecting actions to the group's shared values	Team members know their own personal values and how these may enhance or interfere in working with others; helping the team to stay focused on patient care and their own well-being
"Inspire a shared vision"	Helping the group to see a desired future	Members focus on patient-specified goals and the team considers how to get there; members help each other to bring their ideas together in an agreed-upon plan with the patient
"Enable others to act"	Fostering collaboration and striving to create an atmosphere of trust and human dignity by strengthening each person's capabilities	Members help to guide the team in promoting respect for all members and in arriving at shared goals with patients and team members; members encourage others to take on the leadership role and support clients in their decision-making with the team
"Challenge the process"	Searching for opportunities to change the status quo and look for innovative ways to improve the organization	Carrying out ongoing reflection on how the team works together with patients and based on feedback, make necessary changes related to their provider roles with an interprofessional patient-centred context
"Encourage the heart"	Recognizing contributions of others	Recognizing the positive work of all team members, including the patient, toward achieving shared goals; celebrating achievements of steps toward patient-set goals of care and well-being

Source: Orchard, C., & Rykhoff, M. (2016). Unpublished manuscript.

other's and their patients' work by celebrating successes, reflecting "encouraging the heart" (Kouzes & Posner, 2012).

Further clarity related to collaborative leadership was begun by Rykhoff and Orchard (2019), who completed a concept analysis using Walker and Avant's (2011) eight-step process. The attributes identified are situational interactive process (including mindfulness, complexity of care, and patient-engaged care); collaborative interdependence (including symbiotic relationship, respect, trust for each other's expertise, and shared capacities to achieve goals); shared assets (including information, mental models, decision-making, and collective action); and capacity to lead (including professional competence, knowledge, skills, experience, and credibility in the team). These attributes were then reviewed by Sinclair and Orchard (2018) to consider how the attributes could be objectively measured to assist in developing an instrument to assess collaborative leadership within IP teams. This resulted in slight variations in the previously identified attributes with "situational interactive process" transformed into "symbiotic relationship" and "collaborative interdependence" transformed into the variable "mindfulness." Both "shared assets" and "capacity to lead" were retained. "Symbiotic relationship" was operationally defined as "a collaboration in which both team members have their own well-established roles and mutually adapt to changing demands of the dynamic"; "mindfulness" was defined as "a thoughtful and extended focusing of one's attention on immediate experiences as they transpire"; "shared assets" as "an environment that encourages an openness to distribute knowledge, skill and expertise within a team"; and "capacity to lead" as "a willingness to both lead and accept accountability for the position of leadership" (Sinclair & Orchard, 2018). Thus a new definition of collaborative leadership has been formulated for IP teamwork as a process that occurs when all members of a team, including the patient/family, symbiotically accept their capacity to lead the group by demonstrating mindfulness of the value in working together, and using their shared assets to assist patients to reach achievable and desired health outcomes (Sinclair & Orchard, 2018).

The outcome of this above work was development of the Assessment of Interprofessional Collaborative Leadership Scale (AICLS), which is comprised of 28 items. Initial testing of the instrument has shown good reliability, but it needs further testing. When these shared leadership elements are operationalized in practice, there is believed to be a greater likelihood of effective teamwork and team outcomes. To be effective, though, we need a means to address disagreements within teams, which are a norm for this form of practice.

Interprofessional Conflict Resolution

Effective team functioning and team collaborative leadership are essential for IP collaborative team competence. However, the inherent differences in language and approaches to care across professions within a team can fuel disagreements. How we react to disagreements or conflict situations depends on "relationship[s] within the team (power dynamics); the situation the team is addressing; how other people in the team respond; and whether members are seeking to achieve their own personal or the team's goal" (Adler & Proctor II, 2010, p. 347). Key IP team skill development should focus on each member's capacity to negotiate and work toward collaborative decision-making. Team members' own profession-specific norms of communication and practice are adopted, negotiated, and renegotiated in exchanges they have in IP teams (Foronda et al., 2016). These profession-specific norms and practices are likely to come into conflict when cross-disciplinary approaches to a client's care are being discussed. While conflicts are often perceived as troublesome by professionals, they are healthy and allow for a variety of perspectives to be shared that, when handled well, can result in high-quality comprehensive and collaborative client care planning. To achieve a healthy outcome from IP conflicts, team members need to strive toward finding a win-win solution to any disagreement. If the team does not work to reach this outcome, other options—such as deferring to the other person or compromising with other team members—might be used. This can lead to residual anger or feelings of being undervalued by the person perceiving to have lost. When we perceive we are the loser, residual negative feelings toward those who win persists. To arrive at a collaborative win-win decision necessitates the team using a conflict resolution process. An example of a process is provided below:

- Create an openness to hearing other's views
- Consider all views within your own perspective
- Consider biases that might exist in your viewpoint
- Consider justification for your biases and how you can come to terms with others' views
- Weigh the alternatives in your view, based on others' views in the context of the patient's safety
- Share your thinking with the other team members
- Hear each other's viewpoints
- Come to a shared agreement

An assumption underpinning these process steps is that each team member's contributions have some substantive value to the discussion. If we listen to each other and consider the value of what each team member suggests, then compare it to our own position on the issue, we should be able to see merit in aspects of other viewpoints. These merits can help us to reshape our viewpoint into one that incorporates the richness of all members' shared ideas. Ugirase, Orchard, and Tryphonopoulos (2019) have completed a concept analysis of IP conflict resolution and transformed the attributes into the Interprofessional Conflict Resolution Scale, which is currently in its initial testing phase.

In summary, step 1 in the Collaborative Client-Centred Practice Framework of Getting Ready necessitates team building processes to be undertaken, focusing on the CIHC competency domains of team functioning, role clarification, IP communication, collaborative leadership, and IP conflict resolution. There are programs that have been developed to assist health care organizations/agencies in team development. Three will be mentioned here, but further searching should be done to find one that fits with the needs of an organization or agency. TeamSTEPPS was developed by the US Army to assist teams in their communications and to address adverse events in health care. It also is reported to guide in-patient–centred care implementation. The program is accessible online at https://www.ahrq.gov/programs/index.html?search_api_views_fulltext=&field_program_topics=14172. However, this program is not designed to focus on team building associated with all the CIHC competency domains. The second program is TEAMc, developed by Orchard (2007), which is a licensable online program focusing on a teach-the-trainer model, is underpinned by all the CIHC competency domains, and uses Appreciative Inquiry across its six modules. A unique aspect is the orientation of clients to be members within the development process. A short trailer of this program is available online at www.teamc.ca. A final program is BOOST, provided through the

Centre for Interprofessional Education at the University of Toronto. This program focuses on optimizing outcomes through teamwork. Their website can be viewed at https://ipe.uto-ronto.ca/professional-development/boost-workshops. Each of these programs provides key foci for developing IP Collaborative Teamwork. Presently, there are no published papers that focus on Canadian APNs and their graduate program inclusion of IP collaborative practice learning. This should not be construed as not occurring but just that such measures are not published and may reside in the grey literature.

Step 2: Working Together to Assess, Set Goal, and Plan Care

Step 2 in the Collaborative Patient-Centred Practice Framework refocuses the client's role to being the "driver of their care" and health care professionals as "facilitators of client care." This step is about the competency domain of patient/client/family-centred care/services. This shift reflects the reality that IP client-centred collaborative practice is created to address the care of those clients with complex health challenges and social issues associated with chronic diseases.

Why this shift in focus to the client? Health care professionals provide short, episodic, expert input into how clients and their informal caregivers can address their identified health care issues. Actual outcomes of health care then are dependent on what, how, and when clients choose to address their current health and social challenges. The self-care that clients adopt, based on the information gained and treatments they choose to adopt from the health care professionals, determines their health outcomes, albeit with facilitated guidance from health care professionals. Understanding the impact of the important role that clients and their informal caregivers are being placed in by our health systems necessitates a shift in our thinking from health professionals as "experts" in clients' care to clients as "experts" in their lived experiences. This shift forces a rethinking of how health care professionals relate to their clients and informal caregivers.

To assist in this rethinking, a perspective and three theories will be explored: adult as problem-solver, Jarvis's (2012) Theory of Being a Person in Society, Kline's (2005) Naturalistic Decision Making, and Riegel, Jaarsma, and Strömberg's (2012) Middle-Range Theory of Self-Care in Chronic Illness.

Adult Problem-solving

Adults have long been known for being problem-focused (Knowles, 1984). They seek help from health care professionals to find a solution for an issue they are having difficulty addressing themselves. What is (are) the outer boundary(ies) of what can be achieved beyond clients seeking health professionals' advice for their current problem(s)? While the effectiveness of IP collaborative teamwork depends on its impact in improving clients' health outcomes, the greater the clients' input in shaping their own care, the greater the likelihood of positive outcomes. Enacting step 2 necessitates allowing the client and/or their information caregiver to explain what they are seeking health professionals' help with and why it is important to them. While this approach is often provided in primary care encounters, hospital-based practice's current thinking is that all care should be based on best practices arising from evidence-informed research, which tends to minimize the role of clients and their family members as soon as they state their diagnosis or what they need help with. The weakness of the randomized controlled trial (RCT) gold standard methodology used in evidence-based practice (EBP) to applied health care has been challenged due to the exclusion of confounding variables delimiting large numbers of those with the focused condition because of their comorbidities. Many standards of practice for specific chronic diseases are based on EBM identified through RCT trials. Authors have also reported on limited evidence of positive outcomes when clients are not directly involved in their own care (Adams et al., 2014; Reeves et al., 2009). This in no way undervalues the EBP movement but shifts it from an ideology to a component of care planning that needs to be part of a negotiating process with clients. Further benefits of enacting a client narrative is gaining an understanding of their language and health literacy from their description and creating a dynamic in which they become directly involved in their own care.

Being a Person in Society

The first theory we will explore is Jarvis's (2012) Theory of Being a Person in Society. Within this learning theory, Jarvis reminds us that each individual—whether client, caregiver, or health professional—has a repository of life events, knowledge, skills, and attitudes, including biases, fears, and desires. When we begin the client narrative, each participant will make a choice whether to listen or not to what is being asked, discussed, and suggested based on each person's brain repository. Whatever is stated in the communication interchange will be processed through each person's repository, causing all of these retained views to filter and determine whether what is being shared or suggested will be acceptable or not to the client and team members based on many factors. These factors are often never brought out during client-health professional discussions. Yet fears, previous experiences, etc., influence whether the client will ever follow through with care suggestions. Gathering further information ensures that all aspects associated with the client's issue and how the team members respond will be an interactive process with many factors that must be explored to allow for effective client-centred care. A second theory is important to help ensure that sufficient information is acquired in order to plan care for a client.

Naturalistic Decision-Making

The second theory is Kline's Naturalistic Decision Making (2005). For too long, health care professionals have focused on a linear sequence of activities associated with decision-making. Instead, Kline helps us to consider patterns people adopt in response to a problem. Kline's research focused on members of the American public and noted that decision-making is most often associated with how a person reacts to situations using "patterns of responses." The first pattern is an unconscious response using an automatic, previously learned pattern. An example is the need to put on a pair of shoes. We often do not even think as we take the steps to do this action. However, it is comprised of a pattern of responses that result in the shoes being placed on our feet. If this response does not fully address the need, we then consciously consider what we need to do to achieve the needed outcome. If, for example, we can't find our shoes, we need to consciously consider where we left them last and seek out their location. If we are able to find them in that location, then we move back into an unconscious response in getting the shoes on our feet. Assessment focuses on an alteration in response pattern. If this works, a new pattern is established. However, if we are not able to find the shoes no matter what we do, then we need to seek help from others to find them. While this is a very simple example, it illustrates the three types of patterns a person uses. How does this make sense to client care? First, we need to gain insight into how the client has already tried to address the issue they are seeking our help with. We can then determine what comprised their pattern, what could work if modified for them, and what aspects will not work to overcome the problem. This allows us to build into and modify or expand a pattern they have already formed. Therefore, we use a scaffolding approach starting from what they know to an expanded knowing pattern. IP teamwork then can focus on setting goals and treatment plans to address client/family needs within their capacities, which will lead to a greater likelihood of success. The focus of care then needs to be on what, when, and how our clients can adapt to their patterns of managing their self-care.

Mid-Range Theory of Self-Care in Chronic Illness

The third theory, Mid-Range Theory of Self-Care in Chronic Illness (Riegel et al., 2012), provides a means to consider how to set these adapted patterns. Within this theory there are three foci that the client and/or informal caregiver needs to address: self-care maintenance, which reflects behaviours believed to improve well-being or aid in maintaining physical and emotional health; self-care monitoring, which is their individual process used to observe for changes in normal body functioning through knowing what normal body functioning feels like and then observing for changes and recording observations; finally, self-care management comprising actions the client may or may not take to correct a change in body functioning and return to their own normal state. A measure to test this theory has been developed by Orchard and is in the process of being tested on persons with diabetes. It is hoped that this work may assist health care professionals to seek information about a client's self-care more appropriately. How then should client-centred collaborative practice be enacted where the client is the driver of their own care?

We are adding a new level of health outcomes—those important to the client. These are believed to be most important in enhancing population health by focusing on improving the health of one client at a time. The team members then are fully aware of the client's plan of care; each knows when and what they are responsible for; and how the client will self-monitor to ensure the plan of care is moving forward. When we trialed this process, it actually takes about the same amount of time as patient assessment, but is done only once; can be built onto; and saves tremendous amounts of wasted time trying to connect with other health care professionals to deal with one issue at a time.

Step 3: Delivery Care

In "delivering care," the third step of the Collaborative Client-Centred Framework, the client is made aware of the plan of care, which is shaped around what the client sees as key to their progress markers. While it may be perceived as idealized, we need to keep in mind that 30% of our population in Canada has at least one chronic condition that needs ongoing monitoring, and the number of these conditions increases with age. To keep our health system viable, we need to build into our model for care delivery a fulsome integration of clients so they will be self-care experts of their lived experiences. In step 3 the advanced practice nurse can know what all members of a client's care team are planning to provide and how to support and help the client review progress. This self-care needs to reflect how the client can manage, monitor, and maintain their health within their capacity. Steps 2 and 3 reflect a strength-based approach to care that is very familiar to APNs. Moving to full implementation of step 3 needs to be viewed as valuable in saving time and resources by other health care professionals as well.

There is evidence that when CNSs/NPs/physicians involve other health care providers in discussions around patient care and respect their input, this predominance is mitigated to result in shared planning of care (Gair & Hartery, 2001). Clients' active participation in their own care results in high levels of satisfaction and feelings of empowerment (Adams et al., 2014), and is believed to result in higher self-care management of their health (Hibbard, Mahoney, Stock, & Tusler, 2007).

In step 3 there are markers to determine progress after the goals and treatment/ intervention plan are set. Again, the difference in this step is the direct involvement of a client in working with the team to implement agreed-upon care plans to achieve goals.

Step 4: Reviewing Care

In step 4, the team, the client, and their informal caregiver return to the plan of care and goals to assess progress toward goal achievement from both the client's and the team's perspectives. All the parties carry out a review to determine where achievement has been reached and where there may be further expansion of client treatment goals needed.

In Summary

In summary, the Collaborative Patient-Centred Practice Framework has four steps that enable APNs to consider what is envisioned in this form of practice. It integrates all the CIHC competency domains while also providing the means for including the client and informal caregiver in understanding the goals, the plan of care, and the measures to determine outcomes of the plan. Currently APNs must deliver care within a system that has a "health professional as expert" focus when in reality it is often what the client is doing outside the "expert" direction that makes the difference in their health outcomes.

Advanced Practice Nurses as Members of Interprofessional Collaborative Teams

In the Pan-Canadian Advanced Practice Nurse Framework, it states that APN core competencies "are based on an appropriate depth, breadth and range of nursing knowledge, theory, and research, enhanced by clinical experience" (Canadian Nurses Association [CNA], 2019a, p. 29). Within the core framework, two underlying assumptions associated with collaborative practice are stated: "APN is grounded in client- and family-centred care," and "collaborative relationships with other health care providers and stakeholders whose services impact the key determinants of health involve both independent and shared decision-making, with all parties accountable as per their scopes of practice, educational backgrounds and competencies" (CNA, 2019a, p. 29). Within this set of competencies, one focuses specifically on consultation and collaboration stated as premised on the CIHC competencies. Several of these CNA competencies relate to IP practice competency domains, including:

- Team functioning: Initiate timely and appropriate consultation, referrals, and collaboration with other health care providers
- Team functioning: Practice collaboratively and build effective coalitions and partnerships
- Role clarification and team functioning: Apply theories related to group dynamics, roles, and organization
- IP communication, IP conflict resolution: Use theory to demonstrate knowledge and skill in communication, negotiation, conflict prevention, management and resolution, coalition building, and change management
- Overall collaboration: Coordinate interprofessional, intraprofessional, and intersectoral teams
- Role clarification: Articulate the contribution of APN within the interprofessional health care team and among intersectoral stakeholders

However, none of these collaborative competencies address patient/client/community-centred care, albeit this is an overriding premise of the core APN competencies and collaborative leadership. The only potential direction for APNs associated with collaborative leadership could be their coordination of the team. As has been suggested earlier in this chapter, the nurse may not be the best health professional at key times to be in that team-leading role. Furthermore, the one competency addressing conflict also focuses on conflict prevention, which may undermine ensuring that all team members agree with the advanced practice nurse's directions for client care.

While these revised competencies are moving toward requiring APNs to focus on their collaboration within teams, the question arises: where do APNs learn to be collaborative practitioners within IP teams? A key principle stated is "providing support for interprofessional collaboration without duplication of services by multiple health-care providers" (CNA, 2019a, p. 25), which, while noble, has limited evidence that this is the current norm of delivery of care models in most health care settings. It necessitates collaborative team working and not interdisciplinary teamwork. CNA in the APN framework presents several strategies to support successful implementation, integration, and sustainability. One of the evidence-informed factors for effective integration related to collaborative practice is "interprofessional education and organizations that foster teamwork" (CNA, 2019b, p. 39). This is a significant statement that means all APN graduate education programs, as well as health care organizations, need to ensure the development of the CIHC competency domains to assist in this direction. However, it is not just teamwork as there is a great deal of teamwork occurring, but it is predicated on a multidisciplinary approach to care and not a client-centred collaborative one. To move to such a change in delivery approach, a new framework has been presented above that clarifies the steps needed to transform health teams into client-centred collaborative teams.

Conclusion

APNs, whether a CNS or NP, have the potential to influence the effectiveness of IP collaborative teamwork in either their NP or CNS roles as a group collaborative leader. The NP role has been reported as the bridge in IP teams because of NPs' ability to diagnose and order treatments and drugs (van Soeren, Hurlock-Chorostecki, & Reeves, 2011). The CNS role provides a level of expertise in practice based on both theory and research that can enhance how an IP team considers their collaborative care. However, there is also danger in APNs assuming power in the team based on their advanced education unless they participate collaboratively with other health care professionals in the team who have knowledge, skills, and experiences that complement and enrich their own. More attention to learning about the roles, knowledge, skills, and expertise of other health care professionals is required for APNs to become truly collaborative partners in health care teams. No matter what health care professional role is assumed within IP teams, it must be remembered that the client is the driver and they must be prepared to work with the team to enhance their health to whatever degree is feasible. APNs, like other health care professionals, are simply expert advisors to their clients and their informal caregivers. This is the essence of IP client-centred collaborative practice.

Competence in practice has long been touted as key to being accepted into teams. However, understanding the meaning of competence from a variety of perspectives may have led to differing views of the meaning of competence and competency in roles. This chapter has explored the role of APNs with a focus on both the CNS and NP and how their roles can be integrated into IP client-centred collaborative practice. In essence, APNs have a pivotal role in shifting our practice from provider- and system-centric to being truly client-centred.

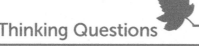

Critical Thinking Questions

1. What changes might you consider making in your practice based on reading this chapter? Within these changes, what alterations will you test based on Roegiers's three elements of "know how to think, know how to respond, and know how to act"?
2. What aspects of your current APN practice would you like to modify based on the discussion of clients as drivers of their own care?
3. How can you articulate your APN role as a health care provider to another health professional? Have you considered the meaning of the communications you use? Are there

words you use that might cause another health care provider to misunderstand your role and message?

4. Consider a conflict situation that you as an advanced practice nurse may have experienced recently in your practice. What role did you assume in this conflict? Were you able to transcend your own viewpoint and hear others' views and come to a positive outcome? Or are you still questioning that outcome?

5. Reflect on the role you can assume within an IP collaborative team and how you might negotiate as its collaborative leader.

6. Reflect on how you as an advanced practice nurse can include your patients and their chosen caregivers in your discussions about their health care. How well have you respected their input into shaping and negotiating their care to fit their needs?

7. To assist you in reflecting on this reconsideration of the client and their family's role in their care, a case study is provided. Please read the case study and return to the Collaborative Patient-Centred Practice Framework's step 2. Then reflect on the questions below the case study.

CASE STUDY

The Story of Mr. Yandry Morales

Mr. Yandry Morales was admitted into the orthopedic ward of your hospital and you have been assigned to him on your 12-hour shift for the first time. You learn that he had a fall and suffered an intertrochanteric fracture of his right hip. He had surgery yesterday and a hip replacement was provided. He also has type 2 diabetes as well as hypertension. Therefore, you now have a patient to care for who has three health issues. You also learn that he lives alone in a house since his wife died two months ago and he has to climb a flight of stairs to get to his bedroom and bathroom. This is a patient who is likely being taken care of by three different medical specialists; and who will need rehabilitation by physiotherapy, post-op recovery from nursing, and counselling as well as planning for when he returns home. These latter issues are likely to need occupational therapy and social work as well as home care transition planning. In a multidisciplinary care model, the nurse would assess his nursing needs, and other health professionals will each focus only on their own respective area. While each will likely receive a referral to consult on this case, each will be done separately and will likely rely on evidence-based practice norms or standard protocols for each health issue. Mr. Morales will likely not be consulted to participate in any planning for his care and the continuity of what the goals should be will not be shared but will be viewed in isolation from each other.

7a. In your reflection on Mr. Morales and his situation, please consider who needs to be on his team at the post-operative level and after he transitions back to his home. These will be health care providers whom Mr. Morales will need to help him shape his care plan and its implementation.

7b. As an advanced practice nurse, reflect on what further information will be needed to help you consider what nursing interventions you can suggest (this reflects the professional action of gathering further information).

7c. As an advanced practice nurse, reflect on what health and social issues Mr. Morales will face when he transitions to home for the first week and then thereafter (this reflects the professional action of determine required health/social needs). Also reflect on which team member is the most appropriate health provider to address each.

7d. As an advanced practice nurse, what goals do you believe Mr. Morales will have, and what nursing interventions might you suggest to address these (this reflects the professional action of set goals and treatment plan to address identified patient/family needs).

7e. As an advanced practice nurse, what might be the markers that Mr. Morales could set for himself to help him determine his progress toward his goal (this reflects the professional action of develop joint outcome measures)? Then consider what these markers reflect in the health team's treatment goals for Mr. Morales. Consider whether you have focused on those important aspects associated with the other team members and the treatments they would likely be providing.

7f. What surprised you the most from working through this case by using the Collaborative Patient-Centred Practice Framework's step 2 professional actions? What did you remind yourself about in the care you have been providing that may have caused you to focus away from your professional APN practice? What might you now trial to begin shifting your client's role to that as driver?

8. How will you now view your role as an IP member of your health care team? Are there changes in your thinking about that role since reading this chapter? If so, what are these changes?

References

Adams, T. L., Orchard, C., Houghton, P., & Ogrin, R. (2014). The metamorphosis of a collaborative team: From creation to operation. *Journal of Interprofessional Care, 28*(4), 339–344. doi: 10.3109/13561800.2014.891571

Adler, R. B., & Proctor II, R. F. (2010). *Looking out looking in* (13th ed.). Boston, MA: Wadsworth Cengage Learning.

Allen, D., Orchard, C. A., Kerr, M., & Adams, T. L. (2019). *The effectiveness of interprofessional role clarification in licensed health care providers in rural and smaller community hospitals.* Unpublished manuscript.

Andregard, A.-C. (2015). The tortuous journey of introducing the nurse practitioners as a new member of the healthcare team: A meta-synthesis. *Scandinavian Journal of Caring Sciences, 29*, 3–14. doi: 10.1111/scs.12120

Axley, L. (2008). Competency: A concept analysis. *Nursing Forum, 43*(4), 214–222.

Balthazard, P., Waldman, D., Howell, J., & Atwater, L. (Eds.). (2004). *Proceedings of the 37th Hawaii International Conference on System Sciences (HICSS): Shared leadership and group interactions styles in problem-solving virtual teams.* Waikoloa, HI: University of Hawai'i.

Canadian Interprofessional Health Collaborative (CIHC). (2010). *A national interprofessional competency framework.* Retrieved from http://www.cihc.ca/files/CIHC_IPCompetencies_Feb1210.pdf

Canadian Nurses Association (CNA). (2019a). *Advanced nursing practice: A pan-Canadian framework.* Ottawa, ON: CNA.

CNA. (2019b). *Position Statement: Advanced practice nursing.* Ottawa, ON: CNA.

Canadian Patient Safety Institute (CPSI). (2014). *The patient safety education program: Module 16: Canadian incident analysis framework.* Ottawa, ON: CPSI. Retrieved from https://www.patient-safetyinstitute.ca/en/education/PatientSafetyEducationProgram/PatientSafetyEducationCurriculum/Documents/Module%2016%20-%20Canadian%20Incident%20Analysis%20Framework.pdf#search=Root%20Cause%20Analysis

Carson, J. B., Tesluk, P. E., & Marrone, J. A. (2007). Shared leadership in teams: An investigation of antecedent conditions and performance. *Academy of Management Journal, 50*(5), 1217–1234.

Chen, A. K., Rivera, J., Rotter, N., Green, E., & Kools, S. (2016). Interprofessional education in the clinical setting: A qualitative look at the preceptor's perspective in raining advanced practice nursing students. *Nurse Education in Practice, 21*, 29–36. http://dx.doi.org/10.1016/j.nepr.2016.09.006

Chinn, P., & Kramer, M. (2018). *Knowledge development in nursing: Theory and process* (10th ed.). St. Louis, MO: Elsevier Mosby.

Cohen, S. G., & Bailey, D. E. (1997). What makes teams work? Group effectiveness research from the shop floor to the executive suite. *Journal of Management, 23*, 239–290.

Cowan, D. T., Norman, I., & Coopamah, V. P. (2005). Competence in nursing practice: A controversial concept—A focused review of literature. *Nurse Education Today, 25*, 355–362. doi: 10.1016/j.nedt.2005.03.002

Defenbaugh, N., & Chikotas, N. E. (2016). The outcome of interprofessional education: Integrating communication studies into a standardized patient experience for advanced practice nursing students. *Nursing Education in Practice, 16*, 176–181. http:/dx.org/10.1016/j.nepr.2015.06.003

Deneckere, S., Robyns, N., Vanhaecht, K., Euwema, M., Panella, M., Lodewijckx, C.,…Sermeus, W. (2011). Indicators for follow-up of multidisciplinary teamwork in care processes: Results of an international expert panel. *Evaluation and the Health Professions, 34*(3), 258–277. doi: 10.1177/0163278710393736

Farrell, K., Payne, C., & Heye, M. (2015). Integrating interprofessional collaboration skills into the advanced practice registered nurse socialization process. *Journal of Professional Nursing, 31*(1), 5–10.

Foronda, C., MacWilliams, B., & McArthur, E. (2016). Interprofessional communication in healthcare: An integrative review. *Nurse Education in Practice, 29*, 36–40. http://dx.doi.org/10.1016/j.nepr.2016.04.005

Gair, G., & Hartery, T. (2001). Medical dominance in multidisciplinary teamwork: A case study of discharge decision-making in a geriatric assessment unit. *Journal of Nursing Management, 9*, 3–11.

Garavan, T. N., & McGuire, D. (2001). Competencies and workplace learning: Some reflections on the rhetoric and the reality. *Journal of Workplace Learning, 13*(4), 144–164. doi: 10.1108/13665620110391097

Gerard, S. O., Kazer, M. W., Babington, L., & Quell, T. (2014). Past, present, and future trends of master's education in nursing. *Journal of Professional Nursing, 30*(4), 326–332.

Giddens, J. F., Lauzon-Clabo, L., Morton, P. G., Jeffries, P., McQuade-Jones, B., & Ryan, S. (2014). Re-envisioning clinical education for nurse practitioner programs: Themes from a national leaders' dialogue. *Journal of Professional Nursing, 30*(3), 273–278.

Gittell, J. H., Godfrey, M., & Thistlethwaite, J. (2013). Interprofessional collaborative practice and relational coordination: Improving healthcare through relationships. *Journal of Interprofessional Care, 27*, 210–213. doi: 10.3109/13561820.2012.73056

Govaerts, M. J. B. (2008). Educational competencies or education for professional competence? *Medical Education, 42*(3), 234–236.

Henderson, S. (2003). Power imbalance between nurses and patients: A potential inhibitor of partnership in care. *Journal of Clinical Nursing, 12*, 501–508.

Hibbard, J. H., Mahoney, E. R., Stock, R., & Tusler, M. (2007). Do increases in patient activation result in improved self-management behaviours? *Health Services Research, 42*(4), 1443–1463. doi: 10.1111/j.1475-6773.2006.00669x

Holmes, D., Murray, S. J., Perron, A., & Rail, G. (2006). Deconstructing the evidence-based discourse in health sciences: truth, power and fascism. *International Journal of Evidence-Based Health Care, 4*(3), 180–196.

Howarth, M., Warner, T., & Haigh, C. (2012). Let's stick together! A grounded theory exploration of interprofessional working used to provide person centred chronic back pain services. *Journal of Interprofessional Care, 26*, 491–496. doi: 10.3109/13561820.2012.711385

Hurlock-Chorostecki, C., Forchuk, C., Orchard, C., Reeves, S., & van Soeren, M. (2013). The value of the hospital-based nurse practitioner role: Development of a team perspective framework. *Journal of Interprofessional Care, 27*(6), 501–508.

Hurlock-Chorostecki, C., Forchuk, C. Orchard, C., van Soeren, M., & Reeves, S. (2014a). Hospital-based nurse practitioner roles and interprofessional practice: A scoping review. *Nursing & Health Sciences, 16*, 403–410. doi: 10.1111/nhs.12107

Hurlock-Chorostecki, C., Forchuk, C. Orchard, C., van Soeren, M., & Reeves, S. (2014b). Labour saver or building a cohesive interprofessional team? The role of the nurse practitioner within hospitals. *Journal of Interprofessional Care, 28*(3), 260–266. doi: 10.3109/13561820.2013.867838

Institute of Medicine. (2001). *Crossing the quality chasm: A new health system for the 21st century.* Washington, DC: National Academy Press.

Jarvis, P. (2012). *Theory of being a person in society.* London, UK: Routledge.

Kilpatrick, K. (2012). Understanding acute care nurse practitioner communication and decision-making in healthcare teams. *Journal of Clinical Nursing, 22*, 168–179. doi: 10.1111/j.1365-2702.2012.04119.x

Kilpatrick, K., Lavoie-Tremblay, M., Ritchie, J. A., Lamothe, L., & Doran, D. (2011). Boundary work and the introduction of acute care nurse practitioners in healthcare teams. *Journal of Advanced Nursing, 68*(7), 1504–1515. doi: 10.1111/j.1365-2648.2011.05895.x

Kline, R. B. (2005). *Principles and practice of structural equation modeling* (2nd ed.). New York, NY: Guilford Press.

Knowles, M. (1984). *The adult learner: A neglected species* (3rd ed.). Houston, TX: Gulf Publishing.

Kouzes, J., & Posner, B. (2006). *Student leadership inventory practices* (2nd ed.). San Francisco, CA: Jossey-Bass.

Kouzes, J., & Posner, B. (2012). *The leadership challenge: How to make extraordinary things happen in organizations* (5th ed.). San Francisco, CA: Jossey-Bass.

Kowitlawakul, Y., Ignacio, J., Lahiri, M., Khoo, S. M., Zhou, W., & Soon, D. (2014). Exploring new healthcare professionals' roles through interprofessional education. *Journal of Interprofessional Care, 28*(30), 267–269. doi: 10.3109/13561820.2013.872089

Lacasse, C. (2013). Developing nursing leaders for the future: Achieving competency for transformational leadership. *Oncology Nursing Forum, 40*(5), 431–433.

Le Deist, F. D., & Winterton, J. (2005). What is competence? *Human Resource Development Internatio-nal, 8*(1), 27–46. doi: 10.1080/1367886042000338227

LeFlore, J. L., & Thomas, P. E. (2016). Educational changes to support advanced practice nursing edu-cation. *Journal of Perinatal Neonatal Nursing, 30*(3), 187–190. doi: 10.1097/JPN/000000000000201

Lowe, G., Plummer, V., O'Brien, A. P., & Boyd, L. (2011). Time to clarify—the value of ad-vanced practice nursing roles in health care. *Journal of Advanced Nursing, 68*(3), 677–685. doi: 10.1111/j.1365-2648.2011.05790.x

Matziou, V., Vlahioti, E., Perdikaris, P., Matzious, T., Megapanou, E., & Petsios, K. (2014). Physician and nursing perceptions concerning interprofessional communication and collaboration. *Journal of Interprofessional Care, 28*(6), 526–533. doi: 10.3109/13561820.2014.934338

McInnes, S., Peters, K., Bonney, A., & Halcomb, E. (2015). An integrative review of facilitators and bar-riers influencing collaboration and teamwork between general practitioners and nurses working in general practice. *Journal of Advanced Nursing, 71*(9), 1973–1985. doi: 10.1111/jan.12647

Morilla-Herrera, J. C., Garcia-Mayor, S., Martin-Santos, F. J., Uttumchandani, S. K., Campos, A. L., Bautista, J. C., & Morales-Asencio, J. M. (2016). A systematic review of the effectiveness and roles of advanced practice nursing in older people. *International Journal of Nursing Studies, 53*, 290–307.

Orchard, C. (2007). Educating a new generation of patient-centred collaborative teams. *Toolkit to En-hance and Assist Maximizing Team Collaboration (TEAMc).* London, ON: Western University.

Orchard, C. A., Anderson, E., & Ford, J. (2018). *Collaborative patient-centred practice framework.* Pre-sentation at All Together Better Health VI, September 3, 2018, Auckland, New Zealand.

Orchard, C. A., Anderson, E., Ford, J., & Moran, M. (2015). *Framework for the interprofessional col-laboration judgement assessment tool.* Unpublished manuscript.

Orchard, C. A., & Rykhoff, M. (2015). Collaborative leadership in the context of interprofessional patient-centred collaborative practice. In D. Forman, M. Jones, & J. Thistlethwaite (Eds.), *Lea-dership and collaboration* (pp. 71–94). Basingstoke, UK: Palgrave Macmillan.

Pearce, C. L. (2004). The future of leadership: Combining vertical and shared leadership to transform knowledge work. *Academy of Management Executive, 18*(1), 47–57.

Pearce, C. L., & Sims Jr., H. P. (2002). Vertical versus shared leadership as predictors of the effectiveness of change management teams: An examination of aversive, directive, transactional, transformatio-nal, and empowering leader behaviors. *Group Dynamics: Theory, Research, & Practice, 6*(2), 172–197. doi: 10.1037//1089-2699.6.2.172

Pettigrew, T. F., & Tropp, L. R. (2008). How does intergroup contact reduce prejudice? Meta analy-tic tests of three mediations. *European Journal of Social Psychology, 38*(6), 922–934. doi: 10.1002/ejsp504

Price, S., Doucet, S., & McGillis Hall, L. (2014). The historical social positioning of nursing and medi-cine: Implications for career choice, early socialization and interprofessional collaboration. *Journal of Interprofessional Care, 28*(2), 103–109. doi: 10.3109/13561820.2013.867839

Reeves, S., Zwarenstrin, M., Goldman, J., Barr, H., Freeth, D., Hammick, M., & Koppel, I. (2009). In-terprofessional education: Effects on professional practice and health care outcomes (review). *The Cochrane Collaboration, 1*, 1–21.

Riegel, B., Jaarsma, T., & Strömberg, A. (2012). A middle-range theory of self-care of chronic illness. *Advances in Nursing Science, 35*(3), 194–204. doi: 10.1097/ANS.0b013e318261b1ba

Robinson, F. P., Gorman, G., Summer, L. W., & Yudkowsky, R. (2010). Perceptions of effective and ineffective nurse-physician communication in hospitals. *Nursing Forum, 45*(3), 206–216. doi: 10.1111/j.1744-6198.2010.00182.x

Roegiers, X. (2007). Curricular reforms guide schools: But, where to? *Prospects, 37*(2), 155–186. doi: 10.1007/s11125-007-9024-z

Roegiers, X. (2016). *A conceptual framework for competencies assessment*. Geneva, CH: UNESCO International Bureau of Education.

Rugen, K. W., Speroff, E., Zapatka, S. A., & Brienza, R. (2016). Veterans affairs interprofessional nurse practitioner residency in primary care: A competency-based program. *The Journal for Nurse Practitioners, 12*(6), e67–e72.

Rykhoff, M., & Orchard, C. A. (2019). *Collaborative leadership: A concept analysis*. Unpublished manuscript.

Sahlsten, M. J. M., Larsson, I. E., Plos, K. A. E., & Lindencrona, C. S. C. (2005). Hindrance for patient participation in nursing care. *Scandinavian Journal of Caring Science, 19*, 223–229.

Salas, E., Cooke, N. J., & Rosen, M. A. (2008). On teams, teamwork, and team performance: Discoveries and developments. *Human Factors, 50*(3), 540–547.

Salas, E., DiazGranados, D., Weaver, S. J., & King, H. (2008). Does team training work? Principles for health care. *Academic Emergency Medicine, 15*(11), 1002–1009. doi: 10.1111/j.1553-2712.2008.00254.x

Schön, D. (1983). *The reflective practitioner: How professionals think in action*. New York, NY: Basic Books.

Sinclair, E., & Orchard, C. A. (2018). *Assessment of Interprofessional Collaborative Leadership (AICLS): Development and initial testing*. Presentation at Research Day, Arthur Labatt Family School of Nursing, May 3, 2018, Western University, London, ON, Canada.

Tardif, J. (1999). *Le transfers des apprentissages [Transfer of learning]*. Montreal, QC: Les Éditions Logiques.

Tutton, E. (2005). Patient participation on ward for frail older people. *Journal of Advanced Nursing, 50*, 143–152.

Ugirase, S., Orchard, D. S., & Tryphonopoulos, P. (2019). *Interprofessional Conflict Resolution Scale (IPCRS): Development & Testing*. Unpublished manuscript, Western University, London, ON.

van Soeren, M., Hurlock-Chorostecki, C., & Reeves, S. (2011). The role of nurse practitioners in hospital settings: Implications for interprofessional practice. *Journal of Interprofessional Care, 25*(4), 245–251. doi: 10.3109/13561820.539305

Walker, L. O., & Avant, K. C. (2011). *Strategies for theory construction in nursing* (5th ed.). Upper Saddle River, NJ: Pearson/Prentice Hall.

Wellard, S. J., Lillibridge, J., Beanland, C. J., & Lewis, M. (2003). Consumer participation in acute care settings: An Australian experience. *International Journal of Nursing Practice, 9*, 255–260.

West, M. A., & Poulton, B. C. (1997). A failure to function: Teamwork in primary health care. *Journal of Interprofessional Care, 11*(2), 205–216. doi: 1356-1820/97/020205-12

Wittenberg, E., Goldsmith, J., & Neiman, T. (2015). Nurse-perceived communication challenges and roles on interprofessional care teams. *Journal of Hospital & Palliative Nursing, 17*(3), 257–262. doi: 10.1097/NJH.000000000000160

Chapter

29 Role Transition

Eric Staples

ERIC STAPLES is an Independent Nursing Practice Consultant. He was a graduate of the first postgraduate Acute Care Nurse Practitioner (ACNP) certificate program in Ontario in 1995 from the University of Toronto, and has held Assistant Professor roles at Dalhousie University, Halifax, Nova Scotia, where he was involved in implementing the Advanced Nursing Practice stream in 1998; McMaster University, Hamilton, Ontario, as NP Coordinator in the Ontario Primary Health Care Nurse Practitioner (PHCNP) Program; and the University of Regina, Regina, Saskatchewan. Eric serves or has served on several CASN committees related to NP education, preceptorship, prescribing, and the development of the position statement on doctoral education in Canada. He was the lead developer and editor for the inaugural edition of *Canadian Perspectives in Advanced Practice Nursing*, published in 2016 and in French in 2017.

KEY TERMS	OBJECTIVES
advanced practice nurses (APNs) nurse practitioner (NP) role transition transition	1. Examine the transition from registered nurse to nurse practitioner (NP). 2. Discuss the stressors facing the novice NP. 3. Discuss recommendations related to advanced practice nursing role transition for practice, education, and policy.

Introduction

Role transition from registered nurse (RN) to advanced practice nurse can be a difficult process. As **advanced practice nurses (APNs)** are already RNs, a **transition** needs to occur that utilizes their previous nursing knowledge in a new way. This involves building on the values and attitudes from baccalaureate level (Cragg & Andrusyszyn, 2005). A level of confidence once known within the RN role may be lost and a sense of belonging may blur as the cohort support diminishes.

Very little evidence related to **nurse practitioners'** (NPs') intent to leave their roles exists in Canada, but in a national survey of NPs, role dissatisfaction was related to a lack of opportunities for professional development and the amount of paperwork and time required to complete documentation (tied at 47%); lack of input into organizational/practice/policies (49%); and salary/remuneration (52%) (Canadian Federation of Nurses Unions [CFNU], 2018). Several studies from the United States (US) have concluded that 27–31% of NPs intend to leave their current positions, and almost 6% intend to leave the nursing profession due to an unsuccessful role transition (DeMilt, Fitzpatrick, & McNulty, 2011; Poghosyan, Liu, Shang, & D'Aunno, 2016).

There is a paucity of Canadian research on clinical nurse specialists (CNSs) as it relates to role transition with the first Canada-wide survey of CNSs conducted in 2014 (Kilpatrick et al., 2014). Kilpatrick et al. found that the reasons for CNSs no longer working in CNS roles were due to lack of role clarity, an inability to find employment as a CNS, and the inability to implement the domains of CNS practice. Currently, there are no mechanisms to identify and track CNSs in Canada due to lack of role protection, education, and regulation. It is clear, from the literature, that it is important for RNs to start the transition to an APN role at the beginning and throughout their graduate studies, as those who fail to successfully make a role transition are unsuccessful in their careers and often return to the RN role (Cragg & Andrusyszyn, 2005; Neal, 2008). Therefore, the purpose of this chapter is to explore the process of transition from RN to NP from a Canadian perspective where possible.

What Is Transition?

The importance of exploring the transition process is relevant for NP practice, but also for the educational programs preparing NPs. It is clear that the process is often stressful and frustrating for the new NP with the loss of role identity, a sense of imposter syndrome, and social isolation appearing to be the most resounding themes among researchers (Brown & Olshansky, 1997; Heitz, Steiner, & Burman, 2004; Kelly & Matthews, 2001). NPs leave a comfort zone of confidence as RNs, who rarely have the final word in decision-making, follow policies and procedures in the hospital setting; respond to orders that originate from other health care practitioners; and enter an unfamiliar territory with an entirely different scope of practice, accountability, and responsibility.

The term *transition* has been defined in many ways by various disciplines. Chick and Meleis (1986) define transition as "passage from one life phase, condition, or status to another, and is a multiple concept embracing the elements of process, time span, and perception" (p. 239). They also explain how the transitional process needs to also include the person's reaction to the transition; their experience, understood from within, adds value to the transitional process.

Despite the perception of the individual who experiences transition, Chick and Meleis (1986) explain that transition is "essentially positive [as it] implies that the person has reached a period of greater stability" (p. 240). Schumacher and Meleis (1994) define transition as passages or movements from one state, condition, or place to another, "which can produce profound alterations in the lives of individuals and their significant others and have important implications for well-being and health" (p. 119). Barton (2007) describes it as a social transition that is a universal process, but each transition remains unique. With the added responsibility, accountability, and autonomy of the novice NP, the experience of the transition process must be explored for the novice NP to understand that their perceptions are like other NPs. The novice NP can be comforted with the knowledge that their feelings are a part of the transition and that their confidence will build.

Research Related to Role Transition

NPs continue to face many barriers within the health care system provincially and nationally. Lack of support at the government level, administrative level, and within primary health care settings themselves all add to the impact and intensity of the transition process from RN to NP (DiCenso et al., 2010; Yeager, 2010). The review of the literature reveals that all but one study related to transition from RN to NP are qualitative.

Kelly and Matthews (2001) studied NP transition from the context of personal experience. The study participants, who were in a transitional phase to their first position after graduation, attended focus groups created to gain their perceptions of preparation, gains/ losses, barriers/facilitators, and strategies for transition. The study's findings identified the following themes during an NP's first position: loss of personal control of time and privacy; changes and losses in relationships; feelings of isolation; and uncertainty in establishing the NP role. An overarching theme, worthy of further discussion, is the loss of privacy discussed by the participants within the study. The study addressed the number of NPs who work in small, rural communities and quickly realized that a trip to the grocery store was also an opportunity for patients to discuss their health care concerns with them. A protective barrier between the new NP and the general public was perceived as a necessity to maintain some form of privacy and normalcy. Another aspect of NP transition was the sense of personal satisfaction with the choice and process toward becoming an NP. Study participants described the positive feelings of transition to the APN role as the "increased self-confidence and changes within themselves; the autonomy and being able to expand their role; but most of all the special bond of trust with their patients" (p. 160). The participants, who perceived they were prepared for their role, also described feeling guilty and being unsure that they may not have the knowledge they should.

Cragg and Andrusyszyn were part of two studies in 2004 and 2005 related to the process of achieving change in knowledge, practice, attitudes, and the processes they perceived and experienced during both NP and CNS graduate education. Graduates (N = 22) of three universities in Ontario participated in a semi-structured interview. Each graduate attended one of the following programs: APN, either acute, community, or specialty based; NP; nursing education; or nursing administration.

Cragg and Andrusyszyn (2004) found that all graduates perceived that they had changed as a result of completing graduate education. Their responses related to the process and outcomes of their education were similar across all three universities. One key process was the influence of faculty on their growth, as they supported and encouraged broader and more in-depth inquiry. Outcomes achieved included greater understanding of the health care system and nursing's place in it; higher level skills in cognition, professional relationships, and research; greater self-confidence; and increased pride in nursing and their role in it. As a result of these changes, the transition to work felt like "entering a new reality." One area of disappointment in returning to new careers, such as NPs or CNSs, was that, although they felt they had changed, much of the health care system had not changed, creating challenges when the new graduates wished to implement innovative and new initiatives (Cragg & Andrusyszyn, 2005).

In a qualitative study on the NP transition, Heitz et al. (2004) interviewed participants who graduated within five years and concluded that full transition to the NP role does not happen in graduate studies but occurs progressively throughout the NP education program and into practice. Key concepts included intrinsic obstacles (i.e., personal sacrifices required), extrinsic obstacles (i.e., learning environment), turbulence, positive intrinsic forces, positive extrinsic forces, and role development. The intrinsic and extrinsic forces are those stressors that are either internal or external and were defined as ones that can be "overcome but not necessarily controlled" (p. 417). The clinical learning environment was an extrinsic obstacle with negative components that hinder the learning experience and included lack of mentoring, staff resistance, and an unhelpful preceptor style. Brown and Olshansky (1997) discussed the effects of a negative learning environment, but focused more on the feelings within each progressive stage. Intrinsic obstacles included the personal sacrifices that are essentially unavoidable throughout the NP education program. Family and friend commitments and special occasions were missed due to academic constraints, which led to feelings of isolation. A "rollercoaster" of emotions that surfaced throughout the obstacles were referred to as "turbulence" (Heitz et al., 2004, p. 417). The findings were compatible to Brown and Olshansky's (1997) model of transition and acknowledge similar feelings of anxiety, confusion of role identity, fear of the unknown, challenges in the work setting, changes in professional identity, and the difficulties of added stressors of personal commitments and sacrifices.

Sullivan-Bentz et al. (2010) conducted a descriptive qualitative study to examine role transition and the supports NP graduates needed in their first year of practice. Ontario NP graduates and co-participants, who included family physicians, NPs, and managers, were interviewed. The interview questions were guided by Brown and Olshansky's Model of Transition (1997; see Table 29.1), and five themes were identified: (1) transition to the NP role, (2) contextual factors affecting NP role transition, (3) interprofessional relationships, (4) provincial policies and politics, and (5) educational preparation (Sullivan-Bentz et al., 2010).

An important part of successful role transition was the familiarity of the NP role and employers and colleagues' scope of practice. Difficult transition for many was due to the lack of preparedness for integrating into practice, and a lack of infrastructure, orientation, mentorship, and awareness of the NP role. One-third of the NP graduates had changed employment during the first year of practice and identified the reasons for the change as interprofessional conflict or problems with acceptance of their role in the practice environment (Sullivan-Bentz et al., 2010). The transition of NP graduates in Ontario was further complicated with perceived changes in primary health care (PHC) delivery and the employment environment not being ready to receive them. The study concluded that necessary strategies include mentorship by a colleague during the NP's first year of practice to integrate new NPs into PHC. Support from family physicians, managers, nurses, and receptionists can assist in NP transition.

Spoelstra and Robbins (2010) conducted a qualitative research study of NP students enrolled in an online roles course in the US. The course's purpose was to provide students with the basic tenets of APN practice prior to progressing to clinical experience. In the course, students compared and contrasted APN domains of practice and competencies of other health care professionals, applied theory to role development, and developed strategies to meet competencies designed to assist in integrating them into the NP role. One central theme and three subthemes emerged. The researchers called the central theme "the essence of nursing." Students demonstrated a commitment to nursing excellence as they focused on their expertise, caring, values, ethics, spirituality, and cultural sensitivity (Spoelstra & Robbins, 2010). This appeared to form the basis for becoming an NP as it was linked to their foundational competencies as RNs. The three sub-themes included the importance of building a framework for nursing practice; the importance of direct patient care; and comprehension of the importance of exemplification of professional responsibilities (Spoelstra & Robbins, 2010). Participant NPs confirmed that information from the course would assist them in understanding and operationalizing their role. The results affirmed that there is a transitional process to becoming an NP and that the process needs to occur, for the benefit of role development, early in the educational program.

Barnes (2015) conducted a descriptive, cross-sectional survey study of practicing NPs to explore factors such as prior RN experience and receiving a formal orientation, and their influence on the transition to the NP role. The survey used the Meleis's Theory of Transitions (2000; see Figure 29.1) as a framework. Participants were asked to rate their agreement/disagreement with statements that included concepts of feeling supported or isolated; patients', physicians', and other staff's understanding of their role; and feeling prepared to manage patients and their time (Barnes, 2015). From the results, 33% of the participants received a formal orientation in their first NP position, which was positively correlated to NP transition. Those with high scores versus lower scores were correlated with a more moderate transition experience. Other outcomes suggested prior RN experience was neither a facilitator nor a barrier of NP role transition, but the type of RN experience gained may have contributed to successful transition. NP role transition may be influenced by one's RN practice setting and subsequent NP role, i.e., in-patient RN role to family/community or in-patient NP role (Barnes, 2015).

Faraz (2016) looked at NP workforce transition and retention in PHC to examine the relationships between novice NP characteristics, role acquisition, job satisfaction, and turnover intention. An online descriptive, cross-sectional survey study was conducted with NPs, all working in PHC and who had graduated in the past 3–12 months. The survey focused on individual characteristics (i.e., educational background, prior work experience, social support, and sense of meaning); role acquisition (i.e., role ambiguity and perceived competence and self-confidence); job satisfaction; and turnover intention (Faraz, 2016). The results indicated that NPs felt their practices had meaning, were moderately confident in their skills and positions, and their turnover intention was moderately low (Faraz, 2016). Factors that were predictive of turnover intention included autonomy and role ambiguity with professional autonomy being the strongest predictor of turnover intention. One of Faraz's conclusions was that a balance of support and autonomy was crucial to job satisfaction and retention.

The most recent integrative review about the first year of NP role transition conducted by Twine (2017) demonstrated three topic areas: role transition, perception of preparedness, and perceived challenges. Having a role identity as an NP, professional socialization, and mentorship were important factors that had a positive impact on transition. The NPs who did not feel prepared, wanted more education, and used past RN experience to fill in knowledge gaps tended to experience a negative transition (Twine, 2017). Perceived challenges included obtaining licensure, developing new professional relationships, and patients who may be unfamiliar with the NP role. Twine concluded that ineffective transition could lead to ineffective delivery of quality health care.

Thompson's study (2018) explored whether an evidence-informed role transition webinar provided to graduate NPs would result in improved transition into their first year of practice. The results demonstrated that the educational webinar was shown to have a positive influence on the participant's reported perceptions of NP role transition related to confidence. There was also a positive correlation between age range of the participant and higher scores in the post-test. This was significant as no other study had ever demonstrated the possibility of age-related differences in NP role transition, and indicated, potentially, that greater life experience may improve coping skills and NP role transition. Other indicators for Thompson's study (2018) showed an improved comfort level with patients, the skills to cope with role transition, and the requirement of less time for role responsibilities. Each of these factors can be important to the NP role practice since they can lead to a shorter and potentially less complicated transition period.

Transition Models

Several models of transition were identified in the literature but only one was specifically developed for the novice NP. It will be discussed at length along with a middle-range theory, which has been applied to NP role transition.

Model of Transition: Limbo to Legitimacy

The Model of Transition (Brown & Olshansky, 1997), which synthesized findings into themes, has been utilized in Canadian role transition research and is explained through four stages (see Table 29.1). Brown and Olshansky's Model of Transition "laid the groundwork for research about NP role transition" (Poronsky, 2012, p. 352) as the authors focused on novice NPs in the primary health care setting during their first year of practice, but their findings are generalizable to any NP role or practice setting.

Their foundational study interviewed NPs throughout their first year of practice at 1 month, 6 months, and 12 months following graduation (Brown & Olshansky, 1997).

TABLE 29.1: Theoretical Model of Transition
Stage 1: Laying the Foundation (0–1 month)
• Recuperating from school • Negotiating the bureaucracy • Looking for a job • Worrying
Stage 2: Launching (1–3 months)
• Feeling like an imposter • Confronting anxiety • Getting through the day • Battling time
Stage 3: Meeting the Challenge (6–12 months)
• Increasing competence • Gaining confidence • Acknowledging system problems
Stage 4: Broadening the Perspective (12 months)
• Developing system savvy • Affirming oneself • Upping the ante

Source: Adapted from Brown, M., & Olshansky, E. (1997). From limbo to legitimacy: A theoretical model of the transition to the primary care nurse practitioner role. *Nursing Research, 46*(1), 46–51.

They found that the transition process could be divided into stages: laying the foundation, launching, meeting the challenge, and broadening the perspective.

Laying the foundation is the time between graduating from an NP program and beginning the first position as an NP. The subcategories of this stage include recuperating from school, negotiating the bureaucracy, looking for a job, and worrying. Upon graduating, most want to enjoy the relief and gratification of completing their degree and the satisfaction of engaging in routine activities such as reading for leisure and spending time with family and friends. While some newly graduated NPs begin to work as soon as possible after licensure, others struggle with role identity and lack of confidence. Those who begin their first positions as NPs experience confusion as to where they socially belong within their organization, whether it be with nurses or physicians. Professional isolation, if not managed well, can lead to feelings of inadequacy and a decrease in one's confidence to perform their role to their highest ability. For novice NPs, this is also a time in which inevitable anxiety about employment and the associated stressors that accompany trying to find a job in a new field of practice will increase.

The NP enters the launching phase once the first job as an NP is secured. Launching is the most stressful stage for many new NPs as feelings of inadequacy are the hallmark of this time. This stage is subdivided into the following categories: feeling like an imposter, confronting anxiety, getting through the day, and battling time. The struggle to develop a professional identity only increases a novice NP's anxiety. When the NP begins independent practice, the necessary knowledge, skills, and abilities that require confidence are often lacking. Feelings of being an imposter can be overwhelming as many feel a lack of significant knowledge to quickly and effectively develop a diagnosis for a patient.

Hill and Sawatzky (2011) found that employer and NP expectations, combined with insufficient opportunities during NP education for socialization, resulted in graduate NPs feeling like imposters. Some NPs become very anxious and wonder if they will ever be a "real NP." Brown and Olshansky (1997) effectively capture the uncertainty of a new NP in the launching stage who is struggling with self-confidence: "pulling the chart off the door, looking at what their chief complaint is, and going, I don't know what this is, I've got to go look this up before I even go in the room …" (p. 48). Time constraints on the new NP are added stress factors. NPs struggle to feel equal to their coworkers but are frequently reminded of their novice inadequacies when they are the only ones "left in the office past closing time on a Friday afternoon" (Brown & Olshansky, 1997, p. 49).

Meeting the challenge is the third stage of transition and can be best described as a time when the NP begins to feel comfortable in their role. The NP gains confidence and slowly develops from the insecure novice. Some begin this stage after six months of practice, but for most, it occurs after 12 months. The subcategories of this stage include increasing competence, gaining confidence, and acknowledging system problems. Patients and diagnoses are now more familiar for the NP. Not every symptom and diagnosis are thoroughly researched prior to opening the door to meet the patient. A solid foundation of acquired skills has been built and the NP feels a part of the advanced, independent role (Brown & Olshansky, 1997).

During the final stage, broadening the perspective, the NP feels significantly more comfortable in their role, in their workplace, and is more confidently providing patient care (Brown & Olshansky, 1997). Self-confidence has reached a level where the NP is prepared to attempt new challenges. At this final stage, when patients express their gratitude for the NP's care, the new NP can see that they played a part in the patients' journey toward meeting their health care goals. The NP has formed a true sense of professional identity and is ready to take on new challenges as the intrinsic and extrinsic forces of the workplace are better understood. NPs also may become involved in the political aspect of their careers through professional development. Although this is clearly not the end of the learning curve for new NPs, this is a stage when they feel more capable and committed to embracing their new role.

Mid-Range Theory of Transitions

Meleis, Sawyer, Im, Messias, and Schumacher (2000) developed the Mid-Range Theory of Transitions, which, although based on the nurse-patient relationship at a time of vulnerability and transition, can conceptually be applied to transitions to practice (see Figure 29.1).

A transition begins before an event and has an end point that is based on many variables. Understanding the nature of and responses to transition; facilitating the process; responding to its different phases; and promoting health and well-being prior to, during, and at the end of the transition comprise the basis for the development of the theory.

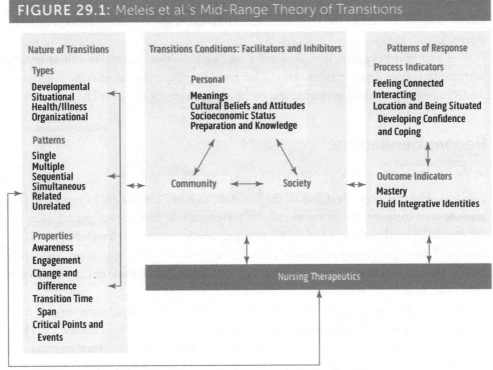

FIGURE 29.1: Meleis et al.'s Mid-Range Theory of Transitions

Source: Meleis, A. I., Sawyer, L. M., Im, E., Messias, D. K., & Schumacher, K. (2000). Experiencing transitions: An emerging middle-range theory. *Advances in Nursing Science, 23*(1), 17.

There are multiple complexities when looking at transitions for this theory. The first part starts with an intervention made to facilitate transition and promote well-being and adaptation to the transition through the utilization of significant others and the health care team. The goals are to clarify what the person may experience by providing knowledge, skills, strategies, and tangible and psychosocial skills to cope with the transition experience and responses.

The second part of the theory is an understanding of the transition experience as the process passes from one phase to another. The four types of transitions include developmental, situational, health and illness, and organizational. These are mediated by whether the person is going through the second concept, patterns of transitions, and can include single or multiple transitions, sequential or simultaneous transitions, or related or unrelated events of transition and the meaning they place on the transition and anything else that may be going on in the person's life.

The third part identifies the properties of the transition experiences and includes awareness, which is the knowledge, perception, and recognition of transition; engagement, which is the degree to which a person engages in the transition process; time span, which is the flow and movement of transition over time; and critical points and events, all of which are key events in the period of transition.

Meleis et al. (2000) further describe additional transition phenomena that may occur. These are actions and events that help or harm the transition (facilitators and inhibitors);

responses during transition (process and outcomes indicators); and nurse and nursing actions that are central to the response and facilitation of the transition process (nursing therapeutics).

The goal of intervention is to facilitate a healthy transition process as well as healthy outcome responses. Interventions can involve providing expertise, identifying milestones, modelling roles, providing resources, and ensuring opportunities for debriefing.

Recommendations

Role Transition

Role transition has been identified in the literature as a key component of transition that needs to start early—in the first semester—of NP education. This is a key period when the NP student leaves the comfort of their RN role, potentially at an expert level with their experience and developed advanced knowledge, skills, and abilities. At the same time, novice NPs need to maintain a sense of connectedness with their colleagues outside of the work setting (Brown & Olshansky, 1997; Heitz et al., 2004; Kelly & Matthews, 2001).

The NP role requires autonomy and advanced decision-making. Autonomy and self-confidence were identified as crucial factors in successful role transition (Twine, 2017). In looking for employment as a novice NP, the literature points to successful transition in practice settings where agencies and facilities were familiar with the NP role, which also promotes further professional socialization. When entering an employment setting where there has previously not been an NP, the novice NP needs to negotiate support for developing the role, which can be accomplished through mentorship (Sullivan-Bentz et al., 2010).

Education and Mentorship

It is clear from the literature that all NP students and novice NPs require formal mentorship, therefore they need to seek and establish linkages to NP organizations and experienced NPs. The NP mentor should be prepared to support the student or novice NP and promote a healthy learning environment. The choice of the mentor should be the decision of the student or NP, as it encourages an increase in self-efficacy and self-confidence. Both a formal, structured, or flexible, informal mentoring relationship between a novice NP and expert NP is "fundamental to a novice NP's learning and growth in the NP role" (Szanton, Mihaly, Alhusen, & Becker, 2010, p. 356). The mentor not only assists with the clinical aspects of practice, but also with the socialization into the role and learning about the organization itself (Harrington, 2011).

The literature also found that faculty mentorship was important in building on core NP competencies (Cragg & Andrusyszyn, 2004, 2005; Hill & Sawatzky, 2011; Twine, 2017). Comparing and contrasting other health care professionals' competencies was also found to be useful in clarifying the NP role, as well as other roles (Spoelstra & Robbins, 2010). Hill and Sawatzky (2011) found that "creating a supportive environment, offering constructive feedback, taking advantage of teachable moments, and allowing the novice NP the time necessary with patients are strategies that mentors can use to promote the growth and development of novice NPs" (p. 166).

Although graduate studies prepare novice NPs with entry to practice knowledge, the reality is that despite where the education is obtained, the duration of the program, or the clinical setting, one simply cannot learn it all. The first year of practice requires a steep learning curve and having a mentor can significantly impact the novice NP's practice (Griffith, 2004).

There is also a benefit for the NP mentor as they find the experience rewarding and it reminds them of how they felt during their first year of practice. Mentors enjoy the opportunity to learn, teach, and remain current. A mentoring program can also reflect positively on NP employers by being recognized as a teaching facility with supportive mentors, and improved recruitment and retention of new graduates (Hill & Sawatzky, 2011). Additionally, NPs need to understand the business aspects associated with the practice setting they are in. Interprofessional education that is inclusive of NPs, physicians, RNs, etc. can assist with successful transition (Sullivan-Bentz et al., 2010).

NP programs can provide practical and assessable educational interventions to optimize NP role transition that result in positive affirmation of the NP role and should help solidify NPs' contributions to health care, to consumers, and to other health care providers (Thompson, 2018).

Employers

Employers have a responsibility to provide a formal orientation with the agency or facility. Position role description, role definitions, and an organizational chart with clear reporting relationships prior to hiring will assist in ensuring a match between the NP and the employer. Organizations hiring NPs for the first time should hire experienced NPs or arrange for the new NP to consult with an experienced NP at another agency or facility to promote successful role transition. Employers need to ensure there is ample space, available resources, clerical support, and policies and procedures that promote full scope of practice in a quickly changing health care environment (Sullivan-Bentz et al., 2010).

Funding

Stable and predictable funding for new NP positions has always been foremost in the Canadian literature. Funds need to be set aside for orientation, mentoring, team building, and continued education that should not be in competition with physician partners (Sullivan-Bentz et al., 2010).

Policy

Where possible, employers and NPs need to advocate for full scope of practice, including prescriptive authority and referral processes. Professional nursing bodies and NP interest groups can be paramount in ensuring that government, employers, and the public are clear about the NP role and practice. Currently, in Canada there is no funding for independent practice nor is there a method for billing for NP services.

Conclusion

Role transition for NPs is "a process consisting of multiple mixed emotions that occurs over time and is a period of great personal development and learning as the NP takes on new autonomy and responsibility for patients" (Barnes, 2015, p. 178). Research suggests the importance of beginning the transition in the first semester of graduate school, or the attainment of a successful transition may be limited. Positive clinical practice experiences and work environments are imperative for students and novice NPs.

Support must be provided as NPs journey through the feelings of inadequacy, professional isolation, and confusion with role identity. A mentorship program can help students and novice NPs make the transition smoothly and can offer a great source of encouragement. Both the mentor and the employer also benefit from mentoring programs as the facility becomes recognized as a positive teaching environment that attracts and retains new NPs. As the role of the NP develops, a positive transition experience is imperative for the success of the NP role.

Determining the factors that contribute to the success of NP role transition, including optimal timing, would be prudent. Therefore, steps need to be taken to facilitate successful transition so that graduates can transform into effective health care providers as soon as possible.

Critical Thinking Questions

1. What has been the impact of your transition from RN to NP in your educational program? Are you happy with the transition? How could you have improved your transition?
2. Have you identified a mentor either from your educational program or from clinical practicums? Have you communicated this to the mentor?
3. How can provincial and professional associations assist you with transitioning into your first NP role?
4. What coping strategies have you found outside of your educational studies that help you with the stress of transition?
5. While the research has focused more on NP role transition, what components do you feel are similar or different for CNS role transition?

References

Barnes, H. (2015). Exploring the factors that influence nurse practitioner role transition. *Journal of Nurse Practitioners, 11*(2), 178–183. doi: 10.1016/j.nurpra.2014.11.004

Barton, T. (2007). Student nurse practitioners—A rite of passage? The universality of Van Gennep's model of social transition. *Nurse Education in Practice, 7*(5), 338–347. doi: 10.1016/j.nepr.2006.11.0522

Brown, M., & Olshansky, E. (1997). From limbo to legitimacy: A theoretical model of the transition to the primary care nurse practitioner role. *Nursing Research, 46*(1), 46–51.

Canadian Federation of Nurses Unions (CFNU). (2018). *Fulfilling nurse practitioners' untapped potential in Canada's health care system: Results from the CFNU pan-Canadian nurse practitioner retention & recruitment study.* Ottawa, ON: CFNU. Retrieved from https://nursesunions.ca/wp-content/uploads/2018/06/CFNU_UntappedPotential-Final-EN.pdf

Chick, N., & Meleis, A. (1986). Transitions: A nursing concern. In P. L. Chinn (Ed.), *Nursing research methodology: Issues and implementation* (pp. 237–257). Rockville, MD: Aspen.

Cragg, B., & Andrusyszyn, M. A. (2004). Outcomes of master's education in nursing. *International Journal of Nursing Education Scholarship, 1*(1), 1–18.

Cragg, B., & Andrusyszyn, M. A. (2005). The process of master's education in nursing: Evolution or revolution? *International Journal of Nursing Education Scholarship, 2*(1), 1–20.

DeMilt, D., Fitzpatrick, J., & McNulty, R. (2011). Nurse practitioners' job satisfaction and intent to leave current positions, the nursing profession, and the nurse practitioner role as a direct care provider. *Journal of the Academy of Nurse Practitioners, 23*(1), 42–50. doi: 10.111/j.1745-7599.2010.00570.x

DiCenso, A., Martin-Misener, R., Bryant-Lukosius, D., Bourgeault, I., Kilpatrick, K., Donald, F., ... Charbonneau-Smith, R. (2010). Advanced practice nursing in Canada: Overview of a decision support synthesis. *Nursing Leadership, 23*(Special Issue), 15–34. doi: 10.12927/cjnl.2010.22267

Faraz, A. (2016). Novice nurse practitioner workforce transition into primary care: A literature review. *Western Journal of Nursing Research, 38*(11), 1531–1545. doi: 10.1177/0193945916649587

Griffith, H. (2004). Nurse practitioner education: Learning from students. *Nursing Standard, 18*(30), 33–41.

Harrington, S. (2011). Mentoring new nurse practitioners to accelerate their development as primary care providers: A literature review. *Journal of the American Academy of Nurse Practitioners, 23*(4), 168–174. doi: 10.1111/j.1745-7599.2011.00601.x

Heitz, L., Steiner, S., & Burman, M. (2004). RN to FNP: A qualitative study of role transition. *Journal of Nursing Education, 43*(9), 416–420.

Hill, L., & Sawatzky, J. (2011). Transitioning into the nurse practitioner role through mentorship. *Journal of Professional Nursing, 27*(3), 161–167. doi: 10.1016/j.profnurs.2011.02.004

Kelly, N., & Matthews, M. (2001). The transition to first position as nurse practitioner. *Journal of Nursing Education, 40*(4), 156–162.

Kilpatrick, K., Kaasalainen, S., Donald, F., Reid, K., Carter, N., Bryant-Lukosius, D., ... DiCenso, A. (2014). The effectiveness and cost-effectiveness of clinical nurse specialists in outpatient roles: A systematic review. *Journal of Evaluation in Clinical Practice, 20*(6), 1106–1123.

Meleis, A. I., Sawyer, L. M., Im, E., Messias, D. K., & Schumacher, K. (2000). Experiencing transitions: An emerging middle-range theory. *Advances in Nursing Science, 23*(1), 12–28. doi: 10.1097/000122 72-2000090000-00006

Neal, T. (2008). *Mentoring, self-efficacy and nurse practitioner students: A modified replication.* Unpublished doctoral dissertation, Ball State University, Muncie, IN.

Poghosyan, L., Liu, J., Shang, J., & D'Aunno, T. (2016). Practice environments and job satisfaction and turnover intentions of nurse practitioners: Implications for primary care workforce capacity. *Health Care Management Review, 42*(2), 162–171. doi: 10.1097/HMR.0000000000000094

Poronsky, C. (2012). Exploring the transition from registered nurse to family nurse practitioner. *Journal of Professional Nursing, 29*(6), 350–358. http://dx.doi.org/10.1016/j.profnurs.2012.10.011

Schumacher, K., & Meleis, A. (1994). Transitions: A central concept in nursing. *Journal of Nursing Scholarship, 26*(2), 119–127.

Spoelstra, S., & Robbins, L. (2010). A qualitative study of role transition from RN to APN. *International Journal of Nursing Education Scholarship, 7*(1), 1–14. doi: 10.2202/1548-923X.2020

Sullivan-Bentz, M., Humbert, J., Cragg, B., Legault, F., Bailey, P. H., & Doucette, S. (2010). Supporting primary health care nurse practitioners' transition to practice. *Canadian Family Physician, 56*(11), 1176–1182. Retrieved from https://www.ncbi.nlm.nih.gov/pmc/articles/PMC2980439/

Szanton, S., Mihaly, L., Alhusen, J., & Becker, K. (2010). Taking charge of the challenge: Factors to consider in taking your first nurse practitioner job. *Journal of the American Academy of Nurse Practitioners, 22*(7), 356–360. doi: 10.1111/j.1745-7599.2010.00522

Thompson, A. R. (2018). *An educational intervention to enhance nurse practitioner role transition in the first year of practice*, presented at Nursing Education Research Conference 2018, Washington, DC. Indianapolis, IN: Sigma.

Twine, N. (2017). The first year as a nurse practitioner: An integrative literature review of the transition experience. *Journal of Nursing Education and Practice, 8*(5), 54–62. doi: 10.5430/jnep.v8n5p54

Yeager, S. (2010). Detraumatizing nurse practitioner orientation. *Journal of Trauma Nursing, 17*(2), 85–100.

Chapter 30

Outcomes Evaluation and Performance Assessment of Advanced Practice Nursing Roles

Joanna Pierazzo and Eric Staples

JOANNA PIERAZZO is an Associate Professor and Assistant Dean, Undergraduate Nursing Programs in the Faculty of Health Sciences School of Nursing at McMaster University, Hamilton, Ontario. She has held advanced practice nursing (APN) roles in regional neurosurgery programs in Ontario, including as an acute care nurse practitioner (ACNP) at Hamilton Health Sciences and APN community outreach at Trillium Health Partners, Mississauga, Ontario. Joanna currently teaches in both the graduate and undergraduate nursing programs. Her research interests have focused on simulation-based learning, self-efficacy, learner anxiety, and the use of CASPer (a measure of non-cognitive abilities) for success in undergraduate programs.

ERIC STAPLES is an Independent Nursing Practice Consultant. He was a graduate of the first postgraduate acute care nurse practitioner (ACNP) certificate program in Ontario in 1995 from the University of Toronto, and has held Assistant Professor roles at Dalhousie University, Halifax, Nova Scotia, where he was involved in implementing the Advanced Nursing Practice stream in 1998; McMaster University, Hamilton, Ontario, as NP Coordinator in the Ontario Primary Health Care Nurse Practitioner (PHCNP) Program; and the University of Regina, Regina, Saskatchewan. Eric serves or has served on several CASN committees related to NP education, preceptorship, prescribing, and the development of the position statement on doctoral education in Canada. He was the lead developer and editor for the inaugural edition of *Canadian Perspectives in Advanced Practice Nursing*, published in 2016 and in French in 2017.

Introduction

Over the last several years, the integration of advanced practice nursing (APN) roles in health care settings in Canada has required continual growth and development through attention to role clarity and other factors enabling role integration (DiCenso & Bryant-Lukosius, 2010). Through advancing awareness of the need for an organized process, introducing APN roles has strengthened role effectiveness and, more importantly, provided evidence related to research-based outcomes. With this professional growth, measuring outcomes has become mandatory as federal and provincial regulatory bodies, institutional guidelines, employers, and the general public advocate for quality health care with enhanced patient care. As pressures to rein in escalating health care costs increases, outcomes are more actively monitored within health care organizations. Monitoring outcomes is useful to guide quality decision-making, while simultaneously attending to accreditation, certification, and competency requirements. To date, evidence has not only highlighted the importance of APN roles in improving patient health outcomes and aspects of quality of life, but also access to primary health care and other health resources (Canadian Nurses Association [CNA], 2019; Shah, Milosavljevic, & Bath, 2017).

Greater discussion on enhancing the quality and safety of health care delivery fuelled early debate regarding which measured outcomes are affected by individual providers, technology, education, and health care systems (Doran, 2003). There has been growing attention to elements of health care services and nurse-sensitive outcomes of patient care (Doran et al., 2010, 2011; Doran, Sidani, & DiPietro, 2010). It is important that outcomes are uniformly and systematically examined to both effectively inform health care policy and guide consumers' choices about their care. Today's consumers are well equipped to ask questions related to their care, particularly in terms of health and well-being. Considering this, it is vital for health care professionals to continue gathering outcome data, evaluating interventions, and identifying issues related to care in order to improve the overall quality and efficiency of health care delivery (Friese & Beck, 2004).

APNs impact both direct patient care and processes within the health care systems in which they practice. As the APN role has evolved, the tracking and documentation of outcomes associated with APN practice have become more prevalent and provide greater clarity and attentiveness to changing health care needs. Outcomes evaluation is considered an essential component of most health care systems' initiatives (Kleinpell & Gawlinski, 2005), and as such, there have been strengthened pockets of quality research across Canada attending to this very focus. The literature supports that APN roles have known and measurable benefits for patients, families, health care, and professional practice, as well as important influences on relationships with collaborative health professionals (CNA, 2006). In addition, the context of health care improvements and evaluations of care interventions have surfaced to support the role of APNs (Crawford, 2019; Kilpatrick, Tchouaket, Jabbour, & Hains, 2020). With this value in mind, Burgess and Purkis (2010) affirm that APNs have risen above tensions related to role development and have become effective providers of care within the community.

This chapter will outline important aspects of the APN role related to evaluating outcomes, performance assessment, and discuss the use of quality indicators to demonstrate APN practice outcomes.

Theoretical Outcomes Framework

Today's health care system is expected to provide efficient and effective care delivery that is both cost effective and has positive outcomes. Trends investigating outcomes begin with a central focus on the result of patient care (Burns & Grove, 2007). In order to comprehensively explain this outcome, it is important to understand both the processes and structures that have contributed to the provision of patient care. Health care providers such as APNs are in a unique position to identify outcomes relevant to the goals of care and matters important to receivers of care (Burns & Grove, 2007; Clancy & Eisenberg, 1997). Using this approach, outcomes-based research may further enhance our understanding of how APN roles impact society and evolve a level of inquiry that considers both the structures and processes within health care.

In considering a comprehensive approach to outcomes evaluation, several structure-process-outcome frameworks have been acknowledged in this area. In the Medical Outcomes Study (MOS; Burns & Grove, 2007; Tarlov et al., 1989), the measurement of quality care outcomes evolved from two-year observational research, replicated at three sites, related to the structures and process of care. The study was designed to distinguish if discrepancies in patient outcomes were related to the system of care, provider specialty, and provider technical and interpersonal styles, and from this, develop tools for monitoring outcomes in patients with one or more of four chronic diseases common to adults (Tarlov et al., 1989).

The MOS's conceptual framework (see Table 30.1) depicts structures of care that include elements of the organization and administration like leadership, tolerance of innovativeness, organizational hierarchy, decision-making processes, distribution of power, financial management, and administrative decision-making processes (Burns & Grove, 2007). Describing these structural elements is an important first step to identifying specific goals for outcomes evaluation. Various theoretical approaches to administration and management further

TABLE 30.1: The Medical Outcomes Study Conceptual Framework

Structures of Care	Process of Care	Outcomes
1. System characteristics (i.e., organization, specialty mix, financial incentives, workload, access/convenience) 2. Provider characteristics (i.e., age, gender, specialty training, economic incentives, beliefs/attitudes, job satisfaction, preferences) 3. Patient characteristics (i.e., age, gender, diagnosis/condition, severity, comorbid conditions, health habits, beliefs/attitudes, preferences)	1. Technical style (i.e., visits, medications, referrals, test ordering, hospitalizations, expenditures, continuity of care, coordination) 2. Interpersonal style (i.e., interpersonal manner, patient participation, counselling, communication level)	1. Clinical end points (i.e., signs and symptoms, laboratory values, death) 2. Functional status (i.e., physical, mental, social roles) 3. General well-being (i.e., health perceptions, energy/fatigue, pain, life satisfaction) 4. Satisfaction with care (i.e., access, financial coverage, quality, convenience)

Source: Adapted from Tarlov, A. R., Ware Jr., J. E., Greenfield, S., Nelson, E. C., Perrin, E., & Zubkoff, M. (1989). The medical outcomes study: An application of methods for monitoring the results of medical care. *Journal of the American Medical Association, 262*(7), 926.

contribute to this initial understanding. The second step is evaluating the impact of these care structures on the process of care (i.e., referrals, test ordering, expenditures, hospitalizations, continuity of care, medications). This step is complicated as it involves comparing different structures of care that provide the same process or outcomes of care (Burns & Grove, 2007). The third step is evaluating outcomes of care (i.e., clinical end points, functional status of patient, general well-being, satisfaction with care), including feedback directly from patients, providers, and records that look at the variations between the structure and process of care.

With a theoretical conceptualization in mind, any number of inquiries can guide the evaluation of APN roles. Since nurse practitioner (NP) and critical nurse specialist (CNS) roles vary in their scope of practice, it is important to critically understand the structure-process-outcome relationship with respect to both roles before embarking on an evaluation study. Although APNs have contributed to capacity and role optimization in the nursing profession (Kaasalainen, 2017), the actual number of CNS roles in Canada has declined over the last several years, and with this mind, one way to strengthen and promote the existence of and need for more CNS roles would be to increase the amount of evidence examining structure-process-outcome relationships in health care settings where the CNS roles exist.

Coupling Role Implementation and Evaluation

Initiating outcomes research and evaluating APN roles has not been an easy feat. With greater attention being given to providing quality, cost-effective care with good outcomes, it is essential for APNs to demonstrate the impact of their roles through outcomes research. Although a theoretical approach to evaluation research has been introduced, it is important to recognize that evaluation is closely coupled with APN role implementation. Often the question of evaluation is a precursor to successfully implementing an NP or CNS role in a health care setting. Unfortunately, this makes the inquiry process more difficult and complicates the development of a good research design. The **Participatory, Evidence-based, Patient-focused Process for guiding the development, implementation, and evaluation of APN (PEPPA)** framework is helpful with role development, implementation, and evaluation of APN roles (Bryant-Lukosius & DiCenso, 2004). This framework is comprised of various steps, including clarifying the patient population, modifying the model of care, and planning role implementation. Finally, evaluation and long-term monitoring of APN roles reinforce the structure-process-outcome approach. APNs should consider outcomes that are sensitive to APN interventions and related to safety, efficacy, and processes of care (Bryant-Lukosius & DiCenso, 2004).

The PEPPA framework has been used to examine implementation and evaluation of APN roles in the health care system. The spread and use of the PEPPA framework in guiding specific elements of APN role development, implementation, and evaluation has been reviewed (Boyko, Carter, & Bryant-Lukosius, 2016). This study examined the uptake of the framework over a 10-year period from 2004 to 2014. Results demonstrated greater use of the framework in the application and role development phases, primarily in Canada, with peak usage in 2010. There has been varying degrees of uptake, ranging from NP role implementation to general use of the framework to guide successful role implementation.

Measurement of Outcomes

Most of the evidence related to measuring outcomes and APN roles has focused on the clinical, consultative, collaborative, and educational dimensions of practice. The body of research has recognized that APNs provide safe and effective health care (DiCenso et al., 2010). Additionally, there are more studies reported for the NP role than for the CNS role in Canada. The following discussion will highlight a number of studies that have reported outcomes research. Although the overview is not exhaustive, it will hopefully provide a broad review of general themes and trends related to measuring outcomes and APN roles.

Since engaging in evaluation research requires the APN to be immersed in the process, Ingersoll, McIntosh, and Williams (2000) surveyed APNs to determine which outcomes they felt were relevant indicators of their practice. The 10 highest ranking indicators were: "satisfaction with care delivery, symptom reduction or resolution, perception of being well cared for, compliance with treatment plan, knowledge of patient and families, trust in the care provided, collaboration among care providers, frequency and type of procedures ordered, and quality of life" (p. 1279). Although these outcomes exemplify vital aspects of the APN role, they do not capture the breadth or depth of APN practice. The evaluation process should strive to identify concrete and measurable outcomes; however, there are disadvantages in using such outcomes to evaluate only the delivery of health care. Depending on the APN role and health care setting, the choice of relevant outcomes, and the time required to measure them may be incompatible. For example, attitudes and satisfaction are two outcomes that cannot be precisely measured, despite the many tools that have been developed precisely to assess this type of outcome variable (Donabedian, 2005). DiCenso et al. (2010) suggested that these underappreciated or even elusive APN contributions "could be made to address important gaps in maximizing the health of Canadians through equitable access to high quality health care service" (p. 32).

Several literature reviews have documented the contribution and impact of APN roles within both Canadian (DiCenso & Bryant-Lukosius, 2010; Sangster-Gormley, 2014) and US health care contexts (Kleinpell, 2009; Newhouse et al., 2011). These resources should be reviewed for a comprehensive understanding of the scope of literature within this field, as they provide an important contribution to advancing knowledge related to APN roles, and the measurement of outcomes. DiCenso et al. (2010) developed a synthesis report examining both CNS and NP roles in Canada. The findings, comprised of over 60 stakeholder interviews and a review of 500 papers, reported on the competencies of these roles, the contexts in which these roles practice, as well as barriers, facilitators, and implications for effective development and utilization of APN roles.

Reported in the findings were a distinct lack of role clarity and ambiguous articulation of the scopes of practice for these APN roles. Furthermore, recommendations included standardizing regulatory and educational standards, developing communication strategies to disseminate the positive outcomes of APN roles, integrating APN roles within human resource planning based on population health needs, and advancing research related to the value of these roles and their impact on health care costs. Bryant-Lukosius, DiCenso, Browne, and Pinelli (2004) identified several factors leading to unsuccessful APN role implementation and evaluation, including the loss of an innovative health system improvement that would benefit all stakeholders from the expertise the APN can provide. In Ontario, unsuccessful APN role implementation in oncology settings has been associated with poor job satisfaction and difficulty recruiting and retaining qualified APNs (Bryant-Lukosius et al., 2007).

The NP role has been well investigated in terms of outcomes research. Sangster-Gormley's (2014) synthesis reports summarized findings related to patient satisfaction with NP care, comparison of NP care with care provided by physicians and other providers, and other health outcomes sensitive to NP interventions. Patient satisfaction and education were found to be the most researched patient-related outcomes associated with NP roles (Kleinpell, 2009; Sangster-Gormley, 2014), and patients reported overall satisfaction with care provided by NPs or in collaboration with other health care providers. NPs contribute to reducing care costs, length of stay, and wait times; they have expert communication skills and empower patients when engaged in patient teaching and health promotion. In terms of NP practice, there were similar, less costly outcomes for models of care integrating NPs or NP-led teams compared to physician-led models (Browne, Birch, & Thabane, 2012; Jacobson & HDR Inc., 2012). APNs were particularly noted to provide effective care in chronic disease management, community care, primary care, and mental health settings, while NP-led initiatives were reported to improve access and continuity of care, education, and disease management.

The impact of NP-Led Clinics, from an NP perception, has included coordination of patient care, interprofessional collaboration, and enhanced understanding of the complexities of patient vulnerability (Heale, James, Wenghofer, & Garceau, 2018).

Outside Canada, the measurement of outcomes has been more extensively discussed, particularly in terms of economic influence. Kleinpell's (2009) textbook on outcome assessment provides a discussion of the literature addressing both the health and economic impact of APN practice. Studies dating from the 1960s to 2008 are integrated in an examination of care-related, patient-related, and performance-related outcomes. Outcome measurements are studied by conducting evaluation research using a process, searching for reliable instruments and measures for APN assessment, and then engaging in research related to more specialized APN roles such as nurse-midwifery and nurse anaesthesia. Outcomes related to clinical end points and patient-specific outcomes are reported, including control of specific diseases, use of diagnostics, cost of care, patient satisfaction, length of stay, complications, prescribing patterns, and quality of life. APN interventions were noted to reduce hospitalization and readmissions, decrease hospital costs, and shorten the average length of stay (Kleinpell, 2009; Sangster-Gormley, 2014).

Another systematic review conducted outside Canada amalgamated all APN outcome studies published between 1990 to 2008 (Newhouse et al., 2011) where the measurable outcomes were primarily related to clinical end points. A synthesis of 37 outcome studies related to the NP role recorded the following outcomes: patient satisfaction, self-reported perceived health, functional status, glucose control, lipid control, blood pressure, emergency department visits, hospitalizations, duration of mechanical ventilation, length of stay, and mortality. Reported outcomes for NPs showed either similarity or improvement on those of a physician. Eleven studies of this synthesis investigated the CNS role, collecting data addressing four outcomes: satisfaction, hospital length of stay, hospital costs, and complications.

Performance Assessment

In terms of individual APN performance assessment, health care organizations are challenged to evaluate the practice competencies of APNs at the advanced practice level. Many current performance assessment methodologies continue to blend a combination of basic nursing competencies with APN competencies or even medical competencies that are based on organizational goals and objectives originating from human resources departments (Scarpa & Connelly, 2011).

A performance assessment must be a meaningful evaluation of practice that meets the needs of APNs across different roles, care specialties, and practice settings (Kenny, Baker, Lanzon, Stevens, & Yancy, 2008). One approach that is both compatible and complementary with the CNA, provincial nursing regulators, and nursing as a profession is peer review.

Peer review is a key component of self-regulation and professional practice. It has been proposed that APNs with similar positions and expertise should participate in peer review. In a quality improvement study, the peer review process was noted by APNs to be an important element in developing their professional practice (Bergum et al., 2017). Peer review of

APNs has existed as part of performance assessment, evaluation of practice patterns, compliance monitoring, and the appraisal of quality indicators (Kenny et al., 2008).

Scarpa and Connelly (2011) utilized a needs analysis approach, including stakeholder focus groups, to develop an APN job description adapted to the Synergy Model. The job description evolved into a "criterion-based performance assessment" and this process produced better-defined APN roles and competencies that were specific to APN practice, ultimately promoting role autonomy, job satisfaction, and quality improvement.

At the Hospital for Sick Children (SickKids) in Toronto, APNs engage in a formal APN performance review process designed to evaluate APN role development and performance against a number of behaviours that delineate the growth of an APN from novice to expert. Through this process, APNs are able to provide a self-review and reflection on professional growth, establish goals and strategies to denote progress and achievement, and identify strengths and areas for growth using quantitative and peer feedback from nursing and other disciplines (SickKids, n.d.).

The US Department of Veterans Affairs utilizes a yearly APN peer review program designed to monitor performance based on clinical competence, practice behaviour, and the ability to perform under approved privileges (Rivera, 2012). This program is a hybrid model, based on recommendations from the American Association of Nurse Practitioners, but it incorporates the medical model integrating peer review between nursing and medicine. APN peers, including physicians, constructively evaluate the candidate on a number of criteria, including the knowledge of biomedical, clinical, and social sciences, and the application of knowledge in providing collaborative patient care and education to stakeholders. Additionally, the APN must demonstrate ongoing professional development and apply research skills that investigate, evaluate, and improve best practices to provide quality, safe, efficient, and effective patient care (Rivera, 2012).

The Yale-New Haven Hospital employs 400 APNs who practice in a wide range of roles and settings, including community health centres and the Yale School of Nursing. A peer review process was used to evaluate APN practice, and a peer review program of ongoing professional practice evaluation (OPPE), based on the medical model, was used by physicians. The hospital's APN council conducted two needs surveys that discovered APNs were practicing under various employment and collaborative practice models. They had little participation in the peer review process, which lacked APN-specific outcome measures, and APNs wanted greater peer advocacy and networking (Davies et al., 2014). In response to these findings, the APN council developed a similar OPPE tool based on the hospital's APN competencies framework and enhanced the peer review process, which included self-evaluation. This initiative was piloted by oncology APNs and presented to hospital-wide stakeholders. Feedback directed the refinement and alignment of the review process with other hospital-wide processes, making it more APN-friendly prior to its implementation across all hospital divisions.

Historically, physician and nursing peer reviews have been separate processes. Emphasizing collaborative practice between physicians and NPs, and expanding care coordination, including expanding clinical NPs' privileges, a unique integrative model for professional peer review was developed in the US to assess, measure, and provide continual quality improvement in practices. This shared structure, along with the processes and practices involved in its development, and the peer review tool were designed to ensure that NPs and physicians are engaged in exemplary provider performance and patient outcomes (Clavelle & Bramwell, 2013).

Conclusion

In reviewing the literature related to outcomes of care, it is evident there are numerous studies that have investigated outcomes related to APN practice for both NP and CNS roles. Measuring APN outcomes is important in defining the scope and practice of APN roles and the impact APN practice has on patient care, health care, costs of care, and other quality indicators, including access, length of stay, and evidence-informed best practices. Through studying various outcomes, strategies can be developed to remove barriers to APN practice by demonstrating its impact on a variety of health care settings and organizations. Promoting the value of APN by implementing new and innovative models of care that evince APN knowledge, skill, and expertise continues to highlight APN roles by identifying their contributions within the health care field.

APNs must ensure that they have a voice in their own performance assessment processes. This will be become more fundamental in Canada as NPs are granted hospital privileges for admission, discharge, and transfer of care. Peer review is one approach that provides a means to monitor and improve professional practice competencies through the evaluations of peers practicing in similar roles and specialties. Like outcome measurements, peer review provides the opportunity for APNs to highlight their contributions to patient care within their employment or practice setting. This essential process supports APN practice and self-regulation while promoting quality patient care and interprofessional collaboration that can stimulate further APN research initiatives.

Critical Thinking Questions

1. Describe a systematic approach that might be utilized for outcomes evaluation of APN roles.
2. How does APN role implementation influence outcomes evaluation?
3. What research inquiries related to outcomes evaluation may further demonstrate the impact of APN roles?
4. How do you distinguish between APN-sensitive outcomes compared to those influenced by other health care professions?
5. What opportunities exist for APNs to be involved in the development of APN-sensitive performance assessment processes?
6. Within your organization, identify any outcome evaluation measures currently in progress or that may be done in the future.

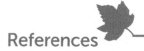

References

Bergum, S., Canaan, T., Delemos, C., Gall, E., McCracken, B., Rowen, D., Salvemini, S., & Wiens, K. (2017). Implementation and evaluation of a peer review process for advanced practice nurses in a university hospital setting. *Journal of the American Association of Nurse Practitioners, 29*(7), 369–374.

Boyko, J., Carter, N., & Bryant-Lukosius, D. (2016). Assessing the spread and uptake of a framework for introducing and evaluating advanced practice nursing roles. *Worldviews on Evidence-Based Nursing, 13*(4), 277–284.

Browne, G., Birch, S., & Thabane, L. (2012). *Better care: An analysis of nursing and healthcare systems outcomes.* Ottawa, ON: CHSRF. Retrieved from http://www.cfhi-fcass.ca/sf-docs/default-source/commissioned-research-reports/Browne-BetterCare-EN.pdf?sfvrsn=0

Bryant-Lukosius, D., & DiCenso, A. (2004). A framework for the introduction and evaluation of advanced practice nursing roles. *Journal of Advanced Nursing, 48*(5), 530–540.

Bryant-Lukosius, D., DiCenso, A., Browne, G., & Pinelli, J. (2004). Advanced practice nursing roles: Development implementation, and evaluation. *Journal of Advanced Nursing, 48*(5), 519–529.

Bryant-Lukosius, D., Green, E., Fitch, M., McCartney, G., Robb-Blenderman, L., Bosompra, K., ... Milne, H. (2007). A survey of oncology advanced practice roles in Ontario: Profile and predictors of job satisfaction. *Canadian Journal of Leadership, 20*(2), 50–68.

Burgess, J., & Purkis, M. E. (2010). The power and politics of collaboration in nurse practitioner role development. *Nursing Inquiry, 17*(4), 297–308.

Burns, N., & Grove, S. K. (2007). Outcomes research. In N. Burns & S. K. Grove (Eds.), *Understanding nursing research: Building evidence-based practice* (4th ed., pp. 272–321). Philadelphia, PA: Saunders.

Canadian Nurses Association (CNA). (2019). *Advanced practice nursing: A pan-Canadian framework.* Ottawa, ON: CNA. Retrieved from https://cna-aiic.ca/-/media/cna/page-content/pdf-en/apn-a-pan-canadian-framework.pdf

Clancy, C., & Eisenberg, J. (1997). Outcomes research at the Agency of Health Care Policy and Research. *Disease Management and Clinical Outcomes, 1,* 172–180.

Clavelle, J. T., & Bramwell, K. (2013). Nurse practitioner/physician collaborative practice: An integrative model for professional peer review. *Journal of Nursing Administration, 43*(6), 318–320.

Crawford, C. (2019). Addition of advanced practice registered nurses to the trauma team: An integrative systematic review of literature. *Journal of Trauma Nursing, 26*(3), 141–146.

Davies, M., Tucker, K., Dest, V., Lyons, C., Fitzsimons, S., & McCorkle, R. (2014). Enhancing peer review to support APN practice. *Oncology Nursing News.* Retrieved from http://nursing.onclive.com/publications/oncology-nurse/2014/October-2014/Enhancing-Peer-Review-to-Support-APN-Practice

DiCenso, A., & Bryant-Lukosius, D. (2010). The long and winding road: Integration of nurse practitioners and clinical nurse specialists into the Canadian health-care system. *Canadian Journal of Nursing Research, 42*(2), 3–8.

DiCenso, A., Martin-Misener, R., Bryant-Lukosius, D., Bourgeault, I., Kilpatrick, K., Donald, F., ... Charbonneau-Smith, R. (2010). Advanced practice nursing in Canada: Overview of a decision support synthesis. *Canadian Journal of Nursing Leadership, 23*(Special Issue), 15–34.

Donabedian, A. (2005). Evaluating the quality of medical care. *The Millbank Quarterly, 83,* 4.

Doran, D. (2003). *Nursing sensitive outcomes: State of the science.* Sudbury, MA: Jones & Bartlett.

Doran, D., Mildon, B., & Clarke, S. (2011). Towards a national report card in nursing: A knowledge synthesis. *Nursing Leadership, 24*(2), 38–57.

Doran, D. M., Sidani, S., & DiPietro, T. (2010). Nursing-sensitive outcomes. In J. S. Fulton, B. Lyon, & K. Goudreau (Eds.), *Foundations of clinical nurse specialist practice* (pp. 35–37). New York, NY: Springer.

Friese, C. R., & Beck, S. L. (2004). Advancing practice and research: Creating evidence-based summaries on measuring nursing-sensitive patient outcomes. *Clinical Journal of Oncology Nursing, 8*(6), 675–677.

Heale, R., James, S., Wenghofer, E., & Garceau, M. (2018). Nurse practitioner's perceptions of the impact of the nurse practitioner-led clinical model on the quality of care of complex patients. *Primary Health Care Research and Development, 19*, 553–560.

The Hospital for Sick Children (SickKids). (n.d.). *APN performance review process.* Retrieved from http://www.sickkids.ca/Nursing/Nursing%20Practice/APN-Performance-Review-Process/index.html

Ingersoll, G., McIntosh, E., & Williams, M. (2000). Nurse-sensitive outcomes of advanced practice. *Journal of Advanced Nursing, 32*, 1272–1281.

Jacobson, P. M., & HDR Inc. (2012). *Evidence synthesis for the effectiveness of interprofessional teams in primary care.* Ottawa, ON: CHSRF. Retrieved from http://www.cfhi-fcass.ca/sf-docs/default-source/commissioned-research-reports/Jacobson-Interprofessional-EN.pdf?sfvrsn=0

Kaasalainen, S. (2017). How has advanced practice nursing influenced the nursing profession in Canada? *Nursing Leadership, 30*(2), 64–70.

Kenny, K. J., Baker, L., Lanzon, M., Stevens, L. R., & Yancy, M. (2008). An innovative approach to peer review for the advanced practice nurse: A focus on critical incidents. *Journal of the American Academy of Nurse Practitioners, 20*(7), 376–381.

Kilpatrick, K., Tchouaket, E., Jabbour, M., & Hains, S. (2020). A mixed methods quality improvement study to implement nurse practitioner roles and improve care for residents in long-term care. *BioMed Central (BMC) Nursing, 19*(1), 1–14. https://doi.org/10.1186/s12912-019-0395-2

Kleinpell, R. (Ed.). (2009). *Outcome assessment in advanced practice nursing* (2nd ed.). New York, NY: Springer.

Kleinpell, R., & Gawlinski, A. (2005). Assessing outcomes in advanced nursing practice: The use of quality indicators and evidence-based practice. *AACN Clinical Issues, 16*(1), 43–57.

Newhouse, R. P., Stanik-Hutt, J., White, K. M., Johantgen, M., Bass, E. B., Zangaro, G., … Weiner, J. P. (2011). Advanced practice nurse outcomes 1990–2008: A systematic review. *Nursing Economics, 29*(5), 1–29.

Rivera, C. (2012). *Advanced practice nurse (APN) peer review program at the Department of Veterans Affairs.* Retrieved from https://prezi.com/q5qespc0kmmt/advance-practice-nurse-peer-review/

Sangster-Gormley, E. (2014). *Nurse practitioner-sensitive outcomes: A summary report.* Halifax, NS: CRNNS.

Scarpa, R., & Connelly, P. E. (2011). Innovations in performance assessment: A criterion based performance assessment of advanced practice nurses using a synergistic theoretical nursing framework. *Nursing Administration Quarterly, 35*(2), 164–173.

Shah, T. I., Milosavljevic, S., & Bath, B. (2017). Determining geographic accessibility of family physician and nurse practitioner services in relation to the distribution of seniors within two Canadian prairie provinces. *Social Science & Medicine, 194*, 96–104. doi: 10.1016/j.socscimed.2017.10.019

Tarlov, A. R., Ware Jr., J. E., Greenfield, S., Nelson, E. C., Perrin, E., & Zubkoff, M. (1989). The medical outcomes study: An application of methods for monitoring the results of medical care. *Journal of the American Medical Association, 262*(7), 925–930. Retrieved from http://www.prgs.edu/content/dam/rand/pubs/notes/2009/N3038.pdf

Chapter 31

Health Policy and Advanced Practice Nursing in Changing Environments

Doris Grinspun

DR. DORIS GRINSPUN is the Chief Executive Officer of the Registered Nurses Association of Ontario (RNAO). She is the founder and visionary of RNAO's internationally renowned Best Practice Guidelines Program and a leading figure in Canadian and international health and nursing policy. Dr. Grinspun served as Director of Nursing at Mount Sinai Hospital in Toronto, Ontario, from 1990 to 1996. She has also worked in practice and administrative capacities in Israel and the United States. Dr. Grinspun holds appointments as Adjunct Professor at several universities. She has been featured in major media outlets and publications in Canada and abroad for her bold and visionary leadership. In 2003, Dr. Grinspun was invested with the Order of Ontario and in 2013 she received the Queen's Diamond Jubilee Medal. Dr. Grinspun is the recipient of three honoris causa doctoral degrees: from the University of Ontario Institute of Technology (2011), the Universitat de Lleida, Spain (2018), and the Universidad de Burgos, Spain (2020). She was inducted as a Fellow of the American Academy of Nursing in 2018.

KEY TERMS

advanced practice nurses (APNs)
Canada's performance
health care system
integrated care model (ICM)
nursing
nursing as a body politic (NBP)
Organisation for Economic Co-operation and Development (OECD)
whole system change (WSC)

OBJECTIVES

1. Discuss and compare Canada's health care system performance nationally and internationally.
2. Understand nursing and advanced practice nursing (APN) as a key solution for Canada's health care system shortfalls.
3. Explore how whole system change happens, and the importance of nursing and nurses' purposeful political engagement to shape healthy public policy.

Introduction

This chapter presents the health policy context in which the role of advanced practice nurses (APNs) is situated. The discussion centres on key health care challenges confronting Canada, and the threats and opportunities that these present for APNs. The need for purposeful and continuous political engagement is centred on integrated care models (ICMs) that necessitate whole system change (WSC), which are discussed as ways to improve Canada's performance overall. These models suggest shifting Canada's heavy reliance on illness care toward robust community care that is anchored in primary care and that focuses on health promotion, disease prevention, mental health, and chronic disease prevention and management. Effective ICMs occur when all health professionals work to their optimal scope of practice in high-performing teams that deliver person-centred and evidence-informed care.

Nursing, being the largest workforce, is key to Canada's health care system transformation. As the profession most trusted by the public, nursing has a duty to speak out and be heard. This chapter concludes with an urgent call to strengthen nursing as a body politic (NBP).

Context: Canada's Health and Health Care Outcomes

International comparisons show that Canada is falling short on key outcome indicators when it comes to delivering health care. For example, the Commonwealth Fund (2017) ranked Canada's health care system ninth out of 11 industrialized countries in terms of quality care, access, efficiency, equity, healthy lives, and expenditures. This is a slight improvement on the ranking discussed in the first edition of this book, when Canada ranked tenth out of 11 countries (Commonwealth Fund, 2014). The Commonwealth Fund report relies on 72 metrics grouped into five distinct categories: care process, access, administrative efficiency, equity, and health care outcomes.

These results, especially in the areas of equity, healthy lives, and expenditures, can be largely attributed to Canada's lower-than-average social spending when compared to other Organisation for Economic Co-operation and Development (OECD) nations. In 2018, total health expenditure accounted for 10.7% of Canada's gross domestic product (GDP), compared to the OECD average of 9.3% (OECD, 2019). In 2018, social spending accounted for 17.3% of Canada's GDP, compared to the OECD average of 20.1% (OECD, 2019). Simply put, if Canada chooses to spend less on upstream investments in programs for determinants of health (both social and environmental), our country will inevitably achieve less equity and less healthy lives and spend more on health care. The solution to improving these specific indicators is investing more in social and environmental programs that will bring increased equity and healthy (or healthier) populations, and will decrease the demand for health care services (see Figures 31.1 and 31.2).

Against this backdrop, nursing holds the key. Through its role as a "body politic" in the space of public and policy debates about the future of Canadian Medicare, and as the

FIGURE 31.1: Total Health Expenditure as a Percentage Share of GDP

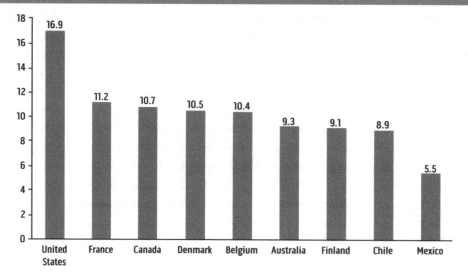

Note: OECD estimated or provisional for 2018.

Source: Adapted from OECD. (2019). *Social expenditure—detailed data.* Retrieved from https://stats.oecd.org/Index.aspx?DataSetCode=SOCX_DET. Reprinted with permission.

FIGURE 31.2: Public Social Expenditure as a Percentage Share of GDP

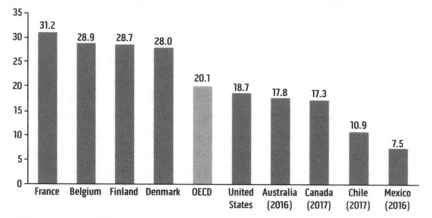

Note: OECD figures are for 2018 unless otherwise specified.

Source: Adapted from OECD. (2018). *Social expenditure database (SOCX).* Retrieved from www.oecd.org/social/expenditure.htm. Reprinted with permission.

largest practice discipline, nursing must be a vigorous influencer as it has much to offer for improving our nation's standing on timely access to quality care, efficiency, and coordinated person-centred care. The role of APNs and an expanded role for registered nurses (RNs) are central to the narrative.

Nursing's Voice: Getting Involved in Health Care System Transformation

On December 19, 2011, the federal government announced that it would not renew the Federal Health Accord. It also announced that the Canada Health Transfer (CHT) growth would continue at 6% per year for three years (2014–2015 to 2016–2017) and then be cut to the rate of growth of GDP. The Canada Social Transfer (CST) would continue to grow at 3% per year. Lastly, equalization transfers would grow at the rate of growth of GDP. The Health Accord was a legal agreement between the federal and provincial/territorial governments on health care funding and spending priorities. It was important as it assured stable funding after the deep cuts of the 1990s, and it leveraged the improved transfer funding to advance common goals. The 10-year plan, signed in 2004, recommitted the federal and jurisdictional leaders to the *Canada Health Act*'s principles of public administration, comprehensiveness, universality, portability, and accessibility. The Accord mandated the federal government to step up to the plate by increasing the CHT payments to 6% per year. At that time, common goals were set around wait times, team-based primary care, home care, and prescription drugs.

Reacting to the news, the Council of the Federation (CoF), composed of the premiers and leaders of all provinces and territories, confirmed in 2012 that the new arrangement, compared to the current one under the Accord, would cost provinces and territories $25 billion. This was the estimate for all jurisdictions except for Alberta, which stood to gain significantly from the new federal arrangement in 2011 (Registered Nurses Association of Ontario [RNAO], 2014).

The 2015 federal election brought with it great optimism as the Liberal Party, headed by Justin Trudeau, promised to strengthen the relationships between the federal government and its provincial and territorial counterparts, and negotiate a new Health Accord, including a long-term agreement on funding (Liberal Party of Canada, 2015). The promise, however, resulted in a series of failed meetings and no new Health Accord. Instead, the federal government signed bilateral agreements with each province, leaving Canadians with no clear vision, goals, or programs to build up our national health care system.

Canada's premiers and territorial leaders issued, at the end of their 2019 Council of the Federation meeting, a call to the federal government to

> increase funding by an annual escalator of 5.2% to the Canada Health Transfer, consistent with independent analysis by the Conference Board of Canada of budget pressures. The Conference Board of Canada also notes the Canada Health Transfer does not factor aging into its payments, and as such, federal transfers are not sufficient to support the additional care needs of Canada's aging population.

The funding challenges are not likely to be resolved anytime soon and will continue to propel system reforms. These, coupled with a clear public preference to receive health services in the community, present a formidable opportunity for nursing to seize its contribution to society at large. This world of possibilities for nursing's contributions will be ever more important after the COVID-19 global pandemic.

Three reports have had a deep impact on health care system transformation in the province of Ontario and have influenced several other Canadian and international jurisdictions. The first, "Primary Solutions for Primary Care" (RNAO, 2012b), outlines a two-phase blueprint to maximize and expand the role of nurses in primary care that includes RN prescribing. RNAO recommends that the move to RN prescribing be based on an enabling framework that improves access to care by recognizing the broad depth of RN expertise. The second report, "Enhancing Community Care for Ontarians (ECCO)," first released in 2012, re-released in its second edition in 2014, and with its third edition issued in 2020, proposes shifting health care from an illness model to a health-oriented one through substantive investments in upstream programs in social and environmental programs, and by repositioning the system to be anchored in primary and community care, as opposed to the current focus on illness and hospital care. This, RNAO argues, will strengthen our publicly funded, not-for-profit health care system and make it more responsive to the public's needs, result in better coordination, be easier to navigate, more efficient, and cost-effective.

Figure 31.3 depicts the ECCO model. Critical areas of focus are health promotion, disease prevention, mental health, and chronic disease prevention and management. These changes must be accompanied by enabling nurses and all other regulated health professionals to work to their full scopes of practice, including RN prescribing, in interprofessional teams, and using evidence to guide clinical and work-environment practices.

The report has already influenced action. The views of Deb Matthews, then Ontario's minister of health, were reflected in her "Action Plan for Health Care" (2012), which supported a continued shift of care delivery to the home and community settings to improve patient outcomes and system cost effectiveness. Similarly, Dr. Eric Hoskins, minister of health from 2014 to 2018, reflected a similar view in his "Patients First: Action Plan for Health Care" (2015), based on a person-centred agenda like ECCO. He referenced ECCO in the Action Plan and stated that it inspired him to bring about this type of reform. Most recently, Christine Elliott, Ontario's current minister of health, announced in 2019 her vision for Ontario based on Ontario Health Teams (OHTs). ECCO 3.0 was released on May 12, 2020, in honour of Florence Nightingale, who once said, "my view you know is that the ultimate destination is the nursing of the sick in their own homes. ... I look to the abolition of all hospitals and workhouse infirmaries. But it is no use to talk about the year 2000" (Baly, 1997, p. 4).

ECCO 3.0 presents the context of Ontario's latest health care system restructuring. We will argue that RNAO's vision of an accessible, equitable, person-centred, integrated, and publicly funded, not-for-profit health care system will be realized only when we have a primary care sector with those same attributes, a goal reachable in the current system reform. In ECCO 3.0, we adapt our model to align with the creation of a single health care system administrator (Ontario Health) and multiple integrated care delivery organizations—OHTs.

Alongside the flurry of reports, we must juxtapose a dose of reality-based action. No substantial improvement in timely access, efficiency, and cost-effectiveness can be achieved without the fulsome participation of nurses, and any barriers that limit such participation

FIGURE 31.3: RNAO ECCO Model Overview

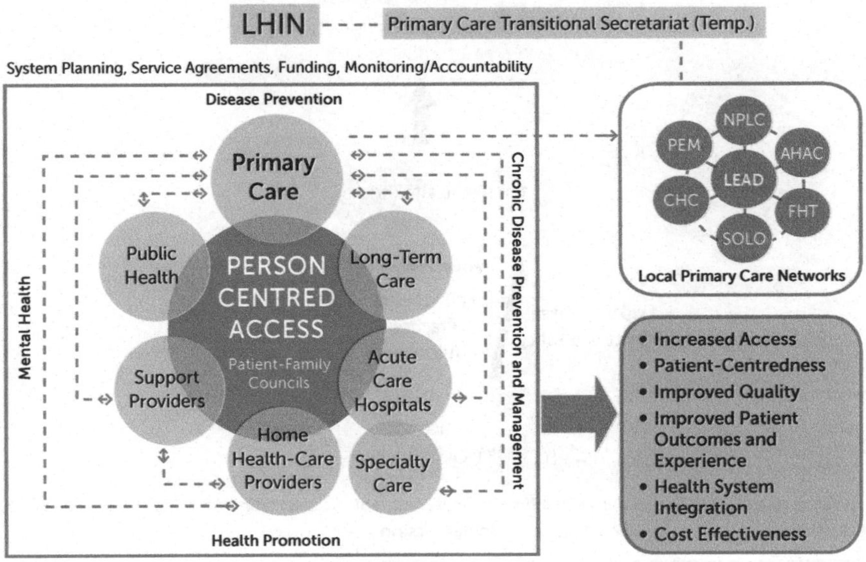

Notes: AHAC = Aboriginal Health Access Centre; CHC = Community Health Centre; FHT = Family Health Team; LHIN = Local Health Integration Network for Ontario; NPLC = Nurse Practitioner-Led Clinic; PEM = Primary Care Enrolment Model; Solo = Solo Practitioner Practice

Source: RNAO. (2012a). *Enhancing community care for Ontarians (ECCO 1.0)*. Retrieved from http://rnao.ca/sites/rnao-ca/files/RNAO_ECCO_WHITE_PAPER_FINAL_2.pdf. Reprinted by permission.

must be torn down (Grinspun et al., 2018). This axiom is as true for Ontario as it is for Canada or any other country where nursing is its largest workforce. Turning the tide from Canada being a lower performer to top performer is within reach; nurses' practice power must be unleashed to its full and expanded potential; APNs must move into the driver's seat; and all must work in high-functioning interprofessional teams that deliver person-centred and evidence-informed practices.

Figure 31.4 shows the three pillars essential for improving timely access to person-centred care, optimizing health outcomes, and achieving health care system effectiveness. These pillars include full scope of practice, interprofessional care, and evidence-based practice. Simply put, timely access to health care services can significantly improve if all health professionals are working to their optimal scopes and in high-functioning interprofessional teams (Grinspun, 2007; Grinspun & Anyinam, 2014; RNAO, 2012a, 2013, 2014, 2020).

The facts speak for themselves. In 2018, there were 287,736 RNs (down from 293,205 in 2014) working in nursing (including nurse practitioners [NPs]) in Canada, and a further 15,410 (up from 12,901 in 2014) not working in nursing or not specified, for a total of 303,146 RNs (Canadian Institute for Health Information [CIHI], 2019; down from 306,106 RNs in 2014 [CIHI, 2015]). Of these, there were 5,335 NPs working in nursing (up from 3,966 in

FIGURE 31.4: Pillars for Health System Effectiveness

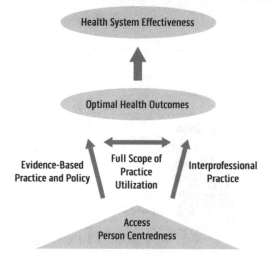

Source: Grinspun, D. (2012). *Healthcare in a time of fiscal restraint: Collaborating for system sustainability*, Keynote address, McMaster University, 2012. Reprinted with permission.

2014), and a further 362 (up from 178) not working in nursing or not specified, for a total of 5,697 (CIHI, 2019; up from a total of 4,144 NPs in 2014 [CIHI, 2015]). Although there is no agreed-upon number of clinical nurse specialists (CNSs) in Canada, the last estimates available, based on self-declared statements, were around 2,200 in 2010, and of these only 800 nurses reporting to be CNSs had a graduate degree (Canadian Nurses Association [CNA], 2012a, 2012b). Just imagine what that would do for timely health care access if members of this robust workforce were utilized to their optimal scopes of practice!

Let us look, as an example, at primary care in the province of Ontario. In 2019, there were 1,882 (up from 1,144 in 2014) working NPs and 4,457 RNs (up from 4,158 in 2014) in the general class, working in primary care in Ontario (from CNO Data Query Tool). As discussed in previous chapters of the textbook, a good percentage of these NPs are not working to their full scope of practice despite having the legislative authority to do so. The same holds true for CNSs. The situation is no better for RNs. Allard, Frego, Katz, and Halas (2010) found in a survey of primary care RNs from across Canada that only 61% of those who responded felt they were practicing to their full practice scope. Likely the percentage of RNs in primary care who are underutilized is even higher given that the nature of the survey—self-reported—may have introduced social desirability bias where the respondents answer in a way that would be seen favourably by others so not to undermine their roles.

The scope of practice underutilization of APNs and RNs poses a substantive cost to Canadians and our health care system, both in terms of timely access and value for service return on their investment as taxpayers. First, timely access: if the majority of NPs, CNSs, and RNs were working to their full scope of practice, it is entirely foreseeable that people would have same-day access to primary care. Meanwhile, only 40% of Ontarians are able to see their family physician on the same day or the next day when ill (Health Quality Ontario, 2018). Secondly, return on investment, the total payments to Ontario's family physicians increased by $1.3 billion or 54% (after inflation) over a period of five years between 2003–2004 and 2009–2010. In 2009–2010, the mean payment per full-time equivalent family physician was $300,100, which equates to anywhere between two and a half to three times the salary of an NP, and five times the current salary of an RN in primary care.

Consumer preferences combined with financially strapped governments are turning their eye to community care to reduce costs. This reality will only increase in the post–COVID-19 era as flaws in the health care system during the pandemic will need to be attended to by cash-strapped governments. The three main sectors that will receive attention are primary health care, home health care, and long-term care. Primary care helps people stay healthy and delay as well as manage chronic conditions. High-quality home care supports them to remain active members of our communities. Long-term care is there for people, as needed, at an advanced aged. Nurses have always played a central role in community care, and NPs and CNSs must assert their clinical and advocacy roles in primary care and home health care.

In Ontario, significant gains have been made in cementing the role of primary care NPs in Community Health Centres, Aboriginal Health Access Centres, Family Health Teams, and NP-Led Clinics, with 27 of the latter being fully operational and providing same-day access to thousands of Ontarians. Ontario also enables NPs, through legislative changes, to treat, transfer, and discharge hospital in-patients, and since 2012, NPs are also able to admit patients to the hospital, a function that has yet to fully materialize. NPs are also taking a lead in long-term care homes, and their numbers and roles are being expanded to that of primary health care provider. What will it take to scale up the NP as a leading role even further within Ontario and across the country? Equally important, how can we ensure the same happens with the invaluable role of the CNS? The case for scaling up NPs' role is being clearly demonstrated as the COVID-19 pandemic unfolds.

Understanding Whole System Change to Spur Innovations and Improve Health Outcomes

It took almost 40 years for NPs to have legislated authority. It will likely take four to five years for RNs to achieve the same regarding RN prescribing. Determining the potential speed of scope expansion adoption lies in understanding the factors that influence the uptake of innovations and the mechanisms that come into play and either accelerate or hinder adoption. The case of NPs in Canada can help illustrate this best.

In a seminal paper on understanding WSC, Edwards, Rowan, Marck, and Grinspun (2011) asked if the vast evidence pointing to the effectiveness of NPs was insufficient to trigger rapid adoption and growth, what else was needed? The authors then mapped out all the factors that influenced the progress of NP adoption, which are summarized in Figure 31.5.

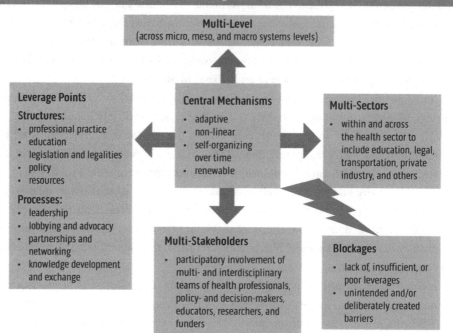

FIGURE 31.5: Whole Systems Change in Health Care: Basic Elements

Source: Edwards, N., Rowan, M., Marck, P., Grinspun, D. (2011). Understanding whole systems change in health care: The case of nurse practitioners in Canada. *Policy, Politics, & Nursing Practice, 12*(1), 4–17. Copyright © 2011 by Sage Publications. Reprinted by permission.

The five lessons that were learned are as follows:

1. WSC is a complex, social, and ecological phenomenon, characterized by dynamic interactions among institutional, political, educational, and at times legislative forces involving multiple stakeholders and multiple sectors within micro-, meso-, and macro-system levels over time (Edwards et al., 2011).

2. Program developers and change agents need to consider potential leverage points and blockages to capitalize on and/or mitigate their interrelated potential to either accelerate or decelerate WSC at varying points in time (Edwards et al., 2011).

3. When introducing health care systems innovations, it is important to assess not only the outcomes of the innovation but also the context of uptake (Edwards et al., 2011).

4. WSC is non-linear and cross-scale, which means that sustainable system changes occur across a panarchy of slower and faster-moving adaptive cycles that transect system hierarchies over time (Edwards et al., 2007; Gunderson & Holling, 2002; Gunderson, Light, & Holling, 1995).

5. Diverse, multi-level, and multi-sectoral forms of leadership are essential to foster whole systems change (Edwards et al., 2011).

These important lessons help us understand the vital importance of active professional organizations. RNAO took upon itself to organize the nursing community with a laser-like focus from 1996 until the proclamation of the NP legislation in 1998. Part of the multi-pronged strategy was strategically meeting with the minister of health to discuss NP initiatives while also orchestrating a letter-writing campaign to the Ontario minister of health, the premier, and opposition leaders to influence their decision regarding the urgent need for NP legislation; a multi-organizational press conference; visits by NPs and RNs with local politicians in their ridings; and media engagement to help the media and public understand NPs as a health care system solution.

Improving the health outcomes of Canadians and our health care system requires the ongoing and persistent engagement of nursing as a collective in the political process. This engagement must be multi-partisan to enrich our democracy and increase the respect we have achieved from the public, politicians, and the media. By targeting specific policies aimed at closing the gap between what Canadians need and what nursing can offer, we can improve our contributions to the health of Canadians and the health and health care performance of our country. Accepting our duty of nursing as an NBP to advance WSC is central to ensuring that Canadians will fully benefit from the APNs' roles and from nurses as a whole. The role of professional associations and labour unions is paramount for this to happen.

In another seminal article, Cohen et al. (1996) delineated four stages of nursing's political development and recommended strategies for implementing the fourth and most complex stage. Nursing in Canada has long evolved from stage 1, the buy-in stage, where the profession recognizes the importance of political activism, but the nature of action is reactive and inward-focused, driven mainly by the interests of nursing. However, we must evolve toward a much more sophisticated stage in order to fundamentally effect change. NBP in Canada must deliberately and skilfully attain what Cohen et al. deem as stage 4, where nursing "leads the way." In stage 4 the profession is envisioned as providing true political leadership on broader policy issues that speak to the public's interests. The profession is proactive in leadership and agenda-setting for a broad range of health and social policy issues, introducing terms that reorder the debate and initiating coalitions beyond nursing for broad policy concerns. At this stage, many nurses are sought to fill nursing and health policy positions because of the value of nursing expertise and knowledge. The authors argue that the further the profession is able to move into this stage, the more the public will benefit from nursing's expertise and the profession's advocacy on behalf of the public (Cohen et al., 1996).

Activism on broader health and social issues does not preclude continued vigilance on professional issues related to nursing practice. Indeed, stage 4 does not rule out pursuit of self-interests; it merely does so within a context that emphasizes the larger public good. Pursuit of stage 4 can be enhanced by building coalitions and constituencies around health and social issues; supporting leadership development as well as visionaries and risk-takers; mobilizing nursing for campaigns; integrating health policy into curricula; developing public media expertise; and gaining increased sophistication in policy analysis and related research (Cohen et al., 1996).

Ennen (2001) defines four spheres for political action that deserve our close attention. Government, the first sphere, plays a critical, far-reaching role in nursing and health care. It defines and regulates nursing practice, sets and influences reimbursement systems for health care and nursing services, and sets the policy agenda related to health care provision. Here the domain of regulation of professional nursing practice is central. Public law defines who nurses care for as well as when, where, and how care is delivered. It also regulates APN educational requirements and certification processes, as well as how they practice within the health care system.

Licensure, a prerogative of the state (in Canada, the provinces and territories), is determined by a legislative process that sets rules and regulations governing licensure and designates an agency responsible for law enforcement (in Canada, the regulatory colleges). The current licensure laws have raised the standards of education, established codes for the ethical behaviour of RNs, and created a state registry of persons meeting these criteria. Workplace is the second sphere for action. The policy and political nuances of the workplace can have a profound impact on the quality of nurses' professional lives. Professional organizations constitute the third sphere. They shape the practice of nursing through political influence and policy-making,

Developing standards of practice, lobbying for changes in the scope of practice, and playing a role in collective action are three services that professional organizations provide their members and the nursing profession as a whole. Strong professional organizations identify issues of concern to nursing and health care and bring them to the attention of the public. Community, the fourth sphere of political action, is more than a practice arena for nursing. It is a social unit involving a variety of special interest groups, community activities, health and social problems, and resources available to solve identified problems.

Advocacy is also essential for nurses at the point of care to impact our practice and the well-being of patients. Tomajan (2012) describes advocacy skills every nurse can employ to advocate for a safe and healthy work environment, and explains how nurses can advocate for nursing as part of their daily activity whether they are point-of-care nurses, nurse managers, or nurse educators. These advocacy practices are applicable, whether in advocating on one's own behalf, for colleagues at the unit level, or for issues at the organizational or system level. It is argued that advocacy requires a set of skills that include problem-solving, communication, influence, and collaboration. These are skills akin to those that nurses use to deliver clinical care. Point-of-care nurses build on their public image of being the most trusted profession by communicating and advocating for a more accurate view of their contributions to health care and society. Managers and administrators advocate in their daily work to obtain required resources for their nursing staff and promote healthy work environments. Nurse educators play a critical role in preparing nurses to strengthen the profession through advocacy. Nurses must be involved in shaping public policy that directly or indirectly affects practice.

Conclusion

Canada's fiscal realities bring challenges and opportunities to the APN role. To thrive, APN roles must be understood and positioned as a key solution to the health and health care imperatives facing the public, both as funders and users of health services. Augmenting the narrative of NPs and CNSs, which already contains remarkable clinical expertise and proven health and system outcomes, with a nursing collective that is leading the way sets the agenda in a purposeful way to benefit the public.

Critical Thinking Questions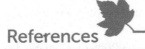

1. Compare and contrast Canada's health and health care performance with other OECD countries.
2. How can a health care system redesign assist in improving Canada's performance?
3. How can APNs (NPs and CNSs) be positioned as a response to solve Canada's health care challenges?
4. What does it take to create a WSC?

References

Allard, M., Frego, A., Katz, A., & Halas, G. (2010). Exploring the role of RNs in family practice residency training programs. *Canadian Nurse, 106*(3), 20–24.

Baly, M. E. (1997). *Florence Nightingale and the nursing legacy* (2nd ed.). London, UK: Whurr Publishers.

Canadian Institute for Health Information (CIHI). (2015). *Regulated nurses, 2014.* Ottawa, ON: CIHI. Retrieved from https://secure.cihi.ca/free_products/RegulatedNurses2014_Report_EN.pdf

CIHI. (2019). *Nursing in Canada, 2018: A lens on supply and workforce.* Ottawa, ON: CIHI. Retrieved from https://secure.cihi.ca/free_products/regulated-nurses-2018-report-en-web.pdf

Canadian Nurses Association (CNA). (2012a). *A nursing call to action: Expert Commission report.* Ottawa, ON: CNA. Retrieved from http://www.cna-aiic.ca/~/media/cna/files/en/nec_report_e.pdf

CNA. (2012b). *Strengthening the role of the clinical nurse specialist in Canada: Background paper.* Ottawa, ON: CNA. Retrieved from https://www.cna-aiic.ca/~/media/cna/page-content/pdf-fr/strengthening_the_cns_role_background_paper_e.pdf

Cohen, S. S., Mason, D. J., Kovner, C., Leavitt, J. K., Pulcini, J., & Sochalski, J. (1996). Stages of nursing's political involvement: Where we've been and where we ought to go. *Nursing Outlook, 44*(6), 259–266.

Commonwealth Fund. (2014). *International profiles of health care systems, 2014: Australia, Canada, Denmark, England, France, Germany, Italy, Japan, the Netherlands, New Zealand, Norway, Singapore, Sweden, Switzerland, and the United States.* New York, NY: Commonwealth Fund. Retrieved from https://www.commonwealthfund.org/publications/fund-reports/2015/jan/international-profiles-health-care-systems-2014-australia-canada

Commonwealth Fund. (2017). *Health care system performance rankings.* New York, NY: Commonwealth Fund. Retrieved from https://www.commonwealthfund.org/chart/2017/health-care-system-performance-rankings

Council of the Federation. (2019, July 19). *Premiers committed to healthcare sustainability, call on federal government to be full partner.* Retrieved from https://www.canadaspremiers.ca/premiers-committed-to-healthcare-sustainability-call-on-federal-government-to-be-full-partner/

Edwards, N., Rowan, M., Marck, P., & Grinspun, D. (2011). Understanding whole systems change in health care: The case of nurse practitioners in Canada. *Policy, Politics, & Nursing Practice, 12*(1), 4–17.

Ennen, K. (2001). Shaping the future of practice through political activity: How nurses can influence health care policy. *American Association of Occupational Health Nurses (AAOH) Journal, 49*(12), 557–571.

Grinspun, D. (2007). Healthy workplaces: The case for shared clinical decision making and increased full-time employment. *Healthcare Papers, 7*(Sp), 85–91.

Grinspun, D. (2012). *Healthcare in a time of fiscal restraint: Collaborating for system sustainability,* Keynote address, McMaster University, 2012.

Grinspun, D., & Anyinam, C. (2014). Leadership. In S. Coffey & C. Anyinam (Eds.), *Interprofessional health care practice* (pp. 131–158). Toronto, ON: Pearson.

Grinspun, D., Botros, M., Mulrooney, L. A., Mo, J., Sibblad, R. G., & Penney, T. (2018). Scaling deep to improve people's health: From evidence-based practice to evidence-based policy. In D. Grinspun, & I. Bajnok (Eds.), *Transforming nursing through knowledge: Best practices for guideline development, implementation science, and evaluation* (pp. 465–494). Indianapolis, IN: Sigmabooks.

Gunderson, L. H., & Holling, C. S. (Eds.). (2002). *Panarchy: Understanding transformations in human and natural systems.* Washington, DC: Island Press.

Gunderson, L. H., Light, S. S., & Holling, C. S. (Eds.). (1995). *Barriers and bridges to the renewal of ecosystems and institutions.* New York, NY: Columbia University Press.

Health Quality Ontario. (2018). *Measuring up 2018.* Toronto, ON: Queen's Printer for Ontario. Retrieved from https://www.hqontario.ca/System-Performance/Yearly-Reports/Measuring-Up-2018

Liberal Party of Canada. (2015). *Real change: A new plan for a strong middle class.* Retrieved from https://www.liberal.ca/wp-content/uploads/2015/10/New-plan-for-a-strong-middle-class.pdf

Organisation for Economic Co-operation and Development (OECD). (2018). *Social expenditure database (SOCX).* Paris, FR: OECD. Retrieved from www.oecd.org/social/expenditure.htm

OECD. (2019). *Social expenditure—detailed data.* Paris, FR: OECD. Retrieved from https://stats.oecd.org/Index.aspx?DataSetCode=SOCX_DET

Registered Nurses Association of Ontario (RNAO). (2012a). *Enhancing community care for Ontarians (ECCO 1.0).* Toronto, ON: RNAO. Retrieved from http://rnao.ca/sites/rnao-ca/files/RNAO_ECCO_WHITE_PAPER_FINAL_2.pdf

RNAO. (2012b). *Primary solutions for primary care: Maximizing and expanding the role of the primary care nurse in Ontario.* Toronto, ON: RNAO. Retrieved from http://rnao.ca/sites/rnao-ca/files/Primary__Care_Report_2012_0.pdf

RNAO. (2013). *Developing and sustaining interprofessional health care.* Retrieved from http://rnao.ca/bpg/guidelines/interprofessional-team-work-healthcare

RNAO. (2014). *Queen's Park day—2014 briefing notes: Renewal of federal health accord.* Toronto, ON: RNAO. Retrieved from http://rnao.ca/policy/briefing-notes/queens-park-day-2014-briefing-notes

RNAO. (2020). *2019–2020 annual report.* Toronto, ON: RNAO.

Tomajan, K. (2012). Advocating for nurses and nursing. *Online Journal of Issues in Nursing, 17*(1), 4. doi: 10.3912/OJIN.Vol17No01Man04

Chapter 32

The Sustainability of Advanced Practice Nursing Roles in Canada

Esther Sangster-Gormley

ESTHER SANGSTER-GORMLEY is an Associate Professor and Associate Dean, Academic in the Faculty of Human and Social Development at the University of Victoria, Victoria, British Columbia. Much of her career has been as a nurse practitioner (NP), practicing in Florida until relocating to New Brunswick. She taught in the NP program at the University of New Brunswick, Fredericton, and currently lives and works in Victoria. Esther has been involved in efforts that contribute to NP role sustainability provincially and nationally. Over the last 10 years, her research focus has been the implementation and integration of NPs.

KEY TERMS

advanced practice nurses
  (APNs)
primary health care
sustainability

OBJECTIVES

1. Develop strategies to sustain the advanced practice nursing (APN) role within an organization.
2. Discuss ways of advocating for APN role sustainability.
3. Discuss contextual factors influencing APN role sustainability.

Introduction

The high cost of health care, aging demographics, and a global shortage of health care professionals are pressuring governments in Canada and worldwide to look for changes in how health care is delivered. Advanced practice nursing (APN) roles are gaining more international attention as an option for meeting health care demands. Currently approximately 50 countries have created or are in the process of creating APN roles (Kleinpell et al., 2014). As APN roles continue to evolve in Canada and around the world, it is important to consider the challenges that exist and the support necessary to ensure that clinical nurse specialists (CNSs), nurse practitioners (NPs), and other **advanced practice nurses (APNs)** are fully utilized and their roles are integrated and sustained within the health care system. In this chapter sustainability of advanced nursing roles means that they are essential to the health care system and will continue to be supported in the future.

Global Emergence of Advanced Practice Nursing Roles

Multiple factors are contributing to the willingness of international governments to recognize the contributions that nurses in advanced roles have made in other countries and consider creating further opportunities to utilize nursing's potential more fully. A shortage of physicians and other health care workers, increasing emphasis on primary health care, and the complexity of hospitalized patients are drivers that are influencing governments and organizations' willingness to extend nursing's capacity within health care. Likewise, nurses' demands for more career choices, along with opportunities to remain in clinical practice, have prompted decision makers to consider advanced nursing roles with increasing responsibility and autonomy (Schober & Affara, 2006). However, for a variety of reasons, there is variation in how APN roles are emerging globally.

A global definition of APN is a starting point toward consistency in how APN roles are described. The International Council of Nurses (ICN) consulted extensively to establish the definition, characteristics, and scope of practice of nurses in advanced roles. ICN defines *advanced practice nurses* as registered nurses (RNs) with expert knowledge, complex decision-making skills, and the clinical competence for practice beyond that of an RN. While a master's degree is recommended for entry to practice, the country and context within which advanced practice nurses are credentialed influences how their practice is enacted (ICN, 2019). This definition allows countries the latitude to adjust APN roles to meet their economic, social, and political context. Consistency in defining the role, regardless of country of origin, contributes to a better understanding of the roles.

Global Challenges to Advanced Practice Nursing Roles

The global emergence of new nursing roles is not without challenges. Most often differences in educational requirements, variation in scopes of practice and titles, and the nursing profession's strength and readiness to advance nursing to a higher level within the health care system impacts the uptake of APN roles (Kleinpell et al., 2014; Pulcini, 2014). Nursing leaders within organizations are vital to the introduction and sustainability of APN roles. At the same time, it must be acknowledged that the nursing profession's power base is stronger in some countries than in others. Consequently, the power differences between nursing and medicine will impact nursing leaders' capacity to launch and sustain APN roles.

Equally important, remuneration for health care services affects APN roles, particularly NPs. The ability to practice to full scope is limited in countries where regulatory and reimbursement structures restrict APNs from being directly reimbursed for the care they deliver. For example, in countries like Canada with universal government-sponsored health care, legislation may limit reimbursement for primary health care services to physicians on a fee-for-service basis. Box 32.1 is a summary of global challenges to APN sustainability.

BOX 32.1

Global Challenges to APN Sustainability

- Lack of uniform scope and standards of practice
- Country-specific regulations and legislation enabling the role varies
- Prescribing privileges differ among countries
- Inconsistent educational standards
- Requirements for physician supervision in some countries
- Reimbursement/remuneration for care provided is not available
- Role recognition and title protection varies with differing titles used
- Independent practice authority does not exist in some countries
- Variation in certification/registration requirements

Source: Adapted from Kleinpell, R., Scanlon, A., Hibbert, D., Ganz, F., East, L., Fraser, D., ... Beauchesne, M. (2014). Addressing issues impacting advanced nursing practice worldwide. *OJIN: The Online Journal of Issues in Nursing, 19*(2), Manuscript 5. doi: 10.3912/OJIN.Vol19NO02Man05; Sheer, B., & Wong, F. (2008). The development of advanced nursing practice globally. *Journal of Nursing Scholarship, 40*(3), 204–211.

It is important for Canadian APNs to be aware of global challenges to sustainability because often those challenges may be the same ones directly impacting Canadian NP and CNS practice.

Motivators for Advanced Practice Nursing Roles in Canada

Reforming the Canadian health care system has been advocated for years (Health Council of Canada, 2005) and can be traced back to 1978 and the World Health Organization's (WHO) meeting in Alma-Ata. The Declaration of Alma-Ata recognized that primary health care (PHC) should be essential care that is universally available to individuals, families, and communities and fosters self-reliance and self-determination (WHO, 1978). Over the years, numerous Canadian reports have highlighted the need for changes to the way PHC is delivered (Health Council of Canada, 2005; Lewis, 2004). National concerns previously identified included inadequate attention to health promotion and disease prevention, lack of continuity of patient care between providers and institutions, patients experiencing difficulty in obtaining access to care, and barriers to integrating primary care providers, such as NPs, into the health care system (Health Canada, 2007, 2012; Health Council of Canada, 2005).

As nursing's nationally recognized professional organization, the Canadian Nurses Association (CNA) has viewed the need to address PHC reform as an opportunity to strengthen nursing's position in the health care system and promote advanced nursing roles (CNA, 2007). CNA's vision for nursing includes nurse leaders using advanced technology to redesign care processes in acute and community care and establishing nurse-led models of care where a health promotion and prevention focus results in engaged patients and families. The CNA exerts influence on policy-makers through published reports and position statements articulating the contributions that all nurses, including NPs and CNSs, make to the health care system (CNA, 2013). Admittedly, increasing public and policy-makers' awareness of nursing's contributions is critically important; regrettably there are other issues that influence role sustainability.

Factors Affecting NP Role Sustainability

Sustaining APN roles is a complex process influenced by socio-political (macro-level), organizational (meso-level), and individual (micro-level) factors that are interconnected and work synergistically to facilitate or hinder sustainability (Champagne, 2002). Ongoing sustainability requires all sectors to work continuously and collaboratively over the long term. NPs provide an illustration of the complex process of implementing and sustaining an APN role.

NPs were introduced into the Canadian health care system almost 50 years ago, yet in 2018, less than 6,000 were registered in Canada (Canadian Institute for Health Information [CIHI], 2019). While the numbers are increasing, up from less than 4,000 in 2013, they still make up a small percentage of health care providers. Initially, in the 1980s and 1990s, NP sustainability was influenced by an oversupply of family physicians, limited public awareness and understanding of the role, and an absence of legislation and regulation legitimizing it. Other factors included the lack of government funding for educational programs, ambiguous support from organized medicine and nursing, and no identified funding models to support NP practice (Calnan & Fahey-Walsh, 2005; de Witt & Ploeg, 2005; Haines, 1993). Fortunately, the Canadian landscape has been changing over the years and many of these impediments have been remedied. Since the mid-1990s, there has been a resurgence of interest in the NP role by federal and provincial governments as a way to influence change in Canada's health care system (Hutchison, Abelson, & Lavis, 2001; Lewis, 2004; Romanow, 2002). Early expectations were that NPs would reduce the costs of health care, provide high-quality care (Sidani & Irvine, 1999), and increase access to health care services (DiCenso, Paech, & IBM Corporation, 2003). The ability of NPs to meet these expectations and thrive in our health care system continues to be influenced by the degree of administrative and physician support, acceptance by other practitioners, a clear rationale for the position, and legislation and regulation to support the role (van Soeren & Micevski, 2001).

Legislative and regulatory changes have occurred incrementally. Alberta led the way by enacting legislation for NP practice in 1996 and Ontario in 1998 (Kaasalainen et al., 2010). The last territory to enact legislation was Yukon in 2009, 13 years after Alberta. However, the early efforts to regulate NP practice were significant because it was the absence of legislation and regulation that, in part, was a major threat to sustainability. These changes have had a favourable influence on sustainable NP roles, but NP remuneration and lack of a legislated funding model continue to be a threat to NP sustainability.

Funding models for NP practice have consistently been identified as a barrier to role sustainability (DiCenso et al., 2010). A brief review of the Canadian Health Act might help to illuminate the NP remuneration issue. The Canadian Health Act ensures that eligible residents in all provinces and territories have reasonable access to necessary hospital, physician, and extended-care services. Extended care includes long-term residential and home care (Health Canada, 2019). Within provincial and territorial governments, ministries of health are responsible for administering health care financial resources. At the federal level, payment for acute and primary health care is limited to services provided through hospitals and by physicians and dentists. However, provincial and territorial governments have expanded the list of providers to include, for example, midwives, optometrists, and acupuncturists.

Currently, no provincial or territorial legislation includes NPs as service providers eligible for payment through their medical services plan. In all Canadian jurisdictions, NPs and CNSs are salaried employees of health authorities. This funding model relies on ministries of health to allocate additional money to health authorities to fund NP positions. In the case of the CNS, the health authority's global nursing budget funds CNS positions (DiCenso et al., 2010). Changes to the current funding model to allow NPs to be recognized and reimbursed are possible, but it will require provinces and territories to enact legislative changes to their Health Act and the political will to do so.

The Shifting Landscape

For more than a decade governments, regulators, educators, employers, and prospective NPs across Canada have expended substantial resources to implement or expand the NP role. For instance, in 2000 the Government of Canada funded the $800 million Primary Health Care Transition Fund (PHCTF; Health Canada, 2007) to support provincial and territorial initiatives to introduce new approaches to PHC delivery, including expanded efforts to integrate NPs in to the health care system. One pan-Canadian project that was funded through the PHCTF was the Canadian Nurse Practitioner Initiative (CNPI). Health Canada provided $8.9 million to the CNA through the PHCTF to fund CNPI. The initiative began in 2003 and was completed in 2006. Consultation with representatives of governments, nursing organizations, regulators, employers, educators, and other health professionals across Canada resulted in a framework for integration and sustainability of the NP role (CNPI, 2006). As a result of the CNPI, efforts to standardize educational programs and consistent NP legislation and regulation across the country have been ongoing (CNPI, 2006; DiCenso et al., 2010). The 2006 recommendations resulting from the CNPI are listed in Box 32.2.

Since 2006 the CNA has continued to collaborate with other professional associations; regulators; federal, provincial, and territorial governments; and health care organizations to implement the CNPI's recommendations. In 2016 CNA published a 10-year retrospective on the status of which CNPI recommendations had been achieved. Now the NP title is protected in all jurisdictions, meaning only those registered as an NP can use the title, a master's degree is required in all provinces, and efforts have been made to provide consistency in scope of practice and registration requirements (CNA, 2016a, 2016b). In 2012, the Canadian

BOX 32.2

2006 CNPI Recommendations

- Develop consistency in federal, provincial, and territorial legislation and regulation pertaining to NPs
- Implement consistent approaches to NP practice federally, provincially, and in territories
- Conduct a pan-Canadian needs-based human resource plan for NPs
- Implement a pan-Canadian approach to NP education
- Adopt the Implementation and Evaluation Toolkit as a guide to support ongoing implementation
- Devise a five-year pan-Canadian social marketing campaign to promote the NP role

Source: Adapted from CNPI. (2006). *Nurse practitioners: The time is now. A solution to improving access and reducing wait times in Canada.* Ottawa, ON: CNA. Retrieved from https://www.cna-aiic.ca/-/media/cna/page-content/pdf-en/01_integrated_report.pdf

Association of Schools of Nursing (CASN) created a national framework and guiding principles for NP education (CASN, 2012b). The education framework came about in response to concerns raised by educators, NPs, and nursing associations for national standards to guide NP education. The framework contributes to national consistency in preparation of NPs in Canada and sets graduate education as a requirement for entry to practice (CASN, 2012b).

Similarly, nursing regulators, working through the CNA, collaborated to develop core entry-level competencies for NP practice (CNA, 2010). The core competencies were used by CNA to develop the national NP registration examination. The landscape for NPs continues to shift toward more harmonization than differences, but the same cannot be said for CNSs.

Factors Affecting CNS Role Sustainability

While the CNS role has existed in Canada for 40 years, the number of CNSs has fluctuated, largely as a result of economic variables. In times of economic constraint, positions were eliminated, only to be reinstated or created when monies were available for reinvestment in health care. Currently, it is difficult to determine the number of CNSs employed in Canada. The CIHI's regulated nurses database includes the CNS role under "other positions," thus rendering the role invisible and difficult to track. Bryant-Lukosius (2010) found that from 2000 to 2008 the numbers of CNSs decreased from 2,624 to 2,222, and the numbers continue to decline (CNA, 2012). Reversing the decline will require policy and decision makers to allocate funding for new positions. However, the role continues to lack support from policy-makers who do not understand CNSs' contributions in the health care system (Bryant-Lukosius, 2010). Without the reallocation of funds for CNS positions, the sustainability of the role in Canada is questionable (CNA, 2012). Other factors are also influencing sustainability of the CNS role.

CNSs were introduced to promote nursing excellence in acute and community care. A primary function of CNSs was to educate and mentor nursing staff in the delivery of high-quality, evidence-informed care. They were expected to be a conduit for the uptake of knowledge generated through research and nursing staff's utilization of evidence to inform their practice (CNA, 2008). There are five key components of the CNS role: clinician, consultant, educator, researcher, and leader (CNA, 2009). Given the declining numbers of CNSs in Canada, the initial intent for the role has not been fully realized for a variety of reasons.

According to the CNA's (2019) advanced practice nursing pan-Canadian framework, CNSs are expected hold a master's or doctorate degree and demonstrate advanced nursing competencies. The CNS role is within the scope of practice of an RN and therefore regulators do not require additional registration or credentialing. In Canada the CNS title is not protected and an RN can assume the title without graduate education. This is currently occurring in Canada as employers have created CNS positions and hired baccalaureate-prepared RNs for them. The mismatch of professional expectations and employer implementation of the role is the result of misunderstanding of the role and minimum requirements for occupants of the CNS role (Kilpatrick et al., 2013). Lack of role clarity is symptomatic of the current Canadian landscape in which there are no standards for CNS education, and only 33% of universities offer CNS-specific educational programs (CASN, 2012a). What's more, there is very little Canadian research demonstrating the benefit of the CNS role or best practices to inform role implementation (Bryant-Lukosius et al., 2010).

Despite what seems to be a bleak outlook for the CNS role in Canada, there are changes occurring that will contribute to improving how the CNS role is understood. In 2014 the CNA began a pan-Canadian initiative to develop a common vision for the CNS role and determine core CNS competencies (Sutherland Boal, 2014). This work is vital to the sustainability of CNSs and will provide guidance and support for regulators, educators, employers, and CNSs. Establishing core CNS competencies is a major step in more precisely identifying the CNS role. However, without title protection, national standards for CNS education and mechanisms for credentialing CNSs' sustainability of the role will continue to be in question.

Conclusion

In reviewing the context of APN roles, it is clear that the future of these roles in the Canadian health care system will continue to be influenced by political and organizational context. APNs will be asked to provide evidence demonstrating their value and cost-effectiveness to patients and the health care system. Box 32.3 outlines strategies that can be undertaken by APNs, regulators, and educators to ensure these roles are sustained and thrive in the changing health care environment. Strategies to promote APN roles highlight work all APNs can undertake to become positive agents of change by advocating for the good of the public and professional growth. As leaders in the nursing profession, APNs cannot afford to passively wait for others to advance their roles. Sustainable roles will require APNs to take every opportunity to participate in policy discussions within their organizations and at provincial and federal levels that determine or affect their professional practice.

BOX 32.3

Strategies to Promote APN Role Sustainability

- Clearly define APN roles
- Standardize regulation and education of APNs
- Use a systematic process to implement new roles that are based on patient needs and stakeholder involvement
- Incorporate APN roles into federal and jurisdictional health and human resource planning
- Increase public awareness of APN roles through media campaigns that describe the value of APN care
- Establish innovative collaborative models to leverage APN knowledge, skills, and abilities
- Fund research into the value-added benefit of APNs
- Educate health ministries, administrative entities, credentialing committees, and medical staff about the practice of APNs to assist in updating hospital bylaws
- Encourage patients cared for by APNs to advocate for them as competent health care providers

Source: Adapted from DiCenso, A., Bryant-Lukosius, D., Martin-Misener, R., Donald, F., Abelson, J., Bourgeault, I.,... Haberman, P. (2010). Factors enabling advanced practice nursing role integration in Canada. *Nursing Leadership, 23*(Special Issue), 211–238; Kleinpell, R., Scanlon, A., Hibbert, D., Ganz, F., East, L., Fraser, D., ... Beauchesne, M. (2014). Addressing issues impacting advanced nursing practice worldwide. *OJIN: The Online Journal of Issues in Nursing, 19*(2), Manuscript 5. doi: 10.3912/OJIN.Vol19NO02Man05

Critical Thinking Questions

1. How has political context influenced APN role sustainability in Canada?
2. What might have happened if APN roles were introduced after a pan-Canadian approach to education, regulation, and legislation had been established?
3. What would you recommend if you were involved in introducing a new APN role to ensure its sustainability?

References

Bryant-Lukosius, D. (2010). The clinical nurse specialist role in Canada: Forecasting the future through research. *Canadian Journal of Nursing Research, 42*(2), 19–25.

Bryant-Lukosius, D., Carter, N., Kilpatrick, K., Martin-Misener, R., Donald, F., Kaasalainen, S., ... DiCenso, A. (2010). The clinical nurse specialist role in Canada. *Nursing Leadership, 23*(Special Issue), 140–166.

Calnan, R., & Fahey-Walsh, J. (2005). *Practice consultation initial report.* Ottawa, ON: CNPI. Retrieved from https://www.cna-aiic.ca/-/media/cna/page-content/pdf-en/02_practice_appendixa.pdf

Canadian Association of Schools of Nursing (CASN). (2012a). *Nursing masters education in Canada final report.* Ottawa, ON: CASN. Retrieved from https://www.casn.ca/2014/12/masters-education-canada/

CASN. (2012b). *Nurse practitioner education in Canada: National framework of guiding principles and essential components.* Ottawa, ON: CASN. Retrieved from https://casn.ca/wp-content/uploads/2014/12/FINALNPFrameworkEN20130131.pdf

Canadian Institute for Health Information (CIHI). (2019). *Nursing in Canada, 2018: A lens on supply and workforce.* Ottawa, ON: CIHI. Retrieved from https://www.cihi.ca/sites/default/files/document/regulated-nurses-2018-report-en-web.pdf

Canadian Nurse Practitioner Initiative (CNPI). (2006). *Nurse practitioners: The time is now. A solution to improving access and reducing wait times in Canada.* Ottawa, ON: CNA. Retrieved from https://www.cna-aiic.ca/-/media/cna/page-content/pdf-en/01_integrated_report.pdf

Canadian Nurses Association (CNA). (2007). *Advanced nursing practice: Position statement.* Ottawa, ON: CNA. Retrieved from http://www.cna-aiic.ca/en/download-buy/nurse-practitioners-clinical-nurse-specialists

CNA. (2008). *Advanced nursing practice: A national framework.* Ottawa, ON: CNA.

CNA. (2009). *Position statement: Clinical nurse specialist.* Ottawa, ON: CNA.

CNA. (2010). *Canadian nurse practitioner: Core competency framework.* Ottawa, ON: CNA. Retrieved from https://www.cna-aiic.ca/~/media/cna/files/en/competency_framework_2010_e.pdf

CNA. (2012). *Strengthening the role of the clinical nurse specialist in Canada: Background paper.* Ottawa, ON: CNA. Retrieved from http://cna-aiic.ca/~/media/cna/page-content/pdf-fr/strengthening_the_cns_role_background_paper_e.pdf

CNA. (2013). *Registered nurses: Stepping up to transform health care.* Ottawa, ON: CNA. Retrieved from http://www.cna-aiic.ca/~/media/cna/files/en/registered_nurses_stepping_up_to_transform_health_care_e.pdf

CNA. (2016a). *Position statement: Clinical nurse specialist.* Ottawa, ON: CNA. Retrieved from https://www.cna-aiic.ca/download-buy/nurse-practitioners-clinical-nurse-specialists

CNA. (2016b). *The Canadian nurse practitioner initiative: A 10-year retrospective.* Ottawa, ON: CNA. Retrieved from https://www.cna-aiic.ca/-/media/cna/page-content/pdf-en/canadian-nurse-practitioner-initiative-a-10-year-retrospective.pdf

CNA. (2019). *Advanced practice nursing: A pan-Canadian framework.* Ottawa, ON: CNA. Retrieved from https://www.cna-aiic.ca/-/media/cna/page-content/pdf-en/apn-a-pan-canadian-framework.pdf

Champagne, F. (2002). *The ability to manage change in health care organizations.* Discussion paper No. 39. Ottawa, ON: Commission on the Future of Health Care in Canada. Retrieved from http://publications.gc.ca/collections/Collection/CP32-79-39-2002E.pdf

de Witt, L., & Ploeg, J. (2005). Critical analysis of the evolution of a Canadian nurse practitioner role. *Canadian Journal of Nursing Research, 37*(4), 116–137.

DiCenso, A., Bryant-Lukosius, D., Martin-Misener, R., Donald, F., Abelson, J., Bourgeault, I., ... Haberman, P. (2010). Factors enabling advanced practice nursing role integration in Canada. *Nursing Leadership, 23*(Special Issue), 211–238.

DiCenso, A., Paech, P., & IBM Corporation. (2003). *Report on the integration of primary health care nurse practitioners into the province of Ontario.* Toronto, ON: MOHLTC.

Haines, J. (1993). *The nurse practitioner: A discussion paper.* Ottawa, ON: CNA.

Health Canada. (2007). *Primary health care transition fund.* Ottawa, ON: Health Canada. Retrieved from https://www.canada.ca/en/health-canada/services/primary-health-care/primary-health-care-transition-fund.html

Health Canada. (2012). *About primary health care.* Ottawa, ON: Health Canada. Retrieved from http://www.hc-sc.gc.ca/hcs-sss/prim/about-apropos-eng.php

Health Canada. (2019). *Canada health act annual report, 2017–2018.* Ottawa, ON: Health Canada. Retrieved from https://www.canada.ca/en/health-canada/services/health-care-system/reports-publications/canada-health-act-annual-reports.html

Health Council of Canada. (2005). *Health care renewal in Canada: Accelerating change.* Ottawa, ON: Carleton University. Retrieved from http://www.healthcouncilcanada.ca/

Hutchison, B., Abelson, J., & Lavis, J. (2001). Primary care in Canada: So much innovation, so little changes. *Health Affairs, 20*(3), 116–131.

International Council of Nurses (ICN). 2019. *Definition and characteristics of the role.* Geneva, CH: ICN. Retrieved from http://international.aanp.org/Practice/APNRoles

Kaasalainen, S., Martin-Misener, R., Kilpatrick, K., Harbman, P., Bryant-Lukosius, D., Donald, F., ... DiCenso, A. (2010). A historical overview of the development of advanced practice nursing roles in Canada. *Nursing Leadership, 23*(Special Issue), 35–60.

Kilpatrick, K., DiCenso, A., Bryant-Lukosius, D., Ritchie, J., Martin-Misener, R., & Carter, N. (2013). Practice patterns and perceived impact of clinical nurse specialist roles in Canada: Results of a national survey. *International Journal of Nursing Studies, 50*(11), 1524–1536.

Kleinpell, R., Scanlon, A., Hibbert, D., Ganz, F., East, L., Fraser, D., ... Beauchesne, M. (2014). Addressing issues impacting advanced nursing practice worldwide. *OJIN: The Online Journal of Issues in Nursing, 19*(2), Manuscript 5. doi: 10.3912/OJIN.Vol19NO02Man05

Lewis, S. (2004). *A thousand points of light? Moving forward in primary health care.* Winnipeg, MB: Primary Care Framework.

Pulcini, J. (2014). International development of advanced practice nursing. In A. B. Hamric, C. M. Hanson, M. R. Tracey, & E. T. O'Grady (Eds.), *Advanced practice nursing: An integrative approach* (5th ed., pp. 133–146). St. Louis, MO: Elsevier.

Romanow, R. (2002). *Building on values: The future of health care in Canada: Final report.* Saskatoon, SK: Commission on the Future of Health Care in Canada.

Schober, M., & Affara, F. (2006). *International Council of Nurses advanced nursing practice.* Malden, MA: Blackwell Publishing.

Sheer, B., & Wong, F. (2008). The development of advanced nursing practice globally. *Journal of Nursing Scholarship, 40*(3), 204–211.

Sidani, S., & Irvine, D. (1999). A conceptual framework for evaluating the nurse practitioner role in acute care settings. *Journal of Advanced Nursing, 30*(1), 58–66.

Sutherland Boal, A. (2014). Strengthening the CNS role. *Canadian Nurse, 110*(6), 19.

van Soeren, M., & Micevski, V. (2001). Success indicators and barriers to acute nurse practitioner role implementation in four Ontario hospitals. *American Association of Critical Care Nursing, 12*(3), 424–437.

World Health Organization (WHO). (1978). *Declaration of Alma-Ata. International conference on primary health care, Alma-Ata, USSR, 6–12, September, 1978.* Retrieved from http://www.who.int/publications/almaata_declaration_en.pdf

Chapter 33

Advanced Practice Nursing from a Global Perspective

Roberta Heale

ROBERTA HEALE is a Professor at Laurentian University, School of Nursing, and a nurse practitioner (NP)-PHC in Sudbury, Ontario. In 2006, Roberta and her NP colleague, Marilyn Butcher, were awarded the development of Canada's first NP-Led Clinic in Sudbury. Roberta's commitment to her profession is evident in her research related to the NP role and her ongoing practice as an NP. She served on the International NP/advanced practice nursing (APN) Network and is a past president of the Nurse Practitioner Association of Canada.

KEY TERMS

advanced practice nursing
   (APN)
barriers to APN roles
jurisdiction
nursing regulation
title protection

OBJECTIVES

1. Develop an understanding of the advanced practice nursing (APN) roles across the globe.
2. Reflect on global variations in educational, regulatory, and credentialing requirements for advanced practice nurses (APNs).
3. Understand the reasons for variation in scopes of practice of APNs across jurisdictions.
4. Review various facilitators and barriers to the development and implementation of APN roles.
5. Consider the role of APNs from jurisdictions with established advanced practice in supporting and promoting nursing globally.

Introduction

The first **advanced practice nursing (APN)** roles to be recognized were in the United States in the mid-1960s. The impetus for this was a shortage of physicians. During this time, registered nurses became authorized to perform some medical tasks (Duffield, Gardner, Chang, & Catling-Paull, 2009). Since then, APN roles have evolved in various forms across the globe

(Heale & RieckBuckley, 2015). APN is an umbrella term, referring to a registered nurse who works at a higher level than basic nursing (Sheer & Wong, 2008). The International Council of Nurses (ICN) defines APN as:

> a nurse practitioner/advanced practice nurse is a registered nurse who has ac-
> quired the expert knowledge base, complex decision-making skills and clinical
> competencies for expanded practice, the characteristics of which are shaped by
> the context and/or country in which s/he is credentialed to practice. A master's
> degree is recommended for entry level. (Nurse Practitioner/Advanced Practice
> Nursing Network [NP/APN Network], 2019a, para 2)

Where they exist, APN roles are operationalized in a unique manner in each jurisdiction. Unfortunately, the wide range of titles, educational and credentialing requirements, and scopes of practice has made it difficult to determine if a role is, in fact, representative of advanced practice. The result is extensive variations, and in many cases, confusion has led to difficulty with understanding the APN role across jurisdictions (Heale & RieckBuckley, 2015).

Evolution of APN Roles

APN roles evolved for a variety of reasons. In most countries, improved access to care was the catalyst for development of APN roles (Delamaire & Lafortune, 2010). The need for enhanced delivery of care to rural and remote locations promoted the initiation of APN roles in both Australia and Canada (Delamaire & Lafortune, 2010). Similarly, although Nicaragua doesn't have a recognized APN role, severe health care shortages in rural areas have resulted in nurses working in an advanced practice capacity (Sequeira et al., 2011).

Unmet health needs have also been a catalyst for APN role development. In Thailand, there were gaps in maternity services, so all advanced practice nurses (APNs) are trained as midwives in order to meet this need (Ketefian, Redman, Hanucharurnkul, Masterson, & Neves, 2001). More recently, aging populations and related increases in chronic diseases were the catalyst for a proposed model of geriatric NP care in Scandinavia to offset a gap in specialized primary health care for this population (Boman, Glasberg, Levy-Malmberg, & Fagerström, 2019).

Many worldwide health care systems have seen rapid expansions in both knowledge and technology. The associated costs of these system changes are high, as are costs in specific services, such as physician remuneration (Furlong & Smith, 2005; Heale & RieckBuckley, 2015). Ultimately, delegation of medical tasks to less expensive APNs has been a viable cost containment mechanism (Delamaire & Lafortune, 2010). In Cyprus, keeping the growth in health care costs in check was a main driver for the development of APN roles (Delamaire & Lafortune, 2010). In many countries, including Canada, improving quality of care is an expected outcome of the introduction of APNs, with the belief that improved quality of care may also result in cost savings to the health system (Delamaire & Lafortune, 2010).

Titles and Roles

There is a plethora of titles and job descriptions for APNs across the globe and even within certain jurisdictions (Heale & RieckBuckley, 2015). Table 33.1 provides a compilation of existing APN roles in a variety of countries. You will notice that the status of APN role development also varies.

TABLE 33.1: Country and APN Roles

Country	Roles
Afghanistan	none
Angola	CNS, NP
Argentina	none
Australia	APN, Clinical Nurse Consultant, CNS, NP
Austria	APN, NS
Bahamas	APN, Nurse Midwife, NP
Bangladesh	none
Belgium	*
Belize	Psychiatric NP
Bolivia	NP
Botswana	NP, NS
Cameroon	Nurse Anaesthetist, Nurse Midwife, Nurse Ophthalmologist
Canada	CNS, NP (Family/All Ages/PHC, Adult, Pediatrics or Neonatal)
Central African Republic	Nurse Anaesthetist
China	APN, CNS, NP
Colombia	*
Costa Rica	*
Cyprus	APN (Diabetic Nurse, Community Mental Health Nurse, Mental Health Nurse for Drug and Alcohol Addiction or Community Nurse)
Czech Republic	NS*
Denmark	NS
Fiji Islands	NP

(Continued)

TABLE 33.1: Continued

Country	Roles
Finland	APN, CNS
France	NS
Gambia	none
Germany	APN*
Greece	NS*
Hong Kong	APN, NS
India	NP*
Islamic Republic of Iran	APN, CNS, NP, NS
Republic of Ireland	Advanced Nurse Midwife, APN, CNS
Italy	CNS, NS
Japan	Certified Nurse Specialist
Kenya	Private Practice NP
Korea	APN
Lithuania	APN
Malaysia	CNS
Mexico	*
Mongolia	NP
Namibia	Midwifery and Neonatology Specialist Midwife, NS (critical care and psychiatry)
Netherlands	CNS, NP
New Zealand	APN, CNS, NP
Nicaragua	*
Norway	APN
Paraguay	none
Poland	CNS*, Nurse Midwife, NS*
Puerto Rico	NS
Russia	none
Samoa	NS

TABLE 33.1: Continued

Country	Roles
Sierra Leone	Nurse Anaesthetist, Nurse Midwife
Singapore	APN
Slovenia	none
South Africa	APN*
South Korea	APN
South Sudan	none
Spain	Specialized Nurse
Sri Lanka	none
Suriname	none
Swaziland	Nurse Midwife, NP
Sweden	APN
Switzerland	APN*
Taiwan	NP
Thailand	APN, CNS, NP, NS
Togo	APN, CNS, NP
United Kingdom	APN, CNS, Matron, Nurse Consultants
United States	CNS, Nurse Anaesthetist, Nurse Midwife, NP

Notes: APN = advanced practice nurse; CNS = clinical nurse specialist; NP = nurse practitioner; NS = nurse specialist; PHC = primary health care; * = under development

Sources: Adapted from Delamaire, M.-L., & Lafortune, G. (2010). *Nurses in advanced roles: A description and evaluation of experiences in 12 developed countries*. OECD Health Working Paper No. 54. Retrieved from https://www.oecd-ilibrary.org/docserver/5kmbrcfms5g7-en.pdf; Heale, R., & RieckBuckley, C. (2015). An international perspective of advanced practice nursing regulation. *International Nursing Review, 62*(3), 421–429. doi: 10.1111/inr.12193; International Advanced Practice Nursing (IAPN). (2017). *The role of advanced practice nursing internationally*. Geneva, CH: ICN. Retrieved from http://internationalapn.org/; Lindblad, E., Hallman, E.-B., Gillsjö, C., Lindblad, U., & Fagerström, L. (2010). Experiences of the new role of advanced practice nurses in Swedish primary health care—A qualitative study. *International Journal of Nursing Practice, 16*(1), 69–74. doi: 10.1111/j.1440-172X.2009.01810.x; Rafferty, A. M., Busse, R., Zander-Jentsch, B., Sermeus, W., & Bruyneel, L. (2019). *Strengthening health systems through nursing: Evidence from 14 European countries*. Health Policy Series, No. 52. Copenhagen, DK: WHO & European Observatory on Health Systems and Policies. Retrieved from https://apps.who.int/iris/bitstream/handle/10665/326183/9789289051743-eng.pdf; Sequeira, M., Espinoza, H., Amador, J. J., Domingo, G., Quintanilla, M., & de los Santos, T. (2011). *The Nicaraguan health system: An overview of critical challenges and opportunities*. Seattle, WA: PATH. Retrieved from https://path.azureedge.net/media/documents/TS-nicaragua-health-system-rpt.pdf; Sheer, B., & Wong, F. K. Y. (2008). The development of advanced nursing practice globally. *Journal of Nursing Scholarship, 40*(3), 204–211. doi: 10.1111/j.1547-5069.2008.00242.x; World Health Organization (WHO). (2019). *Global health workload alliance. Country responses*. Geneva, CH: WHO. Retrieved from https://www.who.int/workforcealliance/countries/countryprofiles/en/

Along with the variation in role titles, there is wide variation in APN practice. The scope of practice of APNs is typically understood to include such things as communicating a diagnosis, prescribing medication, ordering diagnostic testing, admitting to hospital, performing controlled medical acts such as intubation, and practicing independently or autonomously. However, the tasks associated with advanced practice differ considerably across jurisdictions. For example, clinical nurse specialists (CNSs) in Canada do not have separate regulation from the RN. Although several provinces in Canada have introduced limited RN prescribing, the authority to do so is related to specific education beyond the undergraduate degree and not related to their status as a clinical nurse specialist (Canadian Nurses Association [CNA], 2015). Currently, CNSs in Canada do not have the authority to autonomously order tests, diagnose, or prescribe. This is in contrast with CNSs in other countries, such as the United States (US), where many states have regulation that authorizes them to perform many of these tasks independently (Delamaire & Lafortune, 2010).

Not only are there differences in the scope of practice of APNs between countries, there are often differences in the authorized scope of practice for the same APN title in different jurisdictions within an individual country. Regulation for APN roles is developed for each state in the US. Legislation across the country has gone through many changes since the 1970s to a point only in recent years where a number of states now allow APNs independent broader prescribing authority. Despite these changes, only one-third of the states have implemented full practice authority licensure and practice laws for NPs. For example, in most states, NPs must still collaborate with a physician in order to prescribe (Hain & Fleck, 2014). There are slow, painstaking changes with individual lobbies in each state, such as a law that took effect on January 1, 2015, finally allowing NPs in New York State with 3,600 hours of practice experience to work without physician supervision through a collaborative agreement (American Association of Nurse Practitioners [AANP], 2019).

In countries where the APN role is in the developmental stage, nurses are often authorized to perform some, but not all, tasks associated with advanced practice. The recognition of APNs in Belgium, for example, hasn't officially occurred; however, some nursing programs at the graduate level are supporting the development of APN streams and nurses can perform some advanced tasks in hospital or primary health care such as consultation and referral to specialists and management of chronic diseases (Bruyneel, Van den Heede, & Sermeus, 2019).

Roles and responsibilities of APNs vary within a jurisdiction. In the United Kingdom (UK), being a CNS does not necessarily mean that the nurse is able to diagnose, treat autonomously, or use advanced decision-making and judgment in practice (Delamaire & Lafortune, 2010). In addition, all basic nurses in the UK can prescribe medications as long as they have a baccalaureate degree, three years' experience, and successfully completed a program that includes 26 days of theory and 12 days in practice (Delamaire & Lafortune, 2010).

Regulation

There are several methods of regulating health care providers. Two main types of **nursing regulation** are state-based, and profession-based (ICN, 2009). Regulation of health care providers may occur by statute or government decree or through a professional body (Bryant, 2005). In some cases, there is separate legislation for both basic nursing as well as APN roles. In other situations, APN roles are legitimized through credentialing processes, but do not require a separate legislation or licence beyond the basic nursing criteria (DiCenso & Bryant-Lukosius, 2010). Employers, through their organizational objectives and policies, may restrict the APN role and impose a form of regulation (Bryant, 2005). In many cases, changes to existing regulation in a jurisdiction are required to eliminate barriers to the expanded scope of practice of APNs (Delamaire & Lafortune, 2010).

Control over the nursing profession varies. While across Canada, nursing colleges have an important role in the governance of nursing through self-regulation, in many countries powerful governmental influence and political priorities have a strong impact on APN roles both through funding as well as policy development (Heale & RieckBuckley, 2015). The result is that in some countries the nursing profession is managed by a branch of government rather than by an independent nursing college. Thus, while it is within the mandate of the nursing profession to ensure the development of appropriate competencies and standards for APN practice are related to legislation, at times this is not the case.

Where regulation for APNs exists, it typically outlines the specific authority that is granted to the APN. This is often the basis for the scope of practice, or practice standards. Some regulation is very specific and restrictive, while other regulation provides more flexibility in the manner in which the APN role is implemented. The UK has the least restrictive regulation while the US has the most restrictive (Ketefian et al., 2001). In the UK, there is only the basic nursing licence. Nurses are given APN status through training programs, which prepare them for expanded scope of practice (Ball, Rafferty, & Philippou, 2019). In the US, legislation beyond that required for basic RN licensure specifically outlines the tasks that APNs are authorized to perform (Delamaire & Lafortune, 2010; Kruth, 2013).

The existence and type of APN regulation may also include **title protection** for the APN role. Title protection ensures that only those officially authorized to do so are able to practice under an APN title. Although this is the ideal, the reality is that many countries do not have protected titles for APN roles (Heale & RieckBuckley, 2015).

Regulation of the APN role may also be centralized or decentralized. Decentralized regulation often results in different legislation and scope of practice of APNs in different jurisdictions within a specific country. This is the case in both Canada and the US. An APN in one province or state may have difficulty with portability of their licence across jurisdictions. In order to avoid this situation, Australia passed legislation in 2010 that harmonized APN legislation in that country (Delamaire & Lafortune, 2010).

Regulation, or at least official authorization of APN roles, is essential for their successful implementation. This is a difficult objective given that some countries are in the early stages of registering basic nursing and will not be able to develop APN roles for some time. Argentina, for example, only started the process of a national licensing registry for nurses in 2008 (Ministerio de Salud, n.d.).

Inconsistencies in the regulation of APN roles across countries result in differences in clinical practice of the same roles in different jurisdictions. For example, CNSs do not have separate regulation from that of the registered nurse in Canada (DiCenso & Bryant-Lukosius, 2010), while many states in the US have regulated the CNS role, including such things as title protection, diagnosing, and prescribing authority (Delamaire & Lafortune, 2010). Although the focus of practice is similar in both countries whereby the CNS manages disease and promotes health among clients, families, and communities, the regulation of the CNS role in the US offers those practitioners an expanded practice framework and some protection that is not available to their Canadian counterparts.

Educational Requirements

In many circumstances, regulation and/or registration boards determine the practice criteria for APN roles. These boards must ensure that nurses are able to safely and effectively meet the competencies of the role, which points to the need for appropriate educational programs. Also required are processes for review of the quality of education, the development of continuing education opportunities, and if required, procedures for re-licensing and measurement of ongoing competencies (Bryant, 2005).

Educational institutions and nursing organizations that support APN roles have a responsibility to deliver APN programs that will ensure that graduates are able to meet competencies required for safe and effective practice (Furlong & Smith, 2005). Policy and documentation related to the competencies of the APN role should precede the development of educational programs; however, this has often not been the case. One example is the consortium NP educational program in Ontario, which was developed and delivered for several years prior to the enactment of legislation to support nurse practitioner practice (Nurse Practitioners' Association of Ontario [NPAO], 2011).

Many countries and/or jurisdictions do not have graduate preparation for entry to practice for APNs (Delamaire & Lafortune, 2010; Sheer & Wong, 2008). Despite the development of graduate nursing education programs, in some countries, such as Brazil, these are seen to be assigned to those who will conduct research rather than for advanced practice training and there continue to be no clinical advanced practice roles (IAPN, 2017; Ketefian et al., 2001).

Barriers to the Development of APN Roles and APN Practice Internationally

There are many obstacles to the successful development and implementation of APN roles (Heale & RieckBuckley, 2015). Specific barriers to the development of APN roles and growth of APN practice vary considerably; however, some common themes have emerged. The most prominent **barrier to APN roles** has been and remains opposition by physicians (Delamaire & Lafortune, 2010; Heale & RieckBuckley, 2015). In Thailand, physician opposition to NP initiatives squelched the development of APN roles for several years (Ketefian et al., 2001). In 2011 it was reported that the Australian Medical Association had "very deep concerns" about the safety of patient care in a new NP-Led Clinic (Miles, 2011). Physician organizations have blocked and opposed expanding NP regulation in every US state (Hain & Fleck, 2014). Similar examples of physician opposition to APN roles are repeated across the globe. Physicians have authority and are on the top of a hierarchy of power and influence in almost all health care systems (Hain & Fleck, 2014).

There are other barriers to APN roles, which occur independent of, or simultaneous to, physician opposition. Nursing leadership is essential in influencing health care policy, and APN role development and implementation. However, skill level and motivation of nursing organizations to evoke change can be an obstacle to the development and implementation of these roles (Delamaire & Lafortune, 2010; Heale & RieckBuckley, 2015). This is the case in Mexico, where, although nurses are able to specialize in intensive or critical care as of 2013, there was no specific APN role in that country largely due to the lack of nursing leadership in health care (Kruth, 2013).

The development and progress of APN roles is impeded by such things as health policy and decision makers' lack of recognition of the APN contribution (Villegas & Allen, 2012). Restrictive legislation and regulation continue to be an issue in many countries (Delamaire & Lafortune, 2010; Villegas & Allen, 2012). Also, cultural considerations, including the value and role of women in a society, help to shape the expectations for nursing roles (Delamaire & Lafortune, 2010).

Ongoing evaluation of APN roles and research evidence to support the value and quality of APN care is required. Although there is considerable evidence about well-established APN roles, there is little or no evidence about emerging ones. Adding further difficulty is that comparisons with APN evaluation from other countries is difficult given the wide variation in context among APN roles across jurisdictions (Brooten, Youngblut, Deosires, Singhala, & Guido-Sanz, 2012).

In many countries, the numbers of APNs compared to the numbers of nurses are small. During the first decade of the new millennium, CNSs were well established in Canada, and NP roles were being regulated and implemented across the country. However, in 2008 NPs represented 0.6% and CNSs 0.9% of all registered nurses in the country (Delamaire & Lafortune, 2010). Where regulation for an APN role does not exist, the numbers practicing in the role may not be monitored. It is often difficult for APN concerns to be heard and addressed given the low numbers and even more difficult if there is no system for tracking. In the Bahamas, "nurse midwife" is considered an APN role. In other countries, such as Canada, midwifery is not a nursing role but a separate health care provider category altogether.

A poor understanding about the scope of practice of APNs is a barrier. Organizational propensity to view APNs as physician replacement and to limit APN practice inhibits the potential of APNs (Delamaire & Lafortune, 2010; Hain & Fleck, 2014). Role conflict, role overload, and variable stakeholder acceptance are further examples of barriers to the implementation of APN in health care (Heale & RieckBuckley, 2015).

Reimbursement and remuneration of health care providers, including APNs, are other barriers globally (Palumbo, Marth, & Rambur, 2011; Villegas & Allen, 2012). An example is fee-for-service in primary health care, where the introduction of APNs could result in reduced income for the physician, whereas capitation, performance-based, and salaried physician remuneration models are more likely to encourage the development of APN roles (Delamaire & Lafortune, 2010).

Many countries deal with multiple levels of barriers to APN practice. During the development of APN roles in the US, barriers in some states included remuneration of APNs at less than physicians for similar work, professional liability insurance, staff privilege issues, designation as a primary care provider, and prescriptive authority are simultaneously issues affecting APN practice (Ketefian et al., 2001). Many of these barriers to APN practice remain (Hain & Fleck, 2014).

International Focus

The varied nomenclature used to describe APN roles and variation in regulation, educational standards, and scope of practice speak to the need for a common understanding of APN roles, including consensus on competencies (Heale & RieckBuckley, 2015). The need for a consistent approach to the development and implementation of APN roles has been widely acknowledged. Countries across the globe recognize the need for APN roles to have international standards for regulation, education, titles, an identified scope of practice, and core components of practice (Currie, Edwards, Colligan, & Crouch, 2007; Duffield et al., 2009; Heale & RieckBuckley, 2015). At the same time, the ICN (2009) identified the importance for every nurse to enter into policy debates that influence their profession rather than remaining passive and allowing others to determine nursing practice in their country. This will ensure that nurses become constructive change agents for the benefit of the public as well as for professional growth.

There are numerous strategies for the nursing profession to ensure relevance and promote APN roles. Nursing organizations have an opportunity to determine trends and unmet health care needs in their country and mobilize to address these needs through specialized APN services. Examples of these include Japan, which recognized the population was aging and implemented an aging strategy; the care of AIDS patients in the US; or Brazil targeting the younger population and their needs such as smoking cessation (Ketefian et al., 2001). Similarly, NP practice in New Zealand was targeted at aging populations in primary health care (Carryer & Yarwood, 2015).

Nurses and nursing organizations may lack the knowledge and skills to advocate, develop, and implement APN roles. To address this concern, the ICN's NP/APN Network was established in 2000 to facilitate communication among representatives of countries with existing APN roles with those in development (Sheer & Wong, 2008). The NP/APN Network has additional objectives, including making timely and relevant information about NP and APN practice across the globe readily available, providing a forum for sharing knowledge and expertise, and providing support for NPs and APNs (NP/APN Network, 2019b).

As APNs lobby for and implement positive changes to their practices, it's important to consider the role of APNs in supporting the role of nursing in underdeveloped parts of the world. Countries such as Afghanistan, Burkina Faso, and El Salvador have been riddled by conflict for decades. Others, such as Chad, Mali, and Zimbabwe, are some of the poorest in the world. These, along with countless other countries, have enormous physician and nurse to population ratios and few health care resources (WHO, 2019). As leaders and experts not only in clinical health care services but also in education and administration, APNs have an opportunity to provide tangible support for nursing in countries with little to no human health resources. In future, the vision of the NP/APN Network may be to expand the organizational gaze beyond that of the well-developed or well-organized countries who have the resources to participate.

Conclusion

APN roles are recognized in many countries around the globe. Their development and implementation arose for a variety of reasons, most notably to increase access to care in areas with gaps in health care and physician services. These roles vary widely with respect to educational requirements, regulation, and scope of practice. Although many barriers continue to exist in the development and implementation of APN roles, the NP/APN Network provides a forum for nurses and nursing organizations to learn from and support one another in the success of APNs across the globe.

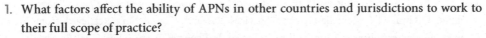

Critical Thinking Questions

1. What factors affect the ability of APNs in other countries and jurisdictions to work to their full scope of practice?
2. Compare and contrast mechanisms that authorize practice for APNs in the UK with NP and CNS roles in Canada.
3. You are a nurse and interested in advocating for the development of an APN role in your jurisdiction. What strategies could you implement to assist in the development of the role? What organizations or institutions would you contact to facilitate your goal? Why?

References

American Association of Nurse Practitioners (AANP). (2019). *State practice environment.* Austin, TX: AANP. Retrieved from https://www.aanp.org/legislation-regulation/state-legislation/state-practice-environment/66-legislation-regulation/state-practice-environment/1380-state-practice-by-type

Ball, J., Rafferty, A. M., & Philippou, J. (2019). England. In A. M. Rafferty, R. Busse, B. Zander-Jentsch, W. Sermeus, & L. Bruyneel (Eds.), *Strengthening health systems through nursing: Evidence from 14 European countries* (pp. 17–30). Health Policy Series, No. 52. Copenhagen, DK: WHO & European Observatory on Health Systems and Policies. Retrieved from https://apps.who.int/iris/bitstream/handle/10665/326183/9789289051743-eng.pdf

Boman, E., Glasberg, A.-L., Levy-Malmberg, R., & Fagerström, L. (2019). "Thinking outside the box": Advanced geriatric nursing in primary health care in Scandinavia. *BioMed Central (BMC) Nursing, 18*(1), 1–9. https://doi.org/10.1186/s12912-019-0350-2

Brooten, D., Youngblut, J. M., Deosires, W., Singhala, K., & Guido-Sanz, F. (2012). Global considerations in measuring effectiveness of advanced practice nurses. *International Journal of Nursing Studies, 49*(7), 906–912. doi: 10.1016/j.ijnurstu.2011.10.022

Bruyneel, L., Van den Heede, K., & Sermeus, W. (2019). Belgium. In A. M. Rafferty, R. Busse, B. Zander-Jentsch, W. Sermeus, & L. Bruyneel (Eds.), *Strengthening health systems through nursing: Evidence from 14 European countries* (pp. 3–16). Health Policy Series, No. 52. Copenhagen, DK: WHO & European Observatory on Health Systems and Policies. Retrieved from https://apps.who.int/iris/bitstream/handle/10665/326183/9789289051743-eng.pdf

Bryant, R. (2005). *Regulation, roles and competency development.* Geneva, CH: ICN.

Canadian Nurses Association (CNA). (2015). *Framework for registered nurse prescribing in Canada.* Ottawa, ON: CNA. Retrieved from https://www.cna-aiic.ca/~/media/cna/page-content/pdf-en/cna-rn-prescribing-framework_e.pdf

Carryer, J., & Yarwood, J. (2015). The nurse practitioner role: Solution or servant in improving primary health care service delivery. *Collegian, 22*(2), 169–174. doi: 10.1016/j.colegn.2015.02.004

Currie, J., Edwards, L., Colligan, M., & Crouch, R. (2007). A time for international standards? Comparing the emergency nurse practitioner role in the UK, Australia and New Zealand. *Accident and Emergency Nursing, 15*(4), 210–216. doi: 10.1016/j.aaen.2007.07.007

Delamaire, M.-L., & Lafortune, G. (2010). *Nurses in advanced roles: A description and evaluation of experiences in 12 developed countries.* OECD Health Working Paper No. 54. Retrieved from https://www.oecd-ilibrary.org/docserver/5kmbrcfms5g7-en.pdf

DiCenso, A., & Bryant-Lukosius, D. (2010). *Clinical nurse specialists and nurse practitioners in Canada.* Ottawa, ON: Canadian Health Services Research Foundation. Retrieved from http://wwwcfhi-cassca/Libraries/Commissioned_Research_Reports/Dicenso_EN_Finalsflbashx

Duffield, C., Gardner, G., Chang, A. M., & Catling-Paull, C. (2009). Advanced nursing practice: A global perspective. *Collegian Journal of the Royal College of Nursing Australia, 16*(2), 55–62. doi: 10.1016/j.colegn.2009.02.001

Furlong, E., & Smith, R. (2005). Advanced nursing practice: Policy, education and role development. *Journal of Clinical Nursing, 14*(9), 1059–1066. doi: 10.1111/j.13652702.2005.01220.x

Hain, D., & Fleck, L. (2014). Barriers to NP practice that impact healthcare redesign. *The Online Journal of Issues in Nursing, 19*(2), Manuscript 2. Retrieved from http://ojin.nursingworld.org/MainMenuCategories/ANAMarketplace/ANAPeriodicals/OJIN/TableofContents/Vol-19-2014/No2-May-2014/Barriers-to-NP-Practice.html

Heale, R., & RieckBuckley, C. (2015). An international perspective of advanced practice nursing regulation. *International Nursing Review, 62*(3), 421–429. doi: 10.1111/inr.12193

International Advanced Practice Nursing (IAPN). (2017). *The role of advanced practice nursing internationally.* Geneva, CH: ICN. Retrieved from http://internationalapn.org/

International Council of Nurses (ICN). (2009). *Regulation 2020: Exploration of the present; Vision for the future.* Geneva, CH: ICN.

Ketefian, S., Redman, R. W., Hanucharurnkul, S., Masterson, A., & Neves, E. P. (2001). The development of advanced practice roles: Implications in the international nursing community. *International Nursing Review, 48*, 152–163.

Kruth, T. (2013). Advanced practice nursing in Mexico. *International Advanced Practice Nursing.* Geneva, CH: ICN. Retrieved from http://internationalapn.org/2013/08/15/mexico/

Lindblad, E., Hallman, E.-B., Gillsjö, C., Lindblad, U., & Fagerström, L. (2010). Experiences of the new role of advanced practice nurses in Swedish primary health care—A qualitative study. *International Journal of Nursing Practice, 16*(1), 69–74. doi: 10.1111/j.1440-172X.2009.01810.x

Miles, J. (2011). Nurse practitioner led clinic to open in Brisbane amid concerns of the Australian Medical Association. *The Courier Mail.* Retrieved from https://www.couriermail.com.au/news/queensland/need-a-doctor-get-a-nurse/news-story/d38f6c9b4d11389579704cdf120a25a3?sv=fa8c-f9c38d02a141a9edfd7362cdaed1

Ministerio de Salud. (n.d.). *Registro unico de profesionales de salud.* Retrieved from https://www.argentina.gob.ar/solicitar-turno-en-linea-al-registro-unico-de-profesionales-de-la-salud

Nurse Practitioner/Advanced Practice Nursing Network (NP/APN Network). (2019a). *Definition and characteristics of the role.* Geneva, CH: ICN. Retrieved from https://international.aanp.org/Practice/APNRoles

NP/APN Network. (2019b). *Network history 1992–2018.* Geneva, CH: ICN. Retrieved from http://international.aanp.org/About/History

Nurse Practitioners' Association of Ontario (NPAO). (2011). *Nurse practitioner history in Ontario.* Toronto, ON: NPAO.

Palumbo, M. V., Marth, N., & Rambur, B. (2011). Advanced practice registered nurse supply in a small state: Trends to inform policy. *Policy, Politics, & Nursing Practice, 12*(1), 27–35. doi: 0.1177/1527154411404244

Rafferty, A. M., Busse, R., Zander-Jentsch, B., Sermeus, W., & Bruyneel, L. (2019). *Strengthening health systems through nursing: Evidence from 14 European countries.* Health Policy Series, No. 52. Copenhagen, DK: WHO & European Observatory on Health Systems and Policies. Retrieved from https://apps.who.int/iris/bitstream/handle/10665/326183/9789289051743-eng.pdf

Sequeira, M., Espinoza, H., Amador, J. J., Domingo, G., Quintanilla, M., & de los Santos, T. (2011). *The Nicaraguan health system: An overview of critical challenges and opportunities.* Seattle, WA: PATH. Retrieved from https://path.azureedge.net/media/documents/TS-nicaragua-health-system-rpt.pdf

Sheer, B., & Wong, F. K. Y. (2008). The development of advanced nursing practice globally. *Journal of Nursing Scholarship, 40*(3), 204–211. doi: 10.1111/j.1547-5069.2008.00242.x

Villegas, W. J., & Allen, P. E. (2012). Barriers to advanced practice registered nurse scope of practice: Issue analysis. *Journal of Continuing Education in Nursing, 43*(9), 403–409. doi: 10.3928/00220124-20120716-30

World Health Organization (WHO). (2019). *Global health workforce alliance. Country responses.* Geneva, CH: WHO. Retrieved from https://www.who.int/workforcealliance/countries/countryprofiles/en/

Chapter 34

Future Directions of Advanced Practice Nursing in Canada

Eric Staples

ERIC STAPLES is an Independent Nursing Practice Consultant. He was a graduate of the first postgraduate Acute Care Nurse Practitioner (ACNP) certificate program in Ontario in 1995 from the University of Toronto, and has held Assistant Professor roles at Dalhousie University, Halifax, Nova Scotia, where he was involved in implementing the Advanced Nursing Practice stream in 1998; McMaster University, Hamilton, Ontario, as NP Coordinator in the Ontario Primary Health Care Nurse Practitioner (PHCNP) Program; and the University of Regina, Regina, Saskatchewan. Eric serves or has served on several CASN committees related to NP education, preceptorship, prescribing, and the development of the position statement on doctoral education in Canada. He was the lead developer and editor for the inaugural edition of *Canadian Perspectives in Advanced Practice Nursing*, published in 2016 and in French in 2017.

KEY TERMS

advanced practice nursing
   (APN) roles
licensure
preceptorship
regulations
remuneration
role development and
   implementation

OBJECTIVES

1. Explore the current key issues impacting on future APN practice in Canada.
2. Identify how APN roles and education are responding to health care system changes across Canada.

Introduction

Since 2011, the first year Canada's baby boomers began turning 65, there has been an acceleration in the number of seniors. In 2018, 17.2% of Canada's population was 65 and older compared to 14.4% in 2011. In 2018, there were 106 adults 65 and over for every 100 children aged 0–14 years (Statistics Canada, 2019). With an aging population, the demand for health care is growing exponentially, driven primarily by rising chronic diseases. Within a health system milieu that continues to see a shortage of both physicians and nurses, increasing complexity, and pressures to contain costs, **advanced practice nursing (APN) roles** can assist in meeting these growing needs. Where nursing shortages exist, the development of more APN roles are occurring. APN role development is considered a factor in increasing and retaining nursing rates because the roles lead to enhancement of nursing career prospects (MacDonald-Rencz & Bard, 2010).

During the last decade, the number of nurse practitioners (NPs) has more than doubled, which has resulted in a 25% increase over a one-year period (Picard, 2018). Between 2017 and 2018, there was an 8% increase, the highest growth among all regulated nursing groups in Canada, to 5,697 NPs in Canada (Canadian Institute for Health Information [CIHI], 2019).

In spite of these positive findings, APN roles must continue to be promoted, integrated, and sustained. New APN roles should only be introduced based on evidence of or in response to the health care needs that have been identified for Canadians. For many years, the Canadian Nurses Association (CNA) has supported the need for a common framework that would include needs-based planning. This framework would anticipate health care needs based on demographic, epidemiological, and cultural factors, and includes benchmarking for regional variation, and a review of specialty mix within and between disciplines (CNA, 2006). This aligns well with models of interprofessional collaboration and practice.

Moving toward the Future

Health care policy-makers and administrators are being required to seek new opportunities that would enhance health care delivery. We are seeing this in many health care sectors where there appears to be a move away from traditional role boundaries toward a mix of health professionals to provide health care (MacDonald-Rencz & Bard, 2010). In Canada, the expansion of nursing roles—for example, registered nurse prescribing—is occurring within regulatory and practice frameworks. Initiatives such as this are occurring in an effort to reorganize health service delivery, increase timely accessibility to health care services, and drive down overall health care costs (CNA, 2015; Canadian Nurses Protective Society [CNPS], 2017).

The PEPPA framework, which is the participatory, evidence-based, patient-focused process for guiding the development, implementation, and evaluation of an APN framework (Bryant-Lukosius & DiCenso, 2004), remains the most well-accepted and supported model in Canada for planning, preparing, and evaluating APN roles. Research data has identified key areas that will further the implementation of APN roles. Positive outcomes from NP practice, such as improved access and timely health care services, have consistently been identified, but more research is required to identify the economic impact of NPs across all health care practice sectors and settings.

The impact of the clinical nurse specialist (CNS) role in Canada, however, remains obscure due to a continued lack of regulation, credentialing, and title protection. With changes occurring in the nursing workforce mix, the CNS role is seen as a collaborative role that will lead interprofessional teams. This may be true as it is becoming even more critical for supporting nurses and providing clinical expertise. As the adoption of health care models based on interprofessional collaboration become more widespread, a unique opportunity exists to identify niches that are best filled by all APNs.

The evolution of APN has aligned with renewed focus in patient-centred care along with demonstrating the expertise required to remain on the leading edge of clinical and technological health care advancements. Clinical leadership, support for nursing staff, and the advancement of research are uniting forces that can lead to improved patient outcomes and satisfaction. Indicators measuring patient outcomes, and the cost benefits of APN, will be influential for developing more APN role opportunities. The variability in CNS specialties continues to make it more difficult to capture the same type of evaluative data that can be found in the NP literature (Bryant-Lukosius, 2010; MacDonald-Rencz & Bard, 2010).

Role Development and Implementation

Successful **role development and implementation** is key to the full integration of APNs across Canada. A pan-Canadian approach has been supported by the investments from the CNA (2008, 2019) and the Canadian Nurse Practitioner Initiative (CNPI; 2006), which coordinate areas of recruitment; interprofessional collaboration and practice; education standards; and legislation and regulation that clarify APN roles, titles, and scopes of practice (DiCenso et al., 2010b). In relation to the CNS, there has been a call not only to establish funding for the role, but also for a research program, to span 10 years or more, that will address implementation and outcomes of CNS practice (Bryant-Lukosius, 2010; CNA, 2012). This would be critical to potential future regulation and credentialing of the CNS role across Canada, but has yet to be operationalized.

Financial investments, including stakeholder commitment required to create, support, and sustain NP roles, as well as those relating to remuneration, have been well described by Donald et al. (2010) and Kilpatrick et al. (2010). For example, in Ontario, to address vacancy rates of NP positions in primary health care (PHC) and as a mechanism to increase the number of PHCNPs, Health Force Ontario in 2006 introduced the Grow Your Own NP, which was updated in 2015 to reflect changes in the health care environment. In this program, government funding, already allocated to organizations for PHCNP positions, could be used to sponsor an RN to complete an approved NP program in return for service upon completion with the sponsoring organization. This program continues to operate (Health Force Ontario, 2015; Health Workforce Planning Branch, 2019). More recently, the Ontario government has launched the Attending Nurse Practitioners in Long-Term Care Homes Initiative (2019) designed to improve the quality of life and care of residents in long-term care homes by funding 75 new PHCNP positions (Health Workforce Planning Branch, 2019).

To address continued barriers for APN role development and integration, DiCenso et al. (2010a) clearly articulated, from what was heard at the Canadian Health Services Research Foundation (CHSRF) roundtable, the need for clearly defined APN roles and titling; role development based on identified client, community, and/or stakeholder needs; stable funding for the role; increased awareness of the role; and ongoing research that demonstrates the value the role brings, which may be critical to sustainability of APN roles.

A shortage of physicians continues to play a role in the growth of the NP as government efforts continue to shift care to the community. Trends suggest that graduates from NP programs will be integrated into new models of PHC delivery. Many are working in community health centres, others in PHC services such as the family health team (FHT) or in NP-Led Clinics, and they remain the backbone of rural and remote PHC services in Canada (Wong & Farrally, 2013).

Although employment in PHC has been important, there are many NPs working in acute care. Sectors identified include cardiology and cardiovascular surgery, geriatrics, medicine, pediatrics, nephrology, trauma, palliative care, oncology, and neonatology. NPs are also employed in emergency departments and are increasingly employed in ambulatory specialty areas, such as oncology, in hospitals (Wong & Farrally, 2013). Thus, the contextual factors that prompted the creation of the acute care nurse practitioner (ACNP) role, including the increased complexity of care, the need for long-term management of chronic conditions, and aging of the population, appear to be influencing a continued need for this type of NP; however for some, the issue of funding/reimbursement models within the acute care sectors continue to challenge full integration in these areas.

Advanced Practice Nursing Education, Practice, and Licensure

NP programs are offered in 28 NP university programs in Canada, graduating over 500 NPs yearly (Canadian Association of Schools of Nursing [CASN], 2017, 2019). The number of NP students increased by 1.8% in 2017/2018 with over 700 students entering programs. Graduates also increased by 1.6% (564) in 2018 compared to the previous year (CASN, 2019). In contrast, it was reported that less than 10 full-time faculty were engaged in teaching graduate-level NP education, and schools reported approximately 45% shortage of NP, graduate, and doctorally prepared nurses seeking academic positions to teach in APN programs (CNA & CASN, 2013).

Although we have consensus in Canada that graduate-level preparation be the minimal standard for APN programs, there continues, at times, to be a mismatch between the education levels obtained and the practice setting where NPs are employed. The data suggest that in fact, many nurses educated in PHC are being employed in specialized areas of acute care.

As NP programs in Canada are at a generalist level, with the exception of neonatology education and specialist education in Quebec, the result is that generalist-prepared NPs may work in specialized areas they were not educated for but are expected to have the competencies to practice in (Martin-Misener et al., 2010).

Some stakeholders in Canada believe that national curriculum standards and a consistent core curriculum for NP programs are required, while others have voiced concern with the rigidity of such an approach (Martin-Misener et al., 2010). Although Canada is a vast country, there are relatively only a small number of APNs in relation to the large number and range of specialty areas, which are a further barrier in how specialist education can be included in educational programs (DiCenso et al., 2010b).

There are, however, course commonalities across Canadian NP programs that include courses in advanced health assessment, pathophysiology, and pharmaco-therapeutic management. There is less consistency in the core graduate courses required in NP programs. In addition, there has been a lack of standardization in the number of clinical placement hours required, and the qualifications that faculty and clinical preceptors should possess (CASN, 2012).

In 2015, the Canadian Council of Registered Nurse Regulators (CCRNR) and Professional Examination Service (ProExam) conducted a practice analysis of nurse practitioners in Canada, which resulted in the creation of the Entry-Level Competencies for Nurse Practitioners currently being used by all regulators in Canada. The NP Practice Analysis Report (CCRNR, 2015) provided a comprehensive description of the entry-level knowledge, skills, and abilities required in three streams of NP practice: Adult, Family/All Ages, and Pediatrics. The analysis demonstrated, among other things, that NP practice appears to be consistent across Canada, and that NPs use the same competencies in their practice in all Canadian jurisdictions across the three streams of practice.

Since that time, CCRNR has continued to explore regulatory options for NP practice, including the possibility of a single generalist entry to practice examination for NPs across Canada with a single national licensure examination (CCRNR, 2019). This initiative, similar to the advanced practice registered nurses (APRNs) movement in the US, is aimed at protecting the public, providing for better access and accessibility to qualified NPs, and being the most feasible and cost-effective approach from a regulatory standpoint (CCRNR, 2015; National Council of State Boards of Nursing [NCSBN], 2008).

There have been attempts, but few graduate programs in Canada focus on CNS education. Hence, CNSs continue to be prepared in generalist graduate programs. Given the lack of credentialing and title protection, any nurse can call themselves a CNS, whether baccalaureate or graduate prepared, therefore there is a need for title protection and a credentialing mechanism (Martin-Misener et al., 2010).

Regulation and Legislation for Practice

In recent years, Ontario legislation has expanded the scope of practice of NPs, allowing for fuller access without physician oversight to prescribing and diagnostic testing as well as admitting, treating, transferring, and discharging both in-patients and community outpatients to and from hospital. Unfortunately, existing regulations in many provinces do not allow NPs to work to full scope of practice, which limits how they practice, including what they can prescribe, which diagnostic investigations they can order, or if they can independently refer to a specialist for consultation.

As stated previously, without regulation or a credentialing mechanism for CNSs in Canada, there is no title protection for the role and any nurse can identify themselves as a CNS in the absence of the requisite education and expertise for the role. CNSs are strongly advocating for title protection not only to strengthen the role, but to ensure those in the role possess the requisite education and experience to enact it. This, in turn, would lead to accurate tracking of the number of CNSs and the roles they are performing across Canada (DiCenso et al., 2010b).

Doctoral Preparation of Advanced Practice Nurses and Faculty Development

Currently, only 18.6% of Canadian universities offer a PhD, and admissions to doctoral programs have remained small but stable over the past five years, although there was a 1% decrease between 2016/2017 and 2017/2018. Likewise, doctoral program graduates decreased by 32.7% over the same period (CASN, 2019).

The CNPI (2006) indicated that faculty who were engaged in clinical practice were best able to teach NPs, but were also expected to have a PhD. Currently, there has been for some time a shortage of nursing faculty who possess both current practice and a PhD (Martin-Misener et al., 2010). Additionally, doctorally prepared NP faculty are challenged in maintaining a practice while meeting the teaching, research, publication, and service criteria for tenure and promotion. However, the practice portion of faculty is often not considered scholarly in relation to tenure and promotion processes.

The Doctor of Nursing (DN) degree will be introduced in the fall of 2021 at the Lawrence S. Bloomberg Faculty of Nursing at the University of Toronto, Toronto, Ontario, which will be the first university in Canada to offer a new choice in doctoral education. How it will be received remains uncertain as there has been a deliberate push away from a professional doctorate in Canada for fear that APNs will choose this alternative over the PhD programs. Further research will be required to explore the need for a practice doctorate and if it can be sustained so that consensus for it is achieved. Otherwise, APNs will continue to seek professional doctoral education elsewhere if it is not available in Canada (Tung, 2010).

Preceptorship of Advanced Practice Nursing Students

Graduate nursing education, specifically for NPs, in Canada relies heavily on **preceptorship** to prepare students for NP practice. Preceptors, acting as role models, provide clinical learning experiences for students that help them apply theory to real life situations, which support role socialization, role transition, and help to develop APN competencies (Staples & Sangster-Gormley, 2017). The literature related to preceptorship is focused primarily on baccalaureate-level education. The CNA (2004), supporting the importance of preceptorship, developed a guide for preceptorship and mentorship. This document, and the literature relating to preceptorship, are equally relevant for APN education in relation to the roles of the student, faculty member, and preceptor.

After the publication of *Nurse Practitioner Education in Canada: National Framework of Guiding Principles & Essential Components* (CASN, 2012), CASN developed the NP Education Interest Group in 2013. From this group, a preceptorship working subgroup was formed in 2014, and they developed a national survey that was administered to all NP programs in 2016 in an attempt to better understand how NP programs are supporting preceptorship, specifically in relation to recruitment and retention of preceptors (Staples & Sangster-Gormley, 2017).

The major problems associated with preceptorship are the recruitment, preparation, and remuneration of appropriate preceptors; competition with similar and other health care students for clinical placements; the clinical setting's ability to provide a supportive learning environment; and evaluation of the students (Ivey, 2006; Martin-Misener et al., 2010; Payne, Heye, & Farrell, 2014; Staples & Sangster-Gormley, 2017).

One of the biggest challenges, which is time consuming, is securing and maintaining a reliable cadre of experienced preceptors across programs, which can be local, provincial, or at a distance. Some programs encourage students to find their own preceptors, but this too can be problematic as it can lead to added competition for limited placement sites (Staples & Sangster-Gormley, 2017).

Although NP programs may have preceptor manuals and guidelines, preceptors often encounter problems, which include managing the duties of their practice expectations while at the same time teaching the student; uncertainty about the expectations of the student and preceptor; and differences in learning styles and personality (Ivey, 2006; Payne et al., 2014; Staples & Sangster-Gormley, 2017). A wider pan-Canadian study of preceptors' perceptions of NP preceptorship programs is being planned over the next two years to explore preceptors' perceptions of their preceptorship role.

Some provinces have developed websites for preceptorship support. Most are broad and support the basics of preceptorship for baccalaureate and NP students, but also for medical students. With a focus on all health care professional placements, the BC Preceptor Development Initiative website (www.practiceeducation.ca/) includes eight modules and e-tips that support preceptors in their role. The University of Saskatchewan hosts the Preceptor Education and Support in Saskatchewan website (www.saskpreceptors.ca), which focuses on the basics of preceptorship, training modules and e-tips, and videos and resources. The only NP-focused preceptorship website was established in 2007 by the Ontario PHCNP program consortium website, which hosts a Resource Centre for Preceptors and Employers, a website still used today (Patterson et al., 2007).

Remuneration and Trends in Employment

Between 2007 and 2011, the CIHI reported that the number of NPs had doubled from 1,344 to 2,777, and by 2015, the number further grew to 3,966 (CIHI, 2015). These increases were due to increased investments in NPs provincially, which led to an increase in data submitted to the CIHI (Picard, 2018). By 2018, CIHI reported that there were 5,697 NPs in Canada, with an 8% increase between 2017 and 2018. Although these increases have been positive, a negative trend began to emerge in relation to where NPs were practicing. Over the five-year period, there was a 10% decrease in NPs working in PHC settings and a 10% increase in NPs working in hospitals and long-term care (LTC; Canadian Nurse, 2012).

The reason for this trend directly corresponds to **remuneration** and benefits in PHC settings, which have not kept up with the salaries in the tertiary care sector, where there is greater perceived job security, increased salary, and a pension plan. In Ontario, for example, NPs in PHC (i.e., FHTs, Community Health Centres, Aboriginal Health Access Centres, and NP-Led Clinics) had seen a wage freeze between 2006 and 2018, which likely contributed to approximately 19% of NP positions remaining unfilled. Many of these NPs are choosing to leave for higher-paying hospital or other health care–setting jobs, which is a concerning trend for the recruitment and retention of Ontario NPs (Association of Ontario Health Centres [AOHC], 2013).

Another reason for this trend is related to the age of NPs. Between 2007 and 2011, the majority of NPs across Canadian jurisdictions were between the ages of 45 and 49. The number of regulated nurses aged 55 and older decreased between 2014 and 2018 with the average age of RNs, including NPs, being 44 (CIHI, 2019). The greatest number (77.9%) of RNs/NPs work in hospitals, 72% in community, and 42.2% in LTC settings. Of this workforce, 56.7% are employed full-time, 32.5% part-time, and 10.5% on a casual basis (CIHI, 2019).

NPs who are leaving PHC are practicing in emergency departments, where they provide triage and care for patients experiencing episodic health-related illnesses/conditions. Others are working in outpatient chronic care clinics that focus on diabetes, renal failure, and cardiac care. If PHCNP positions cannot attract NPs or are left unfilled, problems related to accessibility and wait times will resurface, which will lead to an increase in emergency department visits, resulting in increased health care expenditure and fragmented care delivery (Canadian Nurse, 2012).

To resolve some of these issues, further wage parity with physician colleagues doing the same work needs to be addressed. The option of capturing some NP billing codes for preventative health care and procedures similar to that of other health care professionals may be of value in determining wage parity. Legislation and regulation have allowed NPs to expand outside of non-covered health care procedures (i.e., cosmetic injections), but they are unable to expand their practice to include steroid injections for joint pain and extensive mental health counselling, so remain limited to negotiated agreements with their provinces. On the other hand, physicians have negotiated agreements and are provided with extra billing codes, which allow them to work in walk-in clinics on a fee-for-service basis and shadow billing options that augment their incomes.

As the COVID-19 pandemic has demonstrated, there is a need for a more responsive infrastructure in relation to hotlines and telehealth video options that are user friendly for patients. For health care professionals like APNs, these platforms allow for screening by phone; providing virtual visits, referral, and testing to public health, a health care clinic, or emergency department; and in-person considerations for ongoing clinical practice (i.e., non-infectious complaints, prenatal/immunizations, allergy injections; CNA, n.d.; College of Nurses of Ontario [CNO], 2017).

Conclusion

The roles of health care providers, including APNs, must be optimized to sustain the health system. Increases in chronic diseases related to an aging population will create challenges for many Canadians and health care providers who will have to anticipate these demands within the health system. The continued shift away from illness to health has seen health care consumers become more educated and engaged in participating in maintaining their functional health status.

A pan-Canadian approach will ensure continuity and consistency in education, legislative, and regulatory mechanisms, and systematic planning to guide APN role development and practice at all three levels of government.

While APNs continue to face barriers, a major facilitator is that they remain part of the solution to health care system challenges, change, and reform that are occurring at a rapid pace. New approaches to health care provision, based on interprofessional collaboration and practice, will improve access to timely health care services, and meet the health care needs of individuals, groups, and communities in Canada.

Critical Thinking Questions

1. What are the opportunities for APNs to build on their role today and into the future?
2. Looking at the current practices for APNs, what do you think is the biggest challenge, and what strategies will be needed to address it at local, provincial/territorial, and/or federal levels?
3. Where do you see the APN role in Canada in 1 year, 5 years, 10 years, or even 20 years and why? Compare and contrast the difference between where you live and other provinces and territories.

References

Association of Ontario Health Centres (AOHC). (2013). *Towards a primary care recruitment and retention strategies for Ontario: Compensation structure.* Toronto, ON: AOHC. Retrieved from http://www.aohc.org/sites/default/files/documents/PC-Retention-and-Recruitment-Compensation-Structure-for-IPCOs-Report-to-MOHLTC-June-2013.pdf

Bryant-Lukosius, D. (2010). The clinical nurse specialist role in Canada: Forecasting the future through research. *Canadian Journal of Nursing Research, 42*(2), 19–25.

Bryant-Lukosius, D., & DiCenso, A. (2004). A framework for the introduction and evaluation of advanced practice nursing roles. *Journal of Advanced Nursing, 48*(5), 530–540.

Canadian Association of Schools of Nursing (CASN). (2012). *Nurse practitioner education in Canada: National framework of guiding principles & essential components.* Ottawa, ON: CASN. Retrieved from http://casn.ca/wp-content/uploads/2014/12/FINALNPFrameworkEN20130131.pdf

CASN. (2017). *Registered nurses education in Canada statistics, 2015–2016: Registered nurse workforce, Canadian production: Potential new supply.* Ottawa, ON: CASN. Retrieved from https://www.casn.ca/wp-content/uploads/2017/12/2015-2016-EN-SFS-FINAL-REPORT-supressed-for-web.pdf

CASN. (2019). *Registered nurses education in Canada statistics: 2017–2018.* Ottawa, ON: CASN. Retrieved from https://www.casn.ca/wp-content/uploads/2019/12/2017-2018-EN-SFS-DRAFT-REPORT-for-web.pdf

Canadian Council of Registered Nurse Regulators (CCRNR). (2015). *Nurse practitioner practice analysis project.* Beaverton, ON: CCRNR. Retrieved from http://www.ccrnr.ca/np-practice-analysis.html

CCRNR. (2019). *2018–2019 highlights.* Beaverton, ON: CCRNR. Retrieved from http://www.ccrnr.ca/assets/2018-2019-ccrnr-highlights-en.pdf

Canadian Institute for Health Information (CIHI). (2015). *Regulated nurses, 2014.* Ottawa, ON: CIHI. Retrieved from https://secure.cihi.ca/free_products/RegulatedNurses2014_Report_EN.pdf

CIHI. (2019). *Nursing in Canada, 2018.* Ottawa, ON: CIHI. Retrieved from https://www.cihi.ca/en/nursing-in-canada-2018

Canadian Nurse. (2012). *Perspectives: NP numbers up, but employment trends concerning.* Ottawa, ON: CNA.

Canadian Nurse Practitioner Initiative (CNPI). (2006). *Nurse practitioners: The time is now. A solution to improving access and reducing wait times in Canada.* Ottawa, ON: CNA. Retrieved from https://www.cna-aiic.ca/-/media/cna/page-content/pdf-en/01_integrated_report.pdf

Canadian Nurses Association (CNA). (2004). *Achieving excellence in professional practice: A guide to preceptorship and mentoring.* Ottawa, ON: CNA. Retrieved from https://www.cna-aiic.ca/~/media/cna/page-content/pdf-en/achieving_excellence_2004_e.pdf

CNA. (2006). *Toward 2020: Visions for nursing.* Ottawa, ON: CNA.

CNA. (2008). *Advanced nursing practice: A national framework.* Ottawa, ON: CNA.

CNA. (2012). *Strengthening the role of the clinical nurse specialist in Canada.* Ottawa, ON: CNA. Retrieved from https://www.cna-aiic.ca/~/media/cna/page-content/pdf-fr/strengthening_the_cns_role_background_paper_e.pdf

CNA. (2015). *Framework for registered nurse prescribing in Canada.* Ottawa, ON: CNA. Retrieved from https://www.cna-aiic.ca/~/media/cna/page-content/pdf-en/cna-rn-prescribing-framework_e.pdf

CNA. (2019). *Advanced practice nursing: A pan-Canadian framework.* Ottawa, ON: CNA. Retrieved from https://www.cna-aiic.ca/-/media/cna/page-content/pdf-en/apn-a-pan-canadian-framework.pdf

CNA. (n.d.). *Fact sheet: Telehealth.* Ottawa, ON: CNA. Retrieved from https://www.cna-aiic.ca/-/media/cna/page-content/pdf-en/telehealth-fact-sheet.pdf

CNA & CASN. (2013). *Registered nurses education in Canada statistics 2011–2012. Registered nurse workforce, Canadian production: Potential new supply.* Ottawa, ON: CNA & CASN. Retrieved from https://www.cna-aiic.ca/~/media/cna/files/en/nsfs_report_2011-2012_e.pdf

Canadian Nurses Protective Society (CNPS). (2017). *RN prescribing.* Ottawa, ON: CNPS. Retrieved from https://www.cnps.ca/rnprescribing

College of Nurses of Ontario (CNO). (2017). *Practice guideline: Telepractice.* Toronto, ON: CNO. Retrieved from https://www.cno.org/globalassets/docs/prac/41041_telephone.pdf

DiCenso, A., Bryant-Lukosius, D., Bourgeault, I., Martin-Misener, R., Donald, F., Abelson, J., … Harbman, P. (2010a). *Clinical nurse specialists and nurse practitioners in Canada: A decision support synthesis.* Ottawa, ON: CHSRF. Retrieved from http://www.cfhi-fcass.ca/sf-docs/default-source/commissioned-research-reports/Dicenso_EN_Final.pdf

DiCenso, A., Bryant-Lukosius, D., Martin-Misener, R., Donald, F., Abelson, J., Bourgeault, I., … Harbman, P. (2010b). Factors enabling advanced practice nursing role integration in Canada. *Nursing Leadership, 23*(Special Issue), 211–238. doi: 10.12927/cjnl.2010.22279

Donald, F., Martin-Misener, R., Bryant-Lukosius, D., Kilpatrick, K., Kaasalainen, S., Carter, N., … DiCenso, A. (2010). The primary healthcare nurse practitioner role in Canada. *Canadian Journal of Nursing Leadership, 23*(Special Issue), 88–113.

Health Force Ontario. (2015). *Grow your own nurse practitioner.* Toronto, ON: MOHLTC. Retrieved from http://www.healthforceontario.ca/en/Home/Employers/Grow_Your_Own_Nurse_Practitioner_Program

Health Workforce Planning Branch. (2019). *Nursing: Mid career.* Toronto, ON: MOHLTC. Retrieved from http://www.health.gov.on.ca/en/pro/programs/hhrsd/nursing/mid_career.aspx

Ivey, J. B. (2006). Fostering successful preceptorships for advanced practice nursing. *Topics in Advanced Practice Nursing eJournal, 6*(1), 1–4.

Kilpatrick, K., Harbman, P., Carter, N., Martin-Misener, R., Bryant-Lukosius, D., Donald, F., … A. DiCenso. (2010). The acute care nurse practitioner role in Canada. *Canadian Journal of Nursing Leadership, 23*(Special Issue), 114–139.

MacDonald-Rencz, S., & Bard, R. (2010). The role for advanced practice nursing in Canada. *Nursing Leadership, 23*(Special Issue), 8–11. doi: 10.12927?cjnl.2010.22265

Martin-Misener, R., Bryant-Lukosius, D., Harbman, P., Donald, F., Kaasalainen, S., Carter, N., … DiCenso, A. (2010). Education of advanced practice nurses in Canada. *Canadian Journal of Nursing Leadership, 23*(Special Issue), 61–84.

National Council of State Boards of Nursing (NCSBN). (2008). *Consensus model for APRN regulation: Licensure, accreditation, certification & education.* Chicago, IL: NCSBN. Retrieved from https://www.ncsbn.org/Consensus_Model_for_APRN_Regulation_July_2008.pdf

Patterson, C., Staples, E., Davidson, B., Arthur, H., Price, D., Annis, R., … Shuhaibar, E. (2007). *The development of a resource centre for preceptors and employers involved in nurse practitioner education in the COUPN program: Report to MOHLTC interprofessional, mentorship, preceptorship, leadership and coaching fund.* Hamilton, ON: McMaster University.

Payne, C., Heye, M. L., & Farrell, K. (2014). Securing preceptors for advanced practice students. *Journal of Nursing Education and Practice, 4*(3), 167–179.

Picard, A. (2018, May 9). *Nurse practitioners in Canada more than double in five years (updated).* Toronto, ON: The Globe and Mail. Retrieved from http://www.theglobeandmail.com/life/health-and-fitness/nurse-practitioners-in-canada-more-than-double-in-five-years/article1359892/?utm_source=facebook.com&utm_medium=Referrer%3A+Social+Network+%2F+Media&utm_campaign=Shared+Web+Article+Links

Staples, E., & Sangster-Gormley, E. (2017). Supporting NP education: Preceptorship recruitment and retention in Canada. *International Journal of Nursing Sciences (Special Edition April), 5*(2), 115–120. https://doi.org/10.1016/j.ijnss.2018.03.005

Statistics Canada. (2019). *Canada's population estimates: Age and sex, July 1, 2018.* Ottawa, ON: Statistics Canada.

Tung, T. K. C. (2010). In support of doctor of nursing practice education in Canada. *Topics in Advanced Practice Nursing eJournal, 11,* 1–4.

Wong, S., & Farrally, V. (2013). *The utilization of nurse practitioners and physician assistants: A research synthesis.* Vancouver, BC: Michael Smith Foundation for Health Research. Retrieved from https://www.msfhr.org/sites/default/files/Utilization_of_Nurse_Practitioners_and_Physician_Assistants.pdf

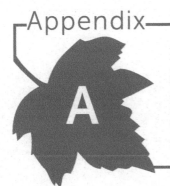

Appendix

A

Canadian Research on the Impact and Outcomes of Advanced Practice Nursing Roles Tables

TABLE A.1: Nurse Practitioners in Primary Health Care

Author	Purpose	Method	Outcomes and/or Impact		
			Patient	Provider	System
Ansell et al. (2017) International	Systematically review the literature to identify interventions designed to ↓ wait times for primary health care (PHC) appointments; secondary objectives were to assess patient satisfaction and to ↓ no-show rates	Systematic review			Open-access scheduling most common intervention; also showed that wait times ↓ by dedicated telephone calls for follow-up consultation; the presence of nurse practitioners (NPs) on staff, nurse, and physician triage, and email consultations
Curnew & Lukewich (2018) New Brunswick, Newfoundland and Labrador, Nova Scotia, Prince Edward Island	Scoping review conducted to examine and synthesize evidence related to nursing roles and resources in PHC settings in Atlantic Canada and associated contributions to patient care	Scoping review	PHC settings with NPs and nurses had positive clinical outcomes and high patient satisfaction		PHC settings with NPs and nurses had improved access to services

Fletcher et al. (2012) Ontario	Measure effect of NP and pharmacist consultations on patients' appropriate use of medications	Randomized control trial (RCT), 120 patients 50+ years old considered at risk for adverse health outcomes in intervention arm	Large ↓ in use of inappropriate medications; baseline 27.2% of medications inappropriate and 77.7% of patients receiving at least one inappropriate medication; at follow-up had dropped to 8.9% and 38.6%, respectively	
Heale & Pilon (2012) Ontario	Patient satisfaction in Sudbury District NP-Led Clinic	Survey	High patient satisfaction with clinic services; areas for review: access to same-day appointment, use of walk-in, and emergency care; most patients had received counselling about a lifestyle issue, resulting in behavioural change	

(Continued)

TABLE A.1: Continued

Author	Purpose	Method	Outcomes and/or Impact		
			Patient	Provider	System
Heale, James, Wenghofer, & Garceau (2018) Ontario	Evaluate care and impact of organizational tools on completeness of care for patients with diabetes and multimorbidity at NP-Led Clinics	Audit of 30 charts at 5 NP-Led Clinics (n = 150)	Overall, care was complete; no significant associations between patient or organizational characteristics and extent to which diabetes care was complete		
Hunter et al. (2016) Alberta	Benefits and challenges of community-led project to introduce NP in rural primary care	Mixed methods, participatory action	Patient outcomes were generally positive; patients expressed satisfaction with care		Increased access to cost-effective, quality PHC
Lawson, Dicks, Macdonald, & Burge (2012) Nova Scotia	Evaluate effect of enhanced collaborative care model, which included team building and addition of NP	Observational, retrospective audit of 392 patient charts (197 pre, 195 post)	↑ of chronic disease management among patients with targeted chronic conditions, particularly diabetes; better preventive health care among all patients		

Lovo et al. (2019) Saskatchewan	Investigate experiences of practitioners and patients during an interprofessional model with urban-based physical therapist using video conferencing to virtually join a rural NP and rural patient with chronic back pain	RCT patient surveys (n = 64) and interviews with practitioners and patients	Most patients "very satisfied" (62.1%) or "satisfied" (31.6%) with the overall experience, and "very" (63.1%) or "somewhat confident" (36.9%) with the assessment	
MacDougall, Cunningham, Whitney, & Sawhney (2019) Ontario	Reduce pediatric pain as evidenced by pain scores at time of vaccination at North Bay nurse practitioner–led clinic	Quasi-experimental utilizing descriptive statistics and quality improvement tools	Improved pain scores during vaccinations' use of topical anaesthetic; ↓ pain scores with use of standardized sucrose water	Nurses agreed to ongoing use of documenting form to sustain use of the guideline
Martin-Misener et al. (2015) International	Determine cost-effectiveness of NPs delivering primary and specialized ambulatory care	Systematic review	NP care equivalent to medical doctor (MD) care in all but seven outcomes favouring NP care	NP care equivalent to MD care in all but four outcomes, one favouring NP care and three favouring MD care; meta-analysis of two studies of NP care resulted in lower mean health care services costs per consultation

(Continued)

TABLE A.1: Continued

Author	Purpose	Method	Outcomes and/or Impact		
			Patient	Provider	System
Martin-Misener et al. (2016) International	Identify recommendations for determining patient panel per caseload size for NPs in community-based primary health care settings	Scoping review			Average number of patients seen by NPs per day varied within and between countries; an average of 9 to 15 patients per day was common; patient characteristics appear to influence patient panel per caseload size
Oosman et al. (2019) Saskatchewan	Evaluate client and provider perspectives on impact of enhancing access to physical therapy services offered by physical therapist (PT) and NP in PHC community-based setting	Qualitative data through interviews and online discussion board	People experiencing homelessness and poverty face barriers to accessing physical therapy; those who accessed PT perceived a positive impact on overall health, function, and wellness		

Rayner & Muldoon (2017) Ontario	Examine perceptions of staff groups about team functioning in mature, community-governed, interprofessional PHC practices	Online survey of 674 staff in 58 of 75 (77%) community health centres (CHCs) Team Climate Inventory Organizational Justice Scale Organizational Citizenship Behaviour Scale		Overall positive perceptions of team function; physicians and NPs rated procedural justice lower than nurses and administrators
Roots & MacDonald (2014) British Columbia	Identify outcomes associated with NP role in collaborative primary health care practice	Case studies with interviews, documents, and before-and-after data		↑ physician satisfaction; improved staff workplace relationships and satisfaction	↑ access to the practice with ↑ availability of appointments; ↑ access to PHC improved for harder-to-serve populations; ↓ emergency use and admissions to hospital
Sun, Jackson, Dunne, & Power (2015) British Columbia	Identify impact of NPs in fee-for-service (FFS) PHC practices	Case study of NP roles in three FFS clinics	↑ patient satisfaction	Positive physician experience; their expenditures increased 12% after NP was implemented

(Continued)

TABLE A.1: Continued

Author	Purpose	Method	Outcomes and/or Impact		
			Patient	Provider	System
Ward et al. (2013) Alberta	Determine if community-based NP-Led Clinic would ↑ management of First Nations people at risk of developing chronic kidney disease	Qualitative description	Reported ↓ HbAlc, ↓ BP, ↓ low-density lipoprotein	↑ prescription of ASA, angiotensin-converting enzyme inhibitor or angiotensin receptor blocker, or statin medications	
Weaver et al. (2014) Alberta, British Columbia, Manitoba, Saskatchewan	Describe barriers to PHC, including care from allied health professionals, for adults with chronic conditions	Survey of 1,849 (79.8%) western Canadians, 40 years or older, who had hypertension, diabetes, heart disease, or stroke about access to PHC and other use of health care	Most (87.3%) indicated they would be willing to see an NP if a physician was unavailable		6.1% indicated that allied health professionals were involved in their care

TABLE A.2: Impacts and Outcomes of Nurse Practitioners in Acute Care

Author	Purpose	Methods	Outcomes		
			Patient	Provider	System
Donald et al. (2015) International	Determine cost-effectiveness of NPs delivering hospital-to-community transitional care	Systematic review of RCTs	Similar patient outcomes to the physician group		Similar resource use to physician group, i.e., rehospitalization
Goldie et al. (2012) British Columbia	Compare the effectiveness of acute care NP-led care to hospitalist-led care in a post-operative cardiac surgery unit in a tertiary care hospital	RCT	Measures of patient satisfaction relating to teaching, answering questions, listening, and pain management were higher in the NP-led group		After discharge, more patients in hospitalist-led group had visited their family doctor within a week ($p \leq .02$)
Hurlock-Chorostecki & Acorn (2017) Ontario	Hospitals require identification of the most responsible provider (MRP) for care of admitted patients; little evidence illustrating adoption of NP-as-MRP model in Ontario	Implementation		NP leadership needed to prepare all affected for new model	In one hospital model used to maximize access to care for senior patients

(Continued)

TABLE A.2: Continued

Author	Purpose	Methods	Outcomes		
			Patient	Provider	System
Kilpatrick et al. (2013) Quebec	To describe how acute care NPs affect perceptions of team effectiveness	Descriptive multiple case study		Team effectiveness ↑ through decision making, communication, cohesion, care, coordination, problem solving, and focus on patients and families	
Kilpatrick et al. (2015) International	Synthesize the evidence of effectiveness and cost-effectiveness of clinical nurse specialists (CNSs) and nurse practitioners (NPs) working in in-patient settings	Systematic review of three RCTs			In two studies, NPs were equally effective with equal-to-higher resource use and equal costs
Li et al. (2017) Alberta	Determine benefits of diabetes through NP intervention on glycemic control, quality of life (QoL), and diabetes treatment satisfaction in patients with type 2 diabetes admitted to cardiology in-patient unit	Baseline and three-month HbA1c and lipid levels (LDLs); Audit of Diabetes-Dependent Quality of Life (ADDQoL); and treatment satisfaction	Significant decrease in HbA1c; improved ADDQoL; no difference in satisfaction		

Nixon et al. (2020) Ontario	NP-led lymphoma rapid diagnosis clinic (LRDC) with the goal of reducing wait times to definitive diagnosis	Examined initial 30-month experience of the LRDC; results compared with before implementation of clinic	Of 126 patients evaluated, 66 (52%) had lymphoma diagnosis; median time to diagnosis was 16 days for LRDC patients and 28 days for historical controls	
Rietze et al. (2016) Ontario	Explore Ontario NPs' knowledge, beliefs, and level of implementation of advanced care planning (ACP)	Survey		NPs in hospitals more likely than NPs in primary care to engage in ACP with patients; no significant differences in beliefs, attitudes, or comfort in initiating ACP
Sawatzky et al. (2013) Manitoba	Explore outcomes of an NP-managed cardiac surgery follow-up intervention	Prospective RCT with 200 elective cardiac surgery patients	Two weeks post discharge, NP-care group had ↓ symptoms and ↑ physical functioning; post discharge two and six weeks, NP-care group was more satisfied with amount of help and quality of services	No statistically significant differences in health care resource use
Singh et al. (2019) British Columbia	Evaluate effectiveness of the first Fracture Liaison Service (FLS) program implemented in British Columbia	Controlled before and after		↑ investigation and treatment for osteoporosis after fracture

(Continued)

TABLE A.2: Continued

Author	Purpose	Methods	Outcomes		
			Patient	Provider	System
Smigorowsky et al. (2017) International	Study protocol to assess effect of NP-led care on health-related quality of life (HRQoL) of adult patients with atrial fibrillation	RCT protocol	Planned outcomes are: difference between groups at six months in change in quality of life scores; satisfaction with NP-led care		Difference between groups at six months in composite outcomes of death, hospitalization, and emergency department visits
Smigorowsky et al. (2020) International	To assess RCTs evaluating the impact of NP-led cardiovascular care	Systematic review (five RCTs, including two from Canada)	No difference between NP-led and usual care for health-related quality of life		No difference between NP-led and usual care for 30-day readmissions and length of stay
Spence et al. (2019) International	Conduct literature review of NPs in orthopedic surgical settings to determine if a need exists for NPs	Literature review	↑ improved patient satisfaction; NPs meet patient needs while surgeons are operating	↑ team communication; ↑ quality of care; positive impact on resident surgeon education	↑ access to care; ↓ length of stay
Stahlke et al. (2017) Alberta	What is known about patient satisfaction with NP care from the perspective of breast cancer patients followed by an NP	Interpretive description	Patients appreciated benefits of NP care and were highly satisfied with physical care and holistic support received during treatment		

TABLE A.3: Impacts and Outcomes of Nurse Practitioners in Long-Term/Home Care

Publication	Purpose	Methods	Outcomes		
			Patient	Provider	System
Carter et al. (2016) National	To explore the role and activities of NPs working in long-term care (LTC) to understand concepts of access to primary health care for residents	Directed content analysis method to analyze data from a pan-Canadian study of NPs in LTC			Availability and accessibility of NP positively impacted access to primary and urgent health care for residents
Donald et al. (2013) International	To report quantitative evidence of effectiveness of advanced practice nursing roles, CNSs, and NPs in meeting needs of older adults living in long-term care (LTC) residential settings	Systematic review: 4 prospective studies conducted in the US and reported in 15 papers were included	LTC settings with advanced practice nurses had ↓ rates of depression, urinary incontinence, pressure ulcers, restraint use, and aggressive behaviours; ↑ in residents experiencing improvement in meeting personal goals and family members who expressed more satisfaction with medical services		

(Continued)

TABLE A.3: Continued

Publication	Purpose	Methods	Outcomes		
			Patient	Provider	System
El-Masri et al. (2015) Ontario	Evaluate effectiveness of NP-led outreach program on health care outcomes, emergency department (ED) transfers, and hospital admissions of LTC residents	Observational prospective cohort study			ED transfers by NPs 27% less likely to be non-urgent than transfers made by MDs; ED transfers by NPs were 3.23 times more likely to be admitted to hospital than transfers by MDs
Kaasalainen et al. (2013) National	Explore the NP role in providing palliative care in LTC	Qualitative descriptive design; data collected from five LTC homes across Canada		Build capacity and help others in LTC learn about NP role in palliative care; optimize palliative care practices by providing consultation and education; build capacity within organizations	Improve accessibility of care and number of hospital visits
Kaasalainen et al. (2016) Ontario	Evaluate effectiveness of NP-led, interprofessional pain management team	Controlled before-and-after study	Significantly ↓ residents' pain; ↑ functional status compared to usual care without access to NP		

Kilpatrick et al. (2020) Quebec	To identify how NPs in LTC influence care quality and inform the wider implementation of these roles in Quebec	Mixed methods; six LTC facilities	↓ number of medications per resident; ↓ falls; less restraint use	↓ transfers to acute care
Lacny et al. (2016) Nova Scotia	Examine the cost-effectiveness of an NP-family physician model of care compared with family physician–only care in a Canadian nursing home	Cost-effectiveness analysis using a controlled before-and-after design		Using willingness-to-pay threshold of $1,000 CAD per emergency department transfer, the probability the NP-physician model was cost-effective compared with internal, external, and combined control groups was 26%, 21%, and 25%
Ploeg et al. (2013) National	Explore the perceptions of residents and family members regarding the role of the NP in LTC homes	Qualitative descriptive approach with individual and focus group interviews with 35 residents and family members from 4 LTC settings	Perceived to provide resident and family-centred care; ↑ quality of care; ↑ informational and emotional support; ↑ facilitation of participation in decision making	Perceived to ↑ availability and timeliness of care and help prevent unnecessary hospitalization

(Continued)

TABLE A.3: Continued

Publication	Purpose	Methods	Outcomes		
			Patient	Provider	System
Sangster-Gormley et al. (2013) National	Examine nursing staff's perceptions of how working with an NP affected their knowledge and skill, ability to provide care, and function as a team	Focus groups that were part of case studies conducted in sequential, two-phase mixed-methods study		Multiple approaches used to increase staff knowledge and skills and improve quality of care	
Tung et al. (2012) Saskatchewan	Discuss potential impact of NP-provided care on ED use for home-care patients in Canada	Two-group prospective design			Number of ED visits reduced at two and four weeks in intervention group; no significant difference in the death rates between the two groups

TABLE A.4: Clinical Nurse Specialists in Care Settings

Publication	Purpose	Methods	Outcomes		
			Patient	Provider	System
Abela-Dimech et al. (2017) Ontario	To develop and implement search protocol to improve patient, staff, and visitor safety by preventing unsafe items from entering a locked in-patient unit	Guided by a CNS, develop and implement a search protocol to improve patient, staff, and visitor safety by preventing unsafe items from entering a locked in-patient unit			Standardized search protocol developed and piloted on one unit; statistical difference between the number of incidents before and after search protocol; safety on an in-patient unit
Bryant-Lukosius et al. (2015) International	Evaluate the clinical effectiveness and cost-effectiveness of CNS transitional care	Systematic review of RCTs	Post-cancer surgery, CNS care was superior in ↓ patient mortality; for patients with heart failure, CNS care ↑ treatment adherence and patient satisfaction; for elderly patients and caregivers, CNS care improved caregiver depression; for high-risk pregnant women and very low birthweight infants, CNS care ↑ infant immunization rates and maternal satisfaction with care		For patients with heart failure, CNS care ↓ death or re-hospitalization; ↑ in treatment adherence and patient satisfaction; ↓ in costs and length of re-hospitalization stay; for high-risk pregnant women and very low birthweight infants, CNS care ↓ maternal and infant length of hospital stay and costs; for elderly patients and caregivers, CNS care improved caregiver depression and ↓ hospitalization, re-hospitalization, length of stay, and costs

(Continued)

TABLE A.4: Continued

Publication	Purpose	Methods	Outcomes		
			Patient	Provider	System
de Mestral et al. (2011) Quebec	Assess impact of tracheostomy team (surgeon, surgical resident, respiratory therapist, speech-language pathologist, and CNS) on downsizing and decannulation times, incidence of speaking, valve placement, and tracheostomy-related complications	Thirty-two patients in pre-service group and 54 patients in post-service group	Reduced incidence of tube blockage and calls for respiratory distress on wards; ↑ in proportion of patients receiving speaking valves; apparent ↓ in time to first tube downsizing and decannulation		
Desrochers et al. (2016) Quebec	Explore perceptions of cancer patients or their family about their telephone-triage assessment conducted by a CNS for a psychosocial oncology program	Qualitative descriptive design; interviews with nine cancer patients and family members	Felt supported by CNS's actions to foster therapeutic relationship; valued different paths to tailored care, i.e., individualized strategies targeted to participant's unique needs		

Fabbruzzo-Cota et al. (2016) Ontario	Reduce hospital-acquired pressure ulcers using evidence-based practice	Quality improvement project, guided by Donabedian model, was based on the Registered Nurses' Association of Ontario's Best Practice Guideline *Risk Assessment and Prevention of Pressure Ulcers*		80% ↓ in hospital-acquired pressure ulcers
Jackson et al. (2018) Ontario	Protocol to explore efficacy of CNS-delivered trauma-informed cognitive behavioural therapy (CBT) on maternal and child health outcomes for pregnant women with post-traumatic stress disorder (PTSD), depression, or anxiety symptomatology resulting from intimate partner violence	Mixed-methods approach grounded in intersectional feminist framework	↓ in expected outcomes in mental illness symptomatology, ↑ in maternal-infant attachment, maternal coping, and maternal quality of life	

(Continued)

TABLE A.4: Continued

Publication	Purpose	Methods	Outcomes		
			Patient	Provider	System
Kilpatrick et al. (2013) National	Identify the practice patterns of CNSs in Canada	National survey	How CNSs influence patient satisfaction, comfort level, quality of life (health and well-being), patient knowledge, and family knowledge varied by clinical specialty	CNSs perceived they influence staff knowledge, multidisciplinary co-operation, staff skill, and improved interdisciplinary communication	
Kilpatrick et al. (2014) International	Describe a systematic review of randomized controlled trials (RCTs) evaluating the cost-effectiveness of CNSs delivering outpatient care	Systematic review of 11 RCTs	Similar or improved patient outcomes to usual care		Mostly similar health care system outcomes to usual care; some evidence of reduced resource use and costs
Kilpatrick et al. (2015) International	Synthesize the evidence of effectiveness and cost-effectiveness of CNSs and NPs working in in-patient settings	Systematic review of three RCTs			In one study, compared to physician care, CNSs were equally effective with equal resource use; in two studies, NPs were equally effective with equal-to-greater resource use and equal costs

Moore & McQuestion (2012) International	Critical review of the literature to better define and understand the CNS role related to patients living with chronic illnesses (cardiovascular and oncology)	Literature review	CNSs provide high-quality care to patients with chronic diseases; CNSs had positive impact on patient and family outcomes	Positive impact on health care team outcomes	Cost-effective care to patients with chronic disease
Stilos & Daines (2013) Ontario	Highlight the clinical leadership role of the CNS as triage leader for a hospital-based palliative care consulting team	Quality improvement			Changes to the team's referral and triage processes are improvements to team efficiency and timely access to care for patients and families
St-Louis & Brault (2011) Quebec	Describe formal assessment, consultation, and follow-up process made by CNS in medicine to facilitate transition between intensive care unit and medical wards	Evaluation of quality initiative	150 patients are assessed annually by CNS; 15% of these are at high risk for complications on transfer; for patients and families, verbalized intervention is helpful	Staff members indicated the initiative is useful in planning patient transfers	

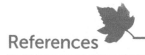

References

Abela-Dimech, F., Johnston, K., & Strudwick, G. (2017). Development and pilot implementation of a search protocol to improve patient safety on a psychiatric inpatient unit. *Clinical Nurse Specialist, 31*(2), 104–114. doi: 10.1097/NUR.0000000000000281

Ansell, D., Crispo, J. A. G., Simard, B., Bjerre, L. M. (2017). Interventions to reduce wait times for primary care appointments: A systematic review. *BioMed Central (BMC) Health Services Research, 17*, 1–9. doi: 10.1186/s12913-017-2219-y

Bryant Lukosius D., Carter, N., Reid, K., Donald, F., Martin-Misener, R., Kilpatrick, K., ... DiCenso, A. (2015). The clinical effectiveness and cost-effectiveness of clinical nurse specialist-led hospital to home transitional care: A systematic review. *Journal of Evaluative Clinical Practice, 21*(5), 763–781. doi: 0.1111/jep.12401

Carter, N., Sangster-Gormley, E., Ploeg, J., Martin-Misener, R., Donald, F., Wickson-Griffiths, A., ... Schindel Martin, L. (2016). An assessment of how nurse practitioners create access to primary care in Canadian residential long-term care settings. *Canadian Journal of Nursing Leadership, 29*(2), 45–63. doi: 10.12927/cjnl.2016.24806

Curnew, D. R., & Lukewich, J. (2018). Nursing within primary care settings in Atlantic Canada: A scoping review. *Sage Open,* 1–17. https://doi.org/10.1177/2158244018774379

de Mestral, C., Iqbal, S., Fong, N., LeBlanc, J., Fata, P., Razek, T., & Khwaja, K. (2011). Impact of a specialized multidisciplinary tracheostomy team on tracheostomy care in critically ill patients. *Canadian Journal of Surgery, 54*(3), 167–172. doi: 10.1503/cjs.043209

Desrochers, F., Donivan, E., Mehta, A., & Laizner, A. M. (2016). A psychosocial oncology program: Perceptions of the telephone-triage assessment. *Supportive Care in Cancer, 24*(7), 2937–2944.

Donald, F., Kilpatrick, K., Reid, K., Carter, N., Bryant Lukosius, D., Martin-Misener, R., ... DiCenso, A. (2015). Hospital to community transitional care by nurse practitioners: A systematic review of cost-effectiveness. *International Journal of Nursing Studies, 52*(1), 436–451. doi: 0.1016/j.ijnurstu.2014.07.011

Donald, F., Martin-Misener, R., Carter, N., Donald, E. E., Kaasalainen, S., Wickson-Griffiths, A., ... DiCenso, A. (2013). A systematic review of the effectiveness of advanced practice nurses in long-term care. *Journal of Advanced Nursing, 69*(10), 2148–2161. doi: 10.1111/jan.12140

El-Masri, M. M., Omar, A., & Groh, E. M. (2015). Evaluating the effectiveness of a nurse practitioner-led outreach program for long-term-care homes. *Canadian Journal of Nursing Research, 47*(3), 39–55.

Fabbruzzo-Cota, C., Frecea, M., Kozell, K., Pere, K., Thompson, T., Tjan Thomas, J., & Wong, A. (2016). A clinical nurse specialist-led interprofessional quality improvement project to reduce hospital-acquired pressure ulcers. *Clinical Nurse Specialist, 30*(2), 110–116.

Fletcher, J., Hogg, W., Farrell, B., Woodend, K., Dahrouge, S., Lemelin, J., & Dalziel, W. (2012). Effect of nurse practitioner and pharmacist counseling on inappropriate medication use in family practice. *Canadian Family Physician, 58*(8), 862–868.

Goldie, C. L., Prodan-Bhalla, N., & Mackay, M. (2012). Nurse practitioners in postoperative cardiac surgery: Are they effective? *Canadian Journal of Cardiovascular Nursing, 22*(4), 8–15.

Heale, R., James, S., Wenghofer, E., & Garceau, M. L. (2018). Nurse practitioner's perceptions of the impact of the nurse practitioner-led clinic model on the quality of care of complex patients. *Primary Health Care Research & Development, 19*(6), 553–560. doi: 10.1017/S1463423617000913

Heale, R., & Pilon, R. (2012). An exploration of patient satisfaction in a nurse practitioner-led clinic. *Nursing Leadership, 25*(3), 43–55.

Hunter, K. F., Murphy, R. S., Babb, M., & Vallee, C. (2016). Benefits and challenges faced by a nurse practitioner working in an interprofessional setting in rural Alberta. *Nursing Leadership, 29*(3), 61–70.

Hurlock-Chorostecki, C., & Acorn, M. (2017). Diffusing innovative roles within Ontario hospitals: Implementing the nurse practitioner as the most responsible provider. *Nursing Leadership, 30*(4), 60–66. doi: 10.12927/cjnl.2017.25448.

Jackson, K. T., Parkinson, S., Jackson, B., & Mantler, T. (2018). Examining the impact of trauma-informed cognitive behavioral therapy on perinatal mental health outcomes among survivors of intimate partner violence (The PATH Study): Protocol for a feasibility study. *Journal of Medical Internet Research (JMIR) Research Protocols, 7*(5), e134. doi: 10.2196/resprot.9820.

Kaasalainen, S., Ploeg, J., McAiney, C., Schindel-Martin, L., Donald, L., Martin-Misener, R., ... Sangster-Gormley, E. (2013). Role of the nurse practitioner in providing palliative care in long term care homes. *International Journal of Palliative Nursing, 19*(10), 477–485.

Kaasalainen, S., Wickson-Griffiths, A., Akhtar-Danesh, N., Brazil, K., Donald, F., Martin-Misener, R., ... Dolovich, L. (2016). The effectiveness of a nurse practitioner-led pain management team in long-term care: A mixed methods study. *International Journal of Nursing Studies, 62*, 156–167. doi: 10.1016/j.ijnurstu.2016.07.022

Kilpatrick, K., DiCenso, A., Bryant Lukosius, D., Ritchie, J. A., Martin-Misener, R., & Carter, N. (2013). Practice patterns and perceived impact of clinical nurse specialist roles in Canada: Results of a national survey. *International Journal of Nursing Studies, 50*(11), 1524–1536.

Kilpatrick, K., Kaasalainen, S., Donald, F., Reid, K., Carter, N., Bryant Lukosius, D., ... DiCenso, A. (2014). The effectiveness and cost effectiveness of clinical nurse specialists in outpatient roles: A systematic review. *Journal of Evaluation in Clinical Practice, 20*(6), 1106–1123.

Kilpatrick, K., Reid, K., Carter, N., Donald, F., Bryant Lukosius, D., Martin-Misener, R., ... DiCenso, A. (2015). A systematic review of the cost effectiveness of clinical nurse specialists and nurse practitioners in inpatient roles. *Canadian Journal of Nursing Leadership, 28*(3), 56–76.

Kilpatrick, K., Tchouaket, É., Jabbour, M., & Hains, S. (2020). A mixed methods quality improvement study to implement nurse practitioner roles and improve care for residents in long-term care facilities. *BioMed Central (BMC) Nursing, 19*(6). doi: 10.1186/s12912-019-0395-2

Lacny, S., Zarrabi, M., Martin-Misener, R., Donald, F., Sketris, I., Murphy, A., ... Marshall, D. A. (2016). Cost-effectiveness of a nurse practitioner-family physician model of care in a nursing home. *Journal of Advanced Nursing, 72*(9), 2138–2152.

Lawson, B., Dicks, D., Macdonald, L., & Burge, F. (2012). Using quality indicators to evaluate the effect of implementing an enhanced collaborative care model among a community, primary healthcare practice population. *Nursing Leadership, 25*(3), 28–42.

Li, S., Roschkov, S., Alkhodair, A., O'Neill, B. J., Chik, C. L., Tsuyuki, R. T., & Gyenes, G. T. (2017). The effect of nurse practitioner-led intervention in diabetes care for patients admitted to cardiology services. *Canadian Journal of Diabetes, 41*(1), 10–16. doi: 10.1016/j.jcjd.2016.06.008

Lovo, S., Harrison, L., O'Connell, M. E., Trask, C., & Bath, B. (2019). Experience of patients and practitioners with a team and technology approach to chronic back disorder management. *Journal of Multidisciplinary Healthcare, 18*(12), 855–869. doi: 10.2147/JMDH.S208888

MacDougall, T., Cunningham S., Whitney, L., & Sawhney, M. (2019). Improving pediatric experience of pain during vaccinations: A quality improvement project. *International Journal of Health Care Quality Assurance, 32*(6), 1034–1040. doi: 10.1108/IJHCQA-07-2018-0185

Martin-Misener, R., Harbman, P., Donald, F., Reid, K., Kilpatrick, K., Carter, N., ... DiCenso, A. (2015). Cost-effectiveness of nurse practitioners in ambulatory care: Systematic review. *British Medical Journal (BMJ) Open 5*, e007167 doi: 10.1136/bmjopen-2014-007167

Martin-Misener, R., Kilpatrick, K., Donald, F., Bryant-Lukosius, D., Rayner, J., Valaitis, R., ... Lamb, A. (2016). Nurse practitioner caseload in primary health care: Scoping review. *International Journal of Nursing Studies, 62*, 170–182.

Moore, J., & McQuestion, M. (2012). The clinical nurse specialist in chronic diseases. *Clinical Nurse Specialist, 26*(3), 149–163. doi: 10.1097/NUR.0b013e3182503fa7

Nixon, S., Bezverbnaya, K., Maganti, M., Gullane, P., Reedijk, M., Kuruvilla, J., Prica, A., ... Crump, M. (2020). Evaluation of lymphadenopathy and suspected lymphoma in a lymphoma rapid diagnosis clinic. *Journal of Clinical Oncology (JCO) Practice, 16*(1). doi: 10.1200/JOP.19.00202

Oosman, S., Weber, G., Ogunson, M., & Bath, B. (2019). Enhancing access to physical therapy services for people experiencing poverty and homelessness: The lighthouse pilot project. *Physiotherapy Canada, 71*(2), 176–186. doi: 10.3138/ptc.2017-85.pc

Ploeg, J., Kaasalainen, S., McAiney, C., Martin-Misener, R., Donald, F., Wickson-Griffiths, A., ... Taniguchi, A. (2013). Resident and family perceptions of the nurse practitioner role in long term care settings: A qualitative descriptive study. *BioMed Central (BMC) Nursing, 12*, 24. doi: 10.1186/10.1186/1472-6955-12-24.

Rayner, J., & Muldoon, L. (2017). Staff perceptions of community health centre team function in Ontario. *Canadian Family Physician, 63*(7), e335–e340.

Rietze, L., Heale, R., Hill, L., & Roles, S. (2016). Advance care planning in nurse practitioner practice: A cross-sectional descriptive study. *Nursing Leadership, 29*(3), 106–119.

Roots, A., & MacDonald, M. (2014). Outcomes associated with nurse practitioners in collaborative practice with general practitioners in rural settings in Canada: A mixed methods study. *Human Resources for Health, 12*(69). doi: 10.1186/1478-4491-12-69

Sangster-Gormley, E., Carter, N., Donald, F., Martin-Misener, R., Ploeg, J., Kaasalainen, S., ... Wickson-Griffiths, A. (2013). A value added benefit of nurse practitioners in long-term care settings: Increased nursing staff's ability to care for residents. *Canadian Journal of Nursing Leadership, 26*(3), 24–37.

Sawatzky, J. A., Christie, S., & Singal, R. K. (2013). Exploring outcomes of a nurse practitioner-managed cardiac surgery follow-up intervention: a randomized trial. *Journal of Advanced Nursing, 69*(9), 2076–2087. doi: 10.1111/jan.12075

Singh, S., Whitehurst, D. G., Funnell, L., Scott, V., MacDonald, V., Leung, P. M., ... Feldman, F. (2019). Breaking the cycle of recurrent fracture: Implementing the first fracture liaison service (FLS) in British Columbia, Canada. *Archives Osteoporosis, 4*(1), 116. doi: 10.1007/s11657-019-0662-6

Smigorowsky, M. J., Norris, C. M., McMurtry, M. S., & Tsuyuki, R. T. (2017). Measuring the effect of nurse practitioner (NP)-led care on health-related quality of life in adult patients with atrial fibrillation: Study protocol for a randomized controlled trial. *Trials, 18*(1), 364. doi: 10.1186/s13063-017-2111-4

Smigorowsky, M. J., Sebastianski, M., & Norris, C. M. (2020). Outcomes of nurse practitioner-led care in patients with cardiovascular disease: A systematic review and meta-analysis. *Journal of Advanced Nursing, 76*(1), 81–95. doi: 10.1111/jan.14229

Spence, B. G., Ricci, J., & McCuaig, F. (2019). Nurse practitioners in orthopaedic surgical settings: A review of the literature. *Orthopedic Nursing, 38*(1), 17–24. doi: 10.1097/NOR.0000000000000514

Stahlke, S., Rawson, K., & Pituskin, E. (2017). Patient perspectives on nurse practitioner care in oncology in Canada. *Journal of Nursing Scholarship, 49*(5), 487–494.

Stilos, K., & Daines, P. (2013). Exploring the leadership role of the clinical nurse specialist on an inpatient palliative care consulting team. *Nursing Leadership, 26*(1), 70–78.

St-Louis, L., & Brault, D. (2011). A clinical nurse specialist intervention to facilitate safe transfer from ICU. *Clinical Nurse Specialist, 25*(6), 321–326. doi: 10.1097/NUR.0b013e318233eaab

Sun, L., Jackson, R. A., Dunne, H., & Power, V. A. (2015). Impact of nurse practitioners in primary healthcare fee-for-service practice settings. *Healthcare Management Forum, 28*(1), 24–27.

Tung, T. K., Kaufmann, J. A., & Tanner, E. (2012). The effect of nurse practitioner practice in home care on emergency department visits for homebound older adult patients: An exploratory pilot study. *Home Healthcare Nurse, 30*(6), 366–372. doi: 10.1097/NHH.0b013e318246dd53

Ward, D. R., Novak, E., Scott-Douglas, N., Brar, S., White, M., & Hemmelgarn, B. R. (2013). Assessment of the Siksika chronic disease nephropathy-prevention clinic. *Canadian Family Physician, 59*(1), e19–e25.

Weaver, R. G., Manns, B. J., Tonelli, M., Sanmartin, C., Campbell, D. J., Ronksley, P. E., … Hemmelgarn, B. R. (2014). Access to primary care and other health care use among western Canadians with chronic conditions: A population-based survey. *Canadian Medical Associate Journal (CMAJ) Open, 2*(1), E27–E34. doi: 10.9778/cmajo.20130045

Appendix

B1

Spotlights on Unique
Advanced Practice Roles
in Canada

Medical Cannabis

Sara Ryan

SARA RYAN is an NP-PHC at the cannabis clinic, North Star Wellness, in Toronto, Ontario. She has extensive experience in cannabinoid therapy and pain management. She has been practicing in the medical cannabis field for two years and is committed to improving the management of patients with chronic pain. Sara is committed to supporting and educating health care practitioners in medical cannabis and has helped lead the development of clinical practice guidelines for the assessment and management of patients using medical cannabis for symptom management.

Introduction

I started my nursing career as a surgical oncology nurse for five years, which is where I found my role in pain management. I cared for patients who had undergone extensive surgeries and required specialized pain management. Early in my career I joined the nursing unit council and our process improvement initiatives focused on improving post-operative pain management and rehabilitation. I completed my Master of Nursing with an initial plan to become a CNS. Although leadership and research were a passion of mine, I valued patient interaction and felt that becoming an NP would allow me to fulfill both the CNS and NP role. As a CNS/NP, I have specialized my practice in pain management to include cannabis-based medicine.

History of the Role

I started specializing in cannabis-based medicine before cannabis became legal in October 2018. I have seen cannabis evolve through complex regulatory and industry changes. As a pioneer in this new field of nursing, I feel obligated to use my past experiences and support all nurses in this exciting new clinical practice. Unfortunately, patients often get lost in the medical cannabis system and I feel that nurses can play a pivotal role in helping patients access education and support. In my current role, I have helped develop a large medical cannabis program that is proudly led by NPs.

Competencies

The pathophysiology related to the endocannabinoid system is highly evolutionary and critically important to the development, function, and control of our entire nervous system and many bodily functions, yet the endocannabinoid system and cannabis have not been historically taught in undergraduate nursing programs. With advanced knowledge and skills, NPs have the academic credentials, clinical experience, and competence to establish standards of care and develop clinical practice guidelines that are needed in cannabis-based medicine. Nurses have seen first-hand the physiological and psychological impact that chronic conditions have on patients and their families and understand how big of an impact "10 extra minutes" can have with their patients.

System Challenges

One of the biggest challenges of legalizing adult-use cannabis has been that medical patients are being overlooked. Medical patients pay taxes on their cannabis-based medicine, and many insurance plans do not cover cannabis as a paid benefit. Unfortunately, most patients with chronic conditions cannot afford medical cannabis and are often pushed to other medications such as opioids. There is a lack of high-quality evidence to support the use of medical cannabis, and this is where I see a key role for NPs. As clinical and academic leaders, we have the knowledge to support and facilitate studies that advocate for safe and effective care for patients looking to use medical cannabis.

Regulatory Considerations

The Cannabis Act (2018) gives provincial governing bodies control to regulate NP practice standards. The College of Nurses of Ontario's (CNO; 2019) NP practice standard permits an Ontario NP who has completed approved controlled substances education to authorize medical cannabis. Every province is unique, so it is very important to check with your regulatory body's practice standards before you consider authorizing medical cannabis.

Conclusion

The last three years have been filled with many exciting and new opportunities as an NP, but there have also been many anticipated and unanticipated challenges. With every challenge, there is opportunity for growth. Overall, I plan to use my research, education, and clinical experience to advocate for adult-use medical cannabis and expand the role of nursing in this field of expertise.

References

College of Nurses of Ontario (CNO). (2019). *Practice standard: Nurse practitioner.* Toronto, ON: CNO. Retrieved from https://www.cno.org/globalassets/docs/prac/41038_strdrnec.pdf

Government of Canada. (2018). *The Cannabis Act: The facts.* Ottawa, ON: Health Canada. Retrieved from https://www.canada.ca/en/health-canada/corporate/contact-us.html

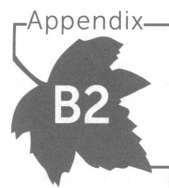

Appendix B2

Spotlights on Unique Advanced Practice Roles in Canada

Cosmetic Injection

Jennifer Fournier

JENNIFER FOURNIER is an NP-PHC based in Sudbury, Ontario. She has worked in a variety of clinical settings and teaches in the Laurentian University School of Nursing. She has been trained at the advanced level in cosmetic injection and is proprietor of AllureRX, a clinical cosmetic business in Sudbury, Ontario.

Introduction

I considered this role for myself when I came to understand that nurse practitioners (NPs) in Ontario could obtain, order, and administer the medications needed to deliver cosmetic services. In many jurisdictions NPs can also provide direct orders and/or medical directives to registered nurses and registered practical nurses while acting as clinical directors. I opened my own skin treatment and cosmetic injection clinic in Sudbury, Ontario, in 2018. This service is in high demand and has proven to be quite rewarding.

History of the Role

Nurse practitioners have been providing clinical cosmetic services within their scope of practice in Canada for over two decades. Clinical cosmetic services include items such as neuromodulator medications (i.e., Botox, Xeomn, Dysport) for facial wrinkles, dermal fillers with lidocaine, sclerotherapy for varicose veins, and medical-grade skin treatments, such as chemical peels and deep micro-needling. These NPs work in a variety of clinical and medi-spa settings. While NPs in some jurisdictions practice independently in prescribing and administrating cosmetic medications, other jurisdictions have chosen to restrict these practices to varying degrees (Canadian Nurses Protective Society [CNPS], 2016).

Competencies

Expanded NP prescribing authority in some Canadian jurisdictions has facilitated NP involvement and practice in medical cosmetic services. In Ontario, for example, NPs have the authority to order and prescribe all medications, including neuromodulators (College of Nurses of Ontario [CNO], 2019a, 2019b).

NP education and a broad array of clinical experiences have provided me with the necessary knowledge and skill base for this role. Advanced knowledge of the intricate features of facial anatomy provides a broader understanding of injection outcomes and danger zones. Education in pharmacology and prescribing best practices permits me to use a holistic approach in devising safe and effective treatment plans for my patients. As well, advanced education in adult teaching and learning principles, and health behaviour change have permitted me to teach patients about various treatments, preventative skin care, and potential complications to watch for in a way they say they haven't experienced in other settings.

Work in the clinical cosmetic field can be very satisfying. Patients who present to my clinic are usually seeking improvement for themselves. While there are risks and requisite skills related to the various treatments, they are usually quite successful, and patients leave satisfied with their care. Often results are immediate, such as with the administration of dermal fillers. Delivery of this service can be rewarding for both myself and the patient due to the quick result. Work in this clinical area can also satisfy when it serves as a welcomed addition to the clinical practice of an NP who needs a change. This work can rejuvenate an interest in learning new knowledge and skills that incorporate existing competencies. The role also offers the opportunity to own a business, which might be appealing to some NPs like myself who have business training and entrepreneurial interests and aptitudes.

System Challenges

The fact that cosmetic aesthetic nursing generally exists within a for-profit system provides cultural and ethical tensions for NPs. Canadian NP education programs focus on preparing generalists, usually in primary health care, grounding teaching in principles consistent with public health care systems. This is one of the few areas of practice where NPs apply relevant clinical knowledge and competencies to provide service to patients in exchange for money. Regulations and practice standards address many areas of independent practice across jurisdictions and set parameters for ethical business practice. For example, professional organizations in some jurisdictions preclude nurses and NPs from offering discounts. Some jurisdictions also disallow prepayment for nursing services, which leads one to question the sale of gift certificates (CNO, 2019a, 2019b). Meanwhile, spas and clinics in the retail environment sometimes offer aggressive discounts, gift certificates and package purchases, therefore making NP business ownership and profitability more challenging. In addition, many clinical cosmetic businesses market themselves on social media. Meanwhile, NP business owners could be at risk legally and in terms of regulation if posting patient photos on social media or communicating with patients or potential patients on such platforms. Regulators and insurers across jurisdictions have produced a variety of documents that address these areas. Standards and guidelines differ greatly among jurisdictions and change often.

Regulation

Regulatory bodies have taken diverse positions on NPs providing clinical cosmetic services as part of their practice. In some jurisdictions NPs can provide orders for and administer cosmetic medications and treatments (i.e., medications and dermal fillers), while in others, approval by specific committees is required. Some jurisdictions have prohibited NPs from engaging in cosmetic aesthetic medical practice, arguing that the associated procedures are not part of primary health care. Meanwhile, NPs move into a variety of other specialty areas within the not-for-profit system. This phenomenon may point to turf challenges among various professions interested in dominating this profitable area of practice.

Conclusion

Clinical cosmetic practice is growing in popularity among NPs in jurisdictions where it is permitted, partly due to the satisfying nature of the work. NPs are well positioned for growth in this industry with graduate-level education and the broad prescribing authority they have in some provinces. I have found that my NP education and clinical experience provided an excellent foundation for advanced education and practice in this area. Meanwhile, work in the for-profit sector has posed some unique challenges. Practice guidelines and codes of conduct prohibit some promotional and advertising activities generally associated with work in this market. Meanwhile, other kinds of businesses can be more creative with their use of these tools. Nonetheless, there are many examples of successful role integration both as front-line clinicians and clinic directors in jurisdictions where delegation is permitted. I have thoroughly enjoyed applying my skills to this new area, working as an autonomous business owner and providing quality care to the patients I see. I look forward to seeing how NP roles in clinical cosmetic services evolve in coming decades.

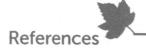

References

Canadian Nurses Protective Society (CNPS). (2016). *Considerations for providing cosmetic services.* Ottawa, ON: CNPS. Retrieved from https://www.cnps.ca/cosmetic

College of Nurses of Ontario (CNO). (2019a). *Practice guideline: Independent practice.* Toronto, ON: CNO. Retrieved from https://www.cno.org/globalassets/docs/prac/41011_fsindepprac.pdf

CNO. (2019b). Can nurses in independent practice administer Botox? *The Standard,* July. Toronto, ON: CNO. Retrieved from https://www.cno.org/en/learn-about-standards-guidelines/magazines-newsletters/the-standard/july-2019/nurses-independent-practice-administer-Botox/

Appendix

B3

Spotlights on Unique Advanced Practice Roles in Canada

Forensic Mental Health and Youth Justice

Joanna Dickinson

JOANNA DICKINSON is an NP-PHC, Wellness Lead at the Syl Apps Youth Centre in Oakville, Ontario.

Introduction

Looking to further explore a role within a mental health specialty, I accepted a position as nurse practitioner (NP) within a forensic mental health and youth justice facility. I took on this role with trepidation as I was also asked to create it. Shortly after I began in the role, I was immersed in the unlimited needs of each client and recognized that the scope of practice and competencies of an NP had prepared me to take on this challenge.

History of the Role

Our in-patient facility admits youth with mental health issues who have been in contact with the law, at risk for harm to self or others, or have been found not criminally responsible and/ or unfit to stand trial (KINARK, 2019). Like many NP roles, this position was developed out of a service gap that couldn't be filled by a physician. The chief nursing officer, an NP, and the chief of psychiatry recognized that the diverse medical and psychiatric needs of the client population would benefit from the broad scope of practice of an NP.

Competencies

NPs in Ontario are registered under broad specialty areas and are not limited in their clinical areas of work (CNO, 2019). The entry to practice competencies such as collaboration, consultation and referral, and health promotion (CNO, 2018) is integral to working with our complex clients and the communities and populations that they will return to. The youth who need this in-patient facility live in such communities and within populations that give rise to adverse childhood experiences known to increase the frequency of high-risk behaviours and psychiatric illnesses (CDC, 2019). Advocating for community follow-up through engagement with community programs and stakeholders is an important role of this NP position. The collaboration skills necessary to work with the youth and the interprofessional team are part of an NP's core competencies and strengths. An NP values the consultative and collaborative process and adds significant contributions with effective communication and clinical skills.

Our youth present with both acute and chronic medical and psychiatric conditions that are often interrelated. Utilizing advanced assessment skills, it is essential to develop and layer management plans toward optimizing health. Recognizing that no treatment is linear, there is a need to remain flexible and adapt the plan as the youth responds. Central to effectively working with this population is acknowledging their lived experiences and their own goals. Assisting them to identify their own health needs and facilitate motivation for change are the art and science of NP care. The scope of NP practice was enhanced in April 2017 with the changes to the *Nursing Act*, which permitted prescribing of controlled substances (CNO, 2019), especially the psychostimulants, which has allowed for greater independent practice and working more seamlessly with the youth.

System Challenges

The youth face significant challenges as they navigate complex systems in the community. For those of us working with these youth, we too face these challenges with them. Many of the community mental health programs have strict admission criteria that are difficult to meet, inflexible, and have long wait lists. This creates barriers to ensuring community follow-up on discharge and takes considerable time for the NP to make multiple referrals. The lack of appropriate community housing for youth involved in the forensic mental health and youth justice systems often means that they will be discharged to a shelter.

Regulatory Considerations

Currently in Ontario there is no mechanism for NPs to bill OHIP for services. This change could allow NPs like myself to be compensated for seeing clients on a transitional basis as they wait for community support. There are several regulatory laws within the *Mental Health Act* (1990) that limit the practice of NPs, thereby reducing timely care for clients. An example of this is NPs' inability to place a client on a Form 1 for involuntary assessment and authorizing community treatment orders to ensure the safety of clients and their home community.

Conclusion

At the centre of my unique practice are the youth who have survived dire life circumstances and trust me enough to share their lived experiences. These youth motivate me daily to learn, practice, and continue to work toward excellence in practice. Collaborating with other mental health NPs across Ontario to become a community of practice within the Nurse Practitioner Association of Ontario and developing a mental health certificate for NPs are exciting opportunities.

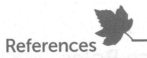

References

Center for Disease Control and Prevention (CDC). (2019). *Adverse childhood experiences.* Atlanta, GA: CDC. Retrieved from https://www.cdc.gov/violenceprevention/childabuseandneglect/acestudy/aboutace.html

College of Nurses of Ontario (CNO). (2018). *Entry-to-practice competencies for nurse practitioners.* Toronto, ON: CNO. Retrieved from www.cno.org/globalassets/docs/reg/47010-np-etp-competencies.pdf

CNO. (2019). *Practice standard, nurse practitioner.* Toronto, ON: CNO. Retrieved from www.cno.org/globalassets/docs/prac/41038_strdrnec.pdf

Government of Ontario. (1990). *Mental health act, R.S.O. 1990, c. M.7.* Toronto, ON: Government of Ontario. Retrieved from https://www.ontario.ca/laws/statute/90m07/v

Kinark Child and Family Services (KINARK). (2019). *Forensic mental health and youth justice.* Markham, ON: KINARK. Retrieved from www.kinark.on.ca/programs-and-services/clinical/forensic-mental-health-and-youth-justice/

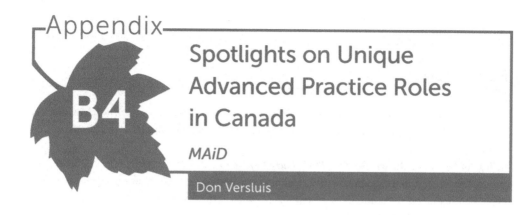

Appendix B4

Spotlights on Unique Advanced Practice Roles in Canada

MAiD

Don Versluis

DON VERSLUIS is an NP-PHC working in General Internal Medicine at Niagara Health System and specializes in MAiD. He received the 2018 President's Award for extraordinary performance. Don is also a Clinical Instructor in the Ontario Primary Health Care Nurse Practitioner (PCHNP) Program at McMaster University, Hamilton, Ontario.

Introduction

I had been a nurse practitioner (NP) for approximately two years when I first became involved in medical assistance in dying (MAiD). At that time, I knew very little about the legislative changes that had recently taken place in Canada, and I had never considered MAiD as part of the NP role. With ongoing experience and practice in MAiD, I quickly discovered how well positioned I was to fulfill this important need of patients with unendurable suffering.

History of the Role

The Supreme Court of Canada ruled in favour of criminal liability exemption on February 6, 2015 (Department of Justice, 2015) for health care professionals participating in delivering MAiD, provided they follow the mandated process for determining eligibility. This legislation was enacted in June 2016 (Parliament of Canada, 2016). Shortly thereafter, the public became increasingly aware and curious about this option.

Having completed my NP educational training in 2014, prior to these legislative changes, I was not prepared with the knowledge, emotional resilience, or etiquette for entering a patient's room with a conspicuous bag of large syringes to assist them in ending their life. The role of the NP has progressively grown in this area. Given the NPs' philosophy of holistic, person-centred care, NPs have proven to be an invaluable resource in exploring this option and offering compassionate provision to eligible patients.

Competencies

MAiD broadly encompasses the NP entry-to-practice competencies (CNO, 2018). The client care competency, encompassing advanced holistic assessment skills that examine the client as a person, and knowledge of therapeutic options available ensure that the client is well informed of their options before deciding on MAiD. Health promotion is accomplished by achieving a goal of minimizing suffering in this instance. The ongoing legislative changes have made good use of the leadership and quality improvement competencies acquired in my NP education and practice. My role as an NP has empowered me to conduct a qualitative study regarding MAiD within my practice. Having expertise in practice and policy has also put me in a position to educate colleagues and students. The NP competency of educator has benefited my interprofessional team in developing a comprehensive understanding of the MAiD process and regulatory factors.

System Challenges

There have been multiple system barriers that made accessing MAiD a challenge. The time required to perform a comprehensive assessment is substantial. Completing a provision is also very involved, requiring support from an interprofessional team. The flexibility of the NP role is helpful in addressing these challenges and can help simplify the process. Currently in Ontario, there is no compensation mechanism for NPs to bill OHIP for these services, which has led to a reduction in those willing to perform this work. All NPs in Ontario can perform assessments and provide MAiD, but do so voluntarily while covering all the costs, including insurance, transportation, and record storage on their own if they are doing so outside their role in an organizational setting. The Canadian Association of MAiD Assessors and Providers (CAMAP, 2019) is one of few resources for those participating in MAiD that can provide emotional and peer support. There is also ongoing development of a care coordination service that supports patient access to clinicians who participate in MAiD (MOHLTC, 2019).

Regulatory Considerations

Data collection and reporting have been a challenge. Currently, there are both provincial data collection for all deaths and federal data collection for MAiD-specific statistics. A single stream for data collection and reporting would facilitate accurate statistics. Previously there was conflict between death certificates containing the word "suicide" potentially voiding policies, but this has been overruled and pursuing MAiD is not a valid reason for denying such benefits (Manulife, 2019; Sakkejha, 2016).

Conclusion

MAiD was something that I had thought little about prior to my involvement in 2016. I have never felt so appreciated in my career saving someone's life as I have helping them avoid further suffering. It took one patient, asking me in a time of desperation, and I found a passion that became very meaningful and even fulfilling once I gave myself permission to release myself of the guilt of providing medications to end someone's life.

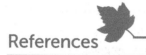

References

The Canadian Association of MAiD Assessors and Providers (CAMAP). (2019). *The Canadian Association of MAiD Assessors and Providers.* Victoria, BC: CAMAP. Retrieved from https://camapcanada.ca/

College of Nurses of Ontario (CNO). (2018). *Entry-to-practice competencies for nurse practitioners.* Toronto, ON: CNO. Retrieved from http://www.cno.org/globalassets/docs/reg/47010-np-etp-competencies.pdf

Department of Justice (2015). *Supreme Court of Canada ruling.* Ottawa, ON: Department of Justice. Retrieved from https://www.justice.gc.ca/eng/cj-jp/ad-am/scc-csc.html

Manulife. (2019). *Medical assistance in dying.* Waterloo, ON: Manulife. Retrieved from https://www.manulife.ca/business/news/legislative-updates/medical-assistance-in-dying.html

Ministry of Health and Long-Term Care (MOHLTC). (2019). *Medical assistance in dying.* Ottawa, ON: MOHLTC. Retrieved from http://health.gov.on.ca/en/pro/programs/maid/#accessing

Parliament of Canada. (2016). *Bill C-14: An act to amend the criminal code and to make related amendments to other acts.* Ottawa, ON: Government of Canada. Retrieved from http://www.parl.ca/DocumentViewer/en/42-1/bill/C-14/first-reading

Sakkejha, Y. (2016). *How will life insurance claims be impacted by medical assistance in dying in Canada?* Toronto, ON: CAMAP. Retrieved from https://beneplan.ca/how-will-life-insurance-claims-be-impacted-by-medical-assisted-dying-in-canada/

Appendix

B5

Spotlights on Unique Advanced Practice Roles in Canada

Transgender Care

Andrew Sharpe

ANDREW SHARPE is an NP-PHC at the Transgender Health Clinic at the London InterCommunity Health Centre (LIHC) in London, Ontario, and specializes in transgender care. He has worked as a Lecturer at Fanshawe College, London, Ontario, in the Internationally Educated Nurse Bridging Program and at Nipissing University, North Bay, Ontario, as a Lecturer and Clinical Instructor.

Introduction

After completing the nurse practitioner (NP) program, I worked for several years in primary health care managing the care for patients of all ages. I was approached by a physician colleague to help start a transgender clinic. I did not realize the enormous lack of health care providers who were qualified or had an interest in providing care to transgender patients. This area of health care is rife with societal, cultural, religious and personal biases, judgments, and discrimination.

The need for inclusive, non-judgmental and affirming health care was clear as 21% of transgender patients avoid the emergency department when they need it because of discrimination in the health care setting. Additionally, there are higher levels of depression and suicide, poverty, exclusion from public spaces, and homelessness among the transgender population (Bauer & Scheim, 2015).

History of the Role

In Ontario, transgender patients have the option of going to an endocrinologist, their primary health care practitioner, or a gender/transgender clinic for assistance and guidance with medical transition. Prior to 2016, all transgender patients requesting transition-related surgeries (TRS) had to be referred to the Centre for Addiction and Mental Health in Toronto, Ontario, and be subjected to psychiatric, psychological, and social assessments before a referral to a surgeon was made.

In 2016, in response to long wait times and barriers to access care, the Ontario government permitted endocrinologists and primary health care providers, with training in gender medicine, to make referrals directly to TRS surgeons. As an NP, I am able to assess these patients and provide the diagnosis of gender dysphoria needed to access trans care. I am also able to provide hormone therapy, refer for counselling and psychotherapy, if required, refer for TRS as appropriate, monitor outcomes, and support clients throughout their transition. As NPs, we are well suited for this role as we have experience in holistically assessing patients using the bio-psycho-social-spiritual model of care and can spend more time with the patient than in traditional medical models of care.

Competencies

Transgender care encompasses many of the NP entry-to-practice competencies (CNO, 2018). Relationship building is a key competency for members of this population who have been discriminated and excluded in the past, so it is important to demonstrate an empathetic and caring approach to the therapeutic relationship. Demonstrating cultural competence and safety toward this group goes a long way in building trust. Utilizing advanced holistic assessment skills, along with the ability to diagnose and prescribe therapeutics, decreases the barriers to care. Transgender patients no longer have to wait years for a specialist to assist with transition since NPs are able to utilize and build upon their competencies. Given that this is an evolutionary field, NPs are able to utilize research and translate this knowledge into practice. As leaders and advocates, NPs can push for more equity, fewer barriers, and easier access to care for this patient population.

System Challenges

One of the system challenges that exists is the number of health care providers who are willing to provide care to transgender patients. There are areas in Ontario where transgender patients can access care quite easily, but in rural areas, care is often difficult to obtain. Some TRS are publicly funded (genital and masculinizing chest surgery); however, many surgeries need to be paid out of pocket. These surgeries, such as facial feminization, breast augmentation, tracheal shave, and voice/pitch can cost thousands of dollars and put a strain on an already impoverished population. In Ontario, NPs cannot bill OHIP and therefore cannot have their own transgender clinics. They must work in a practice such as a Community Health Centre, Family Health Team, Nurse Practitioner-Led Clinics and persuade management that transgender care is important enough to dedicate time and resources for a program.

Conclusion

Transgender care is a very rewarding area of NP practice. I am able to use my advanced practice skills to the full extent, from supporting patients with their medical and mental health and social needs to navigating an often confusing bureaucracy for getting their identification and documentation changed. For me, developing a trusting therapeutic relationship with a marginalized group and breaking down barriers to care is the epitome of nursing practice.

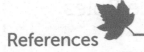

References

Bauer, G. R., & Scheim, A. I. (2015). *Transgender people in Ontario, Canada: Statistics from the trans PULSE project to inform human rights policy (2005–2018)*. London, ON: TransPulse. Retrieved from https://www.researchgate.net/publication/277558920_Transgender_People_in_Ontario_Canada_Statistics_from_the_Trans_PULSE_Project_to_Inform_Human_Rights_Policy

College of Nurses of Ontario (CNO). (2018). *Entry-to-practice competencies for nurse practitioners*. Toronto, ON: CNO. Retrieved from http://www.cno.org/globalassets/docs/reg/47010-np-etp-competencies.pdf

Appendix

B6

Spotlights on Unique Advanced Practice Roles in Canada

Nurse Clinician-Scientist

Sandra Lauck

SANDRA LAUCK is a Clinical Associate Professor and holds the inaugural St. Paul's Hospital and Heart & Stroke Foundation Professorship in Cardiovascular Nursing at the University of British Columbia, Vancouver, British Columbia.

Introduction

The role of the nurse clinician-scientist is gaining interest in addressing the gap between front-line nurses, who require new knowledge in their practice, and academic nurses, who have the tools to produce evidence. Nursing has a rich history of promoting the pursuit of scientific inquiry in practice. In the early days of our discipline, Florence Nightingale pioneered research informed by nursing expertise to implement evidence-informed practice and improve patient outcomes.

History of the Role

I hold the St. Paul's Hospital and Heart & Stroke Foundation Professorship in Cardiovascular Nursing at the University of British Columbia (UBC), a role established in 2017 to strengthen the contributions of PhD-prepared advanced practice nursing (APN) to improve patient outcomes, systems of care, and bridge the research to evidence-informed practice gap. This is one of the few university-appointed cardiovascular nurse clinician-scientist roles in Canada. It is primarily positioned in-house at St. Paul's Hospital Heart Centre, Vancouver, British Columbia, but is held to the academic standards of promotion, including research, teaching, and service. The vision is that the position will be locally, nationally, and internationally recognized as a hub of excellence, strengthen clinical and academic partnerships to improve the health of people with heart disease, and foster the visibility and contributions of cardiovascular nurses. The position was awarded after following the conventional UBC appointment process. I report to the Chief Nursing Officer and Head, Division of Cardiology at St. Paul's Hospital, and a Nurse Clinician-Scientist at St. Paul's Hospital. The distribution of this unique role is 75% clinical practice and 25% university based.

Competencies

My role centres on the triple mission of conducting original research, contributing to a clinical culture that embraces scientific inquiry, and advocating for the uptake of knowledge and its application to practice and innovation. My goal is to demonstrate that my visibility and availability in the clinical setting, the clinical expertise and credibility I have gained over my career, including a decade of APN, and the competencies I bring to accelerate the contributions of nurse-led research, can help achieve the vision of the role.

I obtained my PhD in Nursing at UBC under the mentorship of exceptional nurse scholars and was fortunate to participate as a trainee in a strategic training initiative for health research for cardiovascular nurse scientists led by McMaster University, Hamilton, Ontario. I credit the rigour of my academic preparation for acquiring the research skill set required to fulfill the role of scientist. I also benefited from being included and championed by the interprofessional research group at the Centre for Heart Valve Innovation at St. Paul's Hospital. The combination of expert clinical practice, exceptional scientific training, and membership in a network of clinical and scientific leaders are foundational to the competencies of the nurse clinician-scientist.

System Challenges

The role of the nurse clinician-scientist remains unevenly perceived within both academic and clinical settings, and the term lacks precision. In contrast to our colleagues in medicine, nursing does not have a defined path to employment in the role of university-affiliated and clinically positioned clinician-scientists. The system gaps between the university and health authorities present barriers to standardized models of appointment, distribution of responsibility, promotion, accountability, and funding. In this context, my position remains unique and is a tribute to the dogged determination of all parties to the agreement that supports my role.

Regulatory Considerations

One of my challenges is to articulate what makes me a clinician. It is challenging for a nurse to find opportunities to practice clinically due to labour agreements, the maintenance of competencies, and other employment factors. The academic metrics of my success, scientific impact and productivity, successful competition for grant funding, supervision of graduate students, and knowledge translation activities do not account for the importance of clinical visibility and participation in nursing practice leadership. This conundrum presents additional challenges that require ongoing discussions in our discipline to create a model for recruitment and sustained success.

Conclusion

Nurse clinician-scientists can play an integral role in shaping a supportive culture of inquiry in the clinical setting, providing expert mentorship, and facilitation of "practice close" research and dissemination of science in collaboration with advanced practice nurses and direct health care providers, while championing nurses' roles in improving patient outcomes in measurable and sustainable ways.

Appendix

C

Resources for Advanced Practice Nurses in Canada

National

Canadian Council of Registered Nurse Regulators (CCRNR)
The purpose of the CCRNR is to promote excellence and serve as a national forum and voice regarding provincial, national, and global regulatory matters for nursing regulation.
http://www.ccrnr.ca/

Canadian Nurses Association (CNA/AIIC)
The CNA is the unified voice for RNs in Canada by advancing the practice and profession of nursing to improve health outcomes and strengthen Canada's publicly funded health care system. CNA speaks for RNs and represents Canadian nursing to other organizations and governments nationally and internationally.
http://cna-aiic.ca/

Canadian Nurses Protective Society (CNPS)
The CNPS offers legal advice, risk management services, and professional liability protection relating to nursing practice to eligible RNs and NPs.
http://www.cnps.ca/index.php

The Clinical Nurse Specialist Association of Canada (CNS-C)/Association des infirmières et infirmiers cliniciens spécialisés du Canada (ICS-C)
The CNS-C/ICS-C recognizes that the CNS is an essential component of a sustainable health care system. It provides a leadership platform through which CNSs impact and influence cost-effective health care system change to support safe, quality care and superior outcomes.
http://cna-aiic.ca/

Nurse Practitioner Association of Canada (NPAC)/Association des infirmières et infirmiers praticiens du Canada (AIIPC)
The NPAC/AIIPC is the national voice for NPs. Its goal is to advocate for and reduce barriers to NP practice.
https://npac-aiipc.org/about-npac-aiipc/

Provincial/Territorial

British Columbia

Association of Registered Nurses of British Columbia (ARNBC)
The ARNBC is the professional association representing RNs in British Columbia. It was launched and incorporated under the *BC Society Act* in 2010. Its strategic directions for 2014–2017 include engaging effectively with RNs and NPs in BC; advocating for evidence-informed policies to promote the health and health care of British Columbians; and developing and sustaining professional practice support structures and services for all RNs and NPs in BC.
http://www.arnbc.ca/

British Columbia Nurse Practitioner Association (BCNPA)
BCNPA is a non-profit, volunteer-based professional organization that supports and advances the professional interests of nurse practitioners, nurse practitioner students, and nurses who have an interest in NP practice. Its efforts support enabling NPs to provide accessible, efficient, and effective health care that meets the highest standards across NP practice.
https://bcnpa.org/

Clinical Nurse Specialist Association of BC (CNSABC)
The CNSABC supports the expert role of the CNS by promoting an environment in which members can network, contribute to knowledge, and access support that meets the highest professional standards of practice.
http://cnsabc.ca/

College of Registered Nurses of British Columbia (CRNBC)
The CRNBC is the regulatory body that governs the regulation of RNs and NPs in BC.
https://www.crnbc.ca/Pages/Default.aspx

Alberta

College & Association of Registered Nurses of Alberta (CARNA)
CARNA is the professional organization and regulatory body for nurses in Alberta.
http://www.nurses.ab.ca/

Nurse Practitioner Association of Alberta (NPAA)
NPAA's mission is to advocate and advance NP practice to build a healthier Alberta.
https://albertanps.com/

Saskatchewan

Saskatchewan Association of Nurse Practitioners (SANP)
SANP is the voice of NPs in Saskatchewan through promoting and advancing NP roles. Part of its mission is to contribute to the quality of life and health of communities.
https://www.facebook.com/pg/sanp.sasknp/about/?ref=page_internal

Saskatchewan Registered Nurses' Association (SRNA)
The SRNA is the profession-led regulatory body for the province's RNs and RN(NP)s and has professional practice groups for both NPs and CNSs working in Saskatchewan.
http://www.srna.org/

Manitoba

Association of Registered Nurses of Manitoba (ARNM)
The newly formed ARNM is the result of a transition in the CRNM membership position with CNA and is the professional voice of RNs in Manitoba.
http://arnm.ca/

Clinical Nurse Specialists of Manitoba Interest Group (CNSMB)
The CNSMB serves as a provincial voice to enhance and promote the valuable contributions of the CNS to the health and well-being of patient populations.
http://www.cnsmb.ca/

College of Registered Nurses of Manitoba (CRNM)
CRNM is the professional regulatory body for registered nurses in Manitoba. Its vision is to maximize health for all Manitobans through excellence in registered nursing practice.
https://www.crnm.mb.ca/

Nurse Practitioner Association of Manitoba (NPAM)
NPAM is a non-profit, volunteer-run group that serves as a voice for NPs in Manitoba as a specialty practice group within the CRNM. It endeavours to support and advance the professional interests of NPs in order to provide accessible and effective health care to the public of Manitoba.
http://www.nursepractitioner.ca/

Ontario

Clinical Nurse Specialist Association of Ontario (CNS-ON)
The CNS-ON supports the role of APN in Ontario through the provision of professional networking opportunities and educational development activities for its members by clarifying and promoting the role of APN within the nursing profession and among other health care professionals, health care employers, consumers and policy-makers.
http://rnao.ca/connect/interest-groups/cns_association_of_ontario

The Clinical Nurse Specialist Association of Ontario
This is an interest group of the RNAO.
http://cns-ontario.rnao.ca/

College of Nurses of Ontario (CNO)
The CNO is the regulator for RNs, RPNs, and NPs in Ontario. Its role is to carry out entry to practice requirements, communicating and enforcing practice standards, overseeing its

QA program, and acting in the public's interest by participating in legislative processes and sharing information about Ontario nurses.
http://www.cno.org/

Nurse Practitioners' Association of Ontario (NPAO)
NPAO is the professional association for NPs in Ontario.
https://npao.org/

Registered Nurses Association of Ontario (RNAO)
The RNAO is the professional association representing RNs, NPs, and nursing students in Ontario.
http://rnao.ca/

Quebec

L'Association des infirmières praticiennes spécialisées du Québec (AIPSQ)
The AIPSQ ensures the development, enhancement, sustainability, and uniformity of the role of specialized nurse practitioners in Quebec.
https://aipsq.com/

Ordre des infirmières et infirmiers du Québec (OIIQ)
The OIIQ is the regulatory body for nursing in Quebec. It is mandated with protecting the public by administrating professional practice set out in the regulations of Quebec's Professional Code. Under the *Nurses Act*, there are regulations for classes of specialization for NPs and CNSs.
http://www.oiiq.org/
http://www2.publicationsduquebec.gouv.qc.ca/dynamicSearch/telecharge.php?type=3&file=/I_8/I8R8_A.HTM

New Brunswick

Nurse Practitioners of New Brunswick (NPNB)
The NPNB are partners of the NANB and affiliated with CAAPN. Their goal is to promote sustainable, integrated, and comprehensive NP practice; enhance NP professional development; support ongoing development of APN; and promote the health of New Brunswickers.
http://npnb.ca/

The Nurses Association of New Brunswick (NANB/AIINB)
The NANB/AIINB is the professional regulatory organization in New Brunswick. It acts to protect the public and to support nurses by ensuring standards of practice for nursing education and practice are maintained, and through support of healthy public policy.
http://www.nanb.nb.ca/

Nova Scotia

College of Registered Nurses of Nova Scotia (CRNNS)
The CRNNS is the professional body that regulates the practice of RNs and NPs to protect and serve the public interest in Nova Scotia.
http://crnns.ca/

Nurse Practitioners' Association of Nova Scotia (NPANS)
The NPANS' goal is to enhance the health of Nova Scotians through advocacy, support, and the development of the NP role.
http://www.npans.ca/

Prince Edward Island

The Association of Registered Nurses of Prince Edward Island (ARNPEI)
The ARNPEI is the professional organization and regulatory body for RNs in PEI.
http://www.arnpei.ca/

Prince Edward Island Nurse Practitioner Association (PEINPA)
The PEINPA's mission is to promote a social, economic, and political climate that supports NPs in the provision of accessible, patient-centred, and sustainable health care services.
http://peinpa.ca/

Newfoundland and Labrador

The Association of Registered Nurses of Newfoundland and Labrador (ARNNL)
The ARNNL is the regulatory body and professional association for all RNs and NPs and advocates for healthy public policy in the public interest.
https://www.arnnl.ca/

Newfoundland & Labrador Nurse Practitioner Association (NLNPA)
The NLNPA represents the professional interests of NPs by advocating for accessible, high-quality health care for all citizens throughout NL.
http://www.nlnpa.ca/

Northwest Territories and Nunavut

Registered Nurses Association of Northwest Territories and Nunavut (RNANT/NU)
The RNANT/NU is the regulatory body and professional association for RNs and NPs in both Northwest Territories and Nunavut. Its functions serve to protect the public and it strives to enhance the roles of RNs and NPs through professional advocacy and promotion.
http://www.rnantnu.ca/

Yukon

Yukon Registered Nurses Association (YRNA)
The YRNA is the regulatory body and professional association for RNs and NPs in Yukon and exists to ensure public protection with regard to nursing practice.
http://yrna.ca/

International

International Council of Nurses (ICN)
ICN is a federation of more than 130 national nurses associations, representing more than 16 million nurses worldwide. ICN works to ensure quality nursing care, sound health policies globally, the advancement of nursing knowledge, and the presence worldwide of a respected nursing profession and a competent and satisfied nursing workforce.
http://www.icn.ch/

ICN Nurse Practitioner/Advanced Practice Nursing Network
The Network is an international resource and forum for NPs and APNs, and others who are interested in the roles such as policy-makers, educators, regulators, and health planners.
http://international.aanp.org/

National Organization of Nurse Practitioner Faculties (NONPF)
NONPF is a US-based organization specifically devoted to promoting quality NP education at the national and international levels. NONPF has evolved as the leading organization for NP faculty sharing the commitment of excellence in NP education and represents a global network of NP educators.
http://www.nonpf.org/

Index